Problem-Based Behavioral Science and Psychiatry

Daniel Alicata • Negar Jacobs • Anthony Guerrero
Melissa Piasecki
Editors

Problem-Based Behavioral Science and Psychiatry

Second Edition

Springer

Editors
Daniel Alicata
John A. Burns School of Medicine
University of Hawai'i
Honolulu
Hawai'i
USA

Anthony Guerrero
John A. Burns School of Medicine
University of Hawai'i
Honolulu
Hawai'i
USA

Negar Jacobs
School of Medicine
University of Nevada
Reno
Nevada
USA

Melissa Piasecki
School of Medicine
University of Nevada
Reno
Nevada
USA

ISBN 978-3-319-23668-1   ISBN 978-3-319-23669-8 (eBook)
DOI 10.1007/978-3-319-23669-8

Library of Congress Control Number: 2015959569

Springer Cham Heidelberg New York Dordrecht London

Printed on acid-free paper

Springer International Publishing AG Switzerland is part of Springer Science+Business Media (www.springer.com)

Foreword

Learning behavioral science is a critically important part of becoming a physician. More and more, professional and accrediting organizations are explicitly endorsing the necessity of physicians being skilled and well trained in these areas.

Physicians themselves are increasingly aware of the importance of behavioral health and psychiatric issues in their practices. Whether one intends to practice in a primary care or subspecialty area, an appreciation of behavioral health issues and basic principles of psychiatry is critically necessary. In addition to topics that are more specific to the practice of psychiatry, the authors of this textbook have chosen to cover a range of topics important to all aspects of clinical medicine, including culture, violence, physician–patient relationships, adherence and substance abuse. Almost any practicing physician will admit that effectively addressing these types of behavioral issues is among the more challenging tasks they face.

Teaching and learning about psychiatry and behavioral sciences can be difficult. Basic textbooks do not easily connect their lessons with the complexity of clinical reality. Students cannot easily find the clinical importance from classroom lectures. Even clinical clerkships in psychiatry have difficulty exposing students to the breadth of clinical experiences they need to learn about.

This valuable book has realized the promise of becoming a solution to these challenges. The study of psychiatry and the behavioral sciences is perfectly matched with the problem-based learning methods utilized in this book. Problem-based learning (PBL) is a widely utilized approach to learning that involves the detailed study of patient cases, with a primary goal of identifying topics for self-study relevant to the cases. This approach helps students find meaning in learning a wide variety of topics, and provides an opportunity to apply new knowledge to clinical situations. Through understanding the cases, they learn psychiatry.

This second edition of *Problem-Based Behavioral Science and Psychiatry* has found a way to improve itself from the first edition. In addition to updating the material in each of the chapters, the additional attention to the most recent editions of the content maps of the United States Medical Licensing Examination (USMLE) Step 1 and Step 2 CK will provide additional value to medical students and those responsible for organizing medical student curricula.

For those familiar with the PBL process, this book offers a welcome resource in the area of behavioral sciences and psychiatry. Students are sometimes reluctant to vigorously pursue a study of behavioral issues. They often cite difficulty in finding reliable, evidence-based resources for their independent learning. Unlike the biological and clinical sciences, where there are scores of readily available textbooks, review articles and web-based resources, students often report frustration with the relative dearth of medical student-friendly resources in the behavioral sciences. This book represents a significant addition to student learning resources in behavioral health, and should become a familiar and well-worn companion to students in PBL environments.

For those new to the PBL process, this book will also serve as a useful guide to approaching clinical problems. By working through the case studies in this book, the reader will not only be able to learn important material related to psychiatry and the behavioral sciences but also develop a systematic approach to lifelong learning that will serve them well in their clerkships and beyond.

In addition to providing opportunities to work through clinical vignettes in a problem-based learning format, the authors incorporate other useful and practical learning tools such as *mechanistic case diagramming* and the *bio-psycho-social-cultural-spiritual formulation.* In the long term, readers will benefit as much from these exercises as they will from learning the content within the pages of this book. So, in many ways, this book represents a learning tool as much as a content resource.

I am also particularly encouraged to see that a number of the contributors to this book are themselves graduates of PBL medical schools. Their experiences should provide them with a unique and valuable perspective in what they have chosen to offer on the pages that follow.

Readers will find the methodology and approaches offered in this book to be refreshing and educationally rewarding. I hope that this text will prove to be the first of a number of books that skillfully and thoughtfully blend authoritative content with effective problem-based learning exercises.

Richard T. Kasuya, MD, MSEd
Associate Dean for Medical Education
Professor of Medicine
John A. Burns School of Medicine
University of Hawai‘i at Mānoa

Contents

Contributors

Iqbal Ahmed Department of Behavioral Health, Tripler Army Medical Center, Honolulu, HI, USA

Daniel A. Alicata Department of Psychiatry, John A. Burns School of Medicine, University of Hawai'i, Honolulu, HI, USA

David Antonuccio Private Practice, Reno, NV, USA

Timothy Baker School of Medicine, University of Nevada, Reno, NV, USA

Lisa A. Calvo Psychiatry and Behavioral Sciences, University of Nevada School of Medicine, Reno, NV, USA

University of Nevada School of Medicine, Reno, NV, USA

Frederick Duennebier Department of Psychiatry, John A. Burns School of Medicine, University of Hawai'i, Kaneohe, HI, USA

Michael H. Fukuda Department of Psychiatry, University of Hawai'i John A. Burns School of Medicine, Honolulu, HI, USA

Gretchen Gavero Department of Psychiatry, University of Hawai'i John A. Burns School of Medicine, Honolulu, HI, USA

Asad Ghiasuddin Department of Psychiatry, John A. Burns School of Medicine, University of Hawai'i, Honolulu, HI, USA

Deborah A. Goebert Department of Psychiatry, University of Hawai'i John A. Burns School of Medicine, Honolulu, HI, USA

Anthony P. S. Guerrero Department of Psychiatry, John A. Burns School of Medicine, University of Hawai'i, Honolulu, HI, USA

Department of Psychiatry, University of Hawai'i John A. Burns School of Medicine, Honolulu, HI, USA

William F. Haning Department of Psychiatry, University of Hawai'i John A. Burns School of Medicine, Honolulu, HI, USA

Brandon Harsch Department of Psychiatry, University of Nevada School of Medicine, Reno, NV, USA

Amber Hayes Renown Medical Group, Sparks, NV, USA

Debra J. Hendrickson Northern Nevada Pediatrics, Reno, NV, USA

Earl S. Hishinuma Department of Psychiatry, University of Hawai'i John A. Burns School of Medicine, Honolulu, HI, USA

Kimiko Ishibashi School of Medicine, University of Nevada, Reno, NV, USA

Negar Nicole Jacobs Psychiatry and Behavioral Sciences, University of Nevada School of Medicine, Reno, NV, USA

Brian Kirkpatrick Department of Psychiatry and Behavioral Sciences, University of Nevada School of Medicine, Reno, NV, USA

Aubrey Klaich Department of Psychiatry, Tufts-New England Medical Center, Boston, MA, USA

Barbara Kohlenberg Reno, NV, USA

June C. Lee Department of Psychiatry, University of Hawai'i John A. Burns School of Medicine, Honolulu, HI, USA

Shaye Lewis Boise, ID, USA

Lance Hartmut Linke Saint Louis, MO, USA

M. Nathan Mason Department of Psychiatry, University of Arizona College of Medicine, Rocklin, CA, USA

Jeremy Matuszak Willow Springs Center, Reno, NV, USA

Catherine McCarthy Department of Family and Community Medicine, University of Nevada School of Medicine, Reno, NV, USA

Alex A. Morrison University of Nevada School of Medicine, Reno, NV, USA

Russ S. Muramatsu VA Pacific Islands Healthcare System, Honolulu, HI, USA

Lori Murayama-Sung Honolulu, HI, USA

Justin B. Otis University of Arizona College of Medicine at South Campus Psychiatry, Tucson, AZ, USA

Latha Pai Psychiatry, Mental health services (116), Veterans affairs Sierra Nevada health care system, Reno, NV, USA

Hy Gia Park Arahant Health Services, LLC, Denver, CO, USA

Melissa Piasecki Department of Psychiatry and Behavioral Sciences, University of Nevada School of Medicine, Reno, NV, USA

Jason Reinhardt Department of Psychiatry, University of Nevada School of Medicine, Reno, NV, USA

Jared T. Ritter Florida State University College of Medicine, Holly Hill, FL, USA

Erika Ryst Department of Psychiatry, School of Medicine, University of Nevada, Reno, NV, USA

M. Anand Samtani Department of Commerce and Consumer Affairs, Public Utilities Commission, Honolulu, HI, USA

Andrea Sorensen Department of Psychiatry and Behavioral Science, Reno, NV, USA

Maria-Christina Stewart Berkeley, CA, USA

Maya Strange Reno, NV, USA

Jeanelle J. Sugimoto-Matsuda Department of Psychiatry, Research Division, University of Hawai'i John A. Burns School of Medicine, Honolulu, HI, USA

Junji Takeshita Department of Psychiatry, University of Hawai'i John A. Burns School of Medicine, Honolulu, HI, USA

Ole J. Thienhaus University of Arizona College of Medicine at South Campus Psychiatry, Tucson, AZ, USA

Steven R. Williams Honolulu, HI, USA

Paula Yoshioka The Queen's Health Systems, Honolulu, HI, USA

Steven J. Zuchowski Department of Psychiatry, University of Nevada School of Medicine, Reno, NV, USA

Chapter 1
How to Use This Book

Anthony P. S. Guerrero and Melissa Piasecki

Welcome to the second edition of *Problem-Based Behavioral Sciences and Clinical Psychiatry: A Review for Medical Students*! In this chapter, our aim is to illustrate how the problem-based learning (PBL) process works so that you can apply it to the other cases in this textbook.

The goals of this chapter are:

1. To provide the readers with a guided experience on "how to use this textbook."
2. To review basic principles of problem-based learning, and the rationale for why this approach is used.
3. To illustrate, with a sample case, the processes of:
    a. "Progressive disclosure"
    b. Identifying facts/problems, hypotheses/differential diagnoses, additional clinical information needed, and learning issues
    c. Thinking about underlying neurobiology and other physiological mechanisms to understand the signs and symptoms of a case
4. To review the more generic process of bio-psycho-social-cultural-spiritual formulation in order to understand the various perspectives offered by patient cases.

Because a textbook is not the same as a patient encounter or face-to-face small group discussion, we are not claiming to represent PBL in a pure or "authentic" form (Barrows 2000). However, we hope to integrate many of the principles and potential benefits of PBL into this textbook.

A. P. S. Guerrero (✉)
Department of Psychiatry, John A. Burns School of Medicine, University of Hawai'i,
1356 Lusitana Street, University Tower 4th Floor, Honolulu, HI 96813, USA
e-mail: GuerreroA@dop.hawaii.edu

M. Piasecki
Department of Psychiatry and Behavioral Sciences, University of Nevada School of Medicine,
1664 N. Virginia Street, MS 0426, Reno, NV 89557-0426, USA
e-mail: mpiasecki@medicine.nevada.edu

D. Alicata et al. (eds.), *Problem-based Behavioral Science and Psychiatry*,
DOI 10.1007/978-3-319-23669-8_1

PBL, as described by Norman and Schmidt (1992), aims to endow learners with the skills of clinical reasoning, cooperative learning, and patient-based integration of knowledge. In its ideal form, it begins with a free-inquiry process, in which learners explicitly discuss hypotheses and additional lines of investigation. This is followed by a period of self-directed learning and a synthesis and application of information back to the case. The student then has an opportunity to critically evaluate the initial clinical reasoning process. Because PBL attempts to integrate information from multiple disciplines, all phases of the process emphasize attention to the biological, behavioral, and populational aspects of the case. Several articles (Guerrero 2001; Guerrero et al. 2003) have discussed how certain learning tools can be used to ensure that beneficial PBL processes actually occur in the course of studying a case. We will illustrate these tools, including "mechanistic case diagramming" as part of this sample case.

When compared to traditional learning methods, PBL may enhance the application of concepts to clinical situations, long-term retention of knowledge, and lifelong interest in learning (Norman and Schmidt 1992). It has been shown to improve student and faculty satisfaction and educational outcomes in numerous clinical disciplines, including family medicine, pediatrics, obstetrics, and psychiatry (Washington et al. 1999; McGrew et al. 1999; Kaufman and Mann 1999; Curtis et al. 2001; Nalesnik et al. 2004; McParland et al. 2004). Furthermore, we believe that psychiatry and the behavioral sciences, because of the inherently integrative and holistic approaches of these subject areas, are particularly well suited for the study in a PBL format (Frick 2005; Zisook 2005; Skokauskas et al. 2011). Peters et al. (2000) report on the longitudinal outcomes of a randomized controlled trial and conclude that the New Pathways Program at Harvard Medical School—of which PBL is one important component—improved students' interpersonal skills and humanistic approach to patient care, with no loss in medical knowledge.

We will illustrate the PBL process as applied to a case in this textbook. Typically, each chapter will begin with the first paragraph introducing a case. For example:

Case Vignette 1.1.1 Presenting Situation: Melanie Crystal

Melanie Crystal is a 39-year-old woman who is the single mother of a 17-year-old boy. She was referred for psychiatric assessment at the local emergency room because a police officer on foot patrol found her crying and confused in a nearby parking lot. She was tearful and hostile. She told the screening nurse that she would kill herself "at the first opportunity." On screening for substance use, she stated that she used "dope." Needle marks were visible on both arms.

At this point, the student will see the following sign, which is a prompt to "Proceed with the PBL process" before moving on to the remainder of the case.

STOP	Please proceed with the problem-based approach using the worksheet located in the appendix of Chap. 1!

Please fill in the facts, your hypotheses, further information needed, and learning issues for Learning Issue Table 1.1.1.

Learning Issue Table 1.1.1

FACTS	HYPOTHESES	INFORMATION NEEDED	LEARNING ISSUES

Learning from these cases will be maximized if the student carefully digests all components of the case and engages in the clinical reasoning processes that a clinician uses to effectively evaluate and manage the case. For example, in the case above, it may be worthwhile to:

1. Highlight or underline the facts
2. Specifically identify the clinical signs and symptoms that are present, as these are likely to be the relative "endpoints" of a mechanism that must be subsequently understood. Below we show a graphical way of identifying signs and symptoms through use of italics

Melanie Crystal is a 39-year-old woman who is the single mother of a 17-year-old boy. She was referred for psychiatric assessment at the local emergency room because a police officer on foot patrol found her *crying* and *confused* in a nearby parking lot. She was *tearful* and *hostile*. She told the screening nurse that she *would kill herself* "at the first opportunity." On screening for substance use, she stated that she used "dope." *Needle marks* were visible on both arms.

3. Organize these findings in a grid shown below in appendix A (blank samples are provided for photocopying).
4. Use this grid to guide the clinical reasoning process that will guide further evaluation and management of the case.

Obviously, there will be variations in the specific items one will choose to put under each of the columns. The main principles to follow are as follows:

1. To come up with specific hypotheses, ask the question: "What are the possible *mechanisms* (biological or otherwise) behind the signs and symptoms present in the case?" In this text, we emphasize the neurological and physiological mechanisms that are known to be associated with normal and pathological behavior.
2. Additional clinical information ("What do you want to know next?") reflect your hypotheses and should follow a logical clinical organization.

In this textbook, the use of the clinical reasoning process will prompt or answer many of the questions in the right-most column. Each clinical case includes text coverage of the learning issues likely to be most relevant to medical student learners. Therefore, if this sample chapter were an actual textbook chapter, it would contain sections on:

- The mechanisms behind abnormal mood and confusion
- The mechanisms of action of common illicit drugs
- Definitions of child abuse and neglect

Some chapters offer high-density tables and figures to illustrate mechanisms of action. Examples include the mechanism of psychotic symptoms (see Chap. 20) and the mechanism of action of common substances of abuse (see Table 19.1 in Chap. 19).

With an effective clinical reasoning process, the subsequent sections of the case will address items in the "what do you want to know next" column. A sample continuation of the case vignette is shown below:

Case Vignette 1.1.2 Continuation
Ms. Crystal was uncooperative with further questioning. Attempts to reach collateral informants were unsuccessful. On examination, vital signs were as follows: temperature 100.3°F, pulse 106/min, blood pressure 142/88, respiratory rate 22/min. The remainder of the physical examination was unremarkable except for thin appearance, poor dentition, and needle marks on her skin. Mental status examination (MSE) was remarkable for poor cooperation and eye contact, mumbled rapid speech, labile and tearful affect, tangential thoughts, possible auditory hallucinations, and suicidal ideations.

Please proceed with the problem-based approach using the worksheet located in the appendix of Chap. 1!

Please fill in the facts, your hypotheses, further information needed, and learning issues for Learning Issue Table 1.1.2.

Learning Issue Table 1.1.2

FACTS	HYPOTHESES	INFORMATION NEEDED	LEARNING ISSUES

Once again, this will be a prompt to analyze the case and complete the table as shown above.

Case Vignette 1.1.3 Conclusion

After admission to an inpatient unit, Ms. Crystal went to sleep and remained asleep for almost 14 h. She was ravenously hungry and only marginally cooperative with measurements of vital signs or attempts at interview. She remained irritable and was verbally abusive to staff for the next day.

Three days later, Ms. Crystal became conversant with staff. On the fourth day, she was pleasant and social. She described her history of methamphetamine use disorder beginning in her 20s, with 10 years of abstinence. She stated that she stopped going to meetings and "it only took one guy" who showed her the drug at his home. She reported that as soon as she saw and "smelled" methamphetamine, she began to have intense cravings and immediately relapsed. She has used daily for the last month or so and is not sure where her adolescent son is. She thinks that he will be graduating from high school "one of these days."

The case and text discussion cover core curricular material relevant to the general subject matter. For example, if the goal of the chapter were to review methamphetamine use disorder (refer to Chap. 19 on substance-related disorders), the following learning issues would be covered:

- Epidemiology (including the recent epidemic, age groups affected, mortality statistics)
- Differential diagnosis (including mood, psychotic, and other substance disorders)
- Etiology and neurobiological mechanisms
- Clinical findings (including cognitive changes, psychotic symptoms, motor symptoms, acute and secondary drug effects, and craving)
- Treatment (psychosocial and pharmacological)
- Social, cultural, and legal factors
- Prognosis

1.1 Bio-Psycho-Social-Cultural-Spiritual Model

In all our teaching, we invite students to conceptualize patients' problems by using a bio-psycho-social-cultural-spiritual formulation. This model is used throughout the psychiatric curriculum at the authors' institutions. The goal of these patient formulations is to consider the complexities of patient presentations and to drive treatment planning. Formulations help explain, "how did this patient get to this psychiatric state at this time?"

What follows is a description of the components of the bio-psycho-social-cultural spiritual formulation (adapted from Kohlenberg and Piasecki 2006). We have added prompts for the students to help them think about and organize clinical material. Students are encouraged to include each component in formulations.

This model generally includes the following:

1.1.1 Biological

1.1.1.1 Past

Genetics:

- Consider whether any blood relatives have had psychiatric problems, substance use problems, or suicide attempts/suicides. Is there a history of close relatives who have been hospitalized for psychiatric reasons? What kind of treatments did they get, and how did they respond?

History of Pregnancy and Birth:

- Consider pregnancy variables: Was there in utero exposure to nicotine, alcohol, medications, or illicit substances? Was there anything unusual about pregnancy?
- Note birth complications, such as prematurity, birth trauma, and extended periods of hospitalization.

Relevant Previous Illnesses

- Consider any history of head injury, endocrine disorders (e.g., thyroid and adrenal), seizures, malignancies, or neurological illnesses.
- Consider potential lasting effects of past substance use on brain functions such as cognition, affective regulation, etc.

1.1.1.2 Present

Current Illnesses:

- Identify current illnesses and any direct impact they may have on psychiatric presentation.

Medications:

- Assess current medication regimen. Consider whether these medications have psychoactive effects. (e.g., steroids, beta blockers, pain medications, benzodiazepines, serotonin-selective reuptake inhibitors, and antipsychotics). Consider possible side effects of current medications and pharmacogenomic profiles that influence how medications are metabolized. Note any noncompliance with medications.

Substances:

- Consider the influence of nicotine, alcohol, and illicit drugs on current psychiatric symptoms.
- Consider the possible effects of substance withdrawal.

Endocrine/hormonal:

- Consider the impact of onset of adolescence.
- Consider the impact of the menstrual cycle, pregnancy, postpartum period, and menopause.

1.1.2 Psychological

Past

- Comment on any past history of trauma (child abuse, combat, rape, serious illness, etc.), as well as resiliency (how the patient coped with trauma, for example, through friends, family, and religion).
- Consider the sources of positive self-image and positive role models.
- Comment on the patient's experience with loss.

- Comment on the patient's quality of relationships with important figures, such as grandparents, friends, significant teachers, and significant employers.
- Comment on how past medical problems, substance use, or psychiatric problems impacted the patient's development and their relevance to the patient today.

Present

- Describe the recent events and experiences that precipitated the admission or appointment.
- What are the current stressors? Do they have any symbolic meaning?
- Assess and comment on coping skills, defense mechanisms, and presence or absence of cognitive distortions.
- Consider current developmental demands on the person, such as marriage, divorce, birth, children leaving home, loss, and aging. At what stage of development is the patient now? Is it appropriate to chronological age?
- What is the developmental impact of the patient's illness?

1.1.3 Social

- How adequate is the patient's current support system?
- What is the current status of relationships with important figures?
- What are the possible peer influences?
- Consider the patient's current housing arrangement.
- Comment on vocational/financial status.
- Comment on any relevant legal problems.
- Consider the role of agencies (e.g., Veteran's Administration, Child Protective Services, and Criminal Justice System) on the patient.

1.1.4 Cultural

- Comment on cultural influences and acculturative pressures that may impact the current situation.
- Comment on cultural influences on understanding of illness and/or help-seeking behavior (including language issues).

1.1.5 Spiritual

- Comment on the role of spirituality in the patient's life.
- Is the patient affiliated with some sort of spiritual community?
- How does spirituality contribute to the patient's ability to hope, their position on suicide if relevant, or their contact with a supportive community?

A sample bio-psycho-social-cultural-spiritual formulation for Ms. Crystal would be as follows:

This is a 39-year-old woman with acute psychiatric symptoms. Biological factors that contribute to her presentation include the acute effects of methamphetamine on her mood and behavior. Methamphetamine is likely also contributing to her abnormal vital signs. There is no history of current or previous medical problems, family history of substance use disorder/mental illness, or current medication use.

Psychologically, this patient has recently experienced a relapse. Cues for drug use included the sight and smell of the drug. She apparently lacked coping skills for resisting relapse. There is no information about recent stressors, past trauma, or relationship history. Her role as the mother of a 17-year-old has been seriously compromised, but there is little information about how she perceives this. Her relationship with a man appears to be superficial and based on mutual drug use.

Socially, we have little information about her employment status, housing, legal situation, or social supports. She appears to have benefited from meetings in the past and may have been lacking the social support she needed to remain abstinent prior to her relapse.

Spiritually, we have little information about her history and current beliefs.

In addition, we believe that both pre-clerkship behavioral science students and clerkship psychiatry students can benefit from seeing a "big-picture" graphic representation of the formulation: which uses arrows to detail how one aspect of the case leads to another and ultimately results in her presenting concerns; which shows how the biological, psychological, and social/spiritual/cultural aspects are ultimately related; and suggests how all knowledge learned (including basic neurobiological mechanisms) can be used to benefit the patient in the form of specific treatments (shown as circled items, connected to the rest of the diagram using dotted arrows). An example is shown below (Fig. 1.1):

While it is up to the readers to decide on the degree to which such an exercise suits their learning needs, the textbook chapters will attempt to provide such diagrams on some of the cases, in order to integrate knowledge learned in the chapter and to provide closure to the case vignettes, particularly those that cover major psychiatric illnesses and symptoms (e.g., substance-related and addictive disorders, bipolar and related disorders, depressive disorders, anxiety disorders, neurocognitive disorders, and feeding and eating disorders) We hope that this feature of the textbook will enhance the clinical relevance of topics learned in behavioral science and clinical psychiatry and will stimulate interest in further learning about fundamental neurobiological mechanisms behind behavioral symptoms.

It is now time to learn about other specific topics in this textbook. Once again, welcome aboard and happy learning!

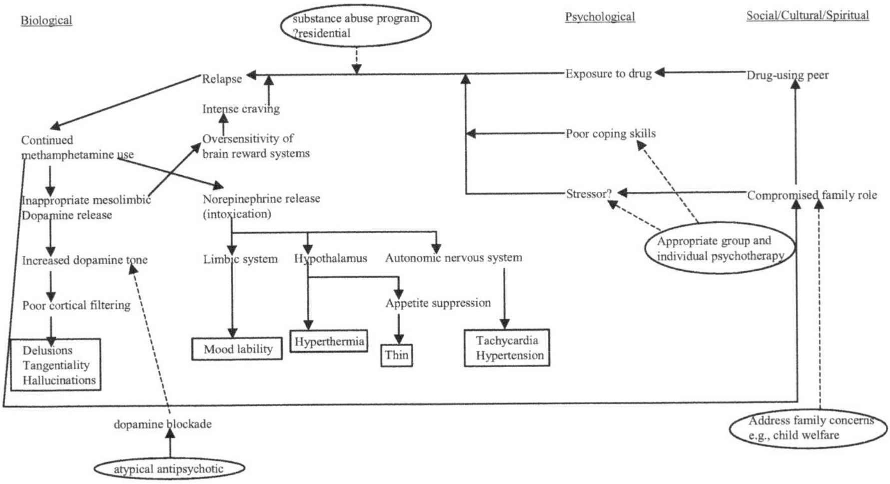

Fig. 1.1 Sample diagram to integrate knowledge and provide closure to case vignettes

Self-Study Questions

For reflection:

1. Problem-based learning is gaining popularity in medical schools. What are three of the documented outcomes that contribute to this popularity?

Appendix A: PBL Worksheet to Guide Case Studies

What are the facts?	What are your hypotheses?	What do you want to know next?	What specific information would you like to learn about?
		HPI: PMH: FH: SH: Exam: Labs:	

Appendix B: Tables with Possible Answers to the Vignettes

Case Vignette 1.1: Presenting Situation Melanie Crystal

Learning Issue Table 1.1

What are the facts?	What are your hypotheses?	What do you want to know next?	What specific information would you like to learn?
39-year old woman Single mother of a 17-year old boy Referred for psychiatric assessment at her local ER Found by police officer at a nearby parking lot Crying/tearful Confused Hostile Stated she would kill herself Used "dope" Needle marks	Drugs: ? Cocaine or methamphetamine ? Heroin (IV) Other psychiatric disorders Abnormal brain activity: • Limbic system • Other places? Sadness Possible neglect of the 17-year old minor Delirium ↑ Endocarditis	<u>HPI:</u> What exactly does she mean by "dope?" Was she having any symptoms even before using drugs? Does she have any other symptoms – disturbed sleep, disturbed appetite, hallucinations <u>PMH:</u> Other medical illnesses HIV test? <u>FH:</u> Other psychiatric illnesses <u>SH:</u> Can anyone else care for the 17-year old son? <u>Exam:</u> Vital signs (tachycardic? Hypertensive?) Heart murmur? Mental status: 1. Speech 2. Thought process 3. Perceptions 4. Is she homicidal? <u>Lab:</u> urine tox	What are the mechanisms behind confusion and abnormal mood? Which drugs can be used intravenously? What defines neglect or abuse of a 17-year old minor?

Appendix C: Online resource for additional PBL worksheets

http://www.laney.edu/wp/environmental_control_tech/ect-nsf-initiative/ect-nsf-labs/pbl/worksheets/#overview

References

Barrows, H. S. (1986). A taxonomy of problem-based learning methods. *Medical Education, 20,* 481–486.

Barrows, H. S. (2000). Authentic problem-based learning. In L. H. Distlehorst, G. L. Dunnington, & J. R. Folse (Eds.), *Teaching and Learning in medical and surgical education: Lessons learned for the 21st Century*. Mahwah: Erlbaum.

Curtis, J. A., Indyk, D., & Taylor, B. (2001). Successful use of problem-based learning in a third-year pediatric clerkship. *Ambulatory Pediatrics, 1,* 132–135.

Frick, E. (2005). Teaching somatoform disorders in a "nervous system and behaviour" course: The opportunities and limitations of problem-based learning. *Education for Health (Abingdon, England), 18,* 246–255.

Guerrero, A. P. (2001). Mechanistic case diagramming: A tool for problem-based learning. *Academic Medicine: Journal of the Association of American Medical Colleges, 76,* 385–389.

Guerrero, A. P., Hishinuma, E. S., Serrano, A. C., & Ahmed, I. (2003). Use of the mechanistic case diagramming technique to teach the biopsychosocial-cultural formulation to psychiatric clerks. *Academic Psychiatry: The Journal of the American Association of Directors of Psychiatric Residency Training and the Association for Academic Psychiatry, 27,* 88–92.

Kaufman, D. M., & Mann, K. V. (1999). Achievement of students in a conventional and Problem-Based Learning (PBL) curriculum. *Advances in Health Sciences Education: Theory and Practice, 4,* 245–260.

Kohlenberg, B., & Piasecki, M. (2006). Bio Psycho Social Spiritual Model, personal communication.

McGrew, M. C., Skipper, B., Palley, T., & Kaufman, A. (1999). Student and faculty perceptions of problem-based learning on a family medicine clerkship. *Family Medicine, 31,* 171–176.

McParland, M., Noble, L. M., & Livingston, G. (2004). The effectiveness of problem-based learning compared to traditional teaching in undergraduate psychiatry. *Medical Education, 38,* 859–867.

Nalesnik, S. W., Heaton, J. O., Olsen, C. H., Haffner, W. H., & Zahn, C. M. (2004). Incorporating problem-based learning into an obstetrics/gynecology clerkship impact on student satisfaction and grades. *American Journal of Obstetrics and Gynecology, 190,* 1375–1381.

Norman, G. R., & Schmidt, H. G. (1992). The psychological basis of problem-based learning: A review of the evidence. *Academic Medicine: Journal of the Association of American Medical Colleges, 67,* 557–565.

Peters, A. S., Greenberger-Rosovsky, R., Crowder, C., Block, S. D., & Moore, G. T. (2000). Long-term outcomes of the New Pathway Program at Harvard Medical School: A randomized controlled trial. *Academic Medicine: Journal of the Association of American Medical Colleges, 75,* 470–479.

Skokauskas, N., Guerrero, A. P., Hanson, M. D., Coll, X., Paul, M., Szatmari, P., Tan, S. M., Bell, C. K., & Hunt, J. (2011). Implementation of problem-based learning in child and adolescent psychiatry: Shared experiences of a special-interest study group. *Academic Psychiatry: The Journal of the American Association of Directors of Psychiatric Residency Training and the Association for Academic Psychiatry, 35,* 249–251.

Washington, E. T., Tysinger, J. W., Snell, L. M., & Palmer, L. R. (1999). Implementing problem-based learning in a family medicine clerkship. *Family Medicine, 31,* 306–307.

Zisook, S., Benjamin, S., Balon, R., Glick, I., Louie, A., Moutier, C., Moyer, T., Santos, C., & Servis, M. (2005). Alternate methods of teaching psychopharmacology. *Academic Psychiatry: The Journal of the American Association of Directors of Psychiatric Residency Training and the Association for Academic Psychiatry, 29,* 141–154.

Chapter 2
Child Development

Andrea Sorensen, Aubrey Klaich and Maya Strange

Changes in the developing child make normal behavior a moving target. It is important for clinicians to understand normal developmental stages in order to appreciate the bounds of normal behavior. The clinical vignettes in this chapter illustrate a few of these developmental stages that may present as a challenge to parents and professionals.

At the end of the chapter, the readers will be able to:

1. Describe normal cognitive, social, emotional, and adaptive functioning of a preschool age child, latency age child, and adolescent youth.
2. Describe protective and parental factors that can help foster normal development.
3. Identify ways in which development, personality, family, culture, and society influence development, adaptation, and coping.
4. List risk factors that may contribute to developing psychopathology at various stages.
5. Relate to how a child's developmental stage influences the physician–patient interview.

A. Sorensen (✉)
Department of Psychiatry and Behavioral Science, 401 W. Second Street, Suite 216, Reno, NV 89503, USA
e-mail: asorensen@medicine.nevada.edu

A. Klaich
Department of Psychiatry, Tufts-New England Medical Center, 800 Washington Street, Box #1007, Boston, MA 02110, USA
e-mail: aklaich@tuftsmedicalcenter.org

M. Strange
4820 Turning Leaf Way, Reno, NV 89519, USA
e-mail: Mstrange@gmail.com

D. Alicata et al. (eds.), *Problem-based Behavioral Science and Psychiatry*,
DOI 10.1007/978-3-319-23669-8_2

Vignette 2.1.1 Presentation Situation: Caleb

You are a resident in a pediatric clinic where 34-month-old Caleb is brought in by his parents with the concern of distressing tantrums. The parents describe that the child can “rage.” He may lie on the floor and flail around for what seems like an hour. He may also run away from his parents in the home and slam doors, then yell at them. He sometimes stands with stiff arms and legs and cries inconsolably. With further discussion, Caleb’s mother shares that her sister has been diagnosed with Bipolar Disorder and that she is concerned that he may have attention deficit hyperactivity disorder “like his cousins.”

Table 2.1.1

FACTS	HYPOTHESES	INFORMATION NEEDED	LEARNING ISSUES

Vignette 2.1.2: Continuation

The parents note that Caleb can generally rage up to 10 min, but they can give an example when it lasted over 30 min. They both agree that triggers for the episodes may be when he does not get what he wants, when they may not be understanding what he says, and when he is tired or hungry. The father states that he speaks clearly to Caleb and sits him in a chair for a couple of minutes. Caleb usually is able to calm down when this happens. The mother admits that she becomes frustrated with him and usually ends up yelling at him. She gives an example from that morning: She gave Caleb some crayons and paper but he only colored for a few minutes and then wanted to play with blocks. She redirected him to the coloring and he sat on the floor and “raged” for at least 5 min. She yelled “stop it” and then felt guilty; so, she gave him the blocks and walked away.

You ask for more history. The parents state that Caleb was the product of a full-term first pregnancy. There were no in utero exposures or complications. He was of easy temperament. He has fed well, slept well, and has always loved to be held. He responded to social games such as peek-a-boo. He shared references with his parents as a toddler as he would point at objects and look at them to share experiences frequently. He spoke his first words by age one and three-word sentences by age 30 months. He walked at 13 months, rode a tricycle at 30 months, can color a circle, and potty trained just recently, though he does wear a pull-up at night. Generally, Caleb is a “happy kid” when he is not having an episode.

You ask to see Caleb alone, and he agrees to let the parents leave the room to meet with you. He is shy initially, but after looking at toys he picks out a toy truck and starts to push it around the room. He looks at you and smiles, then he tells you about his big green and red trucks that he has at home. You prompt him to draw and he colors lines and circles. He asks for his mother a few times during the exam, but he is reassured that she is in the waiting room and then continues to play. He denies that anyone has ever hurt him. He does state that he can get mad and he imitates standing up with a stiff posture, clenching his fists and holding his breath. He then laughs and returns to playing with the truck.

Table 2.1.2

FACTS	HYPOTHESES	INFORMATION NEEDED	LEARNING ISSUES

Vignette 2.1.3: Continuation
Caleb has attended day care 3 days a week for the past 6 months. The teacher told Caleb's mother that he did have difficulty sharing with other kids and following rules initially. He would throw a tantrum and even hit a couple of kids during these episodes. The teacher initiated time-outs. The teacher then used counting to three to give him time to make a choice. Initially, he required several time-outs per day and had difficulty making the right choice. The past month they have not noted any concerns.

2.1 Learning Issues

Reviewing the Denver Developmental Screening Test-II in the pediatric clinic, you note that Caleb has normal development for a boy of his age (Frankenburg et al. 1992). Nearly 3 years of age, he is able to perform social, motor, and adaptive skills for his age. He communicates socially, appreciates personal boundaries, and shares affect (Smidt 2006). His play and conversations remain self-centered, but this is expected of toddlers and preschoolers. This self-centered perspective of the young child can be frustrating for many adults. For example, Caleb is only focused on his interests and does not ask the examiner of her opinion. His attention span during activities may only be 5 min; so he tends to change activities frequently. It is clear, however, that the examiner's presence is important to Caleb. The adult provides a reference for the child and can serve to share experiences and encourage appropriate exploration, communication, and expansion of the child's own self-awareness and learning during his play.

The child's desire for social and environmental interaction is paramount to learning and early brain development. As the child experiences life, neurons undergo dendritic branching and form synapses to create complex networks that allow the child to integrate their understanding of their environment and gain control over their own abilities. This process is also important as the less useful dendritic and synaptic connections undergo the process of pruning (Higgins and George 2007). Approximately one-fifth of neurons are effectively programmed by the age of 2 years, and it is through exploration, and to some extent testing limits, that allows the child to gather the data needed to program the other 80 % of the brain.

Most parents understand that they serve a critical role in providing a safe and interesting environment as well as rules and structure to help children learn without physical injury. Emotional development and learning affective (emotional) regulation also require such interactive parenting. For instance, when Caleb pushes the limits of behavior (throws a tantrum or puts himself at risk) in an attempt to further engage in exploration, the caregiver can acknowledge this desire to learn and then identify acceptable alternatives for the child. For example, Caleb runs across the street to watch the garbage truck at work. The caregiver can acknowledge that this is interesting but he cannot run across the street or stand near the truck as it is unsafe. The caregiver may offer alternatives such as "We can stand on our sidewalk and watch the truck from across the street or we may go home and read a book about trucks." Offering the child options and time to make a decision helps the child develop self-awareness and problem-solving skills. When children resist and retaliate, it may be time for a brief and respectful consequence. If the child makes a good choice, then it is helpful to immediately praise the child. Consistency in these ongoing interactions models appropriate emotional and behavioral regulation and also nurtures the child's security and attachment with the caregiver.

There are a number of developmental theorists who have contributed to the understanding of child and adolescent development. For example, Piaget (1964) noted that the preschooler is in the preoperational phase of development; this phase is egocentric from a cognitive, affective, perceptual, and social standpoint. According to Erik Erikson (1950), a child of this age is navigating through the developmental phase of autonomy versus shame and doubt. The young child becomes more aware of being a separate individual differing from wishes and needs of the parents. "No!" is a common refrain heard by parents of toddlers and preschoolers. There can be a battle of the wills as the child attempts to exert control. Effective communication and established trust between the child and the caretaker are essential for healthfully resolving this stage. Parents who learn to apply supportive interactions will have ongoing rewards, as the child's efforts toward greater separation may begin during this phase but will continue throughout childhood (Wiener and Dulcan 2004). Sociocultural theorists describe that children at this age use significant social referencing. They offer the concept of scaffolding, in which problem-solving for the young child occurs with helpful adults who are the child's primary tool for learning (Lewis 2007).

Vignette 2.1.4: Conclusion
You reassure Caleb's parents that he is normal, bright, and healthy. You offer your favorite resource for parenting the preschooler: 1,2,3 Magic! (Phelan 2003) and Your Child (Pruit 2000), and the website by the American Academy of Pediatrics (AAP)—healthychildren.org. You strongly recommend that both parents observe the preschool teacher's techniques so that they can see what works at school and what would be consistent at home. A local resource for parenting classes is reviewed. They are encouraged to return to the clinic if these initial recommendations are not effective for the family within the next few months.

Vignette 2.2.1 Presenting Situation: Susana
Susana is a 10-year-old Hispanic girl brought to your outpatient clinic by her mother, who is worried that she has been having difficulty concentrating and crying spells for the past few weeks. The girl sits politely next to her mother with a sad expression and wide-opened eyes. She is holding a rubber toy dinosaur close to her chest with her right hand and is touching her mother's arm with her left hand. Susana is the only child and has not had any major health problems in the past.

Table 2.2.1

FACTS	HYPOTHESES	INFORMATION NEEDED	LEARNING ISSUES

Vignette 2.2.2: Continuation
Susana's mother tearfully tells you that her husband, Susana's father, passed away from cancer last month. He had been in hospice care at their home for the last couple of months of his life. She says that even before he died, Susana was having difficulty completing her work at school and her homework. Susana's teacher sent a note home that her worksheets are covered with clouds and the sky. Her mother tells you that Susana has been crying for about 20 min a few times a day for the past several weeks. One time she became frantic when she could not find the toy dinosaur that she has been carrying with her for the past 2 months—a gift from her father on her ninth birthday. She also has awakened her mother at night in a panic, needing to find a particular T-shirt that her father used to wear. Once she finds the shirt, she goes back to sleep. Her mother notes that even though her sleep has been disturbed, her appetite and overall energy level have been fine. You glance at the chart and see that Susana has remained slightly above the 50th percentile for weight.

Table 2.2.2

FACTS	HYPOTHESES	INFORMATION NEEDED	LEARNING ISSUES

Vignette 2.2.3: Continued

When asked about their support system, Susana's mother tells you that they do not have much family, but they do attend a grief group at their church and they have a community of friendships. They have been able to talk about the impact of her father's death.

You ask to speak to Susana alone. Susana appears intelligent in conversation and is open to discussion about the sadness associated with the loss of her father. She admits that she cries for him and that she misses him. She holds the dinosaur closely. During the interview you find that she has several good friends and she has talked to them about her sadness and loss. She continues to ride bikes with them, play at recess, and notes that overall her grades are still good though she recognizes that she finds herself daydreaming about the sky. She feels that looking out the window at school and seeing the clouds and the sky remind her of heaven and she is comforted by the belief that he is "up there" and always with her. She has shared this belief with her mother and her pastor.

Table 2.2.3

FACTS	HYPOTHESES	INFORMATION NEEDED	LEARNING ISSUES

2.2 Learning Issues

Grief is an emotional pain or anguish that one feels after the loss of a loved one. Anticipatory grief is a similar emotional pain that occurs before the impending loss. Three categories, based on age and maturity, of a child's understanding of death have been described (Lewis 2007). Preschoolers look at death as a sleep or a long journey. Five- to nine-year-olds accept that someone can die; however, they do not believe it happens to everyone and especially not to themselves. By 10 years of age, children can understand that death is inevitable and that it may happen to them.

Normal bereavement is not considered a disorder, and loss of a close friend or relative occurs in up to half of all youth by the age of 21. Loss of a parent occurs in approximately 4% of children by the age of 18 (Lewis 2007). Refer to Chap. 16 for a more extended discussion on grief.

Susana's developmental phase has been described by Erik Erikson (1950) as industry versus inferiority. This is a time during which a child develops a sense of competence and focuses on self-worth. The child learns how to become a friend and to identify with others. He or she also gains satisfaction in experiencing hard work that leads to success and also learns to compensate for their weaknesses in some areas by noting accomplishments in other areas. Piaget (1964) describes this stage of development as concrete operations. The child is able to conceptualize rather than simply perceive, but is not able to utilize their own abstract thinking. Thus, Susana can understand the irreversibility and inevitability of death, but may have difficulty applying the concept generally. Mastery of these concepts may then be seen in the themes of dreams or play. Susana pictures heaven as the clouds and the sky and finds this comforting that her father is "up there." She does not expand past this concept.

Complicated bereavement in children does occur and is important to recognize to minimize morbidity later in life. Symptoms of complicated grief are longing and searching for a loved one, preoccupation with thoughts of the loved one, purposelessness and futility about the future, numbness and detachment from others, difficulty accepting death, lost sense of control and security, and anger and bitterness over the death (APA 2013). A study by Melham et al. (2007) indicated that these symptoms could lead to difficulties in schoolwork, friendships, relationships, and other activities. Even 2 years after the death of a parent, preadolescent girls were noted to have increased rates of depression, anxiety, and aggressive behaviors. Adolescent boys were noted to be more withdrawn and have more social problems. Adolescent girls and preadolescent boys seemed to have no differences from their matched controls. Overall, 20% of children who suffered the death of a parent had serious problems at 1 year that could benefit from treatment (Melham et al. 2007).

Vignette 2.2.4: Conclusion

You reassure Susana's mother that Susana is experiencing normal grief or bereavement. This can present in a myriad of ways—some children cry, avoid, deny, or have serious anger when a death occurs. Susana and her mother are commended for their open communication and participation with the community and spiritual supports. It will be important for Susana to continue to express feelings and discuss memories of her father as she works through the process of grief. You advise Susana's mother to have an awareness of the complicated signs of grief. You provide her with a reference to the local grief center that provides support groups for kids that have lost a parent, as Susana may benefit from being with a peer group that have had the same experience.

Vignette 2.3.1 Presenting Situation: Brian

Brian is a 15-year-old male with a history of insulin-dependent diabetes who comes to your family medicine clinic with his mother. He is currently in the 10th grade and lives with his mother, 17-year-old sister, and 11-year-old brother. Brian's parents divorced when he was 9. His father, who lives in town, sees Brian and his siblings every week. His mother brought him to see you due to concerns about changes in his behavior. She states that over the past 6 months, he has changed from a "sweet, loving, and attentive son" to a "stranger." He spends most of his time in his room, on the phone with friends, or on the computer. He used to be a conscientious student, but recently has been doing his homework at the last minute. His grades have fallen from his usual 4.0-grade average to a 3.2 on his last report card. He has been staying up late and sleeping in on the weekends. His taste in music and dress has changed. She describes that he used to be very neat, but more recently has been wearing "skater clothes." He also pierced his ear and eyebrow. He has been talking about wanting a tattoo. His eating habits have changed and he has been more casual about managing his blood glucose levels.

Table 2.3.1

FACTS	HYPOTHESES	INFORMATION NEEDED	LEARNING ISSUES

Vignette 2.3.2: Continuation

You meet with Brian without his mother. He is soft-spoken and cooperative, with brown shaggy hair, a large hooded sweatshirt, and baggy jeans. He tells you he does not know why his mother brought him in and that she "overreacts" to everything. Brian reports that he was diagnosed with diabetes when he was 10 years old. He says, "I know I should do better (managing his diabetes), but sometimes I just want to eat without thinking about it, and it's a pain carrying my insulin around all of the time." Brian used to spend more time at home in middle school because "I didn't have anyone my age to hang out with, so I hung out with my mom." He states that his mother is fairly strict. "It's unfair, my sister would never do anything my mom wouldn't like, so she now does not know what to do with me." He does not tell his mother too much about his girlfriend or friends because "it usually turns into a lecture." Brian also has positive things to say about his family: "My mom is an awesome cook, and she would do anything for us. My sister is kind of a dork, but she always looks out for me."

Brian tells you that school has been going overall well, though he could try harder. He admits to skipping school a few times when the weather was warmer to go skateboarding with friends. He also has a girlfriend and says it is a serious relationship. He had few friends when he was younger, and until a couple of years ago, he was one of the shortest kids in his class. Since starting high school, he has grown 11″ and is now 5′9″ tall. In high school, he has established a large group of friends. He says he has tried alcohol and marijuana at parties, but "they are not for me." He denies discipline problems in school and denies any conduct issues such as a history of stealing, destruction of property, or other high-risk behaviors. He has no legal history.

He notes his mood has been good; he sleeps well, has a good appetite, and overall enjoys his activities and feels he is still performing well in school. When his parents divorced, he remembers that he was easily frustrated and somewhat angry at his father. He denies a history of mania, psychosis, self-harm, or suicidal ideation. In addition to skateboarding, he likes to write, listen to music, and play guitar. He works at an ice cream shop 10 h per week. Brian's ultimate goal is to become a professional skateboarder, but if that does not work out he may eventually open up a skate shop or become an accountant "like his dad."

You invite Brian's mother to talk to you alone. Brian was diagnosed with diabetes after presenting to the emergency room in diabetic ketoacidosis. Brian's mother strictly managed his diet and blood glucose levels. Recently, Brian has wanted more responsibility, and his last hemoglobin A1C was 7 (previous levels had been in the normal range). She tells you that Brian is a "great kid," but points out that her own brother had behavioral difficulties when younger and started using substances in high school. Brian's mother was raised in a very religious household, and her brother regularly had conflict with the family. Her brother continues to abuse substances, has irregular contact with the family, has spent some time in jail related to his drug use, and has been unable to maintain steady employment. Brian's mother says, "I may be completely off base, but I just don't want to see what happened to my brother happen to Brian."

Table 2.3.2

FACTS	HYPOTHESES	INFORMATION NEEDED	LEARNING ISSUES

At this point, the differential remains quite broad. Brian's change in behavior including being more isolative, declining school performance, and change in sleep patterns could be consistent with normal development but may also indicate a substance abuse disorder or depression. It would be important to understand how Brian's change in behavior is affecting his function in other areas, such as with friends and work, as well as his overall level of functioning. A commonly used screening tool is the HEADSS (Home/health, Education/employment, Activities, Drugs, Depression, Safety, Sexuality) Assessment (Stephens 2006).

Adolescence is a period of development during which one discovers one's identity versus suffers identity diffusion (Erikson 1950). The adolescent's goal is to answer the question "Who am I?" As the adolescent tries to figure this out, they may experiment with different identities and rebel against some adult expectations. This stage accompanies significant physical changes and further development of gender and sexual identity. The teen's social network increases in importance. The adolescent engages in various activities as he or she determines his or her own values and goals. The adolescent will begin separating and reconciling their feelings for the family of origin. They will develop romantic relationships, explore interests, and work on mastering one's bodily impulses and functions (Weiner and Dulcan 2004). Thus, the normal process of separation and individuation can be a challenging time for parents.

Brain has admitted to substance use. Teenagers at risk for developing serious substance problems include those who have a family history of substance use, depression, are depressed, have low self-esteem, or feel they do not fit into the mainstream (Weinberg et al. 1998). Signs and symptoms of substance use may be physical fatigue, repeated health complaints, red or glazed eyes, and a lasting cough (Stager 2011). Emotional complaints may be personality change, sudden mood change, irritability, irresponsible behavior, low self-esteem, poor judgment, depression, and general lack of interests or motivation. The family may notice the teen argues more, breaks rules, and is more withdrawn. School concerns may include decreased interest, negative attitude, drop in grades, many absences, truancy, and discipline problems. The teen may have new friends who are less interested in standard home and school activities, have problems with the law, and are less interested in conventional styles of dress and music (Stager 2011). To further assess Brain's substance use, you explore these issues with him. You also administer the CRAFFT (Car, Relax, Alone, Forget, Friends, trouble) screening interview and he scores at low probability of abuse or dependence (Knight et al. 1999). Refer to Chap. 19 for more discussion on substance use disorders.

Screening for other mental health disorders is warranted with changes in behavior. Of note, 10–15% of children and adolescents may have symptoms of depression at any one time (Smucker et al. 1986). The prevalence of major depressive disorder among kids 9–17 years of age has been estimated at 5% (Shaffer et al. 1996).

As adolescents approach adulthood, their brains continue to develop in areas of greater complexity. For example, the process of myelination to insulate neurons into greater conductive speed is already finished in the ventral and deep brain structures. This process continues in adolescence in dorsal regions responsible for higher cognitive functions, such as prefrontal cortex. In the peak adolescent years after puberty, the brain matures specific regions devoted to executive function such as integrating senses and reasoning (Blakemore and Choudhury 2006; Toga et al. 2006). This concept of brain development is consistent with Erikson's stage of development, as he discusses learning responses of inhibition, emotional regulation, planning and organization.

Vignette 2.3.3: Conclusion
You discuss with Brian's mother that Brian and she are likely experiencing normal adolescent development. Though Brian may seem to push his family away at times, he needs them to remain present and consistent while allowing him to explore safely. It will be important to continue to express the family's values and expectation to him in a supportive way. Continuing to engage in activities as a family is also helpful to maintain connection and open lines of communication. You refer Brian's mother to the AAP and American Academy of Child and Adolescent Psychiatry (AACAP) websites, particularly to the Normal Adolescent Development series. You also meet a few months later with Brian and his mother to discuss his progress. You allow time for clarification of certain rules that are nonnegotiable. It is helpful for Brian's mother to hear from him his perspective and overall positive feeling about the family.

Review Questions

1. Which of these statements about a 3-year-old child would be developmentally unusual?
   a. The child eats with a spoon or fork.
   b. The child is more interested in others than himself/herself.
   c. The child may ride a tricycle.
   d. The child's attention span may only last 5–10 min.
2. Which developmental task is associated with adolescence?
   a. Industry versus inferiority.
   b. Stage of concrete operations.
   c. Satisfaction in hard work that leads to personal success.
   d. Determining one's own personal goals and values.
3. Cognitive development in middle childhood includes all of the following except:
   a. Genital organs grow relatively little until the end of latency.
   b. A child can consider situations from a less egocentric and more balanced, objective view.
   c. Peak rates of growth of neuronal connections in the prefrontal and temporoparietal cortices occur.
   d. The child can consider another person's feelings.
4. What percentage of the child and adolescent population may have symptoms of depression at any one time?
   a. 1–5 %
   b. 5–10 %
   c. 10–15 %
   d. 15–20 %

Appendix A: Tables with Possible Answers to Vignettes

Vignette 2.1: Caleb

Facts	Hypothesis	What do you want to know next?	Learning issues
34-month-old male	Normal behavior for age	Where/when/how often?	What is normal behavior for 3-year-olds?
Parents concerned about emotional outbursts in which patient lies on the floor, flails, screams, runs away, slams doors	Bio Developmental Pain Autistic disorder	Duration of episodes?	Counseling parents on typical/atypical behaviors for toddler?
These behaviors are accompanied by inconsolable crying and rigidity with stiff arms and legs	Psycho Mood disorder ADHD	Parents' response to outbursts—what types of things have they tried?	Diagnosis of mood disorders in young children?
FHx includes bipolar disorder in maternal aunt and cousins with ADHD and mood disorders	Social Poor parenting interactions/skills Unstable/stressful social environment	Associated behaviors or concerns in the past with Hx/development? Sleep patterns? Feeding schedule/diet/snacks? Daily routine—consistent or variable?	What are typical early signs/symptoms of ADHD and autism?
Rages are up to 10 min in duration	Normal behavior for age	Does mom frequently give in to requests during episodes?	What are typical developmental milestones for 3-year-olds?
Occur several times a day Triggers: denied wants, naptime/bedtime, trouble communicating	Ineffective parenting skills Social instability	Do outbursts occur outside the home?	Importance of thorough birth and developmental history in pediatric patients

Facts	Hypothesis	What do you want to know next?	Learning issues
Dad's response is stern; patient made to spend 1–2 min in chair		Living situation?	Parental guidance, teaching parenting skills and effective disciplinary actions for toddlers
		Occur equally with mom and dad?	
Mom usually becomes frustrated and yells		Does patient attend preschool? If so, what is behavior like there?	
Birth history is uncomplicated			
Eats/sleeps well			
Normal milestones			
Good social development and interactions—points at objects			
Happy temperament			
On exam: secure attachment, interactive play, good eye contact, and social smile			
Denies fear or history of harm			

Vignette 2.2: Susana

Facts	Hypothesis	What do you want to know next?	Learning issues
10-year-old Hispanic girl seen at outpatient clinic	Bio	Any major changes recently in living condition/daily routine?	What are the symptoms of depression in young kids?
	Temperament: shy/timid		
Mom concerned: patient having difficulty concentrating with frequent crying episodes over the past few weeks	Psycho	Any events that coincided with onset of behavioral changes?	How to interview young patients when suspect possible trauma/abuse?
	Depression		
	Attachment disorder		
	PTSD		
Only child	Psychotic disorder	Progression—better or worse since initial symptoms?	How to approach timid/fearful patient?
	Mood disorder	Friends at school? Social interactions? Any possibility of bullying?	
	Adjustment disorder		
No history of health problems	Social	Family history—any psychopathology?	Only child: common issues?

Facts	Hypothesis	What do you want to know next?	Learning issues
Appearance: patient polite, appears sad	Trauma/abuse	Speak with patient alone: What is behavior when mom leaves the room? Does she feel safe at home? Any signs of abuse on physical exam? Does patient have good support system/adults she can talk to/trust?	
Clutching toy dinosaur, and touching mom	Bullying		
Recent death of parent around the same time as symptom onset	Normal grieving behavior	Does patient have good support system/adults she can talk to/trust?	Grief: normal versus pathological?
	Complicated bereavement	How is mom dealing with death at home?	Grief versus depression versus adjustment disorder?
Prolonged hospice care prior to death: trouble with school, completing work/homework since this time	Major depression	What is mom's response to crying episodes?	Counseling parent to help child to grieve/what to expect/what to be worried about
	Adjustment disorder		
Crying episodes last about 20 min, occur a few times a day for the past several weeks	Temperament—sensitive	Other changes in relationships/activities/friends?	What are the long-term consequences/impact of death of a parent at young age?
Attachment to objects linked to her father; at times becomes distressed without them		Still able to enjoy certain activities?	
Appetite is okay			
Mild sleep disturbances			
Mom reports support comes from grief group at their church	Normal grieving behavior	Are mom and Susana interested in psychotherapy or grief counseling to further process their grief?	Anger in young patients who have experienced loss
	Adjustment disorder		Spiritual role in processing grief

Facts	Hypothesis	What do you want to know next?	Learning issues
Susana says she has two close friends with whom she can talk to about her feelings			
Reports she continues to have good grades			
Activities she enjoys: bike riding and computer games			
Angry at the unfairness of losing her father			
Comfort comes from looking at the sky/clouds and knowing her father is with her "up there"			

Vignette 2.3: Brian

Facts	Hypothesis	What do you want to know next?	Learning issues
15-year-old male with IDDM	Normal behavior for age	From mom: her response to changes in behavior, what is she most concerned about?	Normal behavior during adolescence
Mother concerned about behavioral changes in the last 6 months	Bio	From Brian: HEADSS	Identity development
	Hypothyroid	Home environment	Counseling parents: Desire for independence versus need for discipline/boundaries
	Celiac's disease/poor nutrition	School likes/dislikes, easy/difficult?	
		Peer groups	
		Does he work?	
		Diet and exercise?	
Spends most of time in his room, on phone, or on computer	Psycho	Activities he enjoys outside of school	Peer group changes/appearance
School seems to be less of a priority; from all A's to 3 B's on recent report card	Depression	Drugs/EtOH	Conducting adolescent interview
Staying up late and sleeping in	Mood disorder	Sleep patterns	Teens with chronic illness—effects on psychosocial development

Facts	Hypothesis	What do you want to know next?	Learning issues
Changes in appearance	Psychotic disorder	Relationship with mom/dad/siblings	Substance use in risks in teens
Less attentive to management of glucose levels	Personality disorder	Difficulty concentrating/ focusing	
Social: lives with mom, older sister, younger brother	Social	Suicidal thoughts	
Parents divorced when he was 9 years old			
Sees father weekly			
Cooperative with questioning	Friends/girlfriend	n/v/d? Recent weightloss	
	Bullying		
	School more challenging		
	Drug/EtOH use		
	Normal behavior	Would mom/Brian be willing to compromise on some things?	Counseling parents about typical changes to expect in an adolescent
History of IDDM since age 10; admits he knows he "can do better" about glucose monitoring	BIO	Would Brian be willing to check his sugars/keep a log?	Red flags concerning for possible EtOH/ drug use independence versus discipline
	Predisposition for EtOH/drug abuse/ dependence issues		
Talks positively about family			Diabetes management in teenagers
Admits he could try harder in school, but otherwise school is okay	Psycho X		
	SOCIAL		
	Peer-group changes/ pressures		
	Drug/EtOH exposure/ access		
Currently in a "serious relationship" with girlfriend	Spiritual		
	Mom raised in religious setting: possible there is some conflict in current relationship with son—strict rules versus his desire to be independent/form his own identity		
Large peer group			
Recent growth spurt			

Facts	Hypothesis	What do you want to know next?	Learning issues
Experimented with EtOH in the past—did not like			
Denies discipline problems, history of stealing, fire setting, harm to animals, or running away; denies trouble with the law			
Reports good mood; sleeps well, good appetite			
Denies SI or self harming behaviors			
Enjoys skateboarding, writing, listening to music, and playing guitar			
Works part time at ice cream shop			
Goal oriented/future oriented			
FHx: maternal uncle with substance abuse problem			

EtOH ethanol, *IDDM* insulin-dependent diabetes mellitus

Appendix B: Answers to Review Questions

1. b
2. d
3. c
4. c

References

American Psychiatric Association. (2013). *Diagnostic and statistical manual of mental disorders* (5th ed.). Washington, DC: American Psychiatric Association.

Blakemore, S., & Choudhury, S. (2006). Development of the adolescent brain: implications for executive function and social cognition. *The Journal of Child Psychology and Psychiatry, 47*(3/4), 296–212.

Erikson, E. (1950). *Childhood and society*. New York: Norton.

Frankenburg, W. K., Dodds, J., Archer, P., Shapiro, H., & Bresnick, B. (1992). The Denver II: a major revision and restandardization of the Denver developmental screening test. *Pediatrics, 89*(1), 91–97.
Higgins, E. S., & George, M. S. (2007). *The neuroscience of clinical psychiatry*. Philadelphia: Lippincott Williams & Wilkins.
Knight, J. R., Sherritt, L, Shrier L. A., Harris S. K., & Chang (1999). Validity of the CRAFFT substance abuse screening test among adolescent clinic patients. *Archives Pediatrics and Adolescent Medicine Journal, 156*(6), 607–14.
Lewis, M. (2007). *Lewis's child and adolescent psychiatry: A comprehensive textbook* (4th ed.). Philadelphia: Lippincott Willimas and Wilkins.
Melham, N. M., Moritz, G., & Walker, M. (2007). Phenomenology and correlates of complicated grief in children and adolescents. *Journal of The American Academy of Child Adolescent, 46*(4), 493–499.
Phelan, T. (2003). *1-2-3 magic: Effective discipline for children 2-12*. Glen Ellyn: Child Mangement, Inc.
Piaget, J. (1964). *The early growth of logic in the child*. London: Routledge and Kegan Paul Ltd.
Pruitt, D. (2000). *Your child: Emotional, behavioral, and cognitive development from birth through preadolescence*. New York: Harper Collins.
Shaffer, D. (1996). The NIMH Diagnostic Interview Schedule for children, version 2.3 (DISC 2.3): Description, acceptability, prevalence rates, and performance in the MECA study methods for the epidemiology of the child and adolescent mental disorders study. *Journal of The American Academy of Child Adolescent Psychiatry, 25,* 865–877.
Smidt, W. (2006). *Nelson essentials of pediatrics*. Philadelphia: Elsevier Saunders.
Smucker, E. R., Craighead, W. E., & Green, B. J. (1986). Normative and reliability data for the children's depression inventory. *Journal of Abnormal Child Psychology, 10,* 277–284.
Sowell, E. R., Thompson, P. M., & Toga, A. W. (2004) .Mapping changes in the human cortex throughout the span of life. *Neuroscientist, 10*(4), 372–392.
Stager M. M. (2011). Substance abuse. In R. M. Kliegman, B. F. Stanton, J. W. GemeIII St, N. F. Schor, & R. E. Behrman (Eds.), *Nelson Textbook of Pediatrics* (19th ed). Philadelphia: Elsevier Saunders; chap 108.
Stephens, M. B. (2006). Preventive health counseling for adolescents. *American Family Physician, 74*(7), 1151–1156.
Toga, A. W., Thompson, P. M., & Sowell, E. R. (2006). Mapping brain maturation. *Trends in Neurosciences, 29*(3), 148–159.
Weinberg, N. Z., et al. (1998). Adolescent substance abuse: A review of the past 10 years. *Journal of the American Academy of Child & Adolescent Psychiatry, 37*(3), 252–261
Wiener, J., & Dulcan, M. (2004). *The American psychiatric publishing textbook of child and adolescent psychiatry*. Arlington: American Psychiatric Publishing.

Resources

Clark, L. (2005). SOS help for parents bowling green: SOS Programs and Parents Press.
Normal adolescent development part 1, No. 57; updated June 2001. www.aacap.org/cs/root/facts_for_families/normal_adolescent_development_part_i.
Normal adolescent development part 1, No. 58; updated June 2001. www.aacap.org/cs/root/facts_for_families/normal_adolescent_development_part_ii.
Refer to caring for your child parenting books.
When to seek help for your child, No. 24; ;updated July 2004. www.aacap.org/page.ww?section=Facts+for+Families&name=When+To+Seek+Help+For+Your+Child.
www.aacap.org
www.aap
www.healthychildren.org

Chapter 3
Effects of Early Experience on Brain and Body

Debra J. Hendrickson

A devil, a born devil, on whose nature Nurture can never stick; on whom my pain, humanly taken, all lost, quite lost.
-William Shakespeare (1610)

Parents wonder why the streams are bitter, when they themselves have poisoned the fountain.
-John Locke (1689)

The past is never dead. It's not even past.
-William Faulkner (1950)

This chapter explains how early life experiences affect neurodevelopment. A child's early environment influences synapse formation in the cerebral cortex and gene expression in the hypothalamic–pituitary–adrenal (HPA) axis (our stress response system). By altering these pathways, significant childhood trauma can adversely affect a person's ability to cope with later stress, impacting lifelong health, success, and well-being.

By the end of the chapter, the reader will be able to:

1. Describe how the parent–child bond shapes a child's health and success.
2. Identify circumstances or events that create toxic stress for infants and children.
3. Understand how toxic stress in early life leads to epigenetic and synaptic changes.
4. Explain how, through these mechanisms, early exposure to adverse life events can affect emotional and physical health.
5. List factors that increase resilience in the face of early adversity.

D. J. Hendrickson (✉)
Northern Nevada Pediatrics, 75 Pringle Way #301, Reno, NV 89502, USA
e-mail: debrasrb@gmail.com

D. Alicata et al. (eds.), *Problem-based Behavioral Science and Psychiatry*,
DOI 10.1007/978-3-319-23669-8_3

3.1 Introduction: Nature *and* Nurture

What makes us who we are? It is both the simplest and deepest of questions. Was the murderer on death row "born bad," or is his behavior the product of childhood trauma? Is the professor who does life-saving cancer research simply acting out the coding in his own deoxyribonucleic acid (DNA), or did his parents' high expectations push him to succeed? If we could answer these mysteries, the impact on human society would be profound.

For centuries, writers, philosophers, theologians, politicians, and scientists have debated whether biology or learning is most important in shaping human character and abilities. The argument goes back to at least the 1600s, when Shakespeare (in *The Tempest*) introduced the "nature versus nurture" dialectic by describing Caliban as "a born devil," unaffected by Prospero's efforts to "nurture" him into being a better person. A few decades later, English philosopher John Locke took the opposing view, arguing that the mind at birth is a blank slate *(tabula rasa),* formed entirely by experience—that any baby could be turned into any type of person solely through learning. Bad character, in Locke's view, was solely the parents' fault.

The truth, we now know, is that *both* biology and learning shape us through a fascinating, iterative process. While our innate abilities clearly affect our experiences—a child with cerebral palsy cannot explore her environment like a healthy child, for example—the opposite is also true: environment affects our biology. Not just in obvious, macroscopic ways (a nonsmoking home leads to healthier lungs) but also on a fundamental, microscopic level: our early experiences literally shape our brains (neuroplasticity) and even how our genetic code is expressed (epigenetics).

3.1.1 Neuroplasticity

Synapses in the cerebral cortex proliferate rapidly in the first few years of life, creating a complex web of interneuronal connections. These synapses are then either maintained or atrophy, depending on whether they are stimulated by the child's environment (Jacobson 1991). The brain's ability to mold itself in response to stimuli is called *neuroplasticity.* Though it persists to some degree throughout life, neuroplasticity is particularly evident during "critical periods" in early childhood. Critical periods are windows of time (different for each functional region of the brain) in which the cerebral cortex is highly sensitive to environmental input, but after which environmental input has far less impact (Eliot 1999).

The best-studied example of a critical period is in the visual cortex, in the brain's occipital lobe. Hubel and Wiesel won the 1981 Nobel Prize in physiology and medicine for showing that the development of normal sight in cats and monkeys depended on "a rich variety of visual stimuli" reaching the visual cortex after birth (Nobel Assembly at the Karolinska Institute 1981). If an animal's eye was sewn shut for even a few days in early life, synapses in the visual cortex were permanently altered—creating irreversible vision impairment on that side (Wiesel and

Hubel 1963). Their research explained why severe congenital cataracts in humans, if not discovered and removed promptly, lead to blindness. The visual cortex cannot interpret images from the eye (even after cataract removal) because it lacked appropriate stimuli during its critical period—a window of opportunity that, if missed, affects a child for life.

Critical periods also appear to exist for areas of the brain that control auditory processing (Kral 2013), language (Hurford 1991), and emotional regulation (Schore 1994). The implications are clear: The stimulation and nurturance a child receives (or does not receive) early in life can permanently affect brain structure and function.

3.1.2 Epigenetics

Chromosomes consist of thousands of genes (segments of DNA), each encoding for a specific protein in the body. Having a gene does not guarantee that the body will make the protein. Chemical markers (such as methyl or acetyl groups) can be attached to or removed from genes, turning them "on" or "off" by blocking or enabling protein transcription by RNA polymerase. These chemical switches are called the *epigenome* ("above the genes"). Early life experiences shape the epigenome and can affect a person for life.

Much of our understanding of early life experiences' effects began with research by Weaver et al. (2004) on the impact of parenting style in rats. One group of mother rats was observed to be calmer and more nurturing ("high licking-grooming"), the other more anxious and neglectful ("low licking-grooming"). The gene for glucocorticoid receptor protein (GRP) was more methylated in pups of neglectful mothers; methylation turned the gene "off," so the pups made less GRP. GRP binds with cortisol and signals the HPA axis to stop making more cortisol; it tells the body to calm down after a stressful event. With less GRP, pups of anxious mothers tended to be more anxious and slower to calm. Conversely, pups of the nurturing mothers had less methylation of this gene and produced more GRP. They tended to be calmer and returned to baseline more quickly after stress.

Hypervigilance in a stressful environment makes evolutionary sense. Rat pups with neglectful mothers are more likely to avoid predation and other dangers if they are always on alert. Those with protective and ever-present mothers can afford to relax. The pups' early experiences, in other words, activated or deactivated genes based on what was adaptive to the animal's environment.

Research shows that early experience affects human infants similarly. Adult survivors of child abuse have decreased GRP levels, increased HPA activity, and increased risk of suicide (McGowan et al. 2009). The amount and severity of childhood sexual abuse is correlated with the amount of GRP gene methylation in patients with borderline personality disorder and major depressive disorder (Perroud et al. 2011). Survivors of extreme childhood deprivation in Romanian orphanages have significantly higher baseline cortisol than normal children (Gunnar et al.

2001), and infants of depressed mothers have higher GRP methylation and baseline cortisol than other children (Oberlander et al. 2008; Essex et al. 2002).

These findings likely explain why survivors of adverse childhood events (ACEs) have more health problems in adulthood. In a landmark study from the mid-1990s, the Centers for Disease Control (CDC) and Kaiser Permanente found that the more ACEs reported by adult patients, the more likely they were to experience a range of physical, mental, and behavioral health issues, including heart disease, cancer, diabetes, obesity, alcoholism, drug abuse, and depression (Felliti et al. 1998). A history of childhood poverty (which correlates with higher rates of abuse, neglect, and other ACEs) is associated with increased adult health problems, even if the person is financially successful as an adult (Kittleson et al. 2006).

In other words, a child's early life experiences—whether he is in a loving and enriched home or exposed to trauma and deprivation—can determine how the HPA axis responds to stress throughout life. That stress response, in turn, affects many other aspects of a person's health and well-being, as further described in Chap. 11.

The ability of the brain and HPA axis to mold in response to the child's early world creates amazing flexibility but also incredible vulnerability. The following vignettes explore the types of permanent impact left by early life, how some people seem more resilient to childhood trauma than others, and how adverse childhood experiences can affect long-term health.

Vignette 3.1.1 Presenting Situation: Justin Smith

You are a pediatrician with a busy practice in a small city. One afternoon you enter an exam room and meet Anne, a foster mom in her 40s seeking care for an 18-month-old boy named Justin Smith. Anne does not have much medical history on the boy, who was brought to her last week by the county's child welfare agency. She knows he was born full term and went home with his mother at 2 days of life. Whether or not he received routine medical care is unknown; there is no record of him in the statewide immunization database. He was taken from his mother due to methamphetamine abuse and physical neglect. The mother lived in a residential hotel that houses some of the city's poorest families; his father is unknown.

You ask how Anne thinks Justin is doing. "He seems withdrawn," she says, "and doesn't talk as much as other kids his age." She has seen him smile only once, briefly, when she showed him a video of a laughing baby on her iPad. If she points at something she wants him to see, he will look. She has heard him say "ba-ba" (for his bottle) and "mama," but not much else. He runs short distances, Anne says, and can climb stairs if she holds his hand; he plays cautiously and tentatively with toys.

You smile at Justin, who looks you in the eye but does not smile back; his expression is flat. When you offer him a ball, he looks from you to the toy several times but does not touch it. When you encourage him to take it, he starts to cry.

Table 3.1.1

FACTS	HYPOTHESES	INFORMATION NEEDED	LEARNING ISSUES

3.2 Learning Issues

3.2.1 Toxic Stress

Justin's early life exposed him to *toxic stress*—severe, frequent, or prolonged stress created by adverse circumstances. Toxic stress is created when parents are neglectful or absent, abusive, or under extreme pressure themselves (because of poverty, marital strife, domestic violence, illness, drug use, or mental health issues). All humans feel stress, and a certain amount of it—especially when experienced with loving parents who can support the child and teach good coping skills—is important in becoming a healthy, well-functioning adult. Toxic stress differs from normal stress because its intensity and/or duration exceed a child's ability to cope, adversely affecting development, behavior, and health.

Toxic stress impacts both neural development and the epigenetic programming of the HPA axis. For example, brain magnetic resonance images (MRIs) of severely maltreated children from Romanian orphanages show reduced gray and white matter and overall brain volume, even years after institutionalization (Nelson et al. 2013). In addition, numerous studies have shown that children in stressful environments (those with depressed mothers, or who are poor, homeless, or in orphanages or foster care) have altered GRP gene methylation and serum cortisol levels (Dulin-Keita et al. 2012; Dozier et al. 2006; Essex et al. 2002; Fries et al. 2008; Gunnar et al. 2001; Kertes et al. 2008; Lupien et al. 2001; Oberlander et al. 2008).

Because the neural circuitry of Justin's brain has been partially formed in a toxic, impoverished environment, his personality, social skills, and intellectual ability may be permanently affected. His stress response system (HPA axis) has almost certainly been altered by deprivation and emotional trauma, "revved up" to produce higher levels of cortisol and adrenaline in a perpetual "fight-or-flight" state. In addition, critical periods for the orbitofrontal cortex and limbic system (important in the development of self-awareness, emotional regulation, and social skills) and language centers (Wernicke's and Broca's areas) appear to occur in the first 3–5 years of life (Eliot 1999; Hurford 1991; Schore 1994). Justin's early trauma may affect his future social and economic success by altering these pathways in irrevocable ways. As Balbernie (2001) noted, "The more often the baby responds to trauma or neglect in a particular way, the greater the chances of the stress reaction becoming built-in and henceforth being expressed as a personality trait."

3.2.2 Poverty

When taken from his mother, Justin was living in poverty, a significant predictor of toxic stress. Slightly more than one in five (over 16 million) American children live below the federal poverty line. Among children aged under 5 years (the group most vulnerable to toxic stress), the rate is even higher: 25 %. Among African-American children the rate is 37.5 % (the highest of any ethnic group). Children of single mothers have the highest poverty rate, with *nearly half* living below the poverty line—in 2014, an annual income under US$15,730 for Justin and his mother (De-Navas-Walt and Proctor 2014).

Poverty increases the risk of toxic stress for many reasons. Financial stress alone can affect parents' ability to be physically and emotionally present for their children. Malnutrition, deprivation, and squalid living conditions directly affect physical health. Poor parents are more likely to abuse drugs or alcohol (though the majority do not), and poor children are much more likely to be exposed to violence. In the USA, the rate of child abuse is almost 3.5 times higher, and the rate of neglect almost 7 times higher, in poor versus nonpoor families. In addition, child maltreatment in poor families is 6.5 times more likely to be classified as "severe," resulting in significant child endangerment (Office of Planning, Research, and Evaluation [OPRE] 2010).

Poverty also impacts a child's future success by impairing language skills and intellectual development. Hart and Risley (1995) found that the amount and quality of parents' conversation with their young children correlated strongly with family income, with professional parents speaking an average of 3.5 times more words per hour to their children than welfare parents (2100 vs. 600 words/h). As a result, by age 3 a poor child had heard roughly 30 million fewer words than had a child from a professional family, and had a significantly smaller vocabulary and intelligence quotient (IQ) score. Testing at age 9 showed that these differences persisted as the children grew, despite attending school and (in some cases) receiving interventions like Head Start. The persistence of the poor children's language deficit was likely partly due to reduced neuroplasticity in the brain's language centers after age 3, and a continued impoverished environment at home. Given these findings, we can assume Justin's language delay is at least partly due to his mother speaking to him less than needed for normal development.

Childhood poverty has lifelong implications. Adults who spent part of their childhood in poverty are more likely to have increased methylation of the GRP gene and increased serum cortisol; they are also more likely to be poor as adults and to have major, chronic mental and physical health problems. Poverty is a stronger predictor of future intellectual ability and social problems than is in utero exposure to crack cocaine (Betancourt et al. 2011). All these results are rooted in the quiet poison of toxic stress. As Klass (2013) sadly observed, "Toxic stress is the heavy hand of early poverty, scripting a child's life."

Vignette 3.1.2: Continuation

Anne has brought an 18-month "Ages and Stages" (Squires and Bricker 2009) developmental questionnaire that your staff sent her to complete before the visit. It shows that Justin is significantly delayed in communication and problem-solving skills and mildly delayed in personal–social and fine motor skills. His gross motor skills are normal. She also completed a "Modified Checklist for Autism in Toddlers, Revised with Follow-Up" (M-CHAT-R/F) questionnaire (Robins et al. 2009), which shows he does not meet criteria for autism because he has no stereotypic behaviors and demonstrates some reciprocal social behavior.

Anne continues: "He seems small for his age; I have a 1-year-old in my care who is bigger." She reports his mother had nothing but cow's milk and Pepsi to feed him when he was taken, and he needs a lot of help when trying to eat solid food, "almost like he doesn't know how to do it." You look at his growth chart and see that his weight is below the 3rd percentile (the definition of *failure to thrive*); his height is 20th percentile. He is pale and thin and has healing excoriations on his buttocks from a severe diaper rash. His front incisors are brown and decayed (likely from sleeping with a bottle) and he has a soft I/VI systolic ejection murmur. His physical exam is otherwise normal.

The night he was taken from his mother, he was evaluated in the emergency room (ER) of a local hospital. A complete blood count (CBC) showed that he was anemic, with hemoglobin of 8.4 g/dL (the likely cause of his murmur). A comprehensive metabolic panel (CMP) was normal. His urine toxicology screen was negative for methamphetamine (children of meth-abusing parents are often positive because of drug residue and paraphernalia in the house). The ER doctor advised Anne to start a multivitamin with iron to correct his anemia, which she did. You tell her you will order a thyroid panel (thyroid-stimulating hormone and free T4) and venous lead sample to look for other explanations for poor growth and delayed development. You note that he has gained 6 ounces since his ER visit and do not order any other tests for now. You advise her to schedule an appointment with a pediatric dentist, never let him sleep with a bottle, and brush his teeth twice a day.

You refer Justin to your state's Early Intervention Services program for intensive speech and occupational therapy (to improve his language, fine motor, and eating skills) and schedule 1-month follow-up with you.

Table 3.1.2

FACTS	HYPOTHESES	INFORMATION NEEDED	LEARNING ISSUES

3.2.3 Attachment

Though we do not know much about Justin's relationship with his biological mother, her poverty and drug use (and possibly depression) make it likely their relationship suffered from problems with attachment. "Attachment" refers to the basic need of all infants to be emotionally connected to a primary caregiver. Normal intellectual, social, and emotional development depend on a healthy parent–child bond; infants who lack a close, consistent, reciprocal relationship with at least one caregiver tend to have serious developmental and emotional problems.

Attachment is found in every human culture and makes sense for our survival. A baby who is attached to its parent is more likely to remain close and be protected from harm; a parent who is attached to the baby will not abandon it. Despite the intuitively obvious importance of this bond, early psychologists did not always understand the central role the infant–parent relationship plays in normal development. John Watson, a pioneer of behaviorism, argued in a 1928 best-selling parenting book that children might be better off deprived of contact with their own parents, instead raised in "more scientific ways" (Watson 1928).

In subsequent decades, a series of studies on the impact of "maternal deprivation" revolutionized thinking about the importance of a baby's bond with its caregiver and put Watson's argument forever to rest. The revolution began in the 1940s with Rene Spitz's studies of institutionalized infants (babies who had been orphaned or abandoned). In a move that was very unusual for the time, Spitz had the brilliance to film, rather than just describe, the steady, horrifying deterioration of babies deprived of any close caregiver relationship. The images of these profoundly delayed and psychologically disturbed infants, rocking for hours in their orphanage cribs, had an enormous public impact (Spitz 1945, 1946). At about the same time, psychologist John Bowlby (1951) described the devastating phases of grief (protest, despair, detachment) experienced by World War II orphans after losing their parents, and James Robertson (1952) filmed the psychological deterioration of a 2-year-old girl deprived of all contact with her parents for an 8-day hospital stay (as was common practice at the time). These studies eventually led to the closing of orphanages, the establishment of the foster care system (where our patient Justin was placed), and modern hospital policies encouraging parents to stay with their sick children.

In the 1950s, Harry Harlow conducted perhaps the best-known "maternal deprivation" studies using infant rhesus monkeys taken from their biological mothers at birth and provided instead with surrogate cloth and wire or bare wire "mothers." Harlow found that the infant monkeys preferred the cloth surrogate even when only the wire surrogate provided milk. He also found that infants with a cloth surrogate were more willing to explore their environment and less frightened of new stimuli. (However, the babies with surrogate mothers—cloth or wire—were still more psychologically disturbed than those raised by real mothers.) Harlow had demonstrated that the basis of the parent–child bond was contact comfort, not food (Harlow 1958, 1959).

The impact of these studies was profound. They proved that babies were not spoiled by physical contact and emotional attention but in fact depended on it for normal development, and that the formation of an emotional infant–parent bond was a vital part of parenting. All of these findings were later explained by attachment theory.

Bowlby (1969) defined attachment as a lasting emotional bond between human beings. Our earliest bond, with our parent, impacts a child for life. Ainsworth et al. (1978) later refined the definition of attachment through what she called the "strange situation" experiment. This experiment observed a toddler's reaction to being left alone with a stranger and then reunited with his mother. Through these experiments, Ainsworth and others defined four types of attachment: secure, avoidant, ambivalent, and disorganized (the latter three all being types of "insecure" attachment). Securely attached children protest when separated from their mothers but can be comforted by a stranger and quickly return to baseline when mother returns. Insecurely attached children may be indifferent to their mother's departure and return (avoidant); become emotionally dysregulated, angry toward their mother, and have a hard time regaining calm (ambivalent); or some mixture of the two (disorganized).

Justin shows signs of avoidant attachment. This type of attachment is common in infants of neglectful mothers, who are emotionally disengaged and show little response to their child's distress. Justin does not expect his needs to be met and does not cry or reach out; he tends to withdraw and appears cautious, fearful, or indifferent toward caregivers.

Anne wants to know how Justin will do in the future. One of the things you can tell her is that securely attached children are more likely to have basic trust in other people and have more successful relationships, to have a positive self-image and "ego resiliency," and have good coping strategies and skills. Insecurely attached children are more likely to have problems with trust, relationships, emotional detachment or volatility, and confused self-image. But Justin is still very young and is already showing signs of attachment to Anne. If he has a consistent, loving relationship with a primary caregiver from this point on (especially because he is under age 3), it may help him overcome some of his early experiences.

3.2.4 *Screening for Medical Causes*

Though Justin's social history gives us plenty of explanation for his developmental and medical problems, it is important when first evaluating a new patient with developmental delay and poor growth to consider whether medical problems might also be present. The basic labs drawn in this case are a good start: CBC, CMP, thyroid panel, and lead level. If the child grows appropriately with good nutrition, his lab abnormalities (e.g., anemia) correct, and he seems to stool normally, further work-up is not required. If he does not respond in these expected ways to good care and nutrition, evaluation for cystic fibrosis, celiac disease, fat malabsorption syndromes, or metabolic diseases may be warranted, depending on specific symptoms.

If stigmata of a genetic syndrome associated with poor growth (e.g., Russell–Silver syndrome) are present, a karyotype and single nucleotide polymorphism (SNP) microarray analysis would be justified. Autistic features (delayed language, stereotypic behaviors, and impaired social interactions) and positive M-CHAT-R/F screening would also warrant a SNP microarray and genetic screening for fragile X syndrome (the most common genetic cause of cognitive delay in boys, frequently associated with autism). Please refer to Chap. 18 for further discussion of childhood disorders.

A history of prenatal alcohol exposure should raise concerns of fetal alcohol syndrome (FAS). FAS is a clinical diagnosis based on characteristic facial features (e.g., small eye openings, smooth philtrum, thin upper lip) and cognitive and functional disabilities. It is the leading cause of intellectual impairment in the developed world, with up to 2 of every 1000 live US births affected (May and Gossage 2001). Though there is no treatment for FAS, children benefit from early intervention with speech and other therapies.

Justin's mom was a known methamphetamine user. The long-term impacts of methamphetamine exposure on children, whether in utero or through contact in the home with residue and drug paraphernalia, is poorly delineated and still debated. Irritability and anger, attention problems and hyperactivity, and learning disabilities have been suggested by some studies (Smith et al. 2010; Risch 2008). However, many of these children have experienced confounding variables of neglect, abuse, and multiple foster care placements that make it hard to isolate methamphetamine's direct impact.

Children living in poverty are more likely to have elevated lead levels. Lead is common in paint and other materials found in residences built before 1978 and in soils near major roads (deposited by exhaust before the 1996 ban on leaded fuel). Elevated blood lead levels can affect learning, growth, hearing, and behavior. Six percent of poor US children aged 1–2 years have elevated blood lead levels (≥ 5 µg/dL) and are at risk of permanent brain damage (Raymond et al. 2014).

Vignette 3.1.3: Conclusion

A month later, you tell Anne that Justin's thyroid and lead tests were normal. His weight has increased another half-pound and he has had his first appointment with his speech and occupational therapists. Anne reports that he is "warming up a little." You tell her to continue the multivitamin with iron, follow-up with Early Intervention Services, and return for his 2-year well-child check. You stress the importance of him receiving Anne's focused, undivided attention for part of every day, and tell her everyone in the family should talk a lot to Justin about the world around him and the things they are doing ("narrate his day").

When he returns at age 2, Anne is pleased with his progress. She reports that he smiles more, sometimes even giggling briefly when playing with her. He has also occasionally been defiant, throwing tantrums when she switched him from the bottle to a sippy cup. She says he is more affectionate, but still a little "stand off-ish," and often "seems like he's on alert, watching for something bad to happen." (You note that when you entered the room, he did run to her, as a normal child should do when a stranger approaches.) Hemoglobin is normal (12.6 g/dL), his murmur has resolved, and his weight has climbed to the 5th percentile. The dentist removed his decaying front teeth (under general anesthesia), which improved his demeanor. He now says about 15 words—far less than the average of 50 words plus short phrases expected of normal 2-year-olds—but is babbling much more than he did.

Anne tells you she and her husband would like to adopt Justin, since it appears his biological mother will lose custody permanently. She asks what long-term effects his early life might be expected to have on him.

Table 3.1.3

FACTS	HYPOTHESES	INFORMATION NEEDED	LEARNING ISSUES

3.2.5 Resilience

When he was placed in Anne's care, Justin's developmental delays and behavior demonstrated the tragic vulnerability of infants and toddlers to toxic stress. His language and self-help skills were markedly delayed, and he was socially withdrawn. Those findings, combined with his physical condition—malnourished, anemic, with dental decay and excoriated diaper rash—are the marks of physical and emotional neglect. As noted earlier, his HPA axis and the neural circuitry of his limbic system and cerebral cortex may have been permanently affected by the toxic stress he was exposed to in early life.

Despite this traumatic history, Justin is obviously responding to having a loving, consistent, and attentive parent, and is showing improvement only 6 months after placement in foster care. Because he is so young, he has a better chance than an older child of overcoming some of his earliest experiences. We can also hope that Justin is among the fortunate children who are "resilient"—who grow into relatively healthy, well-functioning people despite ACEs. A significant minority of children demonstrates resilience; a third of children from high-risk (poor, mentally or physically ill, drug using, violent, or abusive) families have no significant mental health problems later in life (Werner 1992, 1993; Werner and Smith 1982, 2001).

Why do some children emerge from trauma more intact than others? Both innate characteristics and lucky circumstances seem to play a role. Inborn strengths (intelligence, musical talent, athletic ability) and experiences that foster a sense of mastery are clearly important, as is an even, calm temperament and good executive function. Strong social skills and a supportive faith or cultural community can help a child navigate difficult, inconsistent, or threatening environments. Finally, a strong relationship with at least one adult seems to enable many children to withstand incredible hardships in early life without significant impacts (National Scientific Council on the Developing Child 2015). Hopefully, Justin's growing attachment to Anne and his innate strengths will help reduce long-term impacts of early trauma.

Vignette 3.2.1 Presenting Situation: Leticia Reed
You are a psychiatrist rounding in an aging urban hospital. Your next patient is a 42-year-old woman named Leticia Reed, admitted for peripheral artery disease secondary to diabetes mellitus with peripheral neuropathy. She also has a history of morbid obesity, tobacco smoking, and cervical cancer at age 27. The surgeon called you to speak with her because of a history of post-traumatic stress disorder (PTSD), depression, borderline personality disorder, and parasuicidal behavior. He is worried about how she will cope with the impending partial amputation of her left foot.

Table 3.2.1

FACTS	HYPOTHESES	INFORMATION NEEDED	LEARNING ISSUES

Vignette 3.2.2: Conclusion
You see a very large woman lying in the hospital bed, an elaborate arm tattoo partially covered by her hospital gown sleeve. "Good morning, Mrs. Reed," you begin, before identifying yourself and explaining why you're there.

"Gonna do this dance again, huh?" she says. Her expression is flat, but she does not seem unfriendly. She agrees to speak with you.

Leticia tells you she has "seen a lot of shrinks, but none for too long" and has been "messed up since I was a kid." When you ask her about any history of victimization or maltreatment, she reveals that her stepfather sexually abused her from age 9 to 14, before being arrested and incarcerated. You ask if her mother knew what was happening before the arrest; she looks out the window and says, "My mama in those days pretty much never left her bed.

I barely remember her lookin' at me. I don't think she wanted to face life, or him. He hit her pretty good sometimes." After her stepfather's arrest, her mother had to make ends meet cleaning a neighbor's house, and Leticia had to care for her younger siblings. She struggled to finish high school and has worked in low-wage jobs most of her life.

She was married briefly and has a son who lives in another state. "He was pretty messed up, too, with drugs, but got his act together, more or less." Leticia admits she was very depressed when he was young. "I feel guilty about that," she says, looking down. "His dad was a drinker, he and I were having problems, and I couldn't deal with it. I'd eat, watch TV, sleep. I got fatter and fatter. When his dad left, I started cutting myself"—she rolls her arms over, revealing dozens of thin, white, horizontal scars—"and a couple of times ended up in the hospital 'cause I went a little too deep." She denies suicidal ideation now, but admits, "I can't really remember ever not being depressed, to tell you the truth."

You ask Leticia how she is feeling about her upcoming surgery. She looks out the window again. "It's just one more thing," she says flatly. "What are you gonna do."

Table 3.2.2

FACTS	HYPOTHESES	INFORMATION NEEDED	LEARNING ISSUES

3.3 Learning Issues

3.3.1 Long-Term Impacts of Adverse Childhood Events

As noted earlier, survivors of ACEs have increased odds of mental and physical health problems in adulthood, and there is a strong correlation between the number of ACEs and the odds of these problems. In the CDC/Kaiser ACE data collected in 1995–1997, roughly 17,000 patients were asked to recall the type and number of the following adverse events of their childhood:

- Psychological, physical, or sexual abuse
- Emotional or physical neglect
- Violence against mother
- Parental separation or divorce
- Living with others who were substance abusers, mentally ill or suicidal, or ever imprisoned

The authors found a graded relationship ($p < 0.001$) between the number of ACEs and adult health problems. Leticia has a history of at least three ACEs—sexual abuse, witnessing violence against her mother, and parental divorce. From her narrative, it also sounds as if her mother suffered from depression, a risk factor for emotional neglect (her fourth ACE) and insecure attachment; her stepfather was also incarcerated. The CDC/Kaiser studies found that a history of four or more ACEs quadruples the odds of depression; it increases the odds of a suicide attempt more than 12 times. It increases the risk of obesity and diabetes mellitus 1.5 times and doubles the risk of tobacco smoking and ischemic heart disease (Felliti et al. 1998). Leticia's current health problems, all the suffering they bring her and all the expense to our society, may be rooted in her childhood.

Sadly, Leticia passed on the same kind of childhood experiences to her son. He was exposed to maternal depression and suicidal behavior, paternal alcohol abuse, and parental divorce, and, according to her story, developed mental health issues (drug abuse).

Though not explicitly stated in the narrative, we can assume from their employment histories that Leticia and her mother are also poor. Although the CDC/Kaiser study did not look specifically at poverty as an ACE, they did find that several measures of financial security were strongly correlated with the number of ACEs (e.g., a more traumatic childhood reduced a person's chances of holding a steady job in adulthood). Also, the ACEs that were measured in the study—abuse, neglect, substance abuse, and violence—are all more common in poverty, as noted earlier (OPRE 2010).

Given the correlation between poverty and ACEs, Holzer et al. (2008) concluded that childhood poverty actually costs the US government US$500 billion/year in decreased economic output (1.3 % GDP), increased crime (1.3 %), and increased health-care costs (1.2 % GDP). In short, improving the financial circumstances of families with young children could reduce many chronic adult medical conditions and social problems.

One of Leticia's diagnoses is borderline personality disorder (BPD, see Chap. 24 on personality disorders). BPD is characterized by unstable self-image, relationships, and emotional regulation; parasuicidal behavior (cutting) and suicide attempts are common. A history of childhood sexual abuse is strongly correlated with BPD; some researchers have suggested that as many as 71 % of BPD patients have this history (Ogata et al. 1990). Other forms of childhood abuse and neglect have also been correlated with BPD (Zanarini et al. 1997). As noted earlier, recent studies have shown increased GRP methylation in patients with BPD and those with depression (another of Leticia's diagnoses). An abnormal, exaggerated physiologic response to stress may have been epigenetically encoded in these patients by early trauma, accounting for some of their emotional dysregulation.

Epigenetic programming of the HPA axis (through methylation of the GRP gene) likely explains many of the ACE study results. Trauma leads to reduced GRP and increased cortisol; chronically elevated cortisol is associated with hypertension, hyperglycemia, lowered immune function, increased abdominal fat, impaired cognitive performance, slow wound healing, and other adverse health effects. Because of their lifelong impacts on our brain and stress response system, traumatic childhood events cast a long shadow of suffering.

3.4 Conclusion

Faulkner's famous observation about the impact of past events on our subsequent lives has turned out to be truer than he could have imagined. As shown in this chapter, early life experiences are encoded in the wiring of our brains and the chemistry of our DNA—we literally carry these events with us, every day, as a permanent, physical change in our bodies. Like a stone thrown into a pond, early experiences ripple through the remainder of our lives, influencing our learning, our relationships, and our ability to be good citizens and good parents for the next generation. This knowledge should guide anyone who cares for children and families, as well as policy-makers shaping our economy and society. We must do all we can to reduce childhood poverty and help at-risk families, enrich the learning environments of young children, intervene quickly to protect them from abuse and neglect, and be alert to problems of parenting and attachment that might be amenable to therapy. Despite the known impacts of early adverse events, some children (because of temperament, intelligence, or the presence of a caring adult) are resilient and go on to lead productive lives after even intense suffering; all traumatized children deserve support and intervention, and no child should be considered "a lost cause." But we should be mindful that past trauma often plays a role in the behavior of difficult, chronically ill adult patients who seem unable to change.

In sum, both our biology and our experiences—nature and nurture—interact to make us the people we become, with our earliest experiences (from birth to age 5), having a particularly powerful, lifelong impact. Because of this, prevention of adverse childhood experiences is clearly the most cost-effective way to address many individual ailments and societal ills. Physicians who care for children and families are on the front lines of this preventative effort. In both clinical practice and as members of society, we are obligated to advocate for enriched, secure, and loving environments that brighten the futures of our youngest patients.

Review Questions

1. Early life experiences can have lifelong impacts because of their effect on:
   a. Methylation of the GRP gene
   b. Cortisol levels
   c. Synaptic remodeling of the brain during "critical periods"
   d. The orbitofrontal cortex and limbic system
   e. All of the above
2. Which of the following outcomes has been linked to elevated ($\geq$4) ACE scores?
   a. Hypotension
   b. Infanticide
   c. Substance use disorders
   d. Increased job stability
   e. Smoking cessation

3. Children living in poverty are more likely to experience:
   a. Abuse and neglect
   b. Toxic stress
   c. Mental and physical health problems and early death
   d. Poverty when they become adults
   e. All of the above
4. Attachment is defined as:
   a. A normal infant's strong unwillingness to leave its mother and explore surroundings
   b. A lasting emotional bond between human beings that is essential for normal infant development
   c. An internalized representation of the baby's parent
   d. The infant's need to be with its mother to obtain food
   e. A mother's responsiveness to her baby's social behavior
5. Traits associated with resilience in children include all the following *except:*
   a. Exposure to bullying
   b. Intelligence
   c. Good social skills
   d. A close relationship with at least one caring adult
   e. Involvement with religious or community groups

Appendix A: Tables with Possible Answers to the Vignettes

Vignette 3.1: Justin Smith

Table 3.1.1

Facts	Hypotheses	Information needed	Learning issues
Justin is an 18-month-old boy	Justin may be a victim of physical and emotional neglect	Is he really delayed?	What is toxic stress and how can it affect development?
His biological mother is a single parent, poor, and a methamphetamine user	He may also be a victim of abuse	Does he have a medical condition or neurodevelopmental disorder that causes developmental delays and flat emotional affect?	Why is it important to enrich Justin's emotional and physical circumstances as soon as possible?
His foster mother thinks he is not speaking or interacting the way kids his age should	These circumstances could have exposed him to "toxic stress"		

Facts	Hypotheses	Information needed	Learning issues
Justin and his family's medical histories are unknown			

Table 3.1.2

Facts	Hypotheses	Information needed	Learning issues
Justin has multiple developmental delays	His developmental delays and blunted social responses are likely the result of emotional deprivation, insecure attachment to his biological mother, and an impoverished environment	Does he have a medical condition that could cause failure to thrive (e.g., cystic fibrosis, celiac disease, hypothyroidism, lead poisoning)?	How does attachment affect development? What type of attachment does Justin display?
He does not have autism	He is malnourished due to neglect		How can we distinguish failure to thrive caused by social versus medical problems?
He has "failure to thrive" (weight below 3rd percentile)	His biological mother did not take care of his basic needs		What kinds of treatments and therapies does Justin need to physically, emotionally, and intellectually improve?
He is anemic	His weakened and uncomfortable physical condition has likely interfered with learning and social enjoyment		
He has excoriated diaper rash			
He has dental decay			
He is already gaining weight in foster care			

Table 3.1.3

Facts	Hypotheses	Information needed	Learning issues
No biological cause of his physical and developmental problems was found	Justin is forming a secure attachment to his foster mother	Will Justin be in a stable, nurturing, and enriched environment for the rest of his childhood?	What traits help some children be "resilient" despite early trauma?
His medical and dental problems have been addressed	His response to good nutrition, love, and an enriched environment indicates his problems were rooted in social, not medical problems		Why is poverty a risk factor for child maltreatment?

Facts	Hypotheses	Information needed	Learning issues
His emotional responsiveness, growth and development are all improving with a loving and enriched environment	He may respond differently to stress in the future because of his early experiences, and have lingering problems with trust, attention, and learning		How could our society reduce the incidence and impact of "toxic stress?"
	Or, intervention may have come soon enough to help overcome his early circumstances (especially if he is resilient)		How does love (or its absence) affect health?

Vignette 3.1: Leticia Reed

Table 3.2.1

Facts	Hypotheses	Information needed	Learning issues
Leticia Reed is a 42-year-old woman	Mrs. Reed's lifestyle has led to chronic, disabling health problems	What keeps her from changing her habits and improving her health?	How does mental health affect physical health, and vice versa?
She has peripheral artery disease, diabetes, peripheral neuropathy, obesity, and a history of cervical cancer	Her mental health issues may contribute to her unhealthy lifestyle choices	What is her attitude toward the upcoming procedure, and those trying to help her?	
She is scheduled for a left foot amputation	Her mental health issues may impair coping with her upcoming surgery and rehabilitation	Does she have social and financial support to help her with rehabilitation?	
She is a tobacco user			
She has PTSD, depression, and BPD with a history of parasuicidal behavior			

PTSD post-traumatic stress disorder, *BPD* borderline personality disorder

Table 3.2.2

Facts	Hypotheses	Information needed	Learning issues
Leticia was sexually abused as a child and witnessed domestic violence between her parents	Her traumatic childhood may have affected important brain regions that control insight, empathy, emotion, and language, impairing her ability to cope with stress, maintain stable, trusting relationships, learn and succeed	Does she have traits she could draw upon to improve her health or circumstances?	How do ACEs affect later physical and mental health, high-risk behaviors, and success in relationships and employment?
Her mother was depressed, her stepfather was incarcerated	Her history of adverse childhood events may have altered her HPA axis and cortisol levels, increasing her risks of chronic health problems		How does maternal depression impact children?
She has been poor her entire life and works in low-wage jobs	Her childhood may have impaired her own ability to be an attentive, loving parent, extending trauma to the next generation		
She is divorced and lives alone			
She was depressed when her son was young			
Her son has a history of drug use			

ACEs adverse childhood experiences, *HPA* hypothalamic–pituitary–adrenal axis

Appendix B: Answers to Review Questions

1. e
2. c
3. e
4. b
5. a

References

Ainsworth, M. D. S., Blehar, M. C., Waters, E., Wall, S. (1978). *Patterns of attachment: A psychological study of the strange situation*. New York: Psychology Press.

Balbernie, R. (2001). Circuits and circumstances: The neurobiological consequences of early relationship experiences and how they shape later behavior. *Journal of Child Psychotherapy, 27*(3), 237–255.

Betancourt, L. M., Yang, W., Brodsky, N. L., Gallagher, P. R., Malmud, E. K., Giannetta, J. M., Farah, M. J., & Hurt, H. (2011). Adolescents with and without gestational cocaine exposure: Longitudinal analysis of inhibitory control, memory and receptive language. *Neurotoxicology and Teratology, 33*(1), 36–46.

Bowlby, J. (1951). Maternal care and mental health: A report prepared on behalf of the World Health Organization as a contribution to the United Nations programme for the welfare of homeless children. Geneva: World Health Organization.

Bowlby, J. (1969). *Attachment and loss, Vol. 1: Attachment*. New York: Basic Books.

DeNavas-Walt, C. & Proctor, B. D. (2014). U.S. Census Bureau, Current Population Reports, P 60–249, Income and poverty in the United States: 2013, Washington, DC: U.S. Government Printing Office.

Dozier, M., Manni, M., Gordon, M. K., Peloso, E., Gunnar, M. R., Stovall-McClough, K. C., et al. (2006). Foster children's diurnal production of cortisol: An exploratory study. *Child Maltreatment, 11,* 189–197.

Dulin-Keita, A., Casazza, K., Fernandez, J. R., Goran, M. I., & Gower, B. (2012). Do neighborhoods matter? Neighborhood disorder and long-term trends in serum cortisol levels. *Journal of Epidemiology and Community Health, 66*(1), 24.

Eliot, L. (1999). *What's going on in there? How the brain and mind develop in the first five years of life*. New York: Bantam Books.

Essex, M. J., Klein M. H., Cho, E., & Kalin, N. H. (2002). Maternal stress beginning in infancy may sensitize children to later stress exposure: Effects on cortisol and behavior. *Biological Psychiatry, 52,* 776–784.

Felliti, V. J., Anda, R. F., Nordenberg, D., Williamson, D. F., Spitz, A. M., Edwards, V., Koss, M. P., & Marks, J. S. (1998). Relationship of childhood abuse and household dysfunction to many of the leading causes of death in adults: The Adverse Childhood Experiences (ACE) Study. *American Journal of Preventive Medicine, 14*(4), 245–254.

Fries, A. B. W., Shirtcliff, E. A., & Pollak, S. D. (2008). Neuroendocrine dysregulation following early social deprivation in children. *Developmental Psychobiology, 50*(6), 588–599.

Gunnar, M. R., Morison, S. J., Chisholm, K., Schuder, M. (2001). Salivary cortisol levels in children adopted from Romanian orphanages. *Development and Psychopathology, 13,* 611–628.

Harlow, H. (1958). The nature of love. *American Psychologist, 13,* 673–685.

Harlow, H. (1959). Love in infant monkeys. *Scientific American, 200,* 68–74.

Hart, B., & Risley, T. R. (1995). *Meaningful differences in the everyday experience of young American children*. Baltimore: Brooks Publishing.

Holzer, H. J., Whitmore-Schanzenbach, D., Duncan, G. J., & Ludwig, J. (2008). The economic costs of childhood poverty in the United States. *Journal of Children and Poverty, 14*(1), 41–61.
Hurford, J. R. (1991). The evolution of the critical period for language acquisition. *Cognition, 40*(3), 159–201.
Jacobson, M. (1991). *Developmental neurobiology* (3rd ed.). New York: Plenum.
Kertes, D. A., Gunnar, M. R., Madsen, N. J., & Long, J. D. (2008). Early deprivation and home basal cortisol levels: A study of internationally adopted children. *Development and Psychopathology, 20*(02), 473–491.
Kittleson, M. M., Meoni, L. A., Wang, N. Y., Chu, A. Y., Ford, D. E., & Klag, M. J. (2006). Association of childhood socioeconomic status with subsequent coronary heart disease in physicians. *Archives of Internal Medicine, 166*(21), 2356–2361.
Klass, P. (13 May 2013). Poverty as a childhood disease. *New York Times*. http://www.nytimes.com/.
Kral, A. (2013). Auditory critical periods: A review from system's perspective. *Neuroscience, 247,* 117–133.
Lupien, S. J., King, S., Meaney, M. J., & McEwen, B. S. (2001). Can poverty get under your skin? Basal cortisol levels and cognitive function in children from low and high socioeconomic status. *Development and Psychopathology, 13*(03), 653–676.
May, P. A. & Gossage, J. P. (2001). Estimating the prevalence of fetal alcohol syndrome: A summary. *Alcohol Research and Health, 25*(3), 159–167.
McGowan, P. O., Sasaki, A., D'Alessio, A. C., Dymov, S., Labonté, B., Szyf, M., Turecki, G., & Meaney, M. J. (2009). Epigenetic regulation of the glucocorticoid receptor in human brain associates with childhood abuse. *Nature Neuroscience, 12*(3), 342–348.
National Scientific Council on the Developing Child. (2015). Supportive relationships and active skill-building strengthen the foundations of resilience: Working Paper 13. http://www.developingchild.harvard.edu.
Nelson, C. A., III., Fox, N. A., & Zeanah, C. H., Jr. (2013). Anguish of the abandoned child. *Scientific American, 308*(4), 62–67.
Nobel Assembly at the Karolinska Institute. (9 October 1981). Press release: The Nobel prize in physiology or medicine 1981. http://www.nobelprize.org.
Oberlander, T. F., Weinberg, J., Papsdorf, M., Grunau, R., Misri, S., & Devlin, A. M. (2008). Prenatal exposure to maternal depression, neonatal methylation of human glucocorticoid receptor gene (NR3C1) and infant cortisol stress responses. *Epigenetics, 3*(2), 97–106.
Office of Planning, Research, and Evaluation (OPRE). (2010). Fourth national incidence study of child abuse and neglect (NIS-4): Report to congress. http://www.acf.hhs.gov/programs/opre/.
Ogata, S. N., Silk, K. R., Goodrich, S., Lohr, N. E., Westen, D., & Hill, E. M. (1990). Childhood sexual and physical abuse in adult patients with borderline personality disorder. *American Journal of Psychiatry, 147*(8), 1008–1013.
Perroud, N., Paoloni-Giacobino, A., Prada, P., Olie, E., Salzmann, A., Nicastro, R., Guillaume, S., Mouthon, D., Stouder, C., Dieben, K., Huguelet, P., Courtet, P., & Malafosse, A. (2011). Increased methylation of glucocorticoid receptor gene (NR3C1) in adults with a history of childhood maltreatment: A link with the severity and type of trauma. *Translational Psychiatry, 1*(12), e59.
Raymond, J., Wheeler, W., & Brown, M. J. (2014). Lead screening and prevalence of blood lead levels in children aged 1–2 years–child blood lead surveillance system, United States, 2002–2010 and National Health and Nutrition Examination Survey, United States, 1999–2010. Morbidity and mortality weekly report. Surveillance summaries (Washington, DC: 2002), 63, 36–42.
Risch, E. C. (2008). *Effects of prenatal methamphetamine exposure on arousal regulation in toddlers*. Tulsa: University of Tulsa.
Robertson, J. (1952). *A 2-year-old goes to hospital*. United Kingdom: Concord Video and Film Council.
Robins, D. L., Fein, D., & Barton, M. (2009). Modified Checklist for Autism in Toddlers, Revised, with Follow-Up (M-CHAT-R/F) TM.

Schore, A. N. (1994). *Affect regulation and the origin of the self: The neurobiology of emotional development*. Psychology Press.
Smith, L., LaGasse, L., Derauf, C., Newman, E., Shah, R. (2010). Motor and cognitive outcomes through three years of age in children exposed to prenatal methamphetamine. *Neurotoxicology and Teratology, 33,* 176–184.
Spitz, R. A. (1945). Hospitalism—An inquiry into the genesis of psychiatric conditions in early childhood. *Psychoanalytic Study of the Child, 1,* 53–74.
Spitz, R. A. (1946). Hospitalism—A follow-up report on investigation described in volume I, 1945. *Psychoanalytic Study of the Child, 2,* 113–117.
Squires, J., & Bricker, D. (2009). *Ages & stages questionnaires. Third Edition. (ASQ-3): A parent-completed child-monitoring system*. Baltimore: Paul Brookes.
Watson, J. B. (1928). *Psychological care of infant and child*. New York: Norton.
Weaver, I. C., Cervoni, N., Champagne, F. A., D'Alessio, A. C., Sharma, S., Seckl, J. R., Dymov, S., Szyf, M., & Meaney, M. J. (2004). Epigenetic programming by maternal behavior. *Nature Neuroscience, 7*(8), 847–854.
Werner, E. E. (1992). The children of Kauai: Resiliency and recovery in adolescence and adulthood. *Journal of Adolescent Health, 13,* 262–268.
Werner, E. E. (1993). Risk, resilience, and recovery: Perspectives from the Kauai longitudinal study. *Development and Psychopathology, 5,* 503–515.
Werner, E. E., & Smith, R. S. (1982). *Vulnerable but not invincible: A longitudinal study of resilient children and youth*. New York: McGraw Hill.
Werner, E. E., & Smith, R. S. (2001). *Journeys from childhood to midlife*. Ithaca: Cornell University Press.
Wiesel, T. N., & Hubel, D. H. (1963). Single cell responses in striate cortex of kittens deprived of vision in one eye. *Journal of Neurophysiology, 26,* 1003–1017.
Zanarini, M. C., Williams, A. A., Lewis, R. E. Reich, R. B., Vera, S. C., Marino, M. F., Levin, A., Yong, L., & Frankenburg, F. R. (1997). Reported pathological childhood experiences associated with the development of borderline personality disorder. *The American Journal of Psychiatry, 154,* 1101–1106.

Chapter 4
Learning Principles of Human Behavior

David Antonuccio and Amber Hayes

A failure is not always a mistake; it may simply be the best one can do under the circumstances. The real mistake is to stop trying.
-B.F. Skinner

4.1 Introduction

The purpose of this chapter is to highlight key learning principles that apply to human behavior. Human behavior responds to punishment and reinforcement in predictable ways. Understanding these relationships can help physicians guide their patients to modify their behavior to achieve desirable outcomes.

4.2 Objectives

At the end of the chapter, the reader will be able to:

1. Define the following behavioral terms: classical conditioning, operant conditioning, reinforcement, reward, punishment, reinforcement schedule, antecedents, consequences, stimulus control, modeling, self-efficacy, motivational interviewing, and functional analysis
2. Apply behavioral principles to understand some common behavioral problems observed in medicine

D. Antonuccio (✉)
Private Practice, 3732 Lakeside Dr., #200, Reno, NV 89509, USA
e-mail: oliver2@aol.com

A. Hayes
Renown Medical Group, 202 Los Altos Drive, Sparks, NV 89436, USA
e-mail: Alhayes81@gmail.com

D. Alicata et al. (eds.), *Problem-based Behavioral Science and Psychiatry*,
DOI 10.1007/978-3-319-23669-8_4

3. Utilize behavioral principles to begin to develop treatment plans for some common behavioral problems

Vignette 4.1.1 Presenting Situation: Ronald

Ronald is a 58-year-old male who came to his primary care physician for an annual physical exam. Through routine interviewing, Ronald is asked about tobacco use because the doctor employs the 5 A's approach (see boxed list below) advocated by the USPHS (U.S. Public Health Service) (Fiore et al. 2008). He admits to being a smoker and smoking two packs of cigarettes per day for the past 40 years. Ronald expresses to the physician that he wishes he could "quit this nasty habit" but has had difficulty in the past. The doctor adopts a *motivational interviewing* (Lai et al. 2010; Hettema and Hendricks 2010) approach that involves helping the patient explore his worries about trying to quit and what he hopes to accomplish by quitting. This approach is a gentle strategy of asking the patient what he or she would like to know about quitting rather than forcefully telling the patient to quit.

Please proceed with the problem-based approach using the worksheet located in the appendix of Chap. 1!

Table 4.1.1

FACTS	HYPOTHESES	INFORMATION NEEDED	LEARNING ISSUES

Vignette 4.1.2 Continuation

When the physician asks Ronald why he wants to quit now, Ronald says that he has been hearing about all of the bad health effects smoking can have. His wife has been nagging him whenever he smokes because she is worried about his health, so he has been sneaking cigarettes behind her back, and he feels guilty about this. He is soon to be a grandfather and is worried about the potential effects of secondhand smoke on his newly arriving grandchild. He also wants to make sure he is around to enjoy his grandchildren and vice versa. In the past, Ronald says he has tried stopping "cold turkey," but the withdrawal symptoms and cravings drove him back to smoking after about 3 days.

4.2.1 Learning Issue: Functional Analysis

The doctor then requests that the patient perform a *functional analysis* of his smoking. A functional analysis is a systematic way to characterize a behavior by examining events that happen prior to (i.e., *antecedents*) the unwanted behavior (in this case, smoking) and the consequences of acting out that behavior. The doctor will have Ronald start to record each cigarette he smokes and the activities leading up to the cigarette to find out what types of triggers or *antecedents* cause him to want to smoke. Smoking a cigarette has been paired with some environmental stimuli many hundreds of times, causing them to become *classically conditioned.* For example, a patient who smokes after a meal to satisfy a craving may find that he has an urge to smoke after all meals. The doctor also asks Ronald to make a list of the *consequences* of smoking to help understand the role of *operant conditioning*. Not all consequences are bad, for example, the feeling of relief after having smoked. Some consequences are powerful *reinforcers,* that is, increase the probability of smoking.

Vignette 4.1.3 Continuation
Ronald returns to his physician 1 week later with a daily log of cigarettes and activities. The table below lists some antecedents and consequences for this patient's smoking and identifies them as punishing (any consequence that makes smoking less likely) and reinforcing (any consequence that makes smoking more likely). The doctor notices that Ronald has a cigarette upon waking, with morning coffee, after every meal, while driving, while on the phone, and while visiting with other smoking friends. He notices that in all cases except for one cigarette, he smokes out of the presence of his wife. Though her nagging serves as a punisher for his smoking, he feels resentful and tends to avoid her. The physician points out that by definition, punishment decreases the probability of a behavior but does not encourage appropriate alternatives, makes him angry, and causes him to avoid his wife. The physician brings the wife into the session to educate her about the downside of nagging and other punishment and encourages her to be supportive or at least neutral when he is struggling with his smoking (Table 4.1).

Table 4.1 Functional analysis of smoking

Antecedent	Consequence	Punishing versus reinforcing
Waking	Feeling relieved	R
On phone	Wife nags him	P
Coffee	Costly	P
After meal	Smoker's cough	P
Driving	Satisfies boredom	R
Visiting	Feeling socially accepted	R

R reinforcing, *P* punishing

Please proceed with the problem-based approach using the worksheet located in the appendix of Chap. 1!

Table 4.1.2

FACTS	HYPOTHESES	INFORMATION NEEDED	LEARNING ISSUES

4.2.2 *Learning Issue: Stages of Change*

The stages of change can be seen in just about any behavior that one wants to modify including behaviors such as eating habits, compliance with treatment, addiction, and much more (Zimmerman et al. 2000). The stages are divided into five phases: precontemplation, contemplation, preparation, action, and maintenance (DiClemente et al. 1991). It is important to note that a person may fluctuate back and forth between stages as they consider changing a particular behavior, and knowing which stage a person is in will guide the assistance the practitioner provides. Most smokers will exhibit the stages of change as they attempt to quit smoking.

Precontemplation Stage In this stage, one is not even considering changing the behavior. To assist people in this stage, it is appropriate to recognize and validate their unwillingness to change at this time, provide personalized reasons that the behavior puts them at risk, and provide an opportunity to revisit the idea of changing the behavior in the future.

Contemplation Stage In the contemplation stage, the idea of the behavior being a problem has crossed the person's mind more than once, but currently they lack the commitment to take action. To assist people in this stage, it is often helpful to make a list of *pros and cons* for continuing the behavior versus changing it. It is also important to highlight the benefits of changing.

Preparation Stage A person in the preparation stage has begun to "test the waters" and is much more serious about changing and developing a plan to change in the near future. A person in this stage will actually set some specific goals or target dates. To assist a person in this stage, it is important to help him or her identify possible roadblocks to changing the behavior, set up a support system, and identify steps that will assist the person in changing the behavior.

Action Stage The action stage has begun when the person begins modification of the behavior. This may require assistance in changing the normal cues for the undesired behavior, continuing to enhance the support system, and identifying obstacles to maintaining the change. It is important to note that persons in this stage may begin to feel a sense of loss for the old behavior.

Maintenance Stage In the maintenance stage, the behavior has been modified for some time but requires continued work to prevent a relapse. The practitioner's role is to help identify the situations in which a relapse could occur and as a team decide on how best to overcome the triggers. It is important for the practitioner to stress that the occurrence of a relapse does not mean instant failure, and more than likely it provides a learning opportunity for the future (Table 4.2).

Table 4.2 Smoking cessation tools: 5 A's approach

The 5 A's approach
The US Public Health Service recommends the "5 A's approach" to treatment of smoking (Fiore et al. 2008):
*A*sk about tobacco use. This also involves addressing myths about quitting. For example, it is a myth that past attempts decrease ability to quit or that older smokers don't benefit from quitting
*A*dvise users to stop. Provide the patient with information on the medical benefits of quitting smoking
*A*ssess willingness to quit. An important factor is to match the intervention with the stage of quitting (see below)
*A*ssist in quitting
*A*rrange for follow-up
(This 5-step program could easily be adapted to any kind of habit change a physician is encouraging in a patient)

Vignette 4.1.4 Conclusion

Ronald asks the doctor what he should do next. The doctor keeps the 5 A's in mind as he advises his patient. The doctor asks the patient if he is ready to pick a target quit date. The patient says he is and chooses his wife's birthday in 3 weeks. The doctor tells him to get some practice at not smoking before his quit day by eliminating smoking during one of the easier situations he has identified. Ronald decides to become a nonsmoker while driving his car. He plans to keep his cigarettes in the trunk of his car and to put sugarless candy in his ashtray as a substitute to help him achieve this goal. This is called a **"stimulus control"** strategy, that is, altering the environment to make it easier to disconnect the stimulus of driving from the behavior of smoking. By altering some of the environmental stimuli, hopefully he can reduce his smoking (Antonuccio 1992).

Ronald comes back to see his physician weekly to evaluate his progress and for support. On his wife's birthday, Ronald begins using the nicotine patch prescribed by the doctor. He chooses to reduce his patch each week so that 3 weeks after his quit date (e.g., Bolin et al. 1999) he is totally nicotine free. He feels proud of himself and his wife tells him it is the best birthday present she has ever received.

Vignette 4.2.1: Presenting Situation: Sally

Sally is 48-year-old female who comes to the clinic today because of sleeping problems. She states that over the last 3 months she has not been sleeping well at all and wonders if there is anything that can be done.

Please proceed with the problem-based approach using the worksheet located in the appendix of Chap. 1!

Table 4.2.1

FACTS	HYPOTHESES	INFORMATION NEEDED	LEARNING ISSUES

Vignette 4.2.2: Continuation

The doctor takes a sleep history using the BEARS (Bedtime, Excessive daytime sleepiness, Awakenings, Regularity and duration of sleep, Snoring) acronym (Ward 2011).

First the doctor reviews bedtime rituals and what happens at sleep onset. He reviews intake of alcohol, nicotine, caffeine, and medications. He asks about how tired she gets during the day. He asks about how well she sleeps through the night and how many hours of sleep she typically gets. He also asks about snoring to rule out some sort of sleep apnea.

The doctor asks Sally to keep a log of her daily activities, emphasizing her nightly rituals before, during, and after sleep. Her log shows that she is having difficulty falling asleep and staying asleep. She details that it takes her over an hour to fall asleep and then she wakes up a short time later. An average evening for Sally includes getting home from work at approximately 6 p.m. Then she usually goes to the gym and exercises on the elliptical machine for an hour. When she returns home, it is usually about 8:30 p.m., and she will have her dinner. At dinner, she usually tries to unwind by having a glass of wine. After dinner, she showers and retires to bed, but notes that every night she feels as though she is not tired and often lies in bed thinking of tomorrow's duties and errands. To try to fall asleep, she will turn on the television and have another glass of wine. After approximately 1 h she will fall asleep, but later at 3 or 4 a.m. she will be wide awake and have difficulty falling back asleep. Her alarm usually goes off about 6 a.m.

Please proceed with the problem-based approach using the worksheet located in the appendix of Chap. 1!

Table 4.2.2

FACTS	HYPOTHESES	INFORMATION NEEDED	LEARNING ISSUES

Vignette 4.2.3: Continuation

Sally's doctor explains to her that there are many causes of insomnia and that often they are the result of our own choices (antecedents) during the day. She is given a handout on Sleep Hygiene that explains which choices, such as exercising late and alcohol use, can lead to the adverse consequence of insomnia. He also tells Sally that her mood can influence her sleep. He asks her about her mood lately and if she has had any feelings that are consistent with depression. Sally answers no, except to a question on worrying often. Instead of worrying about the next day while lying in bed, the doctor suggests setting aside some "worry time" in which she can think over tomorrow's events and current stresses before she starts her bedtime rituals. The doctor also asks her not to go to bed until she is actually sleepy in order to restrict her time in bed to actual sleep time or for sex. This is a *stimulus control* strategy to help make the bed a stimulus primarily for sleep. He asks her to get out of bed if she is unable to fall asleep within 20 min and to read quietly until sleepy. He asks her to get up at the same time each morning no matter what time she falls asleep the night before to help condition her body to waking up on a regular pattern. In fact, he would like her to look toward the horizon (not directly at the sun) each morning to get her biological clock started with broad spectrum light. In addition to limiting her alcohol intake, he asks her to avoid caffeine after 6 p.m. He also asks her to keep her bedroom cool, dark, quiet, and conducive to sleep. He asks her to get regular exercise but never less than 3 h before she is planning to go to sleep. The doctor reassures the patient that most people do not actually need a full 8 h of sleep per night to function adequately and even after a night of insomnia the patient is not likely to feel impaired all of the next day.

Sally decides to start her exercise routine in the morning. She also makes a commitment to limit her alcohol consumption to no more than one glass of wine before 7 p.m. on any given evening. She returns to the clinic after 1 month of adjusting her choices throughout the day, and the result is that she now is sleeping much better.

Vignette 4.3.1: Dennis

Dennis is a 4-year-old boy with lots of energy. He is smart and is the only child in a loving family of older parents who are grateful to have him after years of infertility interventions. He is their miracle baby. His parents have expressed the desire not to spoil him, but they fear that they already have. He plays well with other children at preschool and his preschool teachers do not report any behavioral problems. Dennis's parents are happy he is adjusting well to preschool, but they are concerned about some of his behavior when he is at home. They report that about twice a week he will have a "melt down" during which he will throw a verbal and physical tantrum, often rolling on the floor screaming.

Please proceed with the problem-based approach using the worksheet located in the appendix of Chap. 1!

Table 4.3.1

FACTS	HYPOTHESES	INFORMATION NEEDED	LEARNING ISSUES

Vignette 4.3.1: Continued

The doctor then requests that the parents perform a *functional analysis* of their son's tantrums. After tracking the behavior for a week, the parents discover that he had two tantrums at the supermarket. A careful analysis of the tantrums revealed that it is common for Dennis to go shopping with his mother at the local supermarket and find a toy or small candy that he wants. When his mother tries to say no, he will cry. If she continues to say no, he will escalate and start to throw a tantrum. If she continues to resist, he will often escalate to falling on the ground and screaming. At this point, his mother feels acute embarrassment and will do anything to make it stop, including giving him the toy or candy. He then quickly calms down and a smile returns to his face. Then his mother quickly leaves the store red faced with her purchases.

What are the antecedents and consequences of their son's behaviors? What consequences would be properly characterized as punishers or rewards? How would you characterize the *reinforcement schedule* for the tantrums?

Table 4.3.2

FACTS	HYPOTHESES	INFORMATION NEEDED	LEARNING ISSUES

Vignette 4.3.2: Continued

Dennis's parents learn that they *continuously reinforce* their son's tantrums by giving him what he wants until he calms down. This is a pattern they would like to change. They also learn that Dennis is *negatively reinforcing* his mother's giving in to him by stopping the tantrum as soon as she gives in to his demand. In other words, the child stops the aversive tantrum (negative) whenever the mother gives him what he wants, thereby increasing the mother's behavior of giving in, by definition reinforcing the mother's behavior. The parents learn from his preschool that they use a system called 1-2-3 Magic (Phelan 2004). This system involves giving the child a warning when his behavior is disruptive by telling him, "you are on one." If he does not comply with the request, he is told, "you are on 2." If he still does not comply with the request, he is told, "you are on 3," and there is a negative consequence of some kind. At school the negative consequence is sitting quietly by himself in a time-out room for a few minutes. His parents unobtrusively observe the teachers *model* these techniques in the classroom. One of the teachers is an especially good *model* because she herself also struggled with fertility issues and can relate to the parents' struggles. This teacher had to work at learning the system with her own child by practicing it repeatedly in the classroom. In that sense, she is a *coping model* (i.e., someone who had to learn to cope), an even more powerful *model* than a *mastery model* (i.e., someone for whom reward and time-out comes naturally). *Models* are also more effective if they are similar to the person observing, they are skillful in their implementation of the target behavior, they are attractive, and there is opportunity to practice the target behavior.

Dennis's parents decide to use this system and make the consequence time-out in the corner of whatever room they are in. If he comes out of time-out, he will lose the privilege of dessert with the next meal. His parents decide to build in some flexibility for him to earn back dessert with good behavior such as helping mom with a household chore. To reduce some of her embarrassment, Dennis's mother talks to the store manager and lets him know that she is trying to do a better job of setting limits with her son when he is in public. The store manager who is also a parent is completely sympathetic and understanding. He says it is fine with him if her son has a full-out tantrum on the next trip to the store, and he supports her setting appropriate limits. He agrees to alert the cashiers of her plan the next time she comes in. She lets him know she will come in later that afternoon after preschool.

What would you expect to happen the next time Dennis's mother goes shopping at the store with him?

Dennis's mother explained to Dennis the new system of discipline she was planning to implement. She takes him shopping that afternoon as planned. The store manager gives her a wink when she arrives. Sure enough Dennis finds some M&M candy-coated peanuts he would like. They are his favorite.

Within 5 min he is asking his mother for some M&Ms. She says no because it will spoil his dinner. He begins to cry and get louder. She tells him he is "on 1." He escalates to falling on the floor. She tells him he is "on 2." He begins screaming and she tells him he is "on 3" and must stay there on the floor in time-out until he calms down but that under no circumstances can he have M&Ms today. He screams louder and keeps it up for about 3 min, much longer than he usually does when she gives in to his demands. This is called an *extinction burst,* that is, a burst of behavior following the withdrawal of an expected reinforcer. She tells him when he is calm for 30 s, he can come out of time-out. Another mother whispers to her that she is totally supportive and admires her limit setting. Eventually Dennis calms down, and they leave the store together holding hands. The mother, though still somewhat embarrassed, is proud of herself for sticking to her boundary.

Dennis's mother implements the same strategy the next time she goes to the store and notices that Dennis's tantrum only lasts about 30 s. The third time in the store together he does not tantrum at all. It appears his tantruming behavior is *extinguishing.*

Vignette 4.4.1 Presenting Situation: Nana
Nana is a 75-year-old grandmother who loves to come to Reno to gamble and visit her adult grandson, in that order. Her grandson is concerned because she goes from casino to casino in a bus with her fellow senior citizens but does not even take time out to eat sometimes. Her favorite game is the pull slot machine. She feels she is getting good exercise, but her grandson is concerned that she cannot afford to spend long hours gambling, both physically and financially.

Please proceed with the problem-based approach using the worksheet located in the appendix of Chap. 1!

Table 4.4.1

FACTS	HYPOTHESES	INFORMATION NEEDED	LEARNING ISSUES

Vignette 4.4.2: Continuation
The doctor is concerned that the grandmother's behavior may be indicative of pathologic gambling. He meets with the grandmother and has her keep track of her gambling behavior. He has her write down exactly what games she plays and exactly how much time she is gambling. He also has her write down other activities she enjoys on her trip to Reno. He finds that she gambles as much as 20 h on a 2-day trip to Reno. Although she does not skip any meals, she does delay them sometimes. She also enjoys seeing her grandson and his young children play baseball when they have a little league game scheduled.

Please proceed with the problem-based approach using the worksheet located in the appendix of Chap. 1!

Table 4.4.2

FACTS	HYPOTHESES	INFORMATION NEEDED	LEARNING ISSUES

Vignette 4.4.3: Continuation
In an application of the *Premack principle,* the doctor implements the treatment intervention by encouraging her to engage in her socializing with her grandson and his children before she goes gambling at the casino with her friends. In other words, her gambling forays are contingent on her accomplishing other important tasks first. In order to accomplish this, she stays at her grandson's house instead of the casino. After a morning brunch and afternoon baseball session, her grandson drops her off at a casino with her friends from about 7–9 p.m. After that she is ready for bed. Her tracking shows that she has reduced her gambling from 20 h per weekend visit to only 5 h. She has more quality time with her grandson and great grandchildren in the process. She is not so exhausted.

4.3 Learning Issues

1. Premack principle
   The *Premack priniciple* (named for the theorist David Premack) is that animals have baseline levels of engaging in different behaviors (e.g., eating, drinking, running, playing). The Premack principle postulates that humans and other animals will work at a less probable behavior for the opportunity to engage in a more probable behavior (Danaher 1974). In the above vignette, Nana collaborated with her doctor to arrange to do other things that were important to her, such as spending time with her grandson and great grandchildren, and getting proper nutrition, before she allowed herself her guilty pleasure of gambling. This is an important and simple principle of self-reinforcement, that is, work before play or eating your vegetables before eating dessert.
2. Reinforcement schedules
   The pattern of reinforcement is called a *reinforcement schedule* (Beaton 2001). Reinforcement schedules can vary according to the number of responses before a reward is delivered *(ratio schedule)* or in the time elapsed between rewards *(interval schedule)*. A ratio schedule or an interval schedule can be fixed or variable. In a *fixed ratio schedule,* a reward is delivered after a certain number of responses. For example, a factory worker might receive a bonus for every ten cars manufactured by his or her team. In a *variable ratio schedule,* a reward is delivered after an average number of responses. For example, the slot machines that Nana enjoys are usually set to deliver a payoff after an average number of pulls. Ratio schedules tend to result in a high response rate, and a variable ratio schedule results in a pattern of responding that is the most resistant to extinction (i.e., a dropping off of the response when the reinforcer is removed).
   Receiving a paycheck every 2 weeks is an example of a *fixed interval schedule.* A *variable interval schedule* might involve a fisherman who catches his limit of ten fish over the course of 5 h of fishing. Some of the fish are caught within 5 min of each other, while others might be caught several hours apart.
3. The neurobiology of reinforcement
   The neurobiology of anticipation, reward, and reinforcement has been studied at many levels including molecular, cellular, genetic, systems, behavioral, and computational using many animal and human models. Though there are still many things we do not understand about human neurobiology, research is furthering our knowledge quickly, and one human affliction that spurs research on is drug addiction. The neurobiology of addiction appears to be pathologic use of the same brain structures as normal behavioral adaption (seeking food, water, and opportunity to mate). These structures are collectively referred to as the "mesolimbic reward circuit" and utilize dopamine primarily as the neurotransmitter, though other neurotransmitters such as acetylcholine, 5-hydroxytryptamine, gamma-aminobutyric acid (GABA), and glutamate may play a role (Haynes 2004). This circuit is composed of dopaminergic neurons of the ventral tegmentum that form projections to the nucleus accumbens, amygdala, prefrontal cortex, and other forebrain structures (Vetulani 2001).

In order to better understand normal behavior, the functional systems of the brain can be split into three major categories: arousal, reward, and cognition systems. The arousal system is further subdivided into general arousal (regulating central nervous system (CNS) excitability) located in the ascending reticular system, directed or goal-oriented arousal (providing motivation and emotion) located in the hypothalamus and parts of the limbic system, and peripheral arousal (linking up the brain to other organ systems) made up of the autonomic nervous system and hormonal systems. All of these systems interact to allow the organism to adapt to the environment. The directed arousal system is involved most substantially in addictions. This system provides a ranking of goals and initiates the behavior needed to attain the goal and then processes whether or not the goal was met. If these goals aid in the organism's survival or survival of the species, it is properly rewarded so that such means to achieve that goal are reinforced. In the case of the brain, this reward is dopamine (Vetulani 2001). Hyman (2004) proposes that addiction is a disease of learning and memory and that addictive drugs hijack the reward system. The current body of research has established the rewarding properties of addictive drugs is proportional to its ability to increase dopamine in the ventral tegmental area neurons projecting to the nucleus accumbens (especially the shell region) and other forebrain structures such as the prefrontal cortex and amygdala (Hyman 2004).

Research has also shown that dopamine is released at a basal tonic rate in anticipation of a previously received pleasurable, reinforcing event, such as sugar-water presented to monkeys after a paired stimulus. If the reward is given sooner, it is perceived as "better than expected" and there is a burst of dopamine release. If there is no reward when one is expected, there is a pause in the dopamine release indicating "worse than expected." It is believed that these bursts and pauses of dopamine release encode a "prediction-error signal" that will help the animal to *learn* the new relationship and reinforce behavior that results in the reward. This is termed the "Reward Prediction-Error Hypothesis." It is surmised that with addictive drug intake, the signal is always "better than expected," resulting in an overriding of all other goal-directed behavior (Hyman 2004).

Although we are far from understanding the exact mechanisms driving an organism's behavior, it can be concluded that the main area involved in adaptive behavior and learning is the mesolimbic system, including the ventral tegmental area projections, and that dopamine is the one of the key neurotransmitters involved. Better understanding of these mechanisms may open doors in the future for treatment of drug addiction as a pathologic overlearning.

Vignette 4.5.1 Presenting Situation: Ronda

A 25-year-old female patient named Ronda suffers from extreme social anxiety. She can barely make eye contact with the doctor. She appears to have a limited social network and basically goes to work and goes home.

Please proceed with the problem-based approach using the worksheet located in the appendix of Chap. 1!

Table 4.5.1

FACTS	HYPOTHESES	INFORMATION NEEDED	LEARNING ISSUES

Vignette 4.5.2: Continuation

The doctor decides to have the patient conduct a functional analysis of Ronda's daily social contacts for 1 week. The tracking reveals that she rarely talks with her office mate, and she only has contact with her mother and father outside of work.

Table 4.5.2

FACTS	HYPOTHESES	INFORMATION NEEDED	LEARNING ISSUES

The doctor begins to take the sessions outside of the office. The therapist and patient go for a walk to the local grocery store. Ronda is assigned the task of making eye contact and saying hello to anyone they pass on the way to the supermarket. She is surprised to find that 90% of the people they pass say hello back. She is also assigned the task of asking the grocery clerk where she can find two food items. She gathers the food items and practices making small talk with the clerk using programed questions about the weather and about how business is going today. Ronda does this for several sessions in a row as well as on her own as a homework assignment. After several sessions, the patient can engage in this behavior relatively comfortably and with increased confidence.

The doctor gives her an assignment to practice her small talk skills (e.g., Wadsworth 2012) with her office mate and to invite her office mate to lunch on occasion. As the patient gains confidence, she is experiencing an increase in *self-efficacy (Bandura* 1986*)*, that is, a belief that she can succeed socially. She expresses an interest in dating for the first time in her life, but she does not know where to begin. The doctor helps her develop a tasteful profile for an online dating service. She begins dating for the first time in her life and after about 3 months, she develops a relationship with her first boyfriend. Though she has some anxiety about the risks of falling in love, Ronda is thrilled to be experiencing life more fully.

4.4 Self-Assessment Questions

1. Two new parents wake up quickly to the sound of their 1-year-old baby crying in the middle of the night. Every night when this occurs, they immediately bring the baby to bed with them to comfort her. The baby immediately settles down to sleep. This is an example of:
   a. Intermittent reinforcement
   b. Extinction
   c. Continuous reinforcement
   d. Shaping
   e. Successive approximations
2. A resident observes a skilled surgeon conducting a heart bypass. Based on what you learned about *modeling*, the likelihood of learning and retention is *unrelated* to the:
   a. Attractiveness of the surgeon
   b. Practice opportunities for the resident
   c. Manual dexterity of the resident
   d. Acclaimed skill of the surgeon
   e. Age of the surgeon
3. Pick the *true* statement about punishment:
   a. Punishment teaches appropriate behavior
   b. The punisher (i.e., the person doing the punishing) may model verbal or physical aggression
   c. The punisher may increase the target behavior (i.e., the behavior that is being punished)
   d. People do not learn to avoid the punishment
   e. Punishment tends to reduce emotional behavior
4. In behavioral approaches to treatment, behavior is thought to be *unrelated* to:
   a. Reinforcement history
   b. Current contingencies

c. Genetic endowment
d. Ego functioning
e. Reinforcement schedule

5. A patient notices some anxiety while driving following a serious car accident. She notices some relief of her anxiety if she avoids driving on the freeway, causing her to avoid freeway driving entirely. The relief of anxiety she experiences from avoiding freeways is an example of:

   a. Negative reinforcement
   b. Positive reinforcement
   c. Punishment
   d. Conditioned stimulus
   e. Generalized reinforcer

6. An adult patient comes to you with stomach pain that does not appear to have an underlying biological basis. You decide to use your skills in functional analysis to help correct the problem. You ask the patient to:

   a. Keep track of their dreams
   b. Focus on available punishers in the environment
   c. Keep track of the antecedents of the pain, the pain itself, and what happens after the pain occurs
   d. Take an in-depth history of childhood, focusing on toilet training
   e. Focus on cognitions and reward systems in the environment

7. Behavior analysis is characterized by all *except* one of the following:

   a. Identifying antecendent events
   b. Evaluating consequences
   c. Measuring duration of behavior
   d. Determining a Diagnostic and Statistical Manual of Mental Disorders, 5th Edition (DSM-V) diagnosis
   e. Measuring the frequency of behavior

8. Motivational interviewing:

   a. Shames the patient into changing behavior
   b. Provides a financial incentive for the patient to change
   c. Helps the patient explore reasons and obstacles to change
   d. Involves the physician's enthusiastic support to change
   e. Telling the patient what they need to do from the start

9. Self-efficacy is:

   a. The ability to be successful no matter what
   b. The belief that someone has the skills to be successful
   c. An arrogant approach to life
   d. An inaccurate view of ones own social skills
   e. Humility about oneself

Appendix A: Possible Answers to Vignettes

Vignette 4.1: Ronald

Table 4.1.1

Facts	Hypotheses	Information needed	Learning issues
58-year-old male	Given the patients extensive heavy smoking history, he will need lots of assistance to quit	Why does he want to quit now?	What is the functional relationship between the patient's environment and his smoking?
80 pack-year smoker wants to quit		What has he tried in the past?	What are typical antecedents to smoking for this patient?
		When does he usually smoke?	What are the typical consequences of smoking for this patient?
		What is his longest period of prior abstinence?	How might motivational interviewing help guide this patient to an appropriate goal?
		How does he deal with stress?	

RS reinforcement schedule

Table 4.1.2

Facts	Hypotheses	Information needed	Learning issues
The patient identifies the *antecedents* and the *consequences*	Changing the antecedent behavior may change the consequence	What type of follow-up plan will he need?	What are the stages of change?
			What are smoking cessation tools?

Vignette 4.2: Sally

Table 4.2.1

Facts	Hypotheses	Information needed	Learning issues
48-year-old female complains of insomnia for 3 months	Possible medical reason?	What part of sleeping does she have trouble with?	How do I take a sleep history?

Facts	Hypotheses	Information needed	Learning issues
	Possible stress?	What is her bedtime routine like?	What are typical antecedents for a good or poor night of sleep?
	Mood disturbance?		What are the consequences for a good or poor night of sleep?
	Substance use?		

Table 4.2.2

Facts	Hypotheses	Information needed	Learning issues
Difficulty falling asleep	Changing her routine may have an impact	How does the patient's sleep change after the intervention?	What is sleep hygiene?
Difficulty staying asleep			What are causes of insomnia?
Antecedent behaviors include exercising late			
Eating late			
Alcohol intake			
Stays in bed and worries			
Watches television in bed			
Consequences include feeling fatigued the next morning and unable to concentrate at work			

Vignette 4.3: Dennis

Table 4.3.1

Facts	Hypotheses	Information needed	Learning issues
Dennis is a 4-year-old boy	Parents actions are reinforcing tantrums	What type of activities lead to tantrums (antecedents)?	What are reinforcement schedules?
Parents complain of tantrums		How do the parents react to the tantrums (consequences and reinforcers)?	
No problems in school			
Plays well with peers			

Table 4.3.2

Facts	Hypotheses	Information needed	Learning issues
Antecedents to their son's tantrums: Dennis sees a small toy or piece of candy he wants. Dennis realizes he is in a public place that will be embarrassing for mom if he throws a fit		What happens to the behavior after implementing the intervention?	What are the reinforcement schedules that apply in this situation?
Consequences of his tantrums:	Changing the consequences may alter the behavior		What are some tools to modify behavior in children?
Mom gets embarrassed by Dennis' tantrum			
Mom gives him the toy or candy he wants, and Dennis calms down immediately			

Vignette 4.4: Nana

Table 4.4.1

Facts	Hypotheses	Information needed	Learning issues
75-year-old female	Gambling may be out of control	How much does Nana actually gamble?	How do you diagnose gambling addiction?
Grandson concerned about gambling to point of exhaustion	Reinforcement schedule of slot machines makes it difficult to extinguish the gambling behavior	How much time does she devote to gambling?	Reinforcement schedules of slot machines
		Does she skip meals?	
		What else does she like to do besides gambling?	

Table 4.4.2

Facts	Hypotheses	Information needed	Learning issues
Twenty hours spent gambling during a 2-day trip	Using gambling as a consequence for other activities such as adequate socialization and nutrition will help her have better balance	What happens to Nana's gambling after the intervention?	What is the Premack principle? How can it be applied in this case?

Facts	Hypotheses	Information needed	Learning issues
Delays meals			What are different types of reinforcement schedules?
Enjoys seeing her grandson and watching his young children play baseball			What is the neurobiology of reinforcement?
			What are the DSM 5 criteria for pathological gambling?

DSM 5 Diagnostic and Statistical Manual of Mental Disorders, 5th Edition (APA 2013)

Vignette 4.5: Ronda

Table 4.5.1

Facts	Hypotheses	Information needed	Learning issues
The patient is a 25-year-old woman with extreme social anxiety	She is avoiding social contact due to extreme social anxiety	How many social contacts does she have in a typical day?	What is the functional analysis of this patient's social contacts?
She makes poor eye contact		How many friends does she have?	
She has few friends			
She has never dated			

Table 4.5.2

Facts	Hypotheses	Information needed	Learning issues
Patient only talks with her office mate rarely	Patient lacks social skills to develop social contacts	Can she have some positive experiences in interacting with others?	How can she learn conversational skills?
She has no other contacts besides her father and mother			How can she increase self-efficacy?

Appendix B: Answers to Self-Assessment Questions

1. C The parents are consistently and repeatedly reinforcing their baby's crying every night.
2. E The impact of the model is enhanced by all of the variables except the age of the surgeon.
3. B It is true that the punisher may model verbal or physical aggression. All other choices are false.
4. D Ego functioning is a psychoanalytic concept that is unrelated to behavioral approaches to treatment.
5. A Negative reinforcement has to do with stopping negative stimulation to increase a behavior. Stopping anxiety reinforces driving avoidance behavior in the case example making A the correct choice.
6. C Functional analysis involves tracking antecedents and consequences of behavior, making option C the correct choice.
7. D A behavioral analysis does not rely on a diagnosis.
8. C Motivational interviewing helps the patient explore reasons and obstacles to change. None of the other options are reflective of motivational interviewing.
9. B Self-efficacy is the belief that someone has the skills to be successful. None of the other options are reflective of self-efficacy.

References

American Psychiatric Association. (2013). *Diagnostic and statistical manual of mental disorders* (5th ed.). Washington, DC: American Psychiatric Association.

Antonuccio, D. O. (1992). *Butt out, a compassionate guide to helping yourself quit smoking, with or without a partner*. Saratoga: R & E Publishers.

Bandura, A. (1986). The explanatory and predictive scope of self-efficacy theory. *Journal of Social and Clinical Psychology, 4*(3), 359–373.

Beaton, J. M. (2001). *Learning theory and human behavior in behavior & medicine edited by D. Wedding*. Toronto: Hogrefe & Huber Publishers.

Bolin, L., Antonuccio, D. O., Follette, W., & Krumpe, P. (1999). Transdermal nicotine: The long and the short of it. *Psychology of Addictive Behaviors, 13,* 152–156.

Danaher, B. G. (1974). Theoretical foundations and clinical applications of the Premack principle: Review and critique. *Behavior Therapy, 5*(3), 307–324.

DiClemente, C. C., Prochaska, J. O., Fairhurst, S. K., Velicer, W., Velasquez, W. F., & Rossi, J. S. (1991). The process of smoking cessation: An analysis of precontemplation, contemplation, and preparation stages of change. *Journal of Consulting and Clinical Psychology, 59,* 295–304.

Fiore, M. C., Jaen, C. R., Baker, T. B., et al. (2008). *Clinical practice guideline*. Rockville: U.S. Department of Health and Human Services. Public Health Service. (Treating tobacco use and dependence: 2008 update).

Haynes, T. L. (2004). The neurobiology of addiction and its implications for treatment—drug-seeking behavior and the transition to dependence. http://www.medscape.com/viewarticle/472498. Accessed 22 Dec 2014.

Hettema, J. E., & Hendricks, P. S. (2010). Motivational interviewing for smoking cessation: A meta-analytic review. *Journal of Consulting and Clinical Psychology, 78*(6), 868.

Hyman, S. E. (2004). Addiction: "A Disease of Learning and Memory". *American Journal of Psychiatry, 162,* 1414–1422.

Lai, D. T., Cahill, K., Qin, Y., & Tang, J. L. (2010). Motivational interviewing for smoking cessation. *Cochrane Database System Review, 1,* CD006936.

Phelan, T. W. (2004). *1-2-3 magic: Effective discipline for children.* Glen Ellyn: Parent Magic Inc.

Vetulani, J. (2001). Drug addiction. Part II. Neurobiology of addiction. *Polish Journal of Pharmacology, 53*(4), 303–318.

Wadsworth, M. (2012). *The small talk handbook: Easy instructions on how to make small talk in any situation.* Avon: Adams Media.

Ward, T. M. (2011). Conducting a sleep assessment. In *Sleep disturbances and sleep promotion in nursing practice* (pp. 53–71). New York: Springer. https://books.google.com/books?hl=en&lr=&id=rVyZYcccYwoC&oi=fnd&pg=PA53&ots=kWjvr-DKjm&sig=ruYgUD1QxPzDQB_7x7Ozgoa38Qc#v=onepage&q&f=false.

Zimmerman, G., Olsen, C., & Bosworth, M. (2004). A stages of change approach to helping patients change behavior. AFP Vol. 61/No. 5 (March 1, 2000).

Chapter 5
Sexuality Throughout the Life Cycle

Steven R. Williams and Anthony P. S. Guerrero

There are few topics in medicine that blur the boundaries of science, religion, and morality more than *sexuality*. Less pathologization of gender nonconformity has taken place recently, as has been seen in changes in laws in the military, marriage equality, and changes in diagnostics in the Diagnostic and Statistical Manual of Mental Disorders, Fifth Edition (DSM-5). Gender identity disorder is no longer used, being replaced in the DSM-5 with gender dysphoria; of note, the term "disorder" is not used (American Psychiatric Association 2013). The nomenclature for "intersex" conditions and ambiguous genitalia has been modernized with the use of "disorders of sex development," which is a more logical and applicable classification system, with greater clinical utility.

This chapter aims to provide a basic discussion on sexuality throughout the life cycle. It is hoped that, at the end of this chapter, the reader will be able to:

1. Distinguish between the terms: sex, gender, gender identity, and sexual orientation.
2. Identify normal sexual development in children, adolescents, and adults.
3. Describe the human sexual response cycle.
4. Discuss issues in sexuality for elderly and medically ill patients.

S. R. Williams (✉)
1380 Lusitana Street, Suite 511, Honolulu, HI 96813, USA
e-mail: williamss@dop.hawaii.edu

A. P. S. Guerrero
Department of Psychiatry, John A. Burns School of Medicine, University of Hawai'i, 1356 Lusitana Street, University Tower 4th Floor, Honolulu, HI 96813, USA
e-mail: GuerreroA@dop.hawaii.edu

D. Alicata et al. (eds.), *Problem-based Behavioral Science and Psychiatry*,
DOI 10.1007/978-3-319-23669-8_5

Vignette 5.1.1: Baby Pat

You have been the primary-care physician for several years for a 36-year-old woman who is now 34 weeks pregnant and experiencing severe anxiety, which she associates with the recent information given to her by her obstetrics and gynecology (OB/GYN) physician. The OB/GYN asks you to meet with her in order to address her severe anxiety. Your patient had an amniocentesis performed when she was 16 weeks pregnant and the results were found to be normal with an XY karyotype. She had a repeated prenatal ultrasound yesterday, which indicated the fetus was female, with some uncertainty about this because of the fetal position and the quality of the ultrasound. You meet with your patient and her husband and discuss possible reasons for the discrepancy and correcting any unrealistic fears that are worsening her anxiety. Your patient has no significant psychiatric history and you do not think that a psychiatric medication or psychiatry consult are warranted. Your patient has an uncomplicated delivery at 39 weeks gestation of a newborn girl with normal female genitalia. The parents would like an explanation regarding the karyotype findings and having a baby girl. Baby Pat's serum electrolytes, urinalysis, and other laboratory values are normal. Ultrasound of the pelvic area reveals that there is no uterus and undescended testes are present. You consider the common and uncommon disorders of sex development with a 46XY newborn and the present findings. You know that ambiguous genitalia can be seen in both congenital adrenal hyperplasia and in androgen insensitivity syndrome. You have a higher suspicion of androgen insensitivity because of the normal electrolytes and the ultrasound findings (Donohoue 2011).

Please proceed with the problem-based approach using the worksheet located in the appendix of Chap. 1!

Please fill in the facts, your hypotheses, further information needed, and learning issues for Learning Issue Table 5.1.1.

Learning Issue Table 5.1.1

FACTS	HYPOTHESES	INFORMATION NEEDED	LEARNING ISSUES

Vignette 5.1.2: Continuation

You then request a pediatric endocrinology consult, which leads to genetic testing. The conclusion from the endocrinologist is that Baby Pat has complete androgen insensitivity syndrome (CAIS). This is discussed with the parents, you educate them about this diagnosis, and they have many questions regarding future gender assignment, psychosexual development, and potential medical problems. You inform the parents that as opposed to children who have partial androgen insensitivity syndrome, the vast majority of children with CAIS are raised with the female gender identity. Included in the discussion with the parents is the possible need for surgical removal of the testes before puberty because of the risk of cancer.

What are some of the issues here? How critical is it to assign a gender identity by a particular age? Which psychosexual issues need to be addressed prior to puberty? At what age or developmental stage will the child have powers of assent in order to contribute to decisions regarding treatment such as genital surgery? How much family education needs to occur to facilitate an informed medical decision regarding the child's treatment? What is the role of the family's values in directing medical interventions? How well defined is the "standard of care" regarding treatments related to gender assignment?

The parents have gone to reliable internet sites and educated themselves about CAIS and its treatment. After a few family sessions with the parents, child psychologist, and yourself, the parents have decided to rear Baby Pat as a girl. Family therapy is provided by the child psychologist with close monitoring of the child's psychosexual development and considering at which later stage of cognitive development the issue of her diagnosis should be discussed with her.

You meet with the parents, child psychologist, and Pat, who is now 9 years old. There has been an ongoing discussion with the parents recently as to when to discuss the diagnosis of CAIS with Pat. We all agree that we want Pat to make some of her own decisions regarding treatment sometime during adolescence. Depending on Pat's preferences and anatomical findings, a discussion will be needed regarding options with genital surgery and hormone treatment.

Please proceed with the problem-based approach using the worksheet located in the appendix of Chap. 1!

Please fill in the facts, your hypotheses, further information needed, and learning issues for Learning Issue Table 5.1.2.

Learning Issue Table 5.1.2

FACTS	HYPOTHESES	INFORMATION NEEDED	LEARNING ISSUES

At this point, while a complete discussion of the biology of sex determination is beyond the scope of this chapter, a few basic definitions are worth reviewing, which are summarized in Table 5.1:

While these terms may seem relatively straightforward, sexual development is complex enough to be associated with various concerns and questions that may be presented to the physician throughout the life cycle of a patient.

Vignette 5.2.1: Mike

In your outpatient practice, you see children of all ages. One of your patients is Mike, a 6-year-old boy who is brought in by his mother because of "behavior problems in school that might cause him to get kicked out." According to the principal, he once exposed his penis to a group of his male and female classmates in the playground. While the other children found what he did to be outrageously funny, several parents lodged complaints that they would pull their children out of this school if the teachers could not contain the "immorality" of "other troubled children." He also tends to make "lewd comments" about people depicted in bathing suits in various magazines.

STOP

Please proceed with the problem-based approach using the worksheet located in the appendix of Chap. 1!

Please fill in the facts, your hypotheses, further information needed, and learning issues for Learning Issue Table 5.2.1.

Learning Issue Table 5.2.1

FACTS	HYPOTHESES	INFORMATION NEEDED	LEARNING ISSUES

Table 5.1 Basic definitions

Term	Definition	When determined or manifested	Mechanism of determination	Examples of clinical concerns relevant to this concept
Chromosomal sex	Whether the human is male (XY) or female (XX)	At conception	Fertilization: fusion of mother and father's genetic material	Phenotypic males with multiple copies of either the X or the Y chromosome
				Phenotypic females with either three or more copies of the X chromosome or only one X chromosome
Assigned gender	Whether a baby is identified as a girl or boy, usually based on the appearance of genitalia	Traditionally at birth, though determinable in utero with ultrasound technology	Expression of genes and action of hormones that influence development of sexual organs	Androgen insensitivity syndrome (genetic male with tissues unresponsive to male hormones; hence with female-appearing genitalia)
				Congenital adrenal hyperplasia (genetic female with overproduction of androgens; hence with male-appearing or ambiguous genitalia), illustrated in the case above
				Numerous other intersex conditions: while it had been traditionally taught that sexual reassignment surgery should occur before gender identity (defined below) is established, the implications of this condition are much more complex, because of the reality that sexual behavior is determined by more than just the outwards appearance of one's genitalia
Gender identity	A child's awareness of being male or female	Usually at around age 2 years	Likely complex interplay between awareness of assigned gender, what is taught and reinforced by caregivers, and biological influences on sexual brain development	In gender dysphoria (described further in Chap. 28), there is discomfort with one's own gender; may be seen as early as preschool years and more commonly in boys than in girls
Gender role	Culturally proscribed roles associated with each gender	Usually by preschool age	What is taught and reinforced by caregivers and the community	In gender dysphoria, there may be a preference for the roles associated with the opposite gender
Sexual orientation	Preference for males, females, or both as sexual partners	Usually by adolescence	Genetic and other biologically mediated influences on development; likely an interplay between biopsychosocial factors	Psychological distress around either being in roles that are contrary to one's basic sexual orientation or experiencing the social stigma attached to a nonmajority sexual orientation

Table 5.2 Examples of normal and potentially concerning sexual behavior in a preschool or school age child

Examples of probably normal sexual behavior in a preschool or school-age child	Examples of behavior that suggest either inappropriate exposure to sexual activity or other psychopathology
Fascination and glee with pictures of half-clothed bodies or of people kissing	Detailed knowledge about specific sexual acts
Manually exploring one's own body or attempting to manually explore the bodies of family members and close friends	Attempted or actual sexual behaviors that involve penetration; propositioning strangers and other inappropriate sex talk
Masturbation (possibly aided by toys or other objects) that does not appear to be associated with psychological distress or physical injury and that does not interfere with other developmentally appropriate tasks	Compulsive masturbation associated with psychological distress and/or physical injury and that is so time-consuming as to interfere with other developmentally appropriate tasks

Following awareness of gender identity, and with the further strides in cognitive development that occur at around the preschool age, children become naturally curious about matters pertaining to sex and sexual organs. Common behaviors include sexually themed play, exploration of one's own body and the bodies of others, and enactment of adult sexual roles (e.g., being mommy or daddy), often within the safety of the family. While many of these behaviors are "normal" (as is often the best choice in multiple-choice exams on sexual development), the clinician should certainly consider other conditions and situations that may predispose to behaviors that are either quantitatively or qualitatively inappropriate for the given age of development. Consider Table 5.2.

Vignette 5.2.2: Conclusion
You talk to Mike and his mother. Mike conveys regret over what he had done and says that he will try to be "good" in school. You learn that, while he may have seen some kissing and adult sitcom shows while being babysat by a teenage cousin and her boyfriend a few months ago, he has not had any other exposure to inappropriate sexual material. While your general behavioral screening questionnaire, the 17-item Pediatric Symptom Checklist, suggests that he may have a possible attentional problem, specific questions do not suggest that he has a bipolar, obsessive-compulsive, or autism spectrum disorder. You provide counseling about developmentally appropriate supervision and refocusing on developmentally appropriate tasks.

Obviously, what is "normal" sexual behavior is different for different ages and different stages of development (please refer to Chap. 2 on childhood development). In general, sexual development closely follows development in other areas, including cognitive development, social development, and physical development. Consider the following cases.

Vignette 5.3.1: Mary Jane

Your next patient is Mary Jane, a 14-year-old high school freshman who is brought in by her mother, who requests that Mary Jane be tested for HIV and "anything else that can be sexually transmitted," placed on the "birth control shot," and given "that new cervical cancer vaccine and anything else that can prevent sexually transmitted diseases." The mother learned that Mary Jane slept with a boy classmate at band camp and is now worried that she will catch something from "being promiscuous." Mary Jane explains that she previously had never had sexual intercourse, other than having "experimented" with fondling a close female friend who is lesbian (even though she herself is "straight.") She denies ever having had any other sexual experiences. Mary Jane comes from a "traditional family" that, she believes, would not otherwise condone any premarital sexual activity or any homosexual behaviors.

STOP — Please proceed with the problem-based approach using the worksheet located in the appendix of Chap. 1!

Please fill in the facts, your hypotheses, further information needed, and learning issues for Learning Issue Table 5.3.1.

Learning Issue Table 5.3.1

FACTS	HYPOTHESES	INFORMATION NEEDED	LEARNING ISSUES

Adolescence is a time when hormonal influences lead to the development of secondary sexual characteristics and heightened interest in sexual activity. Key milestones in adolescent development (that often are asked about in standardized tests) are summarized in Table 5.3:

The influence of hormones, primarily testosterone (in both males and females) leads to heightened sexual interest in adolescence. Statistics suggest that sexual activity, including intercourse, is common in adolescence, and should prompt the clinician to assist youth in preventing sexually transmitted disease and unwanted pregnancy. According to the Centers for Disease Control (2013) youth risk behavior surveillance system, 47% of high school students have had sexual intercourse in 2013. A total of 66% of sexually active teen males and 53% of teen females said they had used a condom at last sexual intercourse.

Table 5.3 Highlights of adolescent development

	Male physical development	Female physical development	Cognitive and social development
Early adolescence	Testicular enlargement	Breast bud formation	May still have concrete thinking same-sex peer groups are common
Middle adolescence	Peak in height growth, spermarche	Peak in height growth, generally followed by onset of menses	Emergence of abstract thought, questioning, and risk-taking
Late adolescence	Mature biological sex characteristics	Mature biological sex characteristics	Independence, potential commitment to career, stable partner, etc.

Vignette 5.3.2: Conclusion

You examine Mary Jane and find that she is at sexual maturity rating (SMR) stage 4. You perform a pelvic exam with *Papanicolau* smear and cultures for gonococcus and chlamydia. You also offer blood testing for HIV and syphilis. You insure that her hepatitis B immunizations are up-to-date and administer the first of the human papillomavirus vaccine series. You counsel her on effective methods of preventing sexually transmitted diseases (including abstinence). Even though the mother states she is "still grieving" over the loss of her daughter's "sexual innocence," she is nevertheless very grateful for your care.

Sexual development continues to be influenced by developmental issues at other phases of the life cycle, as illustrated by the following case.

Vignette 5.4.1: Phil Robinson

Mr. Phil Robinson is a 58-year-old male with a history of panic disorder and hypertension. He reports that, for the past 6 months, he and his 49-year-old wife have had sex less and less frequently. While they continued to have a satisfying sex life even after the birth of their three children, they have recently had more difficulties getting "in sync" with each other: either she has little sexual interest (which she relates to "premenopause") or she is sexually interested but he has difficulty maintaining an erection.

Please proceed with the problem-based approach using the worksheet located in the appendix of Chap. 1!

Please fill in the facts, your hypotheses, further information needed, and learning issues for Learning Issue Table 5.4.1.

Learning Issue Table 5.4.1

FACTS	HYPOTHESES	INFORMATION NEEDED	LEARNING ISSUES

While a decline in libido-promoting hormones may occur in later adulthood for both women and men, healthy sexuality remains an important priority for most older adults. Familiarity with Table 5.4 is often helpful when approaching clinical situations involving the human sexual response cycle:

While "normal sexual development" (once again) may be considered in the differential, the above case may suggest the diagnosis of erectile disorder in Mr. Robinson and the possibility of a female sexual interest/arousal disorder in his wife. Given Mr. Robinson's medical history, it would be important to further inquire about the specifics of his health condition and any medications he may be taking. Any health condition or medication that can affect any aspect of sexual physiology (including blood supply and innervation to the sexual organs or anything at all related to brain functioning) could be a culprit in any disorder of the sexual response cycle.

Vignette 5.4.2: Conclusion

In reviewing Mr. Robinson's chart, you discover that he is currently on a beta-blocker for hypertension and a serotonin-selective reuptake inhibitor along with a benzodiazepine for panic disorder. He denies any past history of sexual difficulties, other than what he reports as "premature ejaculation" earlier in his adult life. He thinks it is possible that he had more erectile difficulties ever since his serotonin-selective reuptake inhibitor dose had been increased. He also believes that the increased anxiety symptoms he had been having around that time (hence the dose increase) may have played a more important role and may have contributed to what he feels may be a "vicious cycle" of performance anxiety around sexual intercourse. You work to optimize his medication regimen and insure that he has no new medical problems. At a future visit, you provide education to him and his wife about the various factors that can affect the sexual response cycle. You encourage Mrs. Robinson to follow-up with her physician. In the meantime, you encourage them to focus on enjoying emotional and physical closeness with each other, with a de-emphasis on sexual intercourse. A few months later, he is happy to report that they have enjoyed their sex life once again.

Table 5.4 Characteristics of the human sexual response cycle

Stage of cycle	Characteristics	Examples of conditions involving this stage of the sexual response cycle
Desire	Fantasies	Male hypoactive sexual desire disorder, female sexual interest/arousal disorder
Arousal	Lubrication in female, erection in male	Female sexual interest/arousal disorder, erectile disorder
Plateau		
Orgasm	Intensified pleasure, rhythmic contractions, ejaculation in males	Female orgasmic disorder, premature ejaculation
Resolution		

Sexual issues are encountered in all specialties of medicine, and in patients of all age groups. In this chapter, we have reviewed sexual development throughout the life cycle. A further discussion of clinical disorders that involve sexual behavior is found in Chap. 28.

5.1 Review Questions

1. An adolescent girl who presents with primary amenorrhea and otherwise normal-appearing pubertal development is found to have an XY karyotype. The most likely diagnosis is:

    a. Normal development
    b. Polycystic ovary syndrome
    c. Congenital adrenal hyperplasia
    d. Androgen insensitivity syndrome
    e. Turner's syndrome

2. All of the following patients likely are exhibiting normal sexual development *except* for:

    a. A married couple in the mid-50s who engage in sexual intercourse several times per week.
    b. A 5-year-old male who makes two attempts in the office to peek under his mother's dress.
    c. A 16-year-old female who presents with flight of ideas, seductiveness towards the physician, and her fifth episode of pelvic inflammatory disease, which she said she caught from "sleeping with the whole football team."
    d. A 12-year-old female who is accidentally caught stroking her genital area while in her bedroom

   e. An 18-year-old male who presents with a urinary tract infection, which he believes he might have caught from his male partner, whom he has been with for the past year

3. Which of the following represent the earliest signs of puberty in males and females?

   a. For males: testicular enlargement; for females: breast bud development
   b. For males: spermarche; for females: height spurt
   c. For males: testicular enlargement; for females: menarche
   d. For males: spermarche; for females: breast bud formation
   e. For males: testicular enlargement; for females: height spurt

4. Which of the following represents the correct temporal sequence of the sexual response cycle?

   a. Plateau, desire, arousal, orgasm
   b. Desire, arousal, plateau, orgasm
   c. Arousal, desire, plateau, orgasm
   d. Plateau, arousal, orgasm, plateau
   e. Orgasm, plateau, arousal, desire

Appendix A: Tables with Possible Answers to the Vignettes

Vignette 5.1: Baby Pat

Learning Issue Table 5.1

Facts	Hypotheses	Information needed	Learning issues
36-year-old woman who is 34 weeks pregnant and experiencing severe anxiety	Ambiguous genitalia can be seen in both congenital adrenal hyperplasia and in androgen insensitivity syndrome	Newborn physical and neurological examination	You meet with your patient and her husband and discuss possible reasons for the discrepancy and correcting any unrealistic fears that are worsening her anxiety
Amniocentesis performed at week 16 of pregnancy reveals normal results with an XY karyotype	Higher suspicion of androgen insensitivity because of the normal electrolytes and the ultrasound findings	Labs	Consider the common and uncommon disorders of sex development with a 46XY newborn and the present findings
Repeated prenatal ultrasound at week 34 of pregnancy reveals the fetus was female	How critical is it to assign a gender identity by a particular age?	Pediatric endocrinology consultation	Goals for parent education: address questions regarding future gender assignment, psychosexual development and potential medical problems
Uncomplicated delivery at 39 weeks gestation of a newborn girl with normal female genitalia	Which psychosexual issues need to be addressed prior to puberty?	Genetic testing	How is gender assigned for children with CAIS?
Ultrasound of the pelvic area reveals that there is no uterus and undescended testes are present	At what age or developmental stage will the child have powers of assent in order to contribute to decisions regarding treatment such as genital surgery?	How well defined is the "standard of care" regarding treatments related to gender assignment?	Family therapy is provided by the child psychologist with close monitoring of the child's psychosexual development and considering at which later stage of cognitive development the issue of her diagnosis should be discussed with her

Facts	Hypotheses	Information needed	Learning issues
Pediatric endocrinology consult: genetic testing reveals CAIS	Consider the possible need for surgical removal of the testes before puberty because of the risk of cancer	How much family education needs to occur to facilitate an informed medical decision regarding the child's treatment?	Additional goals of family therapy include, how could Pat be supported to make some of her own decisions regarding treatment sometime during adolescence
After a few family sessions with the parents, child psychologist and yourself, the parents have decided to rear Baby Pat as a girl	What is the role of the family's values in directing medical interventions?		Depending on Pat's preferences and anatomical findings, a discussion will be needed regarding options with genital surgery and hormone treatment
You meet with the parents, child psychologist, and Pat, who is now 9 years old			
There has been an ongoing discussion with the parents recently as to when to discuss the diagnosis of CAIS with Pat			
Family and treatment team agree that Pat should make some of her own decisions regarding treatment sometime during adolescence			

CAIS complete androgen insensitivity syndrome

Vignette 5.2: Mike

Learning Issue Table 5.2

Facts	Hypotheses	Information needed	Learning issues
Mike, a 6-year-old boy who is brought in by his mother because of "behavior problems in school that might cause him to get kicked out"	Normal childhood development	Comprehensive behavioral health evaluation including information from youth, family, and school staff	You talk to Mike and his mother, Mike conveys regret over what he had done
According to the principal, he once exposed his penis to a group of his male and female classmates in the playground	Children become naturally curious about matters pertaining to sex and sexual organs	Comprehensive medical evaluation	You meet with school staff
Several parents lodged complaints that they would pull their children out of this school if the teachers could not contain the "immorality" of "other troubled children"	Developmentally normal behaviors include sexually themed play, exploration of one's own body and the bodies of others, and enactment of adult sexual roles (e.g., being mommy or daddy), often within the safety of the family		You learn that, while he may have seen some kissing and adult sitcom shows while being babysat by a teenage cousin and her boyfriend a few months ago, he has not had any other exposure to inappropriate sexual material
He also tends to make "lewd comments" about people depicted in bathing suits in various magazines	Clinician should certainly consider other conditions and situations that may predispose to behaviors that are either quantitatively or qualitatively inappropriate for the given age of development		You meet with Mike's mother and teaching staff and provide counseling about developmentally appropriate supervision in home and school settings and refocusing on developmentally appropriate tasks

Facts	Hypotheses	Information needed	Learning issues
	Can you consider examples of behavior that suggest either inappropriate exposure to sexual activity or other psychopathology		
	Hypotheses to investigate include abuse, neglect, insufficient financial resources, domestic violence, inadequate supervision, and methods of discipline		

Vignette 5.3: Mary Jane

Learning Issue Table 5.3

Facts	Hypotheses	Information needed	Learning issues
Mary Jane, a 14-year-old high school freshman who is brought in by her mother, who requests that Mary Jane be tested for HIV and "anything else that can be sexually transmitted," placed on the "birth control shot," and given "that new cervical cancer vaccine and anything else that can prevent sexually transmitted diseases"	Adolescent	Comprehensive behavioral health and medical history	Confidentiality
Mary Jane's mother learned that she slept with a boy classmate at band camp and is now worried that she will catch something from "being promiscuous"	Development	Medication history	Special areas of interest for the interview with adolescence patients
Mary Jane explains that she previously had never had sexual intercourse, other than having "experimented" with fondling a close female friend who is lesbian (even though she herself is "straight")	Sexual identity and activity	Routine labs	Statistics suggest that sexual activity, including intercourse, is common in adolescence, and should prompt the clinician to assist youth in preventing sexually transmitted disease and unwanted pregnancy
She denies ever having had any other sexual experiences. Mary Jane comes from a "traditional family" that, she believes, would not otherwise condone any premarital sexual activity or any homosexual behaviors	Normal sexual activity	Sexual history	Offer blood testing for HIV and syphilis

Facts	Hypotheses	Information needed	Learning issues
	Antisocial or delinquent behavior	Physical exam—sexual maturity rating (SMR) stage 4	Insure that hepatitis B immunizations are up-to-date and administer the first of the human papillomavirus vaccine series
	Alcohol and substance abuse	Pelvic exam with Papanicolau smear and cultures for gonococcus and chlamydia	Offer blood testing for HIV and syphilis
	Suicidal ideation or behavior, including non-suicidal self-injury		Counsel her on effective methods of preventing sexually transmitted diseases, including abstinence
	Risks of coercion, sexually transmitted disease, and pregnancy		

Vignette 5.4: Phil Robertson

Learning Issue Table 5.4

Facts	Hypotheses	Information needed	Learning issues
Mr. Phil Robinson is a 58-year-old male with a history of panic disorder and hypertension	Normal sexual development of older adult	Psychiatric and medical history	You work to optimize his medication regimen and insure that he has no new medical problems
For the past 6 months, he and his 49-year-old wife have had sex less and less frequently	Characteristics of the human sexual response cycle	Physical exam	You provide education to him and his wife about the various factors that can affect the sexual response cycle
Recently had more difficulties getting "in sync" with each other, either she has little sexual interest (which she relates to "premenopause") or she is sexually interested but he has difficulty maintaining an erection	Erectile disorder in Mr. Robinson and the possibility of a female sexual interest/arousal disorder in his wife	Medication history	You encourage Mrs. Robinson to follow-up with her physician
He denies any past history of sexual difficulties, other than what he reports as "premature ejaculation" earlier in his adult life	Health conditions	Routine labs	In the meantime, you encourage them to focus on enjoying emotional and physical closeness with each other, with a de-emphasis on sexual intercourse
Mr. Robinson is taking a beta-blocker for hypertension and a serotonin-selective reuptake inhibitor along with a benzodiazepine for panic disorder	Medications he may be taking		
A few months later, he is happy to report that they have enjoyed their sex life once again	Psychosocial stressors and anxiety around sexual intercourse		

Facts	Hypotheses	Information needed	Learning issues
	The increased anxiety symptoms he had been having around that time (hence the dose increase) may have played a more important role and may have contributed to what he feels may be a “vicious cycle” of performance anxiety around sexual intercourse		

Appendix B: Answers to Review Questions

Answers

1. d
2. c
3. a
4. b

References

American Psychiatric Association. (2013). *Diagnostic and statistical manual of mental disorders DSM-5 fifth edition.*

Centers for Disease Control and Prevention. (2013). Morbidity and mortality weekly report youth risk behavior surveillance, 2013. http://www.cdc.gov/yrbs.

Donohoue, P. A. (2011). *Disorders of sex development. Nelson textbook of pediatrics* (19th ed). Philadelphia: Saunders an imprint of Elsevier. (Chap. 582, 1958–1968).

Further Readings

Jellinek M. S., Murphy J. M., Little M., et al. (1999). Use of the Pediatric Symptom Checklist (PSC) to screen for psychosocial problems in pediatric primary care: A national feasibility study. *Archives of Pediatric and Adolescent Medicine, 153*(3):254–260.

Sadock, B. J., & Sadock, V. A. (2015). Kaplan and sadock's synopsis of psychiatry: Behavioral sciences/clinical psychiatry (11th ed). New York: Lippincott Williams & Wilkins.

Chapter 6
Adaptation and Coping in a Medical Setting

Maria-Christina Stewart and Lance Hartmut Linke

Coping in the face of medical adversity is a critical advantage. This chapter illustrates the importance of adaptive coping and how physicians can help patients develop skills. This chapter, like the sample vignette in Chap. 1, uses graphics in the vignette text to help identify key facts for the project-based learning (PBL) process. While this chapter does not cover all of the psychiatric illnesses that may occur following the diagnosis of a medical illness (as these are covered in the specific chapters), it highlights both healthy and potentially unhealthy behaviors.

At the end of this chapter, the reader will be able to:

1. Define and identify methods of coping and adaptation
2. Determine neurobiological, psychological, social, and spiritual variables affecting coping and adaptation
3. Classify and distinguish among functional and dysfunctional methods of adapting to and coping with stressful situations such as medical adversity
4. Identify methods of intervention to facilitate adaptive coping

Case 6.1.1 Presenting Situation: Paul Davis Paul Davis is a 75-year-old African-American male who recently presented with ***"cognitive difficulties."*** Accompanying him at every medical appointment and assisting in decision-making processes is his wife, his "number one supporter" and partner in life. Paul is scheduled today for cognitive testing. Today he arrives with his wife and shares with you his comfort with end-of-life issues, claiming to be "keeping a stiff upper lip" and endorsing generally having a stoic disposition in the face of stress. During the testing process, his

M.-C. Stewart (✉)
3030 Ashby Ave., Ste 115, Berkeley, CA 94705, USA
e-mail: drmariachristina@gmail.com

L. H. Linke
23586 Pershing Avenue Apt. 406, Saint Louis, MO 63112, USA
e-mail: lancelinke@gmail.com

D. Alicata et al. (eds.), *Problem-based Behavioral Science and Psychiatry,*
DOI 10.1007/978-3-319-23669-8_6

wife leaves to run errands and returns to bring him home. Paul is ***silent*** during the majority of the cognitive testing, including after his wife returns to bring him home.

STOP	Please proceed with the problem-based approach using the worksheet located in the appendix of Chap. 1!

Please fill in the facts, your hypotheses, further information needed, and learning issues for Learning Issue Table 6.1.1.

Learning Issue Table 6.1.1

FACTS	HYPOTHESES	INFORMATION NEEDED	LEARNING ISSUES

6.1 Adaptation and Coping Defined

6.1.1 Adaptation

Adaptation refers to efforts and processes aimed at managing demands of stressors. It involves the use of resources, coping, and problem-solving strategies, with the ultimate goal of altering an individual's state of functioning. As we will see, this new state may be positive or negative (e.g., a positive adaptation of using external resources to aid in coping with cancer may become negative if it is the only process of adaptation employed, and the individual does not learn to use inner resources). The process of adapting involves making changes to (Friedman et al. 2003):

- Established patterns of functioning
- Internal resources
- Resources within the family and community
- Appraisal of how demands are being and should be met
- World views
- Problem-solving skills
- Coping methods

6.1.2 *Coping*

Coping refers to problem-specific efforts aimed at preventing, avoiding, or controlling specific external and/or internal stressors that are impairing an individual's well-being (e.g., emotional distress and/or solving problems). More specifically, coping refers to behaviors that can be or are being employed, rather than resources that could be of use (Friedman et al. 2003). As patients adapt to and cope with medical visits, diagnoses, and procedures, it is normal for them to experience transient emotions. When such emotions become persistent or uncontrollable, however, they may hinder adaptive coping and adaptation behaviors and result in a psychiatric disorder.

6.2 Neurobiological Correlates of Adaptation and Coping

As we start to formulate our case conceptualization of Paul and consider which methods of adaptation and coping, if any, he may be employing or from which he may benefit, let us keep in mind the physiology behind two primary emotions often associated with medical adversity: fear and sadness (summarized in Table 6.1; for a detailed review, see Carlson 2006). While a detailed discussion of the physiology of stress is beyond the scope of this chapter and more comprehensively covered in Chap. 11 ("Stress and Health"), it is important to consider the ways in which the primary medical illness being adapted to can, in itself, pose a biological risk to maladaptive coping.

Table 6.1 Examples of neurobiological correlates of persistent fear and sadness

Oversensitive norepinephrine system in the locus coeruleus
Abnormal function of serotonin system
Oversecretion of corticotropin-releasing factor and subsequent long-term reduction in cortisol
Reduction in hippocampal volume

6.3 Effect of Social Support on Adaptation and Coping

Support from external sources such as extended social support networks and the community can significantly aid both in adapting to and coping with major stressors through alleviating much of the associated burden and preventing additional stress and negative consequences (Cohen 2004). Individuals and families with support from social networks tend to cope with medical crises and illness better than individuals or families employing only internal strategies, and absence of social support can engender feelings vulnerability—especially among individuals whose cultural norms include relying on extended kin for assistance (Friedman and Ferguson-Marshalleck 1996). As a result, active participation in and promotion and maintenance of relationships in the individual's immediate and larger social network (neighborhood, town, society) are vital.

6.3.1 *Types of Social Support*

Individuals in crisis may benefit from short-term crisis management or longer-term support for general life issues (e.g., in adjusting to loss of a child or parent). Families often play key roles in providing all types of support, and extended resources aid in meeting those needs that the family cannot address. Types of social support include (House and Kahn 1985):

- Instrumental support (e.g., offering direct assistance)
- Informational support (e.g., sharing information about the illness)
- Appraisal support (e.g., aiding in assessing the illness and/or decision-making)
- Emotional support (e.g., providing counseling)

6.3.2 *Barriers to Seeking Social Support*

Though empirical literature repeatedly demonstrates the value of employing external sources of support, individuals and/or families, especially in Western cultural contexts, may interpret such use as failure to independently cope with the stressor and a marker of weakness. Additionally, individuals may wish to utilize professional services but be unable to afford them (Walsh 1998).

6.3.3 *Case Conceptualization of Paul*

Now that we have examined the meanings behind *adaptation* and *coping,* the neurobiological underpinnings of fear and sadness, and the role of social support in handling medical adversity, let us take another look at what we know thus far about Paul. His cognitive difficulties may have neurobiological underpinnings that may, in turn, relate to his silence. At this point, however, it is unclear to what extent his quiet presentation is reflective of his personality—he described his wife as a significant source of support, and it is possible that her absence during most of the visit related to Paul's silent disposition. He also claimed to be comfortable with end-of-life issues but did not define "issues" or rate his comfort level on a meaningful scale.

Case Vignette 6.1.2 Continuation

Paul returns to the hospital the following day to continue testing. He arrives again with his wife, who stays during today's visit and anxiously asks several questions about the meaning behind these "cognitive difficulties."

Paul has been healthy for most of his life, with the exception of essential hypertension, currently well controlled with diet and medication, and osteoarthritis. He denies any personal history of a psychiatric illness and assures you with a chuckle that he is not crazy and can hold it together just fine. He denies any definite problems with his sleep or appetite.

Paul is again ***quiet*** and looks at the ground as his wife chastises him about being a difficult patient, says he is to blame for being sick, and lectures him about the necessity of taking better care of himself. You are in the room as they talk to their daughter and overhear Paul ***suddenly start screaming*** at her, shouting, "You can be as cool and comfortable as you want! Why don't you just leave the entire family and never talk to me again if that is what you want!"

6.4 Adaptive and Maladaptive Methods of Adapting to and Coping with Medical Adversity

Emotional, cognitive, and behavioral strategies of adaptively or maladaptively coping with medical adversity are person-, problem-, and situation-specific and can develop within an individual or group or be drawn externally from social networks and the larger community. Having a pool of adaptive strategies from which to select is optimal in effectively coping with stressors. Several such strategies are summarized in Tables 6.2 and 6.3. (For a detailed review, see Friedman et al. 2003; McCubbin and McCubbin 1993).

Table 6.2 Adaptive methods of adapting to and coping with medical adversity

Cognitive coping strategies
Normalizing involves focusing thoughts, attention, and behaviors on the normal aspects of life and may be achieved through maintaining rituals and routines that preexisted the stressor, defining life as normal, participating in activities that reflect the normalcy of the individual and/or family, and minimizing attention to any negative social effects of the stressor (e.g., stigma)
Cognitive reframing describes adjusting the interpretation or meaning of a situation
Passive appraisal indicates not actively thinking about stressors, often because it is believed they will remediate on their own
Joint problem-solving involves identifying and communicating in an effort to isolate, select, carry out, and monitor solutions based on shared input from everyone involved in the problem-solving process
Becoming educated about medical adversity is an easy method for individuals to both increase the feeling of control in uncertain situations and better evaluate situations when making decisions. It offers medical teams a means of communication with patients and families and is associated with effective coping and decreased stress
Effective communication
Sharing ideas and feelings, being honest and clear, and using humor significantly effects coping during medical adversity

Table 6.3 Maladaptive methods of adapting to and coping with medical adversity

Individual methods
Denial is a defense mechanism that allows individuals to disbelieve that a situation or some aspect thereof exists
Emotional distancing describes an inability to cultivate close, emotional relationships and may occur during periods of extreme stress
Creation of myths involves suspension of reality by altering belief systems. Myths are produced when wishes and expectations have not been fulfilled and may serve as reflections of both inner and outer states of an individual
Group methods
Scapegoating involves a group negatively labeling, blaming, and displacing tensions, hostilities, guilt, and stress on one member while appearing to have achieved group harmony and cohesiveness
Triangling gives the illusion of limiting and diminishing group tensions by welcoming additional members on whom the stress is displaced
Threats involving permanent ostracism, self-destructive acts of other members of the group (e.g., suicide), and emotional withdrawal may be posited when one group member appears to display autonomy and independence from the group, and the group fears losing cohesiveness
Dissolution and addiction: During periods of extreme stress, attempts to reduce tension may result in separation from loved ones (e.g., divorce), addiction (e.g., gambling, substance use), or violence

6.4.1 *Adapting to and Coping with Illness in the Context of the Family*

Families can also play a significant role as agents of social change during medical adversity (Burr et al. 1994; McCubbin and McCubbin 1993; Walsh 1998). The success of adaptation is determined by, the family's ability to function and adapt to change; the situational pile-up of demands, transitions, strains, and stressors; and family communication. Those families with affirming and/or stress-reducing communication (e.g., calm, soothing support) are more likely to adapt to stress compared to families with conflict-escalating communication (e.g., yelling, blaming), which elevates tension (Friedman et al. 2003). Adaptive relational methods of coping with medical adversity are summarized in Table 6.4 (For a detailed review, see Walsh 1998).

Table 6.4 Adaptive relational methods of adapting to and coping with medical adversity

Family group reliance involves increasing structure and organization in the family and home (e.g., chores, visits, mealtimes), more cogent time schedules and routines, and increased tasks per family member, and can lead to increased integration, cohesion, strength, and predictability, thereby leading to increased coping with the stressor
Increased family cohesion may be achieved through involvement in shared leisure-time activities and rituals, especially when these rituals maintain and foster shared identity and worldviews among group members and increase integration, cohesion, morale, satisfaction, and resilience. Among families, cohesion is characterized by emotional bonding among family members and considered to be a central attribute to the family unit
Role flexibility describes the ability for family members to share and change roles during times of stress and is essential to maintaining the equilibrium between stability and change and thereby coping with developmental, environmental, and life stressors

6.4.2 Case Conceptualization of Paul

Now that we have discussed how the family can influence a patient's ability to adaptively or maladaptively cope with and adapt to medical adversity, let us take another look at Paul. We cannot yet be sure about the nature of his quiet disposition, but we know that he has been quiet on his own and while being chastised by his wife, who appears anxious. We have also caught a glimpse of him screaming threats at his daughter, suggesting that his and his family's methods of coping and adaptation are not providing the maximal level of support possible. He appears to ascribe to a stigma regarding mental illness, suggesting that he may not be very receptive to acknowledging having difficulty coping with his current medical situation.

Case Vignette 6.1.3 Continuation
Paul was cooperative and forthcoming during a semi-structured interview and mental status exam, during which he exhibited ***blunted affect yet simultaneously was tearful***. He denied any substance use, including coffee and cigarettes. Paul revealed having *served in the Vietnam War* and having *grown up Black in the USA before the Civil Rights Movement*. He indicated having a *troubling relationship with each of his six children* and admitted to being "too hard" on them and unnecessarily screaming at them too often. He *disclosed having a sparse support network outside of his family*. Paul denied feeling suicidal and expressed his hopes to live as long as possible, reiterating feeling comfortable with the concept of death and attributing these feelings to his Christian faith and daily prayer.

Please proceed with the problem-based approach using the worksheet located in the appendix of Chap. 1!

Please fill in the facts, your hypotheses, further information needed, and learning issues for Learning Issue Table 6.1.3.

Learning Issue Table 6.1.3

FACTS	HYPOTHESES	INFORMATION NEEDED	LEARNING ISSUES

6.5 Factors Influencing Coping and Adaptation

6.5.1 *Sociocultural Values*

An important variable in understanding and considering adaptation and coping strategies is culture and society. A significant amount of research has demonstrated wide variation in use of the strategies discussed in this chapter, and it is imperative that medical staff sensitively respond to the patient and family's values and norms. For example, the extent to which individuals rely on internal and external coping and adaptation strategies also varies across cultures, and medical staff is advised to take cultural values and background into account when assisting patients and their families in adjusting to illness (Friedman et al. 2003; Friedman and Ferguson-Marshalleck 1996; Kleinman et al. 2006). Culture additionally informs behavioral patterns (such as diet, relationship styles, and work schedules) that can influence gene expression, diagnosis comprehension, and treatment adherence (Kawgawa-Singer and Kassim-Lakha 2003).

Similarly, many individuals and families may find that spirituality and/or religious beliefs lie at the core of coping with and adapting to medical adversity. Reliance on these beliefs naturally varies across developmental, cultural, and socio-economic groups (Clark and Heidenreich 1995). Failure to consider a client's cultural perspectives can result in inaccurate patient history, non-adherence to treatment regiment, poor continuity of care, use of harmful remedies and fewer prescriptions (Flores 2000). Flores (2000) provides evidence from cross-cultural studies that when culturally sensitive clinical care is provided, quality of care and client satisfaction may be increased.

6.5.2 *Gender Differences*

Methods of coping tend to vary across genders. Women use more strategies that involve closeness and intimacy: reaching out to and sharing concerns with family members and friends, openly expressing emotions, cognitive reframing, delegating, and taking time for self-care; whereas men tend to withdraw more, keep emotions hidden, and use alcohol (Burr et al. 1994).

6.5.3 *Development*

Special consideration and attention should be given to the effect of developmental stage on coping and adapting to medical illness and trauma, particularly in children because their experiences are especially influential in shaping future reactions to hospitals and medical procedures. Further discussion on the role of development in adjusting to various transitions is provided in Chap. 2 ("Normal Human Development").

6.6 Bio-Psycho-Social-Cultural-Spiritual Conceptualization

Now that we have garnered information pertinent to most of our learning issues, let us review the neurobiological, social, psychological, and spiritual information relating to Paul's case conceptualization so that we can identify its impact on his psychiatric presentation.

6.6.1 *Biological*

Past: Genetics (no known history of psychiatric illness in patient or family), history of hypertension
Presenting problem: Cognitive difficulties

6.6.2 *Psychological*

Past

Trauma (US war veteran, history as a racial minority in the USA before the Civil Rights Movement)
Personality (stoic disposition)

Present

Affect (blunted, tearful, quiet/silent)
End-of-life issues (eager to live as long as possible, comfortable with death, no suicidality)
Possible stigma about mental health problems, including cognitive difficulties

6.6.3 *Social/Cultural/Spiritual*

- Married to wife whom he describes as supportive and who appears anxious
- Six children, troubled relationship, none live in same city, use of threats toward them

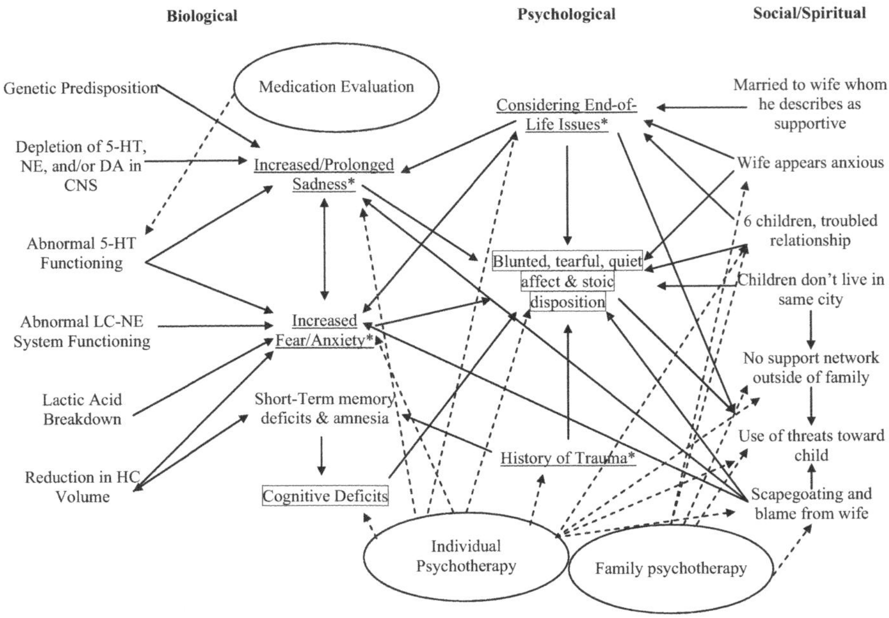

Fig. 6.1 Bio-psycho-social-spiritual case conceptualization model of our sample client Paul. This model demonstrates the interrelated nature of biological, psychological, social, and spiritual variables relevant to case conceptualizations, as demonstrated through the case sample of Paul. *Solid arrows* represent mechanisms underlying clinical hypotheses; presenting symptoms are in *boxes;* potential therapeutic interventions are in *ovals* and linked with *dotted arrows;* and proximal etiological variables are *underlined* and *asterisked*

- No support network outside of family
- Scapegoating and blame from wife
- Christian/prays daily

As we conceptualize Paul's case and consider effective interventions, it may be helpful to continue the inquiry process outlined in Learning Issue Table 6.1 and summarize the current hypotheses in a diagram (Fig. 6.1).

6.7 Psychosocial Interventions to Facilitate Adapting to and Coping with Medical Adversity

Developing and practicing adaptive coping when facing medical crises can be challenging for many patients, especially when they are used to employing maladaptive coping strategies in their daily lives. As a result, psychotherapy for individuals and families is often recommended and has been empirically demonstrated to benefit patients struggling to cope with medical adversity.

Additionally, several psychosocial models have been developed to guide medical staff in addressing maladaptive coping and facilitating in the development of adaptive coping methods. Specific psychosocial strategies include: reviewing the event that led to the injury; processing the sensory experience of the event; assessing beliefs related to the event; using desensitization, relaxation techniques, and pain management for medical interventions; and, with children, using drawings and play to symbolize and elaborate the event further, explaining medical interventions carefully to the child, increasing the child's sense of control over their own bodies, and assisting the parents to manage their own affect relating to the event and subsequent injury.

6.7.1 Case Conceptualization of Paul

When we examine Paul's story, though still incomplete, we can see the great extent to which biological, psychological, social, and spiritual factors interact and influence his presenting symptoms of cognitive deficits and quiet, blunted, and tearful affect. It remains unclear whether these symptoms reflect underlying depression and/or anxiety. However, because Paul's personal history and family presentation reflect the use of both some maladaptive methods of coping with his cognitive deficits (e.g., silence, screaming), it is possible that his daily life and family relations would improve from psychosocial interventions. Let us take a look at a psychosocial assessment conducted 6 months following the end of a psychosocial intervention:

Case Vignette 6.1.4 Conclusion

Following a 3-month intervention of weekly family therapy and individual therapy focused on processing Paul's experience with his cognitive deficits, reviewing previous and current family relations, and increasing family cohesion, reliance on one another, and role flexibility, Paul arrives for a 6-month follow-up assessment. His wife is accompanying him and stays during the entire appointment. Together, they indicate that the amount of screaming in their family has significantly decreased, while the amount of support and communication has increased. They both become tearful and link arms as they admit that they continue to struggle with Paul's cognitive difficulties and unknown diagnosis and sometimes lash out at each other. Overall, though, they express gratitude for their therapy.

6.8 Conclusions

As Paul's case illustrates, adaptive coping with medical illness is influenced by many different factors, especially those related to biology, psychology, social support, and spiritual beliefs (e.g., the type and onset of the illness, individual, and family coping styles). It is imperative to assess patients and, when possible, their family members not only on their medical illness but also their adjustment to the illness.

6.9 Review Questions

1. Maladaptive methods of coping with and adapting to medical adversity include:

   a. Addiction
   b. Triangulating
   c. Threat
   d. All of the above

2. Adaptation involves:

   a. Specific behaviors aimed at preventing, avoiding, or controlling specific stressors
   b. Changing external situations to improve internal responses
   c. Use of internal and external resources, coping, and problem-solving strategies, aimed at managing demands of stressors
   d. Selection of only one effective strategy to adjust to stressors

3. Which of the following is recognized as a specific type of support:

   a. Instrumental
   b. Informational
   c. Appraisal
   d. Emotional
   e. All of the above

4. Assessing beliefs related to medical trauma has been discussed as one method of:

   a. Maladaptive coping
   b. Facilitating adaptive coping
   c. Both of the above
   d. Neither of the above

Appendix A: Tables with Possible Answers to the Vignettes

Case Vignette 6.1: Paul Davis

Learning Issue Table 6.1

Facts	Hypotheses	Information needed	Learning issues
Age 75	1. He relies on his wife for significant support	History of Present Illness (*HPI*)	1. How are adaptation and coping defined?
Male		Medication?	
Married	2. He is facing and considering end-of-life questions and issues	Sleep? Appetite? Hopelessness? Fear?	2. What are the major neurobiological and psychosocial correlates of adaptation and coping?
Cognitive difficulties			
Receiving cognitive testing		Post Medical History (*PMH*)	
Claims to be comfortable with end-of-life issues	3. His silence and stoic disposition may be a sign of underlying difficulties in adapting to and coping with his cognitive deficits	Has he had any previous medical or psychiatric diagnoses, including substance abuse?	3. How do social support, spirituality, and cultural variables affect adaptation and coping?
Stoic disposition		Family History (*FH*)	
Considers wife to be a source of support			
		Any history of psychiatric illness?	4. What are interventions for coping deficits?
Silent	4. His silence and stoic disposition may be related to an underlying medical/neurological or psychiatric condition (e.g., major depression, dementia, etc.)	Social History (*SH*)	
		Social support besides wife?	
		Exam	
		Physical exam? Vital signs?	
	5. Cognitive deficits, in particular, may be particularly difficult for him to accept because of stigma		

Appendix B: Answers to Review Questions

Answers

1. D
2. C
3. E
4. B

References

Burr, W., Klein, S., Burr, R., Doxey, C., Harker, B., Holman, T., et al. (1994). *Reexamining family stress: New theory and research*. Thousand Oaks: Sage.
Carlson, N. (2006). *Physiology of behavior* (9th ed.). Bostan: Allyn & Bacon.
Cohen, S. (2004). Social relationships and health. *American Psychologist, 59*(8), 676.
Clark, C., & Heidenreich, T. (1995). Spiritual care for the critically ill. *American Journal of Critical Care, 4*(1), 77–81.
Flores, G. (2000). Culture and the patient-physician relationship: Achieving cultural competency in health care. *Journal of Pediatrics, 136*, 14–23.
Friedman, M. M., & Ferguson-Marshalleck, E. (1996). Sociocultural influences on family health. In S. Hanson & S. Boyd (Eds.), *Family health care nursing: Theory, practice & research* (pp. 81–98). Philadelphia: Davis.
Friedman, M. M., Bowden, V. R., & Jones, E. G. (2003). Family stress, coping, and adaptation. In M. M. Friedman, V. R. Bowden, & E. G. Jones (Eds.), *Family nursing: Research, theory, and practice* (5th ed.). Upper Saddle Ridge: Prentice Hall Health.
House, J. S., & Kahn, R. L. (1985). Measures and concepts of social support. In S. Cohen & S. L. Syme (Eds.), *Social support and health* (pp. 83–108). Orlando: Academic.
Kawgawa-Singer, M., & Kassim-Lakha, S. (2003). A strategy to reduce cross-cultural miscommunication and increase the likelihood of improving health outcomes. *Academic Medicine, 78*(6), 577–587.
Kleinman, A., Eisenberg, L., & Good, B. (2006). Culture, illness, and care: Clinical lessons from anthropologic and cross-cultural research. *Focus, 4*(1), 140–149.
McCubbin, M. A., & McCubbin, H. I. (1993). Families coping with illness: The resiliency model of family stress, adjustment and adaptation. In C. Danielson, B. Hamel-Bissell, & P. Winstead-Fry (Eds.), *Families, health, and illness: Perspectives on coping and intervention* (pp. 21–63). St. Louis: Harcourt Health Services.
National Center for Health Statistics. (2005). *Health, United States, 2005, with chartbook on trends in the health of Americans*. Hyattsville, Maryland.
Walsh, F. (1998). *Strengthening family resilience*. New York: The Guilford Press.

Chapter 7
Violence and Abuse

Jeanelle J. Sugimoto-Matsuda and Anthony P.S. Guerrero

This chapter reviews conditions that are among the leading causes of morbidity and mortality throughout the life cycle, yet remain under-recognized and under-addressed in clinical practice.

At the end of this chapter, the reader will be able to:

1. Discuss typical presenting signs and symptoms of patients who are victims of various types of violence or abuse.
2. Define the different types of violence and abuse.
3. Discuss resources and treatments for victims of violence and abuse.

Case Vignette 7.1.1 Presenting Situation Mary Infante
Mary Infante is a 32-year-old married woman who is 20 weeks pregnant and having severe cramps. She has had two miscarriages in the past and is worried that she may be having another one. Previous laboratory tests were unremarkable. Upon physical examination, she has bruising on the upper arms and abdomen. The bruising is not noticeable on any areas of the body that are not covered by her clothing.

Ms. Infante is a secretary at a local law firm. Her husband was recently laid off from his position with a management consulting company, and is seeking another company to work with. He has apparently been let go from a

J. J. Sugimoto-Matsuda (✉)
Department of Psychiatry, Research Division, University of Hawai'i John A. Burns School of Medicine, 677 Ala Moana Boulevard, Suite 301, Honolulu, HI 96813, USA
e-mail: SugimotoJ@dop.hawaii.edu

A. P. S. Guerrero
Department of Psychiatry, University of Hawai'i John A. Burns School of Medicine, 1356 Lusitana Street, University Tower 4th Floor, Honolulu, HI 96813, USA
e-mail: GuerreroA@dop.hawaii.edu

D. Alicata et al. (eds.), *Problem-based Behavioral Science and Psychiatry*,
DOI 10.1007/978-3-319-23669-8_7

number of positions since they have been together. They have been married for approximately 3 years, but have not yet been able to have children. A psychiatric consultation was requested by her physician to evaluate the situation.

Please proceed with the problem-based approach using the worksheet located in the appendix of Chap. 1!

Please fill in the facts, your hypotheses, further information needed, and learning issues for learning issue Table 7.1.1.

Learning issue Table 7.1.1

FACTS	HYPOTHESES	INFORMATION NEEDED	LEARNING ISSUES

7.1 Abuse and Neglect of Adults

Although further information must still be gathered from the patient and her husband, spousal abuse should be a strong consideration in this case. All physicians in all specialties must be aware of the physical and emotional signs of violence and abuse. As can be seen in this case study, the obstetrician discovered the symptoms in the context of a recent miscarriage. Injuries and bruising can be discovered during any physical examination, and key statements that may reveal underlying problems can be elicited during any patient interview. It is up to the physician to make the initial identification and refer the patient to an appropriate specialist.

Family violence is a general term that includes acts of violence between family members or other individuals with close relations (Director and Linden 2004). Domestic violence is a specific type of family violence, and includes acts between intimate partners (therefore, the term is also interchangeable with "intimate partner violence"; Director and Linden 2004). It includes acts that may coerce, control, or demean the victim (Director and Linden 2004). The American College of Emergency Physicians outlines domestic violence as, "…part of a pattern of coercive behavior which an individual uses to establish and maintain power and control over another with whom he or she has or had an intimate, romantic, or spousal relationship. Behaviors include: actual or threatened physical or sexual abuse, psychological abuse, social isolation, deprivation, or intimidation" (American College of Emergency Physicians 1995). The Diagnostic and Statistical Manual of Mental Disorders, Fifth Edition (DSM-5; American Psychiatric Association 2013) notates abuse and neglect under, "Other conditions that may be a focus of clinical attention," and categorizes these diagnoses as follows: (1) Child maltreatment and neglect problems (child physical abuse; child sexual abuse; child neglect; child psychological abuse), (2) adult maltreatment and neglect problems (spouse or partner violence, physical; spouse or partner violence, sexual; spouse or partner neglect; spouse or partner abuse, psychological; adult abuse by nonspouse or nonpartner).

According to the 2010 National Violence Against Women Survey, 35.6% of women and 28.5% of men in the USA have at some point experienced rape, physical violence (24.3% of women and 13.8% of men), and/or stalking from an intimate partner. Furthermore, 48.4% of all women and 48.8% of men have at some point experienced psychological aggression by an intimate partner (Black et al. 2011).

The effects of domestic violence are varied and widespread. Not only do the victims suffer physically and emotionally, but family and friends also become involved. The situation is especially taxing on children who may witness the abuse. These secondary victims may in turn show their own signs and symptoms, including behavior changes, sleep disturbances, and increased aggression (Director and Linden 2004). They may also be at risk for post-traumatic stress disorder, acute stress disorder, adjustment disorders, or other specified trauma- and stressor-related disorders (please refer to Chap. 22).

Case 7.1.2 Continuation

You interview Ms. Infante individually. You talk to her about her career. She received a merit-based raise, and her coworkers even put together a small dinner to thank her for such good work. When asked about her husband's career, she comments that he was recently laid off from his job. Apparently, the management consulting company he worked for was restructured. She thinks he feels cheated out of a position, and even wrote an angry letter to the president of the company.

After further inquiry, she reveals that the miscarriages might have been caused by spousal abuse while she was pregnant. You suspect that her husband also abuses her when she is not pregnant. She says that he is a very caring husband when in the presence of others, but his temper "gets the best of him" when they are alone. He relates his temper to the severe physical and emotional abuse he had experienced while growing up.

You then call the husband into the room. Overall, he is cordial and polite and seems attentive to his wife. You note that he often interrupts his wife while she is attempting to answer a question. You politely ask him to refrain from answering questions directed at his wife, but he continues to answer questions for her.

Please proceed with the problem-based approach using the worksheet located in the appendix of Chap. 1!

Please fill in the facts, your hypotheses, further information needed, and learning issues for learning issue Table 7.1.2.

Learning issue Table 7.1.2

FACTS	HYPOTHESES	INFORMATION NEEDED	LEARNING ISSUES

While there are no definitive tests that can determine with 100% accuracy that an individual is a victim of domestic violence, there are certain risk factors and signs/symptoms the physician can consider (Director and Linden 2004).

- Risk factors
  - Being female
  - Being younger
  - Being single, separated, or divorced
- Physical signs and symptoms
  - Initial signs may be vague and nonspecific
  - Injuries
    - Injuries that are not consistent with the patient history, or complaints that are not consistent with the problem
    - Recurrent injuries with increasing severity over time
    - Multiple injuries in different stages of healing
    - Injuries to central body areas (breasts, abdomen, and chest) in addition to the face and extremities
    - Injuries to normally protected areas (inner thigh and inner arm)
    - Injuries suggesting defensive posture

  - General health concerns
    - Higher rates of general health problems (headache, back pain, vaginal infections, and gastrointestinal complaints)
    - Frequent exacerbations of chronic illnesses (asthma, diabetes, and hypertension)
    - Increased use of the health-care system, but delay in seeking treatment for the actual problem
    - Lack of prenatal care
    - Injury during pregnancy

- Emotional signs and symptoms
  - Frequent reporting of emotional symptoms (depression, low self-esteem, increased daily stressors, and anxiety)
  - Feelings of guilt and isolation
  - Possible substance abuse, eating disorders, and post-traumatic stress disorder
  - Possible suicidality

- Characteristics of the abuser
  - Substance abuse
  - Lower educational achievement
  - Intermittent employment
  - Victimization as a child
  - Feelings of inadequacy
  - Personality disorders (antisocial, borderline)
  - Younger
  - Hovering, domineering presence in spite of cordial/attentive appearance to outside parties
  - Verbal abusiveness

The physician's first step toward treatment is screening. The screening process not only pushes all parties toward the end goal, but also lets the patient know that the physician is concerned for his/her welfare and safety. The patient should be interviewed alone and in a supportive, nonjudgmental, confidential setting (Director and Linden 2004). There are a number of protocols available to physicians. Overall, most of the literature suggests using simple, open-ended questions. Below are some suggested questions, ranging from less to more invasive.

- Simple and open-ended (Director and Linden 2004)
  - How does your partner treat you?
  - Are you or have you been in a relationship in which you felt you were treated badly?
  - We all fight at home; what happens when you and your partner fight or disagree?
  - Do you ever feel afraid of your partner?

- Has your partner ever prevented you from leaving the house, seeing friends, getting a job, or continuing your education?
- Has your partner ever destroyed things you care about?

- More direct questions
  - The Partner Violence Screen—65–71 % sensitivity (Feldhaus et al. 1997)
    - Have you been hit, kicked, punched, or otherwise hurt by someone within the past year? If so, by whom?
    - Do you feel safe in your current relationship?
    - Is there a partner from a previous relationship who is making you feel unsafe now?
  - The "StaT" Screening Tool—97 % sensitivity (Liebschutz and Paranjape 2003)
    - Have you ever been in a relationship in which your partner has pushed or slapped you?
    - Have you ever been in a relationship in which your partner threatened you with violence?
    - Have you ever been in a relationship in which your partner has thrown, broken, or punched things?

Case Vignette 7.1.3 Conclusion
You decide to admit Ms. Infante for threatened miscarriage and for further assessment and intervention for domestic violence. You consult a social worker, who meets with her individually and provides her with information on spousal abuse and women's shelters. A safety plan is formulated that includes cash, a cell phone, and keeping the car tank full of gas. You involve Ms. Infante's sister, as well as two of her closest friends. She will stay in the hospital for a few days and then with her sister. The social worker also assists Ms. Infante with a referral to legal counsel, in case she wishes to file a formal restraining order against the husband.

You and the social worker meet with her and her sister about a month later. She states that she and her husband will attempt marriage counseling with a psychologist the social worker recommended. During this period, however, she will still stay with her sister to maintain her personal safety.

After the initial screening, some general steps should be taken to help abuse victims (McLeer and Anwar 1987):

- Obtain history
- Diagnose and treat injuries
- Evaluate the emotional safety of the patient
- Determine the risk to the victim
- Determine the need for legal intervention

- Develop a follow-up plan
- Document findings

Brown (1997) applied the Transtheoretical Model of Change to the process of a victim's emergence from the cycle of violence. This model is discussed in Chaps. 4 (Learning Principles of Human Behavior) and 10 (Adherence in Medicine).

There are many reasons why victims are unable to break out of the cycle of violence. If the physician has a good understanding of the victim's reasoning, he or she is more likely to make an appropriate referral.

Below are some common scenarios.

- Common reasons for the victim staying in an abusive relationship:
  - Nonrecognition that he or she is being abused
  - Fear of the abuser or fear of retaliation
  - Desire to fulfill predetermined cultural or gender roles
  - Fear of losing financial or childcare support
- Common physician-related reasons why the victim may not disclose information to the physician
  - *Failure of the physician to inquire*
  - Discomfort with talking to patients about this topic
  - Lack of confidence in ability to diagnose abuse
  - Perceived inability to offer appropriate referrals if diagnosed
  - Fear of offending the victim or crossing a cultural barrier
  - Lack of time or privacy with the individual
  - Personal experiences with abuse
- Common patient-related reasons why the victim may not disclose information to the physician
  - Low self-esteem
  - Lack of trust toward the physician
  - Fear that disclosure will involve the police or child protective services (CPS)
  - Fear of being judged
  - Language or cultural barriers

The Community Coalition on Family Violence (CCFV) notes that five statements can provide important encouragement to an abuse victim (Williams 2005):

- You are not alone.
- No one has the right to hit you.
- Domestic violence is not your fault.
- It is against the law.
- Help is available and I will be here when you need me.

Physicians should also be aware of other specific types of abuse among adults, including rape or sexual assault and elder abuse.

There are several misconceptions about rape, including: that it involves a sex-deprived young male attacking an attractive female; that it is not a violent crime; and that it is a street crime (rather than one that may even occur between partners and spouses). According to Englander (2007), there are various types of perpetrators, including violent rapists (who may engage in brutal beatings, who view sex as secondary, and who are chronically angry), and power rapists (who typically use only enough force to complete the act and who have underlying feelings of inadequacy). In general, perpetrators of rape often demonstrate a lack of empathy and an acceptance of cognitive misperceptions (e.g., that the victim deserved it or is making too big a fuss about it). Alcohol or substance abuse (on either the part of the perpetrator or victim) can be a risk factor (though by no means an excuse) for rape to occur.

Elder abuse can include physical abuse (including overmedicating, under-medicating, force-feeding, inappropriately using physical restraints, and exposing to the elements) and emotional abuse (including treatment like a child and isolation from family and friends, neglect, sexual abuse, and financial abuse; Muehlbauer and Crane 2006).

Given the unfortunately high prevalence of victimization and the potential serious sequelae, it is critical for physicians of all specialties to screen all patients of all ages for abuse. The next section is focused upon abuse and neglect of children.

Case Vignette 7.2.1: Nicholas Head

An emergency room (ER) physician refers Nicholas Head, a 5-year-old boy, to your care. Nick's mother reported that he was running in the house and tripped and hit his head on the corner of their dining room table. Upon examination, it was clear that Nick's left eye and the left side of his face are badly bruised. During the complete full-body examination, the ER doctor saw bruising on his upper arm and tenderness when palpating his abdomen. He orders several X-rays, one of which indicates that the boy has a healing fractured humerus. His mother reports that he was roughhousing on the playground with some other children at school and fell off the jungle gym. You are called to join the case to perform a psychiatric consultation on the child.

STOP

Please proceed with the problem-based approach using the worksheet located in the appendix of Chap. 1!

Please fill in the facts, your hypotheses, further information needed, and learning issues for learning issue Table 7.2.1.

Learning issue Table 7.2.1

FACTS	HYPOTHESES	INFORMATION NEEDED	LEARNING ISSUES

7.2 Abuse and Neglect of Children

At this point, child neglect and/or abuse is a valid suspicion. Child abuse is one of the leading causes of injury-related mortality in infants and children (Centers to Disease Control and Prevention 2014). Nationally, it is estimated that one in four children experience some form of child maltreatment in their lifetimes. Among the estimated 686,000 children (or 9.2 per 1000) who were victims of maltreatment in 2012, 78 % were victims of neglect, 18 % of physical abuse, 9 % of sexual abuse, and 11 % were victims of other types of maltreatment, including emotional and threatened abuse, caregiver drug/alcohol abuse, or lack of supervision. Furthermore, in 2012 an estimated 1,640 children died from child maltreatment (rate of 2.2 per 100,000 children).

The Child Abuse Prevention and Treatment Act (CAPTA) defines abuse as, "…a recent act or failure to act that results in death, serious physical or emotional harm, sexual abuse or exploitation, or imminent risk of serious harm; involves a child; and is carried out by a parent or caregiver who is responsible for the child's welfare (McDonald 2007)." Child abuse can be categorized as neglect, emotional abuse, physical abuse and sexual abuse, and each of these can be further categorized according to the definitions below (McDonald 2007):

7.2.1 Child Neglect

- Physical neglect—basic needs for food, clothing, shelter, hygiene, protection, and supervision not met
- Emotional neglect—lack of love and affection
- Educational neglect—failure to enroll child in school
- Medical neglect—failure to seek medical assistance to upkeep child's well-being

7.2.2 Emotional Abuse

- Several subtypes, including rejection, isolation, terrorism, ignorance, psychological unavailability, corruption, and inappropriate expectations of or demands on the child

7.2.3 Physical Abuse, of Which Typical Findings May Include:

- Bruises, including
  - Handprints (typically adult-sized)
  - Unusually distributed lesions
  - Lesions at various stages of healing
- Bites (typically adult-sized)
- Burns
  - Cigarette burns
  - Burns with clear demarcation and uniform depth (e.g., submersion burns)
- Fractures
  - Posterior rib fractures
  - Long bone fractures in children under 2 years of age
  - Scapular, spinous process, and sternal fractures
- Abdominal trauma
- Head trauma
  - Retinal hemorrhages
- Trauma that is inconsistent with the reported mechanism of injury

7.2.4 Sexual Abuse

CAPTA defines sexual abuse as, "The employment, use, persuasion, inducement, enticement, or coercion of any child to engage in, or assist any other person to engage in, any sexually explicit conduct or simulation of such conduct for the purpose of producing a visual depiction of such conduct; or the rape, molestation, prostitution, or other form of sexual exploitation of children, or incest with children (McDonald 2007)."

Children who experience any of these types of abuse may demonstrate emotional symptoms, which include: social withdrawal, anger or aggression, feeding disorders, developmental delay, or emotional disturbances.

A number of risk factors for child abuse and neglect have been identified. They can be categorized by caregiver, child, and family/environmental factors (McDonald 2007):

- Caregiver factors
  - Criminal history
  - Inappropriate expectations of the child
  - Mental health history
  - Misconceptions about childcare
  - Misperceptions about child development
  - Substance abuse
- Child factors
  - Behavior problems
  - Medical fragility
  - Nonbiologic relationship to the caretaker
  - Prematurity
  - Special needs
- Family and environmental factors
  - High local unemployment rates
  - Intimate partner violence in the home
  - Poverty
  - Social isolation
  - Lack of social support

Abusive parents or caregivers may demonstrate the following characteristics (Lau et al. 2006; McDonald 2007):

- They may exaggerate the child's behavior or even put blame on the child for the family's problems.
- They have low tolerance of behaviors that would otherwise not be seen as serious.
- They will make few statements or gestures that positively support the child.
- They are more likely to be critical in interactions with the child.
- They possess overall negative impressions of their child and the child's behavior.
- They may describe their child as bad, burdensome, or even "evil."
- They do not explain the child's injuries.
- The history changes over time, or history of self-inflicted trauma does not correlate with development.

Case Vignette 7.2.2 Continuation
You and a hospital social worker interview Nick and his mother. Currently they live in a low-incoming housing complex. Nick's father is not around, and likely left the city before the boy was born. Therefore, the mother is forced

to work two jobs to make ends meet. While she is at her second job in the evenings, the mother's live-in boyfriend watches over her son.

You question the mother about the Nick's living conditions at home. She states that Nick receives the three meals a day that he deserves and has a roof over his head. When asked how many hours of the day she spends with her son, she becomes defensive and goes on about her two jobs and how little sleep she gets each night. When questioned about the incident that produced Nick's black eye, she alleges that she was not home at the time of the accident.

You manage to question Nick independently of his mother. When asked about his home, he says that he usually goes to school without eating breakfast and is lucky to have dinner at night. On certain nights, his mother's boyfriend will order pizza or purchase fast food from the convenience store around the corner from their house and give him a portion. On other nights, however, the boyfriend is not around, and so Nick is forced to fend for himself. On certain mornings, he will see his mother getting ready for work and inquire if any breakfast is available. When probed on what her response is, he looks down at the floor and states that occasionally his mother will become angry at his question so recently he has stopped asking. Nick will not answer any more questions about the boyfriend.

STOP — Please proceed with the problem-based approach using the worksheet located in the appendix of Chap. 1!

Please fill in the facts, your hypotheses, further information needed, and learning issues for learning issue Table 7.2.2.

Learning issue Table 7.2.2

FACTS	HYPOTHESES	INFORMATION NEEDED	LEARNING ISSUES

Because of the apparent neglect and abuse, the assessment of this child requires both medical and legal investigation. Assessment must include history of the alleged abuse, assault, or neglect; a medical history; a psychosocial history (including family composition, substance use in the home, and previous involvement with CPS); a review of systems; a comprehensive physical exam (including an anogenital exam if sexual abuse is possible); and a collection of forensic evidence and forensic interviews (Laraque et al. 2006). Especially in sexual abuse cases, examinations should be done by a health-care professional trained in forensic examination techniques. Documentation is crucial during all assessments (interviews and physical assessments). Comprehensive evaluation is time-consuming, but statistics show that 50 % of abused children will likely be abused again (McDonald 2007).

The following are general guidelines for interviewing and examining youth who are possible victims of abuse or neglect (McDonald 2007; Laraque et al. 2006):

- Setting the tone
  - Initiate general rapport-building.
  - Explain who you are and why you are there.
  - Ask if the child knows why he/she is there.
  - Clearly state that confidentiality will be upheld.
  - Explain any physical exams you will conduct.
  - Allow the child to handle any equipment you will be using.
  - Obtain consent for each part of the exam, including who else will be allowed in the room during the exam (it must be explained to parents/caregivers if the child requests that they not be in the room).
  - Establish ground rules prior to commencing the exam (stop at anytime, etc.).
- Type of environment
  - The examination should be in a safe, neutral place if possible.
  - Only one interviewer should be present; multiple adults and interviews are discouraged.
  - If possible, interview the child separately from the parents/caregivers.
  - Offer the option of writing answers down or making a sketch.
- When speaking
  - Use short and simple sentences, concrete terms, proper names, and direct questions.
  - Do not be biased, leading, and presumptive.
  - Determine the child's language and development.
  - Verify the child's statements; rephrase questions if needed, ask if the child understands the question.

The evaluation process should not further traumatize the child. In certain instances, it may be helpful for a non-offending parent (usually the mother if she is not suspected in the abuse) to be present for the exam (Laraque et al. 2006). Below are the recommended exams and assessments that should be done even in the middle of a hectic ER. While each case will be different and have several contributing factors, failure to conduct an exam properly can, in the end, devastate a criminal case and cause lifelong trauma for the child.

- Photography of all injuries (preferably taken by a forensic investigator or medical photographer)
  - Obtain informed consent if possible, although it is not required in child maltreatment cases.
  - Use a color or digital camera, with the highest resolution possible.
  - Photograph injuries before treatment.
  - Photograph from different angles, and take at least two photos of each injury.
  - Use a ruler or coin to give perspective of the injury's size.
  - Include the patient's face in at least one photograph.
  - Document the patient's name, location of injury, date, photographer, and names of those present on the back of the photo.
  - Place photos in a sealed envelope, mark as confidential, and attach to the medical record. Maintain chain of custody.

Guidelines for further assessment in cases of suspected sexual abuse

- General principles:
  - Should be done by a medical professional trained in forensic examinations.
  - Should be done promptly if child complains of dysuria, anal or vaginal bleeding, vaginal discharge, or pain with defecation or if alleged incident occurred less than 72 h prior to presentation.
  - If the alleged incident occurred more than 72 h prior to presentation, the child can be scheduled for an examination at a center specializing in sexual assault examinations.
  - Most sexual abuse cases do not show findings upon physical examination unless the child is examined within 24 h of the incident; therefore, obtaining an oral history is especially critical.
- Examination should collect:
  - Victim's clothing, debris, stains on skin (dried secretions), oral swabs and smears, vaginal/penile swabs and smears, rectal swabs and smears, pubic hair brushings/combings, head hair combings, genital swab, saliva and blood specimen, reference head and pubic hair, fingernail scrapings or clippings, and nasal mucous
  - Condoms and tampons
  - Tests for sexually transmitted diseases
  - Linens and other clothing

Guidelines for further diagnostic studies:

- Recommended in most cases:
  - Ophthalmologic studies—dilated, indirect ophthalmoscopy performed by an ophthalmologist to detect retinal hemorrhages in children younger than 2 years
  - Radiological studies—head computerized tomography (CT) to detect subarachnoid, subdural, or intraparenchymal injury; skeletal survey radiography (e.g., of the spine, extremities, and skull)—suspected old or new fracture

  - Laboratory studies—evaluation of amylase, complete blood count, hepatic transaminases, lipase, partial thromboplastin time, prothrombin time, fecal occult blood test, urinalysis, and urine toxicology—to detect genitourinary or abdominal trauma and to ensure no underlying blood disorder

- Optional:
  - Abdominal CT—if history, examination, or laboratory results suggest abdominal trauma
  - Bone scan—to find occult fractures up to 2 weeks after injury
  - Dental consultation—if there is a bite present, dentists can determine the source
  - Magnetic resonance imaging of the head—if CT of the head is inconclusive

Case Vignette 7.2.3 Conclusion
The social worker calls CPS and expects a return call. You admit Nick to the hospital pediatrics unit for his safety and to ensure that his immediate medical needs are addressed first, such as possible malnutrition.

You learn later from an "auntie" that Nick has been more disruptive and aggressive in school. You hope that the boy, a victim of violence, does not go on to become a perpetrator of violence as an older child or adolescent. You wonder what interventions could prevent such an outcome.

Of course, the next step is arranging for involvement of a social worker who makes plans with CPS for a safe discharge. The following are some online resources about child abuse that may be helpful to the physician:

- Recognition and management
  - Visual Diagnosis of Child Abuse (available through http://www.aap.org)
  - Tennyson Center for Children (http://www.childabuse.org)
  - Child Abuse Evaluation and Treatment for Medical Providers (http://www.ChildAbuseMD.com)
  - MedlinePlus: Child Sexual Abuse (http://www.nlm.nih.gov/medlineplus/childsexualabuse.html)
  - Child Welfare Information Gateway (http://www.childwelfare.gov)
- Crisis Counseling
  - Childhelp USA (http://childhelpusa.org)
- State Statutes
  - Child Welfare Information Gateway (http://www.childwelfare.gov/systemwide/laws_policies/search/index.cfm)
- Protocols and Forms
  - California Governor's Office of Emergency Services, OES 900 Forms (http://www.oes.ca.gov/Operational/OeSHome.nsf/CJPD_Documents?OpenForm)

In this age of seemingly increased interpersonal youth violence being reported in the media, some consideration must be given to this topic. The literature shows an increased number of youth perpetrators. Therefore, assessment techniques must also adapt to this type of evaluation. The following are statistics from the 2006 Juvenile Offenders and Victims National Report (Snyder and Sickmund 2006):

- More than one-third of juvenile victims of violent crime known to law enforcement are under age 12.
- In 2002, 1 in 12 murders in the USA involved a juvenile offender. One-third of murders committed by a juvenile offender also involved an adult offender.
- On a typical day in 2004, about 7000 persons younger than 18 were inmates in adult jails. Nearly 9 in 10 were being held as adults.
- Law enforcement agencies made 2.2 million arrests of persons under age 18 in 2003. The most serious charge in almost half of all juvenile arrests in 2003 was larceny-theft, simple assault, a drug abuse violation, disorderly conduct, or a liquor law violation.

The following are recommended priorities from the Commission for the Prevention of Youth Violence (2000):

1. Support the development of healthy families.
2. Promote healthy communities.
3. Enhance services for early identification and intervention for children, youth, and families at risk for or involved in violence.
4. Increase access to health-care and mental health-care services.
5. Reduce access to and risk from firearms for children and youth.
6. Reduce exposure to media violence.
7. Ensure national support and advocacy for solutions to violence through research, public policy, legislation, and funding.

Hopefully, with care for this patient's physical and emotional well-being and careful implementation of the above guidelines, this patient will not become one of the above statistics and will not suffer the same fate of the perpetrator in the first case vignette.

7.3 Review Questions

1. Which of the following physical findings would raise the highest degree of suspicion for child abuse or neglect?
   a. Retinal hemorrhages in a 2-year-old with head trauma, reportedly from falling out of bed
   b. Second-degree burns in the shape of a splash mark on the leg of a 9-year-old, who reportedly spilled hot soup on himself
   c. A fractured forearm in a 10-year-old girl who fell on outstretched hands while playing on the jungle gym

d. "Picky eating" and being below the fifth percentile for height and weight in a 3-year-old child
e. A child-sized bite mark on the shoulder of a 5-year-old who claims that the wound was inflicted by the 4-year-old sister during an episode of roughhousing

2. Which of the following are recommended strategies to prevent violent behavior in youth:

a. Increase access to health-care and mental health-care services
b. Reduce access to and risk from firearms for children and youth
c. Reduce exposure to media violence
d. All of the above
e. A and C only

Appendix A: Tables with Possible Answers to the Vignettes

Case Vignette 7.1: Mary Infante
Learning issue Table 7.1

Facts	Hypotheses	Information needed	Learning issues
Mary Infante is a 32-year-old married woman who is 20 weeks pregnant and having severe cramps	Medical conditions	Comprehensive medical evaluation and physical exam	Previous laboratory tests were unremarkable
She has had two miscarriages in the past and is worried that she may be having another one	Substance use disorder	Laboratory tests	Upon physical examination, she has bruising on the upper arms and abdomen. The bruising is not noticeable on any areas of the body that are not covered by her clothing
Ms. Infante is a secretary at a local law firm. The husband was recently laid off from his position with a construction company and is seeking another company to work with	Domestic violence	Obstetric evaluation and prenatal care	Physicians should be aware of physical and emotional signs of violence and abuse
He has apparently been let go from a number of positions since they have been together	Abuse	A psychiatric consultation was requested by her physician to evaluate the situation (information required from patient and husband)	It is the responsibility of the physician to make the initial identification and refer the patient to an appropriate specialist

Facts	Hypotheses	Information needed	Learning issues
They have been married for approximately 3 years, but have not yet been able to have children	The perpetrator of abuse may have experienced abuse while growing up	–	What are certain risk factors and signs/symptoms of domestic violence the physician needs to consider?
After further inquiry, Ms. Infante reveals that the miscarriages might have been caused by spousal abuse while she was pregnant	Psychosocial stressors	–	Physicians need to be aware of other specific types of abuse among adults, including rape or sexual assault and elder abuse
You then call the husband into the room to discuss your concerns with the current pregnancy	–	–	You interview the patent and husband, together and independently
Overall, he is cordial and polite, and seems attentive to his wife	–	–	You note that he often interrupts his wife while she is attempting to answer a question
–	–	–	You politely ask him to refrain from answering questions directed at his wife, but he continues to answer questions for her
–	–	–	What are common physician-related reasons why the victim may not disclose information to the physician?
–	–	–	You decide to admit Ms. Infante for threatened miscarriage and for further assessment and intervention for domestic violence
–	–	–	A safety plan is formulated
–	–	–	A social worker assists Ms. Infante with a referral to legal counsel

Case Vignette 7.2: Nicholas Head

Learning issue Table 7.2

Facts	Hypotheses	Information needed	Learning issues
An ER physician refers Nicholas Head, a 5-year-old boy, to your care	Medical and/or psychiatric illness of patient and parents	Comprehensive behavioral health and medical evaluation	Upon examination, it was clear that Nick's left eye and the left side of his face are badly bruised
Nick's mother reported that he was running in the house and tripped and hit his head on the corner of their dining room table	Parent substance abuse	Physical and neurological examination	During the complete full-body examination, the ER doctor saw bruising on his upper arm and tenderness when palpating his abdomen
His mother reports that he was roughhousing on the playground with some other children at school and fell off the jungle gym	Abuse, neglect, and maltreatment	Baseline labs	The ER physician orders several X-rays, one of which indicates that Nick has a healing fractured humerus
Nick's mother is a single parent and is forced to work two jobs to make ends meet	If abuse is determined, what is the likelihood that Nick experienced repeated episodes of abuse?	Diagnostic imaging (X-ray)	You are called to join the case to perform a psychiatric consultation
While she is at her second job in the evenings, the mother's live-in boyfriend watches over her son	Domestic violence	Psychiatric consultation	The clinician must be aware of identified risk factors for child abuse and neglect (categorized by caregiver, child, and family/environmental factors)
When asked about his home Nick says that he usually goes to school without eating breakfast and is lucky to have dinner at night	Psychosocial stressors	–	You and a hospital social worker interview Nick (independently) and his mother
On certain mornings, Nick will see his mother getting ready for work and inquire if any breakfast is available	Single parent		Because of the apparent neglect and abuse, the assessment of Nick requires both medical and legal investigation, what is the physician's role in the investigation; notification of CPS?

Facts	Hypotheses	Information needed	Learning issues
When probed on what her response is, he looks down at the floor and states that occasionally his mother will become angry at his question so recently he has stopped asking	Limited parent resources and supports	–	What are the general guidelines for interviewing and examining youth who are possible victims of abuse or neglect?
Nick won't answer any more questions about the boyfriend	Nick is experiencing behavioral (aggression) and school problems	–	Nick is admitted to the hospital pediatrics unit for his safety and to ensure that his immediate medical needs are addressed first, such as possible malnutrition
The social worker calls CPS and expects a return call			You hope that Nick, a victim of violence, does not go on to become a perpetrator of violence as an older child or adolescent. You wonder what interventions could prevent such an outcome
You learn from an "auntie" that Nick has been more disruptive and aggressive in school	–	–	–

Appendix B: Answers to Review Questions

Answers

1. a
2. d

References

American College of Emergency Physicians. (1995). Emergency medicine and domestic violence. *Annals of Emergency Medicine, 25,* 442–443.

American Psychiatric Association (2013). *Diagnostic and statistical manual of mental disorders* (5th ed.). Arlington: American Psychiatric Association.

Black, M.C., Basile, K.C., Breiding, M.J., Smith, S.G., Walters, M.L., Merrick, M.T., Chen, J., & Stevens, M.R. (2011). *The national intimate partner and sexual violence survey (NISVS): 2010 summary report*. Atlanta: National Center for Injury Prevention and Control, Centers for Disease Control and Prevention.
Brown, J. (1997). Working toward freedom from violence: The process of change in battered women. *Violence Against Women, 3,* 5–26.
Centers for Disease Control and Prevention. Injury Prevention & Control: Division of Violence Prevention (2014). http://www.cdc.gov/ViolencePrevention/childmaltreatment/index.html. Accessed 22 Feb 2015.
Commission for the Prevention of Youth Violence. (2000) Youth and violence: Medicine, nursing, and public health: Connecting the dots to prevent violence. http://stopdomesticabuse.org/wp-content/uploads/2012/02/Youth-and-Violence-Medicine-Nursing-and-Public-Health2.pdf. Accessed 2 Feb 2015.
Director, T. D., & Linden, J. A. (2004). Domestic violence: An approach to identification and intervention. *Emergency Medical Clinical of North America, 22,* 1117–1132.
Englander, E. (2007). *Understanding violence*. Mahwah: Lawrence Erlbaum Associates.
Feldhaus, K., Kozoi-McLain, J., Amsbury, H., Norton, I., Lowenstein, S., Abbott, J. (1997). Accuracy of 3 brief screening questions for detecting partner violence in the emergency department. *Journal of the American Medical Association, 277,* 1357–1361.
Laraque, D, DeMattia, A, Low, C. (2006). Forensic child abuse evaluation: A review. *The Mount Sinai Journal of Medicine, 73,* 1138–1147.
Lau, A. S., Valeri, S.M., McCarty, C.A., Weisz, J. R. (2006). Abuse parents' reports of child behavior problems: Relationship to observed parent-child interactions. *Child Abuse & Neglect, 30,* 639–655.
Liebschutz, J., & Paranjape, A. (2003). How can a clinician identify violence in a woman's life? In: Liebschutz, J., Frayne, S., Saxe, G., (Eds.), *Violence against women: a physician's guide to identification and management* (pp. 39–69). Philadelphia: American College of Physicians—American Society of Internal Medicine.
McDonald, K.C. (2007). Child abuse: Approach and Management. *American Family Physician, 75*(2), 221–228.
McLeer, S.V., & Anwar, R.A. (1987). The role of the emergency physician in the prevention of domestic violence. *Annals of Emergency Medicine, 16,* 1155–1161.
Muehlbauer, M. 1., & Crane, P. A. (2006). Elder abuse and neglect. *Journal of Psychosocial Nursing and Mental Health Services, 44,* 43–48.
Snyder, H., & Sickmund, M. (2006). Office of justice programs: Juvenile offenders and victims national report. http://www.ojjdp.gov/ojstatbb/nr2006/. Accessed 11 Feb 2015.
Williams, B. (2005). Domestic violence: medicine's response. *Tennessee Medicine, 98,* 477–480.

Chapter 8
The Physician–Patient Relationship

Negar Nicole Jacobs* and Lisa A. Calvo

The relationship between a physician and his or her patient is the heart of medicine. The quality of this relationship is strongly influenced by the doctor's communication skills and in turn has an impact on patient outcomes as well as on physician factors such as satisfaction, burnout, and malpractice risk. This chapter will also explore the importance of patient education and ensuring understanding and will review how to deliver bad news using the SPIKES model. Vignettes that highlight these learning issues will be presented, and readers will be invited to apply the problem-based approach to work through these vignettes.

8.1 Objectives

At the end of this chapter, the reader will be able to:

1. Describe the factors that can affect physician–patient alliance
2. Discuss how the physician–patient relationship can affect outcomes
3. List questions to elicit a patient's explanatory model of illness and apply the LEARN model to guide culturally sensitive encounters
4. Explain the importance of patient education and ensuring understanding
5. Outline how to deliver bad news to patients utilizing the SPIKES model

---

"The good physician treats the disease; the great physician treats the patient who has the disease."—Osler
*Co-first editor of the book

N. N. Jacobs (✉) · L. A. Calvo
Psychiatry and Behavioral Sciences, University of Nevada School of Medicine,
5190 Neil Road, Suite 216, Reno, NV 89502, USA
e-mail: nnjacobs@medicine.nevada.edu

L. A. Calvo
Psychiatry and Behavioral Sciences, University of Nevada School of Medicine,
1155 Mill Street, W-11, Reno, NV 89502, USA

D. Alicata et al. (eds.), *Problem-based Behavioral Science and Psychiatry*,
DOI 10.1007/978-3-319-23669-8_8

Vignette 8.1.1 Mr. Taylor

In the 23rd hour of your call, you are paged to see a patient presenting to the Emergency Department (ED) with complaints of shortness of breath. You feel exhausted and burned out. After glancing at Mr. Taylor's chart, you notice that he has a history of congestive heart failure, with multiple ED visits for exacerbations of his heart failure, which require hospitalization. You joke that Mr. Taylor is a "frequent flyer" and you are irritated that you will now have to stay past your shift to complete his admission. You also notice that he has multiple "no-shows" on his follow-up clinic appointments. You are frustrated about why the patient cannot seem to take care of himself, take his medications, and make it to his clinic appointments. At each hospital visit, due to worsening of his symptoms, Mr. Taylor's medication doses have been increased, and new medications have been added. His current list includes eight medications for his heart failure.

Entering the room and standing before the patient, you state "Good afternoon, Mr. Taylor. You're back again! Need some more medications?" You pull over a stool and sit down, pulling out your prescription pad.

Mr. Taylor begins his story, explaining that since his last hospital discharge 2 months prior, he has had progression of his shortness of breath. You interrupt with many questions about his shortness of breath but he talks over you, saying "This feels just like one of my heart failure flare-ups, doc." After completing the history and performing a physical exam, you order lab tests and imaging that confirm your suspicion: exacerbation of congestive heart failure.

In reviewing the causes of heart failure exacerbations as well as this patient's history of frequent ED visits and missing clinic appointments, you are concerned about possible noncompliance with his medications.

STOP

Please proceed with the problem-based approach using the worksheet located in the appendix of Chap. 1!

Table 8.1.1

FACTS	HYPOTHESES	INFORMATION NEEDED	LEARNING ISSUES

8.2 Learning Issues

The most successful physician–patient relationships are those in which the physician applies good communication skills to gather information from the patient, explain the diagnosis, provide patient education, and jointly work with the patient to develop a treatment plan. A strong physician–patient relationship has been associated with both patient outcomes and satisfaction as well as physician outcomes such as reduction of malpractice risk, improvement of satisfaction, and prevention of burnout.

8.3 Factors Affecting Alliance

Physician Communication Skills A physician's ability to communicate with patients is an essential skill in the practice of medicine. A report from the American Academy on Physician and Patient after the second Kalamazoo conference in 2002 defined communication skills as "specific tasks and observable behaviors that include interviewing to obtain a medical history, explaining a diagnosis and prognosis, giving therapeutic instructions and information needed for informed consent to undergo diagnostic and therapeutic procedures, and providing counseling to motivate participation in therapy or to relieve symptoms" (Duffy et al. 2004). Physician communication skills such as active listening are some of the qualities most highly desired by patients (Matthews et al. 1987).

Poor communication between doctors and patients can be problematic for a number of reasons, including the impediment of information gathering and patient disclosure as well as increases in patient complaints and risk of malpractice. In one study of physician communication, doctors were found to interrupt patients on average of just 18 s into the patient's description of their presenting complaints, and these interruptions were noted to stop patients from disclosing their other important complaints (Beckman and Frankel 1984). Richards (1990) noted that the majority of patient complaints against doctors were centered around the doctors' poor communication skills rather than their clinical competence. Furthermore, it has been found that the majority of malpractice claims against doctors arise from errors in communication (Shapiro et al. 1989).

Physician Interpersonal Skills The interpersonal skills of a physician are another critical element affecting the physician–patient relationship. Duffy and colleagues separated physician's communication skills and interpersonal skills (Duffy et al. 2004). The authors highlighted how communication skills alone are insufficient, and how process-oriented interpersonal skills focus on how the physician's communication skills affect the patient. The report listed important elements of interpersonal skills such as "(1) respect, including treating others as one would want to be treated; (2) paying attention to the patient with open verbal, nonverbal, and intuitive communication channels; (3) being personally present in the moment with the patient, mindful of the importance of the relationship; and (4) having a caring intent, not only to relieve suffering but also to be curious and interested in the patient's ideas, values and concerns" (Duffy et al. 2004, p. 498).

Empathy Empathy is a key element of a quality doctor–patient relationship and has been shown to have a positive impact on patient psychosocial outcomes (such as quality of life and moods) as well as medical outcomes (Neumann et al. 2011). Mercer and Reynolds (2002) define physician empathy as the physician's ability to "(a) understand the patient's situation, perspective and feelings (and their attached meanings), (b) communicate that understanding and check its accuracy and (c) act on that understanding with the patient in a helpful (therapeutic) way." When patients feel understood by their physicians, they may feel more comfortable in disclosing their symptoms and concerns, which could lead to more accuracy in the physician's diagnosis and more patient-centered treatment plans (Neumann et al. 2011).

There may be therapeutic effects of the physician's empathy and support that translate into improvements in the patient's psychosocial well-being. One study of psychiatrists treating patients with depression found that providers who created a strong therapeutic bond with their patients had better treatment outcomes in treating the patients with placebo than did providers who used active medication but did not have a bond with the patient (McKay et al. 2006).

Empathy has been found to be associated with improvements in patient outcomes. One study showed that patient's perceptions of physician empathy predicted the severity and duration of the common cold and were associated with immune system changes in Interleukin-8 and neutrophil counts (Rakel et al. 2011). Another study examined the role of empathy in outcomes with diabetic patients and found that patients of physicians with high empathy scores were significantly more likely to have better control of their hemoglobin A1c as well as better low density lipoprotein-cholesterol (LDL-C) control than patients of physicians with lower empathy scores (Hojat et al. 2011). Furthermore, another study noted that diabetic patients of physicians who were high in empathy had significantly lower rates of acute metabolic complications than patients of physicians rated low in empathy (DelCanale et al. 2012). Clearly, empathy is an important component of the doctor–patient relationship, and the data indicate that it plays an important role in patient outcomes.

8.4 Effects of the Doctor–Patient Relationship on Patient Outcomes

Disease Outcome The quality of the doctor–patient relationship, including the effectiveness of clinical communication as well as the use of patient-centered decision-making and paying attention to contextual factors in patient care, is associated with positive health outcomes for patients. One of the first studies aimed at systematically assessing the effects of clinical communication on health outcome was conducted by Egbert and his colleagues over 50 years ago (Egbert et al. 1964).

The study compared postsurgical outcomes for patients randomly assigned to a control group versus those in a "specialty care" group, who received a preoperative description of the surgery as well as information about the nature of the pain they would experience after the surgery and how they could relieve it through relaxation procedures that they were instructed on. The researchers found that compared to the control group, those in the specialty care group asked for less analgesic medication, were noted to be in better emotional and physical condition, and were discharged 2–3 days earlier from the hospital.

Balint wrote about the importance of the doctor–patient relationship, noting that what was important was "not only the medicine…or the pills, but the way the doctor gave them to the patient—in fact the whole atmosphere in which the drug was given" (Balint 1955). In a review of 25 randomized controlled trials examining the connection between the doctor–patient relationship and patient outcomes, Di Blasi and colleagues found that interpersonal context provided by the physician as the medical treatment is delivered to the patient is critically important. Specifically, they concluded that "physicians who adopt a warm, friendly, and reassuring manner are more effective than those who keep consultations formal and do not offer reassurance" (DiBlasi et al. 2001).

Patient Satisfaction It is well known that patient satisfaction is positively affected by the quality of the doctor–patient relationship. Specifically, what has been found to drive patient satisfaction is a doctor's instrumental as well as affective behavior (Roter et al. 1987; Roter 1989). A doctor's instrumental behavior involves factors such as giving information. Additionally, greater length of interview as well as increased amount of time spent discussing preventative care has been found to be positively correlated with patient satisfaction (Smith et al. 1981). A physician's affective behavior includes aspects like showing interest, nonverbal attention such as eye contact, making encouraging statements, and providing verbal empathy (Bensing 1991). Bensing (1991) concluded that these affective behaviors were the most important factor in driving patient satisfaction. Furthermore, it has been found that doctors who provide patient-centered care, characterized by allowing patients to express all of their reasons for the medical visit, have patients who feel better understood and fall in the highest quartile of patient satisfaction (Henbest and Stewart 1990).

Vignette 8.1.2 Continuation

After learning about how physician skills affect the doctor–patient relationship and how the alliance affects patient outcomes, you decide to apply your best skills to ask Mr. Taylor about what is going on with his health and medication usage. You ask Mr. Taylor about his compliance with his complex (and costly) medication regimen, he admits to missing "a few doses."

"I used to forget to take them when I was at work, but since losing my job last month, I have been trying to space them out so that I won't run out, since

I know I won't be able to pay for them again. That means I usually take them every other day, if I remember."

You empathize with his situation and respond, "I am sorry to hear that you've come in to some difficulties with your finances and are having a hard time affording your medications. We'll talk more about that. But first, I also notice that you haven't made it to many of your clinic appointments. What can you tell me about that?"

Mr. Taylor: "Easy, doc. My co-pay on my insurance was too high that I didn't go to the clinic when I felt well. And now that I've lost my job, I've lost my insurance and there's no way I could afford to pay for an entire clinic visit. That's why I usually end up here. They have to see me, whether I can pay my bill or not."

Please proceed with the problem-based approach using the worksheet located in the appendix of Chap. 1!

Table 8.1.2

FACTS	HYPOTHESES	INFORMATION NEEDED	LEARNING ISSUES

Adherence It is possible that quality physician–patient communication enhances patient outcomes via improved adherence to treatment regimens. Patient adherence has been defined as "the degree to which patients follow the recommendations of their health care professionals" (Haskard Zolnierek and DiMatteo 2009). Effective communication between providers and patients helps patients to better understand their disease as well as the risks and benefits of treatment (Osterberg and Blaschke 2005). Through communication, patients feel encouraged and supported by the physician, and they are offered help in developing the resources needed to adhere (DiMatteo and DiNicola 1982).

A recent meta-analysis of 106 correlational studies and 21 experimental interventions analyzing the effects of adherence on medical outcomes found a strong, positive correlation between physician communication and patient adherence (Haskard Zolnierek and DiMatteo 2009). Specifically, the researchers found that there was a 19 % higher risk of nonadherence in patients of physicians who communicated poorly compared to patients of physicians who communicated well (Haskard

Zolnierek and DiMatteo 2009). The standardized relative risk of nonadherence was 1.47 times greater in patients whose physician was a poor communicator, and the standardized odds ratio of a patient adhering was 2.16 times better if the patient's physician was a good communicator (Haskard Zolnierek and DiMatteo 2009). The meta-analysis also found that training doctors in communication skills led to significant improvements in patient adherence rates, with patients of physicians who had received communication training having a 1.62 times higher odds ratio of adhering to treatment compared to patients of physicians who had received no training (Haskard Zolnierek and DiMatteo 2009). Please refer to Chap. 10 for more information on adherence.

Contextualized Care Outcomes One potential benefit of effective doctor–patient communication is the way in which such communication can facilitate inquiry regarding elements of a patient's environment or behavior that can affect health outcomes. For example, contextual patient factors such as their access to care, caretaker responsibilities, social support, skills and abilities, and economic situation can affect the extent to which they adhere to treatment recommendations and in turn can affect their health outcomes (Weiner et al. 2010). Physician's awareness of these factors is essential to the provision of individualized treatment planning. The term, contextual errors, refers to medical errors that result from a physician's failure to identify and incorporate essential patient contextual factors into the treatment plan (Weiner 2004, 2008).

In order to minimize contextual errors, Weiner and colleagues have suggested the use of patient-centered decision-making (PCDM; Weiner et al. 2013). PCDM has been defined as "the process of identifying clinically relevant, patient-specific circumstances and behaviors to formulate a contextually appropriate care plan" (Weiner et al. 2013). Use of PCDM has been associated with significant improvements in patient health outcomes. In a study comparing encounters in which PCDM occurred versus those in which there was inattention to patient contextual factors, it was found that heath outcomes improved in 71 % of clinical encounters involving use of PCDM compared with health improvements in only 46 % of the encounters that did not involve attention to contextual factors (Weiner et al. 2013).

Vignette 8.1.3 Continuation

Mr. Taylor is admitted to the hospital, treated with oral and IV medications, and his symptoms improve. You take time to thoroughly review his home medication list. You notice several name-brand medications that cost several times what effective generic or alternative but equally effective medications may cost. You discuss with the pharmacist regarding safe, effective options and formulate a new and simplified medication list, which includes only four medications.

On his second hospital day, Mr. Taylor reports his symptoms have resolved and that he feels ready for discharge. Prior to discharge, you print the new list of his medications and enter his room to review them.

"Mr. Taylor, I understand that you are having financial difficulties currently that were, at least in part, preventing you from being able to afford your heart medications and clinic appointments. We have made an appointment for you to see me at the local outreach clinic that takes patients on a sliding scale, meaning that they will work with you to come up with a realistic and manageable charge and payment plan. In addition, I spent some time simplifying your medication list to include only four very important medications that you must take every day, all of which are $4 a month, or less. Is that something that you can afford?"

Mr. Taylor: "It is, doc. I really appreciate you taking the time to make these changes and set up the appointment. Nobody has ever worked so hard to understand my situation and help me so much."

Please proceed with the problem-based approach using the worksheet located in the appendix of Chap. 1!

Table 8.1.3

FACTS	HYPOTHESES	INFORMATION NEEDED	LEARNING ISSUES

Effects of the Physician–Patient Relationship on the Physician Physicians are highly susceptible to professional burnout, defined as a psychological response consisting of emotional exhaustion, depersonalization (treating patients as if they were objects), and reduced perceptions of personal exhaustion (Maslach 1982). Burnout can affect the doctor–patient relationship, communication between doctors and patients, and the quality of care that providers provide to patients. Physician burnout and professional satisfaction have been linked with the likelihood of making medical errors (West et al. 2006) and with patient adherence and satisfaction (DiMatteo et al. 1993). Interventions aimed at reducing burnout, such as teaching physicians mindfulness skills, have been shown to improve burnout as well as mood in physicians (Krasner et al. 2009). Such interventions to reduce burnout have also been found to reduce medical errors and malpractice risk (Jones et al. 1988). Physicians wishing to have an effective relationship with their patients, prevent burnout, and reduce malpractice risk and may benefit by practicing mindfulness and stress management skills.

Vignette 8.1.4 Conclusion

Mr. Taylor showed up for his clinic appointment two weeks later and was feeling well. He brought his new medications with him, indicating that he was able to pick them up and stated that he was taking them as prescribed. He was very encouraged by how well he was doing and expressed appreciation that you had taken the time to work within his financial limitations to treat him as a person, not just a disease. You feel honored to have been able to help Mr. Taylor and watch his health improve. You notice that being empathic with your patients and spending a few extra minutes with them to understand their situation makes you feel more satisfied with your work and less burned out.

Vignette 8.2.1 Mrs. Gebreselassie

As a busy colorectal surgeon, you are seeing Mrs. Gebreselassie, a 73-year-old Eritrean woman in clinic following biopsy of a suspicious colonic mass showing adenocarcinoma. She is strictly Arabic speaking and knows very little English. She is accompanied by her granddaughter. Through an interpreter, the patient reports that she is feeling well and has no complaints. You realize that the patient is not aware of her diagnosis, but you are not sure how to deliver the bad news. Frustrated by the delay in having to use an interpreter, you glance at your watch and realize that you're already 30 min behind.

Please proceed with the problem-based approach using the worksheet located in the appendix of Chap. 1!

Table 8.2.1

FACTS	HYPOTHESES	INFORMATION NEEDED	LEARNING ISSUES

8.5 Learning Issues

Communication and Culture Every culture, including that of the provider as well as that of the patient, has social and cultural norms that prescribe the doctor–patient relationship. Culture and ethnicity have been cited as barriers in establishing a doctor–patient relationship that is effective and satisfying (Schouten and Meeuwesen 2006). Specifically, a review of cultural differences in medical communication in the literature cited the following key predictors of culture-related communication problems: "(1) cultural differences in explanatory models of health and illness, (2) differences in cultural values, (3) cultural differences in patients' preferences for doctor–patient relationships, (4) racism/perceptual biases, and (5) linguistic barriers" (Schouten and Meeuwesen 2006).

Communication between the provider and the patient is highly influenced by cultural factors. Language barriers are an obvious problem, and it is recommended that professional translators be used in favor of asking family members or friends to interpret what the patient says, as this can be highly problematic and inappropriate. Nonverbal communication can also be problematic when working with patients from different cultural backgrounds. While physicians in Western medical schools are taught about the importance of such factors as eye contact and touch, patients from differing cultural backgrounds may be offended by eye contact or touch.

Although it is impossible for providers to learn everything about every culture in order to provide culturally competent care to their patients, they should have some background on general norms and value systems of the cultures of the patients they treat, and they should be careful to regard this information as hypotheses to be tested with the individual patient that stands before them instead of assuming that the stereotypes hold true for every patient from that culture. Modern medical education is steering away from trying to create culturally competent providers, as the term "cultural competence" implies that there is a finite body of cultural knowledge that can be mastered by physicians. The current goal is to create physicians who demonstrate cultural sensitivity as well as cultural humility, in that they appreciate cultural differences, have an awareness of their limitations when working with culturally different patients, demonstrate understanding of health-care disparities and injustices, examine their own belief systems, and are careful to assess each patient's beliefs individually (Lindsey et al. 2003). Please refer to Chap. 14 for more information about culture and health care.

Delivering Bad News Using the SPIKES Model Breaking bad news to patients and their families about diagnosis or prognosis is one of the most difficult tasks of a physician. In the recent past, delivering news about a cancer diagnosis was considered inhumane and detrimental to patients (Baile et al. 2000). However, with modern medicine's value for patient autonomy it has become increasingly important for physicians to hone the complex skill of being able to deliver bad news to patients. Baile and colleagues (Baile et al. 2000) note that the way in which bad news is delivered can affect the patient's understanding of the information, their satisfaction with medical care, how hopeful they are about their condition, and how well they adjust psychologically. Given the complexity yet importance of the task of delivering unfavorable information about a patient's future, Baile and colleagues developed a six-step protocol to guide physicians in the delivery of bad news and named it the SPIKES model (Baile et al. 2000). The model will be described and applied to the case below.

Step 1: S—SETTING Up the Interview Physicians should mentally rehearse what they will say and anticipate the emotional reactions the patient may have. They should also set up the physical environment such that the patient will have privacy, time constraints and interruptions will be managed, and will be accompanied by significant others if they so wish. Physicians should sit down and make a connection with the patient as they deliver the bad news.

> After realizing that Mrs. Gebreselassie was not aware of her diagnosis, you changed her appointment time from the standard 15 min to a full 45 min consultation, in an effort to avoid feeling rushed to move on to the next patient. You worked with the trained interpreter to help you manage the language barrier. You take a few minutes to think about how you will approach the conversation, recalling the SPIKES model. As you enter the room, you see that Mrs. Gebreselassie and her granddaughter, who accompanied her to clinic, are seated. They appear anxious. You greet them by name, shaking each of their hands, and sit down.

Step 2: P—Assessing the Patient's PERCEPTION Before discussing the news, physicians should first use open-ended questions to assess what the patient already knows and understands about their medical situation. This information can be used to correct misinformation and then to tailor the delivery of the bad news.

> You begin: "Thank you both for coming to clinic today. If you can, please explain to me your understanding of where we are at in the process of evaluating these GI symptoms you have been having."
> Mrs. Gebreselassie (through an interpreter): "Well, I know that there are a few things that can cause the symptoms, but the biggest thing that we (looks over at her granddaughter) are concerned about is cancer."

Step 3: I—Obtaining the Patient's INVITATION Because patients vary in the extent of information they desire, physicians should ask patients how much they want to know and how they would like that information to be delivered.

> "It is true that cancer could potentially cause some of the symptoms you are having. The biopsy that you had done last week has given us some more information. Would you like to discuss those results now?" you ask.

Step 4: K—Giving KNOWLEDGE and Information to the Patient To lessen the shock that bad news may engender, physicians should first warn the patient that they have bad news. Information should then be delivered in a manner that is understandable to the patient, and physicians should check in with patients to ensure their understanding.

> Mrs. Gebreselassie and her granddaughter both nod.
> You explain, "As you mentioned, cancer is one of the different possibilities to explain your symptoms. Unfortunately, I'm afraid I have some bad news to deliver. The biopsy you had last week of your colonic mass showed adenocarcinoma." You allow a moment of silence

before proceeding. "The good news is that your CT scan showed that there was no metastatic spread."
A few more moments of silence pass, allowing Mrs. Gebreselassie time to process what you had said. You respectfully ask, "I am sorry to have this news for you. Do you feel as though you understand what I have said?"

Step 5: E—Addressing the Patient's EMOTIONS with Empathic Responses Physicians should observe, name, and identify reasons for any emotions the patient expresses. Physicians can then communicate this understanding to the patient and validate their feelings. If patients are silent, physicians should ask exploratory questions to identify how the patient is experiencing the bad news.

Mrs. Gebreselassie: "I knew this was possible, but hearing that I now carry this diagnosis is really scary. I'm very anxious about how this disease is going to impact my lifestyle and my family."
You reply, "It is very understandable that you feel scared and anxious facing this new diagnosis and how it may affect your quality of life and the lives of those around you."

Step 6: S—STRATEGY and SUMMARY If patients are ready to discuss treatment planning, physicians should present treatment options and inquire about what patients want, in an effort to achieve shared decision-making.

Mrs. Gebreselassie: "What is the next step, doctor?" We want to get as much information on treatments ASAP."
"Since there is no evidence of metastatic spread, surgery may be curative. The first step would be a partial colectomy with temporary colostomy, followed ultimately by surgery to reverse the colostomy. Please know that I am here to address any questions or concerns that come up along the way."

Despite your careful delivery of bad news, Mrs. Gebreselassie declines surgery without offering an explanation. You are frustrated and explain that you have nothing else to offer at this point. You quickly excuse yourself from the exam room.

Vignette 8.2.2 Continuation
A few weeks later, you receive a call from the oncologist who initially sent the patient on referral to your office. She reports to you that the patient was recently admitted for a bowel obstruction, believed to be due to the tumor. A CT scan showed a new lesion in the liver, concerning for metastatic disease. She wanted to discuss with you the details regarding the refusal of surgery.

Please proceed with the problem-based approach using the worksheet located in the appendix of Chap. 1!

Table 8.2.2

FACTS	HYPOTHESES	INFORMATION NEEDED	LEARNING ISSUES

Culturally Sensitive Communication In line with the goal of creating culturally sensitive and humble physicians, the current literature emphasizes the importance of eliciting the patient's explanatory model of their illness, or their understanding about the cause, severity, and progress of the disease, how the illness affects their life, and their expectations about treatment (Eisenberg 1977). Kleinman et al.(1978) developed a number of questions for eliciting a patient's explanatory model, such as "What do you think has caused your problem?, What do you think your illness does to you?, What chief problems has it caused?, How does it work?, How bad do you think your illness is?, What kind of treatment would you like to have?, What are the most important results you hope to get from your treatment?" In order to minimize communication problems and maximize chances of effective treatment, providers should always ask these questions of their patients, especially when they are working with patients from a different cultural background than themselves.

The LEARN model has been proposed to teach physicians the necessary tasks in a culturally sensitive encounter and should be used by physicians in order to maximize treatment outcomes. LEARN is an acronym for the following steps: (1) LISTEN to the patient's explanatory model; (2) EXPLAIN your views and treatment recommendations as the physician, building upon the patient's explanation; (3) ACKNOWLEDGE the similarities and differences in the patient's and provider's ideas; (4) RECOMMEND a course of action, giving options whenever possible; and (5) NEGOTIATE a plan, building upon the patient's ideas and promoting active participation of the patient in the development of the plan (Berlin and Fowkes 1983).

Patient Education and Ensuring Understanding Another important patient–physician communication skill is the ability to explain and ensure that the patient has understanding of their disease and the treatment plan, which can have a direct effect on patient outcome. One of the ways in which clinical outcomes are measured is the hospital readmission rate following discharge, which is also increasingly being tied to provider compensation. A recent study found that up to one third of readmissions related to adverse drug events were due to medication noncompliance (McDonnell and Jacobs 2002). Taking the time to apply the skills of communication outlined in this chapter to explain to patients their medications, for example, has been shown to improve clinical outcome for patients due to increase in compliance

(Dunbar-Jacob 2000). When working toward the goal of providing patient education and ensuring understanding, maintaining a focus on patient-centered care is paramount. A model that has been used by many physicians and health-care teams is the "teach back" method, in which patients are asked to restate in their own words their disease and/or diagnosis and the treatment plan. This method allows for identification of misunderstanding, reinforcement of accurate information and has also been shown to increase compliance as part of patient-centered care (Tarn et al. 2006). Providing a written copy of the overall treatment plan, written at a level the patient can understand, can also be helpful.

Vignette 8.2.3 Continuation

You have a hard time initially recalling the encounter and pull up your documentation from the first clinic visit. Your note is brief, indicating only that the patient refused surgery but does not explain why. The oncologist asked if you had addressed this refusal, knowing that the patient refused potentially curative treatment. You admit that you did not have this conversation with the patient. The oncologist reports, "I asked Mrs. Gebreselassie to explain her reason for refusing the surgery. She explained that she was concerned about being unclean and being unable to partake in Islamic prayer. However, I reiterated the fact that it would be temporary, and we spent time reviewing options for colostomy care and discussing the Islamic community consensus on colostomies and prayer. She was very receptive to receiving treatment once we discussed her reasons for refusal." You realize that you have made a medical error, and you worry about being sued. You wonder whether you should apologize to the patient.

Please proceed with the problem-based approach using the worksheet located in the appendix of Chap. 1!

Table 8.2.3

FACTS	HYPOTHESES	INFORMATION NEEDED	LEARNING ISSUES

Apology Since the extent of medical error was documented in the Institute of Medicine's 1999 report, *To Err is Human* (Kohn et al. 1999), the idea that physicians should make full disclosure of the error to patients has been advocated. One way of addressing the medical error is to offer an apology along with the disclosure. Such disclosure and apology can enhance patient safety and quality of care as well as fulfill ethical commitments around honesty to patients. Apology can be beneficial to patients in that it can make them feel cared for by the physician, help them to regain their sense of self-respect and dignity, make them feel validated, and help to restore their power (Lazare 2006). Apology is also important because it can facilitate communication between the patient and the provider and can strengthen relationships (Lazare 2006). For physicians, apology can heal through diminishing their sense of guilt, shame, and fear of retaliation (Lazare 2006). In addition, apology has also been known to reduce malpractice claims against physicians (Gertner 2005).

Despite the benefits of apology, some physicians are reluctant to offer patients an apology due to fear of losing their jobs or their license. In fact, many attorneys advise their physician clients to avoid apologies in fear that it might be an admission of guilt. However, more than half of US states have adopted "I'm sorry" laws, which render inadmissible for proving liability the comments that physicians make to patients after a medical error (Bender 2007). Other states do not allow physicians to admit fault, but do allow them to express gestures such as caring, regret, and consolation following a medical error.

In spite of the imperative for physicians to offer apologies to patient and the documented benefits of doing so, apology as a clinical skill is not often discussed or taught in medical education. Lazare (2006) offered a framework to use and analyze apologies. He defined apology as "an acknowledgement of responsibility for an offense coupled with an expression of remorse" (Lazare 2006, p. 1401) and divided it into four components: (1) acknowledgement of the offense, including details of the offense and validation that the behavior was not acceptable; (2) explanation for committing the offense, including reasons for what happened or an explanation that the reasons are not clear; (3) expression of remorse, shame, humility, and a commitment to not repeat the offense; and (4) reparation, ranging from such behaviors as early rescheduling of the next appointment to a financial settlement. Lazare (2006) noted that apologies often fail when one of the four components is missing, or when apologies are fraudulent, insincere, or disingenuousness.

Malpractice Risk An additional benefit of quality doctor–patient communication is reduced threat of litigation against the physician. The literature on medical malpractice clearly points to communication between physicians and patients as well as their families as one of the most important factors in the decision to consult an attorney in order to file a malpractice suit against the physician (Killila 1990). Retrospective correlational studies show that physicians who demonstrated more negative communication behaviors were more likely to have been sued for malpractice than those who exhibited more positive doctor–patient relations (Levinson et al. 1997). A randomized experimental design showed empirical evidence for a direct, causal effect of positive communication in the doctor–patient relationship in decreasing malpractice claim intentions toward the physician and the hospital in the event of an adverse medical outcome (Moore et al. 2000). Furthermore, a review of plaintiff depositions in cases involving medical malpractice revealed the following themes when patients were asked about why they were suing: experiencing abandonment, feeling devalued, thinking that information was delivered poorly, and believing that the physician failed to understand the patient and/or their family (Beckman et al. 1994). Thus, strong relationships between patients and providers, including strong communication, are important not only for patient medical outcomes but also for providers.

Vignette 8.2.4 Conclusion
The oncologist tells you that she will no longer refer patients to your practice. You are informed a week later by your office manager that the patient and family are considering legal action against you for poor communication resulting in a negative outcome. You find yourself wishing you had used the LEARN model earlier in the encounter to understand the patient's explanatory model of illness and reasons for declining surgery. This would have helped you to understand that she was declining surgery for religious reasons and could have helped you to talk with her further about surgery or at least suggest alternatives that would not interfere with her religious values. Ensuring clear doctor–patient communication and using cultural sensitivity during the encounter could have prevented the spread of her disease and also could have prevented you from being sued. Next time you will be sure to remember.

8.6 Conclusions

As Osler stated, great physicians treat not only disease but patients who have the disease, and this holistic treatment occurs in the context of a strong doctor–patient relationship. The doctor–patient relationship is significantly affected by the physician's communication and interpersonal skills as well as by cultural factors. The quality of the doctor–patient relationship, in turn, affects not only patient factors such as disease outcome, adherence, and satisfaction but also has effects on the physician such as lowering burnout and malpractice risk.

8.7 Review Questions

1. Based on the chapter reading, improved physician patient communication has been shown to lead to which of the following outcomes?
   (a) Increased patient satisfaction, improved clinical outcomes, longer clinic visits.
   (b) Decreased physician burnout, increased malpractice lawsuits, improved clinical outcomes.
   (c) Improved adherence with treatment plans, longer clinic visits, increased physician burnout.
   (d) Increased patient satisfaction, improved clinical outcomes, improved adherence with treatment plans.
2. As a physician, you are seeing a patient in clinic with heart failure who has a history of dietary noncompliance. He continues to have a poor diet despite extensive education. Based on the chapter reading, what are some appropriate ways in which this may effectively be addressed?
   (a) Telling the patient, "You need to start eating better." One of these times he will listen.
   (b) Asking about contextual factors, such as "How much time do you have to prepare and eat your meals?"
   (c) Applying the SPIKES model.
   (d) Explaining to the patient that if he ends up back in the hospital again, it will negatively affect your rating as a physician.
3. How should a physician approach culturally sensitive issues with patients?
   (a) Don't ask too many questions. The patient will share what they are comfortable discussing.
   (b) Avoid working with patients with cultural beliefs they are unfamiliar with.
   (c) Approach the encounters with sensitivity and humility, with the goal of understanding the patient's perspective and the role their cultural beliefs may play in their health-care choices.
   (d) Learn everything there is to know about as many cultures as possible.

Appendix A: Tables with Possible Answers to the Vignettes

Vignette 8.1: Mark Taylor

Table 8.1.1

Facts	Hypotheses	Information needed	Learning issues
Mr. Taylor has a CHF exacerbation Mr. Taylor has frequent ER visits and clinic no-shows	Mr. Taylor is not adherent to medications, possibly due to	What does the patient understand about his disease?	What are the factors that affect the doctor–patient relationship?
	Financial difficulties	Is he taking his medications? Why not?	How does the doctor–patient relationship affect patient outcomes?
Mr. Taylor's medication doses are increased and new medications are added at each visit	Lack of understanding of disease	Why is he not making clinic appointments?	
You notice that your alliance with Mr. Taylor is poor	Improving the doctor–patient relationship may improve Mr. Taylor's outcomes		

Table 8.1.2

Facts	Hypotheses	Information needed	Learning issues
Mr. Taylor is not compliant with medications due to complexity of medication regimen and contextual factors	Medication compliance could be increased by simplifying the medication regimen and by using less costly medications	How can Mr. Taylor's medication regimen be simplified?	What can physicians do to maximize patient adherence?
		What can Mr. Taylor afford? Can any of his medications be changed to generics so they are more affordable?	How can contextual factors affect patient outcomes?
Financial constraints limit Mr. Taylor's ability to pay for medications	If nothing changes, Mr. Taylor will end up in the ED and hospital again soon		How can contextual factors be addressed?
Mr. Taylor is not following up due to lack of insurance			

Table 8.1.3

Facts	Hypotheses	Information needed	Learning issues
The medication regimen is simplified by cutting the number of medications needed to half	The strong communication skills you used with Mr. Taylor have improved your doctor–patient relationship, which will increase the likelihood of Mr. Taylor's adherence	Does Mr. Taylor take his medications and show up for clinic appointments now?	How does a strong doctor–patient relationship affect the physician?
The remaining medications are switched to generics and the new cost is US$16/month, which Mr. Taylor can afford	More affordable medications are likely to increase adherence	How does taking the time to understand Mr. Taylor's situation and help him affect your judgments about this patient, how you feel about being a doctor, and your level of burnout?	
The next appointment is set up through a local outreach clinic, which Mr. Taylor can afford	Simplified medication regimens are likely to increase adherence		
	Having a follow-up appointment made through a more affordable clinic is likely to increase adherence		

Vignette 8.2: Mrs. Gebreselassie

Table 8.2.1

Facts	Hypotheses	Information needed	Learning issues
Mrs. Gebreselassie is a 73-year-old Eritean woman who speaks Arabic only	Patient may not be aware of her diagnosis or treatment options due to language or cultural barriers	What does the patient understand about her disease?	How does the patient's cultural and religious background affect her treatment considerations?
She is not aware of her cancer diagnosis, and you need to tell her the bad news	Patient may have good reasons for declining surgery, but you have not explored them	Are language or cultural barriers interfering with the patient's understanding?	How should the provider deliver the bad news about the patient's diagnosis?
Her cancer has not spread, and it can be cured by surgery		Why has the patient declined surgery? Are there other forms of treatment she may accept?	
Patient declines surgery without offering an explanation			

Table 8.2.2

Facts	Hypotheses	Information needed	Learning issues
The cancer has spread, possibly as a result of declining surgery	You made a medical error by not exploring the patient's reasons for declining surgery and not offering other treatment options	What was Mrs. Gebreselassie's reason for declining surgery, and is she open to any treatment options?	What questions should the physician ask to understand the patient's explanatory model?
The oncologist wants to know why Mrs. Gebreselassie refused the surgery, and you are now being held accountable by a colleague	Patient may have been open to surgery or other treatment options if you had explored her explanatory model	Does Mrs. Gebreselassie understand her treatment options?	What model could the physician have used to guide a culturally sensitive encounter?
			How can the teach-back method be used to ensure patient understanding?

Table 8.2.3

Facts	Hypotheses	Information needed	Learning issues
You failed to address Mrs. Gebreselassie's refusal in your last visit, and you did not offer alternative treatment options	Mrs. Gebreselassie would have likely agreed to surgery sooner if her concerns had been addressed	Will patient and her family sue you? Will an apology affect your risk of being sued?	Should physicians apologize after a medical error?
The patient had religious reasons for not pursuing the surgery			How should physicians offer an apology?
You made a medical error and are at risk for being sued			How does the doctor–patient relationship affect malpractice risk?
You are not sure whether you should apologize for your medical error			

Appendix B: Answers to Review Questions

1. D
2. B
3. C

References

Baile, W. F., Buckman, R., Lenzi, R., Glober, G., Beale, E. A., & Kudelka, A. P. (2000). SPIKES—A six-step protocol for delivering bad news: Application to the patient with cancer. *Oncologist, 5*(4), 302–311.

Balint, M. (1955). The doctor, the patient, and his illness. *The Lancet, 265*(6866), 683–688.

Beckman, H. B., & Frankel, R. M. (1984). The effect of physician behavior on the collection of data. *Annals of Internal Medicine, 101,* 692–696.

Beckman, H. B., Markakis, K. M., Suchman, A. L., & Frankel, R. M. (1994). The doctor-patient relationship and medical malpractice: Lessons from plaintiff depositions. *Archives of Internal Medicine, 154,* 1365–1370.

Bender, F. F. (2007). "I'm sorry" laws and medical liability. *Virtual Mentor, 9,* 300–304.

Bensing, J. (1991). Doctor-patient communication and the quality of care. *Social Science & Medicine, 32*(11), 1301–1310.

Berlin, E. A., & Fowkes, W. C., Jr. (1983). A teaching framework for cross-cultural health care. *The Western Journal of Medicine, 139,* 934–938.

DelCanale, S., Louis, D. Z., Maio, V., Wang, X., Rossi, G., Hojat, M., & Gonnella, J. S. (2012). The relationship between physician empathy and disease complications: An empirical study of primary care physicians and their diabetic patients in Parma, Italy. *Academic Medicine, 87*(9), 1243–1249.

DiBlasi, Z., Harkness, E., Ernst, E., Georgiou, A., & Kleijnen, J. (2001). Influence of context effects n health outcomes: A systematic review. *The Lancet, 357,* 757–762.

DiMatteo, M. R., & DiNicola, D. (1982). *Achieving patient compliance: The psychology of the medical practitioner's role.* New York: Pergamon Press (Patient Education and Counseling, 5(1), 51–51).

Di Matteo, M.R., Sherbourne, C.D., Hays, R.D., Ordway, L., Kravitz, R.L., McGlynn, E.A., Kaplan, S., & Rogers, W.H. (1993). Physicians' characteristics influence patients' adherence to medical treatment: Results from the Medical Outcomes Study. *Health Psychology, 12*(2), 93–102.

Duffy, F. D., Gordon, G. H., Whelan, G., Cole-Kelly, K., Frankel, R., et al. (2004). Assessing competence in communication and interpersonal skills: The Kalamazoo II report. *Academic Medicine, 79,* 495–507.

Dunbar-Jacob, J., Erlen, J. A., Schlenk, E. A., Ryan, C. M., Sereika, S. M., & Doswell, W. M. (2000). Adherence in chronic disease. *Annual Review of Nursing Research, 18,* 48–90.

Egbert, L.D., Battit, G.E., Welch, C.E., & Bartlett, M.K. (1964). Reduction of postoperative pain by encouragement and instruction of patients: A study of patient-doctor rapport. *New England Journal of Medicine, 270*, 825–827.

Eisenberg, L. (1977). Disease and illness: Distinctions between professional and popular ideas of sickness. *Culture Medicine and Psychiatry, 1,* 9–23.

Gertner, R. (2005). The art of apologizing takes hold in the legal world. St. Louis Daily Record, December 22, 2005.

Haskard Zolnierek, K. B., & DiMatteo, M. R. (2009). Physician communication and patient adherence to treatment: A meta-analysis. *Medical Care, 47*(8), 826–834.

Henbest, R. J., & Stewart, M. A. (1990). Patient-centeredness in the consultation: Does it really make a difference? *Family Practice, 7,* 28–33.

Hojat, M., lLouis, D. Z., Markham, F. W., Wender, R., Rabinowitz, C., & Gonnella, J. S. (2011). Physicians' empathy and clinical outcomes for diabetic patients. *Academic Medicine, 86*(3), 359–364.
Jones, J. W., Barge, B. N., Steffy, B. D., Fay, L. M., Kunz, L. D., & Wuebker, L. J. (1988). Stress and medical malpractice: Organizational risk assessment and intervention. *Journal of Applied Psychology, 74*(4), 727–735.
Killila, B. (1990). Improving communications can prevent malpractice. *Indiana Medicine, 82,* 272–273.
Kleinman, A., Eisenberg, L., & Good, B. (1978). Culture, illness, and care: Clinical lessons from anthropologic and cross-cultural research. *Annals of Internal Medicine, 88,* 251–258.
Kohn, K. T., Corrigan, J. M., & Donaldson, M. S. (1999). *To err is human: building a safer health system*. Washington, DC: National Academy Press.
Krasner, M. S., Epstein, R. M., Beckman, H., Suchman, A. L., Chapman, B., Mooney, C. J., & Quill, T. E. (2009). Association of an educational program in mindful communication with burnout, empathy, and attitudes among primary care physicians. *Journal of the American Medical Association, 302*(12), 1284–1293.
Lazare, A. (2006). Apology in medical practice: An emerging clinical skill. *Journal of the American Medical Association, 296*(11), 1401–1404.
Levinson, W., Roter, D. L., Mullooly, J. P., Dull, V. T., & Frankel, R. M. (1997). Physician-patient communication: The relationship with malpractice claims among primary care physicians and surgeons. *Journal of the American Medical Association, 277,* 553–559.
Lindsey, R. B., Nuri-Robins, K., & Terrell, R. D. (2003). *Cultural proficiency: A manual for school leaders* (2nd ed.). Thousand Oaks: Corwin Press.
Maslach, C. (1982). *Burnout: The cost of caring*. Englewood Cliffs: Prentice Hall.
Matthews, D. A., Sledge, W. H., & Lieberman, P. B. (1987). Evaluation of intern performance by medical inpatients. *American Journal of Medicine, 35,* 936–944.
McDonnell, P. J., & Jacobs, M. R. (2002). Hospital admissions resulting from preventable adverse drug reactions. *The Annals of Pharmacotherapy, 36*(9):1331–1336.
McKay, K. M., Imel, Z. E., & Wampold, B. E. (2006). Psychiatrist effects in the psychopharmacological treatment of depression. *Journal of Affective Disorders, 92,* 287–290.
Mercer, S. W., & Reynolds, W. J. (2002). Empathy and quality of care. *British Journal of General Practice, 52,* S9–S13.
Moore, P. J., Adler, N. E., & Robertson, P. A. (2000). Medical malpractice: The effect of doctor-patient relations on medical patient perceptions and malpractice claims. *Western Journal of Medicine, 173,* 244–250.
Neumann, M., Edelhauser, F., Truschel, D., Fischer, M. R., Wirtz, M., Woopen, C., Haramati, A., & Scheffer, C. (2011). Empathy decline and its reasons: A systematic review of studies with medical students and residents. *Academic Medicine, 86*(8), 996–1009.
Osterberg, L., & Blaschke, T. (2005). Adherence to medication. *New England Journal of Medicine, 353,* 487–497.
Rakel, D., Barett, B., Zhang, Z., Hoeft, T., Chewning, B., Marchand, L., & Scheder, J. (2011). Perception of empathy in the therapeutic encounter: Effects on the common cold. *Patient Education and Counseling, 85*(3), 390–397.
Richards, T. (1990). Chasms in communication. *British Medical Journal, 301,* 1407–1408.
Roter, D. L. (1989). Which facets of communication have strong effects on outcome—a meta-analysis. In M. Stewart & D. Roter (Eds.), *Communicating with medical patients*. Newbury Park: Sage Publications.
Roter, D. L., Hall, J. A., & Katz, N. R. (1987). Relations between physicians' behaviors and analogue patients' satisfaction, recall and impressions. *Medical Care, 25,* 437–451.
Schouten, B. C., & Meeuwessen L. (2006). Cultural differences in medical communication: A review of the literature. *Patient Education and Counseling, 64,* 21–34.
Shapiro, R. S., Simpson, D. E., Lawrence, S. L., Talsky, A. M., Sobocinski, K. A., & Schiedermayer, D. L. (1989). A survey of sued and nonsued physicians and suing patients. *Archives of Internal Medicine, 149,* 2190–2196.

Smith, C. K., Polis, E., & Hadac, R. R. (1981). Characteristics of the initial medical interview associated with patient satisfaction and understanding. *Journal of Family Practice, 12,* 283–288.
Tarn, M. T., Heritage, J., Paterniti, D., Hays, R., Kravitz, R., & Wenger, N. (2006). Physician communication when prescribing new medications. *Archives of Internal Medicine, 166,* 1855–1862.
Weiner, S. J. (2004). Contextualizing medical decisions to individualize care: Lessons from the qualitative sciences. *Journal of General Internal Medicine, 19,* 281–285.
Weiner, S. J. (2008). Contextual error. In M. Kattan (Ed.), *Encyclopedia of medical decision making* (pp. 198–202). London: Sage.
Weiner, S. J., Schwartz, A., Weaver, F., Goldberg, J., Yudkowsky, R., Sharma, G., Binns-Calvey, A., Schapira, M. M., Persell, S. D., Jacobs, E., & Abrams, R. I. (2010). Contextual errors and failures in individualizing patient care: A multicenter study. *Annals of Internal Medicine, 153,* 69–75.
Weiner, S. J., Schwartz, A., Sharma, G., Binns-Calvey, A., Ashley, N., Kelly, B., Dayal, A., Patel, S., Weaver, F. M., & Harris, I. (2013). Patient-centered decision making and health care outcomes. *Annals of Internal Medicine, 158*(8), 573–579.
West, C. P., Huschka, M. M., Novotny, P. J., Sloan, J. A., Kolars, J. C., Haberman, T. M., & Shanafelt, T. D. (2006). Association of perceived medical errors with resident distress and empathy: A prospective longitudinal study. *Journal of the American Medical Association, 296*(9), 1071–1078.

Chapter 9
Clinical Ethics and Professionalism

Kimiko Ishibashi, Shaye Lewis and Timothy Baker

"As physicians, we see the worst and the best of people. At times, they are helpless and angry and make foolish decisions. But when confronting problems that are too large for them people often become heroes."
Lo

The act of confronting problems, helping patients navigate their way through health, wellness, sickness, and dying, and trying to find a balance among conflicting values, beliefs, ethics, and morals can complicate the doctor–patient relationship. The doctor–patient relationship is complex and is built upon trust. That trust can be affected by many different factors, as discussed in Chap. 8. What happens when the ethical principles that create and strengthen the doctor–patient relationship conflict? In this chapter, we address many of the ethical principles that create a foundation for this relationship. Some of the principles that we explore include beneficence, acting in a patient's best interests, and doing no harm. Balancing these principles with a patient's right to make autonomous decisions to guide their own medical care, especially when a patient refuses a recommended treatment, can be difficult. Providing a patient with the appropriate information needed to make informed decisions and give consent to treatment can strengthen the trust held in the doctor–patient relationship, but giving insufficient information or not disclosing health information can harm that relationship, while at other times nondisclosure may be beneficial. Confidentiality is essential in maintaining a trusting relationship; however, there are times when those confidences may need to be broken. Lastly, acting justly and in an unbiased way and treating patients with respect is vital. But, what happens when a physician forms assumptions or biases towards their patient? How do we as

K. Ishibashi (✉) · T. Baker
School of Medicine, University of Nevada, 6600 Marble Canyon Road, Reno, NV 89511, USA
e-mail: kishibashi@medicine.nevada.edu

T. Baker
e-mail: tkbaker@medicine.nevada.edu

S. Lewis
3374 S Canonero Way, Boise, ID 83709, USA
e-mail: sllewis@uw.edu

D. Alicata et al. (eds.), *Problem-based Behavioral Science and Psychiatry*,
DOI 10.1007/978-3-319-23669-8_9

health-care professionals continue to provide quality health care when we are struggling to find a balance between conflicting ethical principles?

9.1 Introduction to Clinical Ethics and Professionalism

Medical ethics is filled with cases that infuse your day with perplexing questions and sometimes even keep you up at night. Most physicians have experiences that, years later, still evoke crisp memories due to the ethical dilemmas faced. Ethical questions in health care are not unique to physicians, and it is clear that medical students have already begun to think about these issues even before matriculation to medical school.

> How and when do you decide that a life is no longer worth living?
> When can the decision be made that suffering or pain or lack of any further effective treatment outweighs the precious gift of a person's life?
> Why must a physician act in their patient's best interest even to their own personal or financial disadvantage?
> Why must physicians act in their patient's best interest even if those actions may put the physicians themselves at personal risk?
> Why must our patients' confidences be held in the strictest sense?

This chapter will provide a foundation with which to approach these dilemmas and will review the introductory ethical principles that will help guide your decisions. In some cases, it may seem that an obvious course of action has to be taken, but in most, there is an equally compelling argument to a different course of treatment, action, or plan. It is the goal of this chapter to give an introduction to clinical ethics and professionalism challenges that can, in turn, help patients struggling with these issues by giving a framework and guidance to students and future physicians in helping to resolve these hard cases that keep us up at night.

> As a doctor you are allowed into the most intimate and important moments in a person's life. From an infant being born, personal secrets, true fears, to a loved one's death, your patients will allow you to see them at their most vulnerable. Your words have the power to change someone's life…As a relative stranger, you automatically become a most trusted confidant just by your title. (Shah 2011)

Patients and society hold physicians to a high professional standard, one that may be too high for any human to meet. This standard though is commensurate with the level of intimacy and trust that must exist between a patient and a physician.

We hope to provide you with the tools needed to begin to think about ethically or professionally difficult situations, how to work with your patients in order to establish a strong rapport and trusting relationship so you can best help to guide them through these dilemmas, and to develop confidence in your decision-making. After all, when the philosophic debates are over, a decision must be made and a physician must act.

"In medical care, dilemmas can not merely be contemplated, they must be resolved" (Jonsen et al. 2006).

By the end of the chapter, the reader will be able to:

1. Illustrate the importance of the study of ethics to clinical practice
2. Introduce the approach of using clinical cases to evaluate, discuss, and resolve ethical dilemmas
3. Define and describe the ethical principles of respect for persons, non-maleficence, beneficence, and justice
4. Evaluate the dilemmas that may occur when these principles conflict
5. Understand the relationship between informed consent and autonomy
6. Understand the professional's contract with society
7. Describe the ethical, legal, and professional standards that give rise to patient rights to privacy and confidentiality and the duties to maintain privacy and confidentiality

Vignette 9.1.1 Presenting Situation: Ann J.
A long-time patient of yours, Ann J., is coming in today to discuss the results of her tests and scans. Ann is a 52-year old who has managed to avoid the typical health problems of her peers through a health-conscious lifestyle. She is postmenopausal and has never been on hormone replacement therapy (HRT). She is well educated, reads up on current health issues, and sees you only for recommended checkups, flu shots, and the occasional sinusitis. A couple of weeks ago, she noticed a lump in her right breast while showering.

Mammogram shows a BI-RADS 4 lesion; a subsequent core needle biopsy confirms an estrogen receptor (ER) + ductal carcinoma. Ann comes in with her husband, apprehensive that you asked for an office visit rather than just giving her results in a phone call. After you confirm that she does in fact have stage II breast cancer, you discuss treatment options and the necessary referrals, arrangements, and benefits/risks for those treatment options, including side effects and likely survival rates. You recommend that Ann be referred to a breast surgeon and an oncologist for a lumpectomy and radiation. Given that her tumor is ER positive, you tell her that the oncologist may recommend that she be on tamoxifen for several years after the tumor is removed. Ann is understandably stunned and overwhelmed by all of the information you just gave her, but you assure her that you will be there for her and are willing to try to answer any questions she might have.

Ann sees the breast surgeon and an oncologist, who recommend lumpectomy and radiation followed by at least 5 years of tamoxifen. She agrees readily to the lumpectomy; however, she has done some research of her own. She and her husband are opposed to her taking unnatural, laboratory-produced chemicals or radiation into her body; they feel that her excellent health to this point has been secondary to her avoidance of such things. She has looked into an alternative natural herbal therapy offered by a physician out of the country. Her insurance will not pay for this treatment; however, she has the means and desire to pursue this treatment on her own. She contacts you to advise you of her plans and asks if you would be willing to research the alternative treatment for her before she goes.

Please proceed with the problem-based approach using the worksheet located in the appendix of Chap. 1!

Table 9.1.1

FACTS	HYPOTHESES	INFORMATION NEEDED	LEARNING ISSUES

9.2 Learning Issues

9.2.1 Basic Medical Ethics Terms

Beneficence:

The obligation of a clinician to provide medical care that benefits their patient (Jonsen et al. 2006). Risks as well as benefits to the patient should be considered, and only treatment that provides a net benefit to the patient should be performed (Lo 2013).

Non-maleficence:

The obligation of a clinician to avoid providing medical interventions that cause harm to their patient, also referred to as "do no harm." The concepts of beneficence and non-maleficence should be considered together.

9.2.2 Medical Decision-Making

The way that treatment and medical decisions have been made has evolved throughout the past 50 years. These medical decision-making modalities often involve trying to find a balance between beneficence and non-maleficence, as well as the concepts of paternalism and autonomy. Historically paternalism was the dominant model and the way that most physicians practiced. Paternalism is best described by the old adage "the Doctor knows best." It is the concept that a person in authority knows best, and therefore their opinion can/should override the patient's preferences. In paternalism, beneficence is valued over autonomy (Jonsen et al. 2006). In the 1960s and 1970s, however, with societal and social changes, patients began to demand more involvement in the medical decision and choices that were made regarding their own bodies, and what is known as the "Age of Autonomy" began.

Autonomy, taken literally, means "self-rule" (Lo 2013). And autonomous decision-making refers to a physician's duty to respect a patient's preferences (Jonsen et al. 2006). Autonomy requires that a patient is, first, informed and, second, can then act on that information and make a decision regarding their treatment plan.

In recent years, a new model of decision-making has emerged—shared decision-making. Shared decision-making combines paternalism and autonomy and involves dialog between physician and patient to make a decision together. In an ideal situation, a clinician gives the patient all of the medical information necessary for the patient to make the best, informed decision for themselves, but, additionally, the physician gives the patient their recommendation as to the medical treatment option that they feel would be best for that patient. The clinician should take into account what they know of the patient's values when giving their professional opinion (Jonsen et al. 2006). Shared decision-making does not necessarily mean that both parties are in perfect agreement; however, it is the clinician's obligation to do their best to ensure that their patient is well informed and allow the patient to participate in and direct their treatment choices.

9.2.3 *Refusal of Medical Treatment*

Ann is an example of an informed patient who is choosing not to follow the advice of her physicians. Her physician researched treatment options and gave Ann as much information possible regarding her treatment options, as well as a recommendation for what he felt was in her best interest, but Ann exercised her right to make an autonomous decision regarding what she was willing and not willing to put into her body. A physician who respects her autonomy should respect Ann's right to make this decision. While there may be times that a physician feels that a patient is making an unwise or bad decision, adults of sound mind may exercise their right to make such a decision.

Vignette 9.1.2: Continuation

You take some time to research ER + breast cancer treatments; however, the majority of the information available with regard to the treatment Ann wishes to utilize is either provided by the treatment center or anecdotal in nature. Given the lack of peer-reviewed clinical research with regard to this treatment, you tell Ann that you are not able to recommend the alternative treatment at this time. You advise her to follow the recommendations of her oncologist and inform her that the studies you found supported the oncologist's recommendations. Ann thanks you for your time, but tells you that she will be leaving the country within the week to obtain the alternative treatment, and she will be looking for a primary care physician who is more on board with alternative medicine. A few days later, your staff notifies you that another physician has requested her records.

Nine months later, you are the attending on the hospital rotation, and Ann is admitted for altered mental status and shortness of breath (SOB). Computed tomography (CT) scans show a single large lesion in Ann's frontal lobe and multiple smaller lesions in Ann's lungs and liver; it appears that her breast cancer has metastasized. Ann is not able to make decisions for herself given her altered mental state, but her husband is desperate to have any and all treatments given to his wife. He is sure that resection of the brain lesion accompanied by radiation and treatment with tamoxifen will result in a return of her mental function and shrinkage of the lung and liver lesions with an ultimate cure. Neurosurgery is consulted; their note states that "surgical resection of Mrs. J.'s brain tumor, given the multiple metastases seen on CT, is futile and not worth the inherent risk of the procedure." Ann's husband is understandably upset and demands that you explain how any treatment that would prolong her life could be futile.

Please proceed with the problem-based approach using the worksheet located in the appendix of Chap. 1!

Table 9.1.2

FACTS	HYPOTHESES	INFORMATION NEEDED	LEARNING ISSUES

9.3 Learning Issues

9.3.1 Futility

Futility has multiple meanings; the simplest of which is termed physiologic futility, which occurs when there is a physiologic impossibility that medical intervention will be effective. Ethically more difficult definitions include probabilistic futility. This is defined as an effort to provide a benefit to a patient, which reason and experience suggest is highly likely to fail. Finally, qualitative futility is the judgment that the goal that might be attained is not worthwhile. Considerations of these latter definitions of futility may include factors such as likelihood of success, quality of life, and use of resources (Jonsen et al. 2006; Lo 2013).

In Ann's case, the neurosurgeon made a decision of probabilistic futility. In his experience, he felt that surgery was likely to fail. In his despair, Ann's husband was requesting medical treatments that to our knowledge are inconsistent with her beliefs, wishes, and goals of care. Are her previous preferences important in knowing how to proceed with her case?

9.3.2 End-of-Life Decision-Making

Ideally, a well-informed patient makes their own decisions about end-of-life care. However, many patients have not and/or would not like to think about end-of-life issues, such as resuscitation, artificial respiration, fluids and nutrition, and withdrawal of life support. It is important for a clinician to explain to their patient what these interventions will be like for them and the risks/benefits associated with each intervention. Unless a patient has indicated their wishes with regard to end-of-life care, the patient may receive interventions that they would not otherwise desire. Advanced directives are a legal means for patients to express their wishes regarding end-of-life care and can speak for a patient after the patient is no longer able to speak for themselves. Without an advance directive, a patient's loved ones are required to make those decisions for them.

Vignette 9.2.1 Presenting Situation: Mr. Jones

You are working on the hospital wards on a Saturday when a patient comes in. Mr. Jones is a 72-year-old male patient with a past medical history of chronic obstructive pulmonary disease (COPD) and no other diagnosed medical conditions, largely due to the fact that he has never really sought medical care before. He presents with chest pain and describes the pain as a feeling of heaviness and pressure that spreads across his chest and up into his jaw. The pain has been occurring with activity for several weeks but has occurred at rest for two nights this past week. He has an impressive smoking history: He has smoked >2 packs per day since he was 15 years old. He quit smoking 7 years ago when he was diagnosed with COPD but has not had any further medical treatment since that time. The electrocardiogram (EKG) is largely normal, and troponins are negative; however, the resting angina is concerning for acute coronary syndrome. You consult the cardiologist, who recommends that the patient go for angiogram and possible stenting. You happen to be outside the room when the cardiologist's staff obtains consent from your patient for the procedure, and you notice that none of the major complications of catheterization are mentioned: myocardial infarction (MI), stroke, or even death. In fact, the procedure is not explained well; it is explained to the patient as a very minor procedure that is necessary to prevent death. After the consent form is signed, you go in to talk to your patient; he is very concerned. He asks you if there is any way that medicine could be tried prior to angiogram and/or stenting. "Is this procedure really safe? Is there any chance I could die?"

Please proceed with the problem-based approach using the worksheet located in the appendix of Chap. 1!

Table 9.2.1

FACTS	HYPOTHESES	INFORMATION NEEDED	LEARNING ISSUES

9.4 Learning Issues

Informed Consent "The willing acceptance of a medical intervention by a patient after adequate disclosure by the physician of the nature of the intervention with its risks and benefits and of the alternatives with their risks and benefits" (Jonsen et al. 2006).

Informed consent does not consist of simply getting a signature on a piece of paper authorizing consent for a procedure. Rather, informed consent is a process; one in which the treating physician presents the relevant facts and information regarding a recommended treatment or procedure to a competent patient so that the patient can make a voluntary choice to accept or refuse treatment. In this process, the physician explains the recommended procedure along with the risks, benefits, and alternatives that accompany the procedure, thus allowing the patient's decision to be an informed one. The patient then shows that they have an understanding of the information presented, assesses the treatment choices, and expresses a preference for one of the options proposed by the physician, either giving informed consent or refusal.

The notion of informed consent originates from the legal and ethical right the patient has to direct what happens to their body and from the ethical duty of the physician to involve the patient in their health care. This can be seen in early court cases dating back to the early 1900s.

"Every human being of adult years and sound mind has a right to determine what shall be done with his own body; and a surgeon who performs an operation without his patient's consent commits an assault for which he is liable in damages" (Schloendorff v. Society of New York Hospitals 1914).

Legal Versus Ethical Requirements for Informed Consent
The legal intention of informed consent documentation is to protect patients from unwanted medical procedures or treatments. The ethical intention of obtaining informed consent is to enable the patient to define their own treatment goals and to protect the patient's autonomy (Hall et al. 2012).

Required Components to Informed Consent

It is difficult to find any single measure of what is required in a conversation obtaining informed consent; however, most agree on the following five basic elements that should be included in the discussion: diagnosis, treatment, risks, and benefits of the treatment; alternative treatments with their risks and benefits; as well as the risks and benefits and expected outcome for a patient if they were to opt for no treatment at all.

Standards for Obtaining Informed Consent

Legal standards for obtaining informed consent and how much information needs to be disclosed in order to inform a patient varies from state to state, and every clinician should be aware of the required components specific to where they work. However, there are some general standards that all physicians should be aware of. In years past, most states used the *reasonable physician standard:* What would a reasonable and prudent physician tell a patient (regarding a specific treatment or procedure)? Today most state laws have changed their requirements to the *reasonable patient standard:* What information would a reasonable patient need to know to make a rational decision? Taking these standards one step further is the *subjective standard or individual preference standard.* This would involve a patient being informed on the basis of his individual attitudes/beliefs/culture/lifestyle/goals of care. The information provided is specifically tailored to a particular patient's need for information and understanding. This standard requires that the physician get to know their patient reasonably well enough to know some of their preferences, beliefs, values, and goals. For example, while a 0.001 % change of numbness and decreased mobility of the patient's pinky finger following a procedure may not be a risk factor that would be important to mention to most patients, if the patient is a world famous concert pianist, using the subjective standard, it may be a risk that needs to be discussed. While the reasonable patient standard may be legally and ethically sufficient, the subjective standard is ethically ideal.

Vignette 9.2.2: Continuation

Mr. Jones obtains an angiogram that shows too many stenosed regions to reasonably place any stents. A quintuple bypass is performed the next day, your day off, and when you come back, Mr. Jones is in the intensive care unit (ICU) recovering from his open-heart surgery. Over the next several weeks, due to his underlying COPD, Mr. Jones is having a difficult time coming off the ventilator, and, out of necessity, has been sedated. All attempts at weaning him off the ventilator have been unsuccessful. Mr. Jones will need a tracheostomy; however, Mr. Jones is unable to consent to any further procedures.

Please proceed with the problem-based approach using the worksheet located in the appendix of Chap. 1!

Table 9.2.2

FACTS	HYPOTHESES	INFORMATION NEEDED	LEARNING ISSUES

9.5 Learning Issues

9.5.1 Informed Consent and Surrogate Decision-Makers

If a patient lacks decisional capacity or becomes incapacitated and is not able to speak for themselves, most states have specific laws specifying who the patient's surrogate decision-maker should be. Traditionally, a patient's spouse is the first surrogate, followed by members of the patient's family: adult children, parents, siblings, and then sometimes will continue to extended family members, friends, or neighbors. If a patient does not have available next of kin, a guardian can be appointed by the court. In all cases, the surrogate is to act in accordance with the patient's wishes, if known (Jonsen et al. 2006).

9.5.2 Informed Consent and Emergencies

As may often occur in an emergency situation, a patient may not be able to give consent, and/or there is not sufficient time to obtain informed consent. In those situations, where a delay in treatment could cause severe disability or even death, it is acceptable for clinicians to presume that the patient would give consent if given the opportunity.

Vignette 9.2.3: Conclusion

Several days after the tracheostomy, Mr. Jones is finally weaned off the ventilator. He is extremely weak and very anxious about the length of time it is taking him to recover and worries about how he will manage at home. You try to reassure him by telling him that home health nursing services can be provided to help him with any of his daily needs. He continues to have difficulty breathing and requires supplemental oxygen, but breathing treatments seem to give him some relief.

Several more weeks later, Mr. Jones is finally discharged. You arrange for home health to come and check on him daily for a few weeks. Two days following discharge, Mr. Jones presents at the emergency department (ED) with SOB and hypoxia. A complete workup reveals that Mr. Jones now has pulmonary edema secondary to congestive heart failure (CHF), and additionally continues to suffer from his preexisting COPD. Mr. Jones's son requests to speak to you privately about Mr. Jones's prognosis prior to disclosing it to his father. You have a long discussion with Mr. Jones's son about the newly diagnosed CHF and his prognosis. His son is understandably upset at this turn of events. He asks about treatment and palliation options. You describe in detail the medical management of CHF along with best and worst case prognoses. At the end of your discussion, Mr. Jones's son implores, "Please don't tell him about this. Dad was having a tough time before all of this happened, and I'm afraid that after hearing the worst case scenario you just described, he might just lose any hope for recovery and will have no motivation to take the medications you prescribe. If you tell him about his condition like you just told me, it would be the same as killing him—it would take away his will to live. Maybe you could just tell him the best case scenario and really stress to him that the medications will help?"

Please proceed with the problem-based approach using the worksheet located in the appendix of Chap. 1!

Table 9.2.3

FACTS	HYPOTHESES	INFORMATION NEEDED	LEARNING ISSUES

Ethics of Nondisclosure—Arguments Both for and Against

In their article addressing therapeutic privilege, Richard et al. (2010) argue that there is an inherent ambiguity present in full disclosure: In respecting the patient's right to the truth and autonomy by fully informing the patient, there is a risk of increasing the suffering of the patient, thus violating the principle of beneficence. They propose a process whereby the benefits of nondisclosure or the disclosure of biased, partial, or altered information is viewed in the context of minimizing the patient's suffering and/or increasing the patient's overall well-being. In the situation with Mr. Jones above, this would entail the clinician asking themselves whether nondisclosure would prevent suffering and then further exploring whether the benefits of nondisclosure outweigh the consequences of withholding the truth. The clinician also needs to consider other courses of action and whether the patient would consider the withheld and/or altered information to be important.

However, as mentioned previously, the doctor–patient relationship is one based largely on trust—the physician is "one who owes to another the duties of good faith, trust, confidence, and candor" (Edwin 2008). Ethically, Edwin argues that the patient's right to autonomy, obligations of fidelity, and the need for trust in the doctor–patient relationship override any argument for nondisclosure (Edwin 2008). Indeed, "trust is fundamental to a moral community and arguably 'the fundamental virtue at the heart of being a good doctor'" (Stirrat and Gill 2005). It is impossible for this trust to be built on untruthfulness. In addition, the argument that full disclosure might upset the patient and impair their ability to make a truly informed decision is flawed, as people will get upset throughout their lives, but this does not mean that they are unable to make a rational decision. Edwin also argues that the assumption that the patient would not like to know the full truth is paternalistic and should therefore be rejected out of hand.

In the case of Mr. Jones, as well as many other similar cases, perhaps a good option might be to ask Mr. Jones how much information he would like to have regarding his illness, prognosis, and treatment options, thus giving him the autonomy to still direct his medical care as much or as little as he desires.

Vignette 9.3.1: Mr. L.

Mr. L. is a 43-year-old male who presented to the ED due to a prolonged unrelenting cough that has recently worsened to hemoptysis. Chest X-ray (CXR) showed a cavitary lesion in the left upper lobe. A sputum sample is sent for acid-fast-bacillus (AFB) smears, and he is presumptively diagnosed with tuberculosis (TB).

Further history reveals that he is currently homeless after the factory he was working in closed just over a year ago. He has been living in various shelters and out of his car, and on occasion with various friends and acquaintances. He has been able to pick up a few odd jobs working as a handyman but has not been able to find any steady work. The ED physician discusses with Mr. L. his diagnosis of TB and the course of treatment that will be required. Mr. L. voices concern over his inability to pay for his medications, particularly because he will need to take medication for 9 months. He does not have a primary care doctor. The social worker comes to meet with him and gives him information about other shelters and places to stay, as well as sets him up with the county TB clinic where he will be able to receive his medications for directly observed therapy (DOT) daily and can follow up with the doctors there with regards to his treatment. He is given his first dose of medications and is discharged from the ED with an appointment at the clinic next morning.

After his discharge, the medical student who was observing the case asks the attending, "How contagious is TB exactly? Do other people who were in the ER tonight including health-care workers need to be concerned about possible exposure? Furthermore, do the shelters where he has been living need to be notified or the friends that he has stayed with? And if the shelters are notified will that make it more likely that he will be turned away and will not have a roof over his head?"

Please proceed with the problem-based approach using the worksheet located in the appendix of Chap. 1!

Table 9.3.1

FACTS	HYPOTHESES	INFORMATION NEEDED	LEARNING ISSUES

9.6 Learning Issues

9.6.1 Confidentiality and the Doctor–Patient Relationship

Confidentiality refers to prevention of disclosure of information that has been provided to the physician and/or other health-care entities by the patient to other parties. Confidentiality is a cornerstone to the doctor–patient relationship and is a longstanding tradition in medicine. Patients reveal sensitive personal information to their health-care providers, including information about emotional problems, drug use, and sexual activity. Keeping this information confidential not only shows respect for patients, it engenders more beneficial treatment for the patient, as the patient will be encouraged to seek medical care and to freely disclose sensitive matters related to their illness. Confidentiality can also help prevent discrimination and/or stigmatization of people with certain medical conditions. Confidentiality is not only an ethical obligation but it is also mandated by state and federal law. However, it is important to remember that while confidentiality is a vital and extremely important aspect of the doctor–patient relationship, confidentiality is not an absolute right. The discussion of confidentiality in the health-care field often focuses on what and when a physician can disclose to third parties.

9.6.2 Legal Requirements of Maintaining Confidentiality

The Health Insurance Portability and Accountability Act (HIPAA) was enacted by the US Congress in 1996. There are many different parts to this act including provisions protecting health insurance coverage for people after losing their jobs and established national standards for electronic health-care transactions. It was one of the first of its kind protecting insurance coverage for people with preexisting medical conditions. But one of the most well-known aspects of HIPAA was that it mandated that the federal government issue health privacy regulations and address the security and privacy of health data. These regulations documented in the HIPAA

Privacy Rule are what most people commonly know as Health Insurance Portability and Accountability Act (HIPAA) regulations.

The HIPAA Privacy Rule involves federal regulations that regulate the use and disclosure of protected health information by virtually all health-care service providers. It requires that health-care providers and businesses that have access to health information protect patients' health information.

In most cases, health-care providers must obtain a patient's written authorization prior to use or disclosure of their health information, with some specific exceptions. HIPAA regulations are not meant to impede access to information that is necessary to provide quality patient care. Patient authorization is not required to use or disclose information for facilitating medical treatment, obtaining payment, and improving health-care operations such as quality improvement, quality assurance, outcome assessments, or educational purposes. However, when in the above instances, any health information is disclosed, every reasonable effort needs to be made to disclose only the minimum necessary information required to achieve its purpose.

It is also important to note that the law may hold physicians liable for unwarranted disclosure of medical information. It provides for civil and criminal penalties for noncompliance.

Vignette 9.3.2: Continuation

The following morning, Mr. L. presents to the county clinic for his DOT. He continues to promptly report daily for 10 days. The last couple of days he has complained to the nurse that he has been having stomachaches, occasional vomiting, and headaches, and he has voiced concerns that these symptoms may be a side effect of his medication. He has also become increasingly upset about these daily appointments, stating that having to drive across town every single day is causing his gas usage to significantly increase. The clinic nurse addresses and treats some of the side effects that he seems to be having, and enrolls him into an incentive program that helps pay for his gas expenses if he continues to show good compliance with the program for one more week. The next day, however, he does not show up for his appointment. The nurse notifies the doctor in charge at the clinic, who decides to give him one to two more days to re-present for his medications. Three days later, he still has not returned for his treatment medication, and the hospital laboratory calls to notify the clinic that Mr. L.'s test results came back. He is not only positive for AFB but it is also a multidrug resistant strain.

The health department is notified, and they begin trying to find Mr. L. in order to resume his treatment and also to notify close contacts of their potential exposure.

Please proceed with the problem-based approach using the worksheet located in the appendix of Chap. 1!

Table 9.3.2

FACTS	HYPOTHESES	INFORMATION NEEDED	LEARNING ISSUES

9.7 Overriding Confidentiality to Protect Others

The ethical principle of non-maleficence requires both patients and physicians to avoid harming other people and prevent harm to others. A patient's right to confidentiality can at times be justifiably overridden by the right of other members of society to be protected. In general, violating a patient's confidentiality is justifiable when the potential harm to third parties is serious, the likelihood of harm occurring is high, there is no alternative for warning or protecting those at risk, breaching confidentiality will prevent harm from occurring, and harm to the patient (by breaching confidentiality) is minimized (Lo 2013).

In some situations, physicians are required by law to break confidentiality in order to report the name of a patient to appropriate public health officials. Physicians, hospitals, and laboratories are required to report specific infectious diseases to public health officials. The diseases that mandate reporting vary by state but most often include highly transmissible infectious diseases such as TB, gonorrhea, chlamydia, syphilis, HIV or AIDS, influenza, and some enteric pathogens.

Aside from infectious diseases and the threat that they pose to maintaining public health, there are several other situations in which confidentiality may be breached to protect others. These include providing warning to persons at risk of being harmed by a patient, wounds and injuries secondary to a weapon or incurred in the course of a crime, conditions that impair a patient's ability to drive, and abuse (child, elder, domestic; Jonsen et al. 2006; Lo 2013; Bourke and Wessely 2008).

Vignette 9.3.3: Conclusion
Due to the severity of having a multidrug resistant strain, the health department felt it was of utmost importance to locate Mr. L., and consequently, when notifying the most recent shelter where he has stayed, they did not keep patient identification confidential and simply notified them of possible exposure and the need to have all contacts tested. They revealed Mr. L.'s name along with a description of his appearance, as well as the nature of his disease. Unfortunately, the shelter director stated that she had not seen Mr. L. in several days,

but she had overheard him talking to some other occupants of the shelter that he was thinking about driving to another state to try to find work. The director of the health department decided that more significant actions needed to be taken in order to find Mr. L. and restart his treatments. He therefore took out an advertisement in the local newspaper as well as ran a segment on the local news showing a picture and the name of Mr. L., pleading to the general public to help locate this man, as he has a potentially deadly, very serious disease.

The next morning the clerk at a motel in a neighboring state called the health department stating that she thinks that the man who was on the news is staying at her motel. The police are called and they escort Mr. L. from his motel room to the nearest hospital. At the hospital, an angry Mr. L. insists that the doctor discharge him, and when the doctor refuses to do so stating that he will be held isolated in the hospital in order to ensure treatment, Mr. L. states that his "constitutional rights" have been violated and he plans on suing the health department for breach of confidentiality when they released his name and diagnosis over the television, as well as suing the hospital for holding him against his will.

Please proceed with the problem-based approach using the worksheet located in the appendix of Chap. 1!

Table 9.3.3

FACTS	HYPOTHESES	INFORMATION NEEDED	LEARNING ISSUES

In recent years there have been several instances involving isolation or quarantine of individuals with contagious illnesses. Specifically this was seen during the severe acute respiratory syndrome virus (SARS) epidemic, cases of multidrug resistant TB, and most recently with the Ebola virus. Additionally, this can and may be seen with the concern for the use of infectious agents for bioterrorism. The use of quarantine and isolation, particularly when done forcibly and against someone's will, can be ethically problematic. Some feel that quarantine measures are necessary in order to protect public health and are essential to prevent and control communicable disease spread; however, others believe that it violates a person's right of liberty, self-determination, and autonomy. The American Medical Association has developed a report addressing this particular issue (American Medical Association 2006). In this report they state, "The medical profession, in collaboration with public health colleagues, must take an active role in ensuring that those interventions are based on science and are applied according to certain ethical considerations." Their recommendations for the medical profession are as follows:

- “Seek an appropriate balance of public needs and individual restraints so that quarantine and isolation use the least restrictive measures available that will minimize negative effects on the community through disease control while providing protections for individual rights.”
- “Help ensure that quarantine and isolation are based upon valid science and do not arbitrarily target socioeconomic, racial, or ethnic groups.”
- “Advocate for the highest possible level of confidentiality of personal health information whenever clinical information is transmitted in the context of public health reporting.”
- “Advocate for the availability of protective and preventive measures for physicians and others caring for patients with communicable diseases.”
- “Encourage patients to voluntarily adhere to scientifically grounded quarantine and isolation measures by educating them about the nature of the threat to public health, the potential harm that it poses to the patient and others, and the personal and public benefits to be derived from quarantine or isolation. If the patient fails to comply voluntarily with such measures, the physician should support mandatory quarantine and isolation for the non-compliant patient” (American Medical Association 2006; Bostick et al. 2008).

Vignette 9.4.1 Presenting Situation: Pat

Pat is a 37-year-old patient who presents to your office to establish care with you as a new primary care physician. The patient was approximately 20 min late for the appointment today. Medical history includes obesity, high blood pressure, diabetes, and chronic lower back pain. The patient reports no new complaints and that the appointment was made primarily because of a need for a refill of pain medications. Social history reveals that the patient is a current smoker (two packs per day), drinks daily, denies illicit drug use, is unmarried, but lives with a significant other of 3 months in the motel down the street. The patient does not currently work and reports to be on disability. New primary care is being sought because “my last doctor and I didn't really see eye to eye.”

Please proceed with the problem-based approach using the worksheet located in the appendix of Chap. 1!

Table 9.4.1

FACTS	HYPOTHESES	INFORMATION NEEDED	LEARNING ISSUES

9.8 Learning Issues

9.8.1 *Drug-Seeking Behaviors and the Ethics of Continuing Their Care*

It is important (and often difficult) to assess if a patient is actually drug seeking versus seeking relief from increasing pain. Further complicating this assessment is the frequent overlap between patients with genuine pain issues *and* coexisting medication misuse. As a health-care provider, it is imperative that you do not facilitate a drug habit; however, it is equally vital that you address any legitimate pain your patient is having. Indeed, pain is a common reason for patients to seek health care. Pain agreements are a way to equitably manage pain issues with patients. Components of a pain agreement may include an agreement to avoid improper use of pain medications, agreements to only obtain pain medication from one provider (you), limitations on replacing medication, agreement for random drug screening, appointment terms, and terms for disciplinary termination of the pain contract (Fishman et al. 1999). As physicians can be liable for both facilitating a drug habit *and* for failure to address a patient's medical issues, a pain contract may help protect them legally. It is important, however, to have equal implementation and enforcement of pain contracts in order to avoid bias. Many patients with uncontrollable chronic pain could benefit from a referral to a pain management clinic, if one is available.

9.8.2 *Making Judgments*

Physicians are taught to assess patients and to use their clinical judgment. As a clinician's judgment plays a significant role in the treatment that each patient ultimately receives, clinicians should recognize that all patients deserve responsible clinical judgment. Responsible clinical judgment does not stem from visceral, knee-jerk reactions to a patient, rather it is deliberative. Clinicians must be careful to avoid "snap" judgments with regard to a patient's race, ethnicity, background, or any other irrelevant characteristic (McCullough 2013).

9.8.3 *Justice Issues that Come from Making Assumptions*

Because there are many potential justice issues that can stem from clinical assumptions, it is vital to make every attempt to take a thorough and objective clinical history and to perform an appropriate physical exam relevant to the patient's complaint. Forming a treatment plan based on subjective assumptions rather than more objective assessments can result in an inappropriate treatment plan. For example, an assumption that a patient is unreliable can deny the patient appropriate, albeit more complicated treatment. An assumption of a patient's motives (such as labeling a patient as just seeking pain medication, as in this case) can deny the patient appropriate and needed treatment. An assumption about a patient's assets and access to health-care resources may result in a patient not being notified of resources available to them. Assuming that a patient will not comprehend technical information about their condition can result in a patient making a less informed treatment decision. At its worst, an assumption about a patient can cause a clinician to dismiss vital physical complaints. Physicians should attempt to refute or confirm their assumptions, prior to any negative impact that can occur with regard to medical decision-making. Clinicians must learn to skillfully navigate the fine line between clinical judgment and assumption (Rhodes 2005).

Vignette 9.4.2: Continuation

Feeling somewhat rushed and irritated by the fact that he was late to his appointment, you hurry through your history, skipping over the nonessential parts such as the social history, and move on to do a quick physical examination. When examining his back, you see a large tattoo and shake your head. As you continue your exam, you come across another tattoo on his upper arm. This one catches your eye, and you notice it is a military rifle, standing upright on the ground next to a pair of soldier's boots and a helmet resting on the end of the rifle.

Further discussion with him reveals that he is a veteran of the US Army where he was a lieutenant. He was wounded while in Afghanistan when an improvised explosive device (IED) was detonated near the vehicle he was in. Two of the four occupants were wounded severely, while the other two died. All were under his command. He suffered a significant back injury, which has left him in chronic pain. Since leaving the army, he has been seeking a job and is excited that he has an interview the next day for a position for which he can use his degree in communications. He is somewhat nervous about the interview, though, since he travels by public transportation and does not want to be late.

STOP

Please proceed with the problem-based approach using the worksheet located in the appendix of Chap. 1!

Table 9.4.2

FACTS	HYPOTHESES	INFORMATION NEEDED	LEARNING ISSUES

9.9 Learning Issues

9.9.1 How Perception of Patients, Misconceptions, and Stereotypes Affect Patient Care

Fiester (2012) states that anywhere from 15–60% of patients are deemed "difficult" patients; patients with more complaints or conditions (this patient in this vignette had multiple) are more likely to be deemed "difficult" by their health-care provider. Interestingly, however, it is physicians who score lower on empathy scales that are more likely to perceive patients as difficult. At a glance, the patient described above could be described as difficult, especially given his less than amicable separation from his previous health-care provider and his stated purpose of seeking narcotics. How would this patient's care have been affected if the provider had not noticed his military-related tattoo and assumed the worst? Patients often complain that doctors do not listen to them; clinicians need be aware of their preconceived perceptions and utilize listening skills that will help clinical facts overcome these preconceived perceptions (Fiester 2012).

9.9.2 All-Around Review of the Doctor–Patient Relationship and Professional Interactions

The doctor–patient relationship is one of implicit trust; it is the obligation of the clinician to provide appropriate treatment in a manner that respects the patient as a person and acts in the patient's best interest, all while utilizing health-care resources appropriately. The clinician is obligated to respect a patient's autonomy, treat patients with empathy and dignity, keep confidences, avoid deceiving their patients, and to be of their word. Treatment plans should be guided by the best interests of the patient and tempered with judicious allocation of limited health-care resources (Lo 2013). Please refer to Chap. 8 for further discussion of the doctor–patient relationship.

9.10 Review Questions

1. Your patient refuses to comply with a recommended treatment regimen due to concerns of potential side effects and the belief that alternative treatment modalities will be as effective as the ones prescribed by you. In respecting their decision to pursue alternative treatments you are respecting their right to:

    a. Practice paternalistic medicine
    b. Make autonomous decisions
    c. Justice and equality in health care
    d. Confidentiality and adherence to HIPAA regulations

2. *Short answer:* The differences between legal and ethical standards for informed consent are:
3. *True or false:* Confidentiality is an important component to the doctor–patient relationship but is only an ethical obligation. It is not legally required of physicians.
4. *Short answer:* What are some things that you as a health-care provider can do in order to try to prevent yourself from falling into the trap of forming biases or opinions about a patient that could adversely affect the care that they receive from you?

Appendix A: Tables with Possible Vignette Answers

Table 9.1.1: Ann J.

Facts	Hypotheses	Information needed	Learning issues
Previously healthy, postmenopausal 52-year-old woman	Given Ann's history of living a very natural lifestyle and her belief that her health until now has been attributed to avoidance of chemicals and toxins, Ann will not agree to radiation, tamoxifen, or chemotherapy if they were indicated	What are the survival rates for stage II breast cancer with the recommended treatment?	What is beneficence and non-maleficence?
ER + stage II breast cancer	Ann will refuse most offered standard medical treatments	What are the survival rates for no treatment at all?	What is a physician's obligation to their patient regarding researching alternative treatments?
Well educated		What is the alternative treatment that she is seeking?	How can medical decisions best be made?
Recommended to have lumpectomy, radiation, and tamoxifen		How much data and research has been done on this treatment?	What are paternalism, autonomy, shared decision-making?
Opposed to taking chemicals or radiation			Is there a difference in physicians' legal vs. ethical duties towards informing their patient about treatment options?
Wants to pursue alternative treatments and has the financial means to do so			

ER estrogen receptor

Table 9.1.2

Facts	Hypotheses	Information needed	Learning issues
Ann's breast cancer has progressed and metastasized due to her lack of standard treatment	If a surgeon or physician feels that an intervention is futile, they cannot be forced to operate	What now are the survival rates for widely metastatic breast cancer?	What does futility mean, and what are the types of futility?
She lacks decisional capacity at this time	Ann will die due to the advancement of her cancer	Does Ann have an advance directive?	End-of-life decision-making
Her husband is making her medical decisions		Have she and her husband discussed whether she would now accept conventional treatments for her cancer?	Termination of treatment against the wishes of a patient or their family
He wants anything possible to be done to save her life		Would surgery be more harmful than helpful? What would radiation and tamoxifen add to her survival at this late date?	
The neurosurgeon feels surgical resection of her brain tumor would be futile			

Table 9.2.1: Mr. Jones

Facts	Hypotheses	Information needed	Learning issues
72-year-old male with COPD and angina	Mr. Jones needs an angiogram for diagnostic purposes and possibly for therapeutic reasons as well	What are all of the risks of angiogram?	What is the definition of informed consent?
Cardiology recommends angiogram, but the procedure and the risks/benefits are not explained	He does not understand fully what the procedure will entail or what the risks may be	What are the benefits of angiogram?	What are the legal and ethical requirements of obtaining informed consent?
		How much information do you need to give a patient to obtain their consent?	What are the components of informed consent?
			What are standards for obtaining informed consent?

COPD chronic obstructive pulmonary disease

Table 9.2.2

Facts	Hypotheses	Information needed	Learning issues
Mr. Jones is intubated and sedated	Someone else will need to authorize and give consent to performing a procedure upon Mr. Jones	Does Mr. Jones have any family members?	Under what conditions can surrogate decision-makers provide informed consent?
His physicians now recommend another procedure (tracheostomy)		What are the medical indications for a tracheostomy tube?	Who are the decision-makers for patients who lack decisional capacity?
		What is his prognosis given his recent major surgery as well as his underlying COPD?	What happens with informed consent in emergency situations?
		What are the risks and benefits of the procedure?	

COPD chronic obstructive pulmonary disease

Table 9.2.3

Facts	Hypotheses	Information needed	Learning issues
Mr. Jones now has pulmonary edema due to CHF	Mr. Jones's physician will need to decide how much information he needs to disclose to Mr. Jones	What is Mr. Jones's prognosis?	What are the ethics of nondisclosure?
He still suffers from baseline COPD	Mr. Jones may have a poor outcome if he learns of his grave prognosis and loses hope in recovery	What is his predicted life expectancy?	Are there cultural components to nondisclosure?
Mr. Jones's son does not think he will do well if he is made aware of the possibility of a very grim prognosis and asks you to refrain from telling his dad the worst case scenario		What is a physician's obligation to informing a patient of their current health status?	How can patient autonomy and right to direct their own medical care be balanced with appropriate care?
		Can informed consent be obtained if a patient is not truly informed about their diagnoses and prognosis?	

CHF congestive heart failure, *COPD* chronic obstructive pulmonary disease

Table 9.3.1: Mr. L.

Facts	Hypotheses	Information needed	Learning issues
43-year-old homeless male diagnosed with tuberculosis	Given his financial and social situation, compliance with a lengthy medical treatment course may be difficult, and his ability to obtain follow-up care may be concerning	How contagious is tuberculosis?	How does confidentiality affect the doctor–patient relationship?
He does not have a primary care physician		Do close contacts need to be tested or treated? Do casual contacts need to be tested or treated?	What are HIPAA laws and confidentiality requirements for health-care providers?
He is unemployed and unable to pay for his medication		What responsibility does a physician have towards protecting their patients' right to privacy and confidentiality?	
		What responsibility does a physician have towards protecting other individuals or society in general when it comes to individuals with infectious diseases?	

HIPAA Health Insurance Portability and Accountability Act

Table 9.3.2

Facts	Hypotheses	Information needed	Learning issues
Mr. L. had been compliant with his medical treatment regimen until he started to experience a number of adverse effects from his medication	The inconvenience of reporting for daily treatment and the adverse effects that the drugs are causing will likely affect Mr. L.'s continued compliance	How can a physician or government agency notify close contacts without violating confidentiality laws?	Where is the overlap between confidentiality and public health notification?
Mr. L. has multidrug resistant TB	Because he has multidrug resistant TB, the health department will want to notify any close contacts to get them tested and treated if needed	What are the "exceptions to the rule?" Are there times when it may be justified to break a patient's confidences or reveal personal health information?	Are there times when breaches in confidentiality may be justified?
Mr. L. has been lost to follow-up			
The health department has been notified			

TB tuberculosis

Table 9.3.3

Facts	Hypotheses	Information needed	Learning issues
Mr. L. has multidrug resistant tuberculosis and not only stopped taking his medication but also was lost to follow-up and moved to another state	His lack of compliance caused a significant concern for the health and welfare of the general public	Have Mr. L.'s rights been violated?	Can a public health agency act ethically while potentially violating an individual's right to autonomy and self-determination?
The health department informs the media in order to locate Mr. L.		Is it the action of the public health officials justified in order to protect the greater good?	Has there been any precedent for this type of action?
			What are the AMA recommendations regarding quarantine and isolation?

AMA American Medical Association

Table 9.4.1: Pat

Facts	Hypotheses	Information needed	Learning issues
37-year-old patient	Possible drug-seeking behavior	How long has the patient been taking pain medications?	What is a pain agreement?
Multiple medical problems	Possible addiction	Which pain medication is the patient taking?	How should physicians approach the care of patients that are concerning for misuse of medications? What ethical issues arise in the care of these patients?
Needs pain medications	Worrisome for mental health disorders	What other medications is the patient taking?	How do the assumptions made about a patient relate to issues of justice?
Previous problems with a physician	"Difficult" patient	Is the patient adherent to the overall medication regimen?	
		What is the patient's gender or ethnicity?	

Table 9.4.2

Facts	Hypotheses	Information needed	Learning issues
US Army veteran with trauma history	Previous assumptions about patient as a "drug seeker" may have been incorrect	What are his current support systems?	How is patient care affected by a physician's perception of patients, misconceptions, and stereotypes?
Back injury was combat related		Why is he not seeking care at the VA?	What influence does physician bias have on patient care decisions?
Actively seeking new employment			
College graduate			

VA Veterans Administration

Appendix B—Review Question Answers with Explanations

Review Questions

1. Your patient refuses to comply with a recommended treatment regimen due to concerns of potential side effects and the belief that alternative treatment modalities will be as effective as the ones prescribed by you. In respecting their decision to pursue alternative treatments you are respecting their right to:

   a. Practice paternalistic medicine
   b. Make autonomous decisions
   c. Justice and equality in health care
   d. Confidentiality and adherence to HIPAA regulations

Answer: B. Your patient is exercising their right to make autonomous decisions regarding their health care. Autonomous decision-making refers to a physician's duty to respect a patient's preferences.

2. *Short answer:* The differences between legal and ethical standards for informed consent are:

Answer: The law requires that patients be informed regarding their illness and recommended treatments or procedures. It in general gives physicians some guidance for minimum standards and information that needs to be provided to patients. Ethical guidelines, however, push those standards a little farther. Ethical ideals recommend that informed consent be individualized to include information that may be considered important to each particular patient based upon what the physician knows about that patient's beliefs, culture, life goals, etc.

3. *True or false:* Confidentiality is an important component to the doctor–patient relationship but is only an ethical obligation. It is not legally required of physicians.

Answer: False. Confidentiality is an essential component to the doctor–patient relationship, and while it is considered an important ethical obligation, it is also mandated by state and federal law with very specific and limited exceptions to the rule.

4. *Short answer:* What are some things that you as a health-care provider can do in order to try to prevent yourself from falling into the trap of forming biases or opinions about a patient that could adversely affect the care that they receive from you?

Answer: Make every attempt to obtain a thorough and objective clinical history. Avoid creating preconceived notions or assumptions based upon gender, race, culture, appearance, etc. Attempt to refute or confirm any assumptions that you may have made prior to any negative impact that can occur with regard to medical decision-making. Finally, be aware of personal biases and perceptions that you may hold, and utilize listening skills that will help clinical facts overcome these preconceived perceptions.

References

American Medical Association. (2006). AMA code of medical ethics, opinion 2.25—The use of quarantine and isolation as public health interventions. http://www.ama-assn.org/ama/pub/physician-resources/medical-ethics/code-medical-ethics/opinion225.page? Accessed 11 March 2015.

Bostick, N., Levine, M., & Sade, R. (2008). Ethical obligations of physicians participating in public health quarantine and isolation measures. *Public Health Reports, 123*(1), 3–8.

Bourke, J., & Wessely, S. (2008). Confidentiality. *The BMJ, 336*(7649), 888–891.

Edwin, A. (2008). Don't lie but don't tell the whole truth: The therapeutic privilege-is it ever justified? *Ghana Medical Journal, 42*(4), 156–161.

Fiester, A. (2012). The "difficult" patient reconceived: An expanded moral mandate for clinical ethics. *The American Journal of Bioethics, 12*(5), 2–7.

Fishman, S., Bandman, T., Edwards, A., & Borsook, D. (1999). The opioid contract in the management of chronic pain. *Journal of Pain and Symptom Management, 18*(1), 27–37.

Hall, D., Prochazka, A., & Fink, A. (2012). Informed consent for clinical treatment. *Canadian Medical Association Journal, 184*(5), 533–540.

Jonsen, A., Siegler, M., & Winslade, W. (2006). *Clinical ethics: A practical approach to ethical decisions in clinical medicine* (6th ed.). New York: McGraw Hill, Medical Pub. Division.

Lo, B. (2013). *Resolving ethical dilemmas: A guide for clinicians* (5th ed.). Philadelphia: Lippincott, Williams, and Wilkins.

McCullough, L. (2013). Critical appraisal of clinical judgment: An essential dimension of clinical ethics. *Journal of Medicine and Philosophy, 38*(1), 1–5.

Rhodes, R. (2005). Justice in medicine and public health. *Cambridge Quarterly of Healthcare Ethics, 14*(1), 13–26.
Richard, C., Lajeunesse, Y., & Lussier, M. (2010). Therapeutic privilege: Between the ethics of lying and the practice of truth. *Journal of Medical Ethics, 36*(6), 353–357.
Schloendorff v. Society of New York Hospitals. (1914). New York court of appeals.
Shah, A. (2011). Jason's journal—Thoughts of an ethically conflicted medical student. 2010 runner-up essay. *AMA Journal of Ethics (formerly Virtual Mentor), 13*(7), 461–465.
Stirrat, G., & Gill, R. (2005). Autonomy in medical ethics after O'Neill. *Journal of Medical Ethics, 31*(3), 127–130.

Chapter 10
Adherence in Medicine

Jared T. Ritter

After gathering an appropriate history and conducting a diagnostic clinical interview, the biopsychosocial formulation for the patient should drive the comprehensive treatment plan. Selecting the right intervention in collaboration with the patient is complex and open for modification over the treatment course. Furthermore, prescribing a treatment in psychiatry is rarely sufficient to cause a particular clinical disorder to quickly enter full remission without relapse. One of the key factors in treatment success is for patients to actually adhere to their agreed upon treatment plans.

At the end of this chapter, the reader will be able to:

1. Understand the burden of nonadherence on the health-care system and treatment
2. Recognize risk factors that decrease a patient's adherence
3. Use the biopsychosocial formulation to conceptualize nonadherence as a manageable clinical problem
4. Discuss approaches to enhance adherence in medicine

Case Vignette 10.1.1 Presenting Situation Lono

Lono is a 13-year-old Hawai'ian and Samoan male eighth grader from Oahu, Hawai'i who has come to your pediatric clinic for a school physical exam and with parental concerns that he has not been focusing well in school. The family recently relocated, so this is your first time meeting with them. Lono is polite and quiet during the first visit, but you notice that he is fidgety throughout the session and frequently plays with medical instruments hanging on the wall next to the examination table. On review of the vitals, he is found to have a height in the 90th percentile and a weight greater than the 98th percentile, which surprised you since he appeared tall for his age but not obese on gross examination.

J. T. Ritter (✉)
Florida State University College of Medicine, 1340 Ridgewood Avenue,
Holly Hill, FL 32117, USA
e-mail: jaredritter@me.com

D. Alicata et al. (eds.), *Problem-based Behavioral Science and Psychiatry*,
DOI 10.1007/978-3-319-23669-8_10

His mother, two younger cousins, and maternal grandmother accompanied him for this appointment. The family moved in with his aunt and uncle after his father had to move back to American Samoa when Lono's paternal grandparents became too ill to manage the family farm. Three of his older brothers went along to help their father leaving Lono with their mother and two younger sisters. His oldest brother is in law school and lives away from the family with roommates.

The past records reviewed indicated that the patient had a history of mild asthma that improved over the years. The family history was significant for diabetes, hypertension, nicotine use disorder, and stroke in the mother; obesity and alcohol use disorder in the father; a paternal uncle with amphetamine use disorder and legal problems; and possible attention-deficit/hyperactivity disorder (ADHD) in two other siblings. The mother smoked cigarettes throughout her pregnancy with Lono and occasionally consumed alcohol in the first trimester before finding out she was pregnant. Lono was born 2 weeks early but did not have any significant delays in development requiring clinical attention. His milestones were met on time. However, he struggled throughout school especially in reading. Among the records received, there were several ADHD questionnaires completed by the parents and teachers at 7 and 8 years of age. The results were consistent with ADHD inattentive type, but at the bottom of the parent questionnaire it was noted, "Family not interested in medication for ADHD."

Please proceed with the problem-based approach using the worksheet located in the appendix of Chap. 1!

Please fill in the facts, your hypotheses, further information needed, and learning issues for Learning Issue Table 10.1.1.

Learning Issue Table 10.1.1

FACTS	HYPOTHESES	INFORMATION NEEDED	LEARNING ISSUES

According to the Diagnostic and Statistical Manual of Mental Disorders, 5th Edition (DSM-5), Nonadherence to Medical Treatment is a category that "…can be used when the focus of clinical attention is nonadherence to an important aspect of treatment for a mental disorder or another medical condition" (APA 2013). It is a common problem, and certain demographic factors and diagnoses are associated with increased risk. An estimated $290 billion is wasted annually in the USA because of poor medication adherence (NEHI 2011). The WHO has reported that an average of 50 % of medications for chronic medical conditions are not taken as prescribed (Zullig et al. 2013). After 3 years of use, children with ADHD take their medication less than 50 % of the time (Charach 2008).

At the very first visit, skilled clinicians should already be assessing for those factors that may place the patient at risk and hence take care to mitigate the risks and promote adherence. Practice guidelines often include recommendations for addressing treatment adherence. As a complex behavioral problem, nonadherence is most frequently multifactorial in its origin and requires a personalized assessment to be fully understood.

Case Vignette 10.1.2 Continuation

A few days later, you review the results from Lono's baseline fasting labs and electrocardiogram (EKG):

Sodium: 138 mEq/l	Bicarbonate: 24 mmol/l	Cholesterol (total): 190 mg/dl
BUN: 18 mg/dl	Glucose: 115 mg/dl	LDL: 175 mg/dl
Creatinine: 0.8 mg/dl	Glycosylated Hb: 5.6 %	Triglycerides: 160 mg/dl
TSH: 1.20 μIU/mL	EKG: unremarkable	

BUN blood urea nitrogen, *LDL* low-density lipoprotein, *Hb* hemoglobin, *TSH* thyroid-stimulating hormone, *EKG* electrocardiogram

Afterwards you call the patient's mother at home and arrange for a follow-up visit.

Based upon the initial lab results and additional history about diet and exercise habits, you make recommendations about cutting back on simple carbohydrates and eating more fiber-rich alternatives. The mother tells the office staff that her son's teachers again sent her an e-mail regarding Lono's poor attention in class, trouble following directions, forgetfulness, making careless mistakes, and getting distracted easily. She thinks his troubles in school might be related to the new school because the teachers at his former school would give him a front row seat in the class, provide afterschool tutoring for reading, allow short breaks during class, and help with organizing his planner. She worries that her son was labelled as "lazy" but does not want him to be on medications that will turn him into a "zombie" or make him addicted.

You ask for Lono's mother and his current teachers to complete ADHD questionnaires and see him back in your office. Lono knows his mother is thinking about trying a medication for him to take to help him focus in school. He wants to do better in school; however, he discloses, "I saw some police come to the school last year and take away a student from the counselor's office. My friends told me they heard that she 'got off her meds' and went to the hospital because 'it made her crazy.'" He does not want to take a medication that will change who he is or that he will have to take for the rest of his life. The mother asks about natural supplements or other diet changes that could be tried. She heard about fish oil being good for the brain during a daytime television program. She observes that since the father (an avid fisherman) moved away they have been eating less fish and more packaged red meats and canned meat products because of convenience and affordability. You discuss the latest evidence and recommendations for omega-3 in treating ADHD in children and adolescents.

When reviewing the most recent ADHD questionnaire results, you point out that the scores were very similar to those completed in the past and demonstrate predominately inattentive ADHD symptoms. You discuss prescription medication treatment options and recommend that he be started on a long-acting Food and Drug Administration (FDA)-approved treatment for ADHD. You explain the common risks and benefits for both stimulant and non-stimulant treatment options. In addition to answering the family's questions about the risks of not treating, you help to dispel common myths about ADHD treatment increasing substance use disorders and explain how treatment is associated with decreased risk for ADHD patients developing legal troubles into adulthood. The family agrees to a trial of a generic long-acting stimulant and schedules a follow-up appointment in 1 month. A medication information sheet is provided to take home.

Please proceed with the problem-based approach using the worksheet located in the appendix of Chap. 1!

Please fill in the facts, your hypotheses, further information needed, and learning issues for Learning Issue Table 10.1.2.

Learning Issue Table 10.1.2

FACTS	HYPOTHESES	INFORMATION NEEDED	LEARNING ISSUES

On the surface, treatment nonadherence does not appear to be a significant problem in this case vignette. However, closer inspection reveals that there were already several years of missed treatment going back to at least age seven based upon historic records. The previous provider even documented that the family was not interested in medication treatment. It is unknown if the family's concerns were previously explored to an appropriate degree or if ample education about ADHD and its treatment were provided in a nonjudgmental and supportive manner. In this particular case, having a broad knowledge base and familiarity with literature (Bloch and Qawasmi 2011; Lichtenstein et al. 2012) related to allaying some of the family's fears proved helpful.

Treatment adherence can be understood as a dynamic process that is subject to modification across a continuum. Gearing et al. (2011) proposed six phases of adherence—treatment initiation, treatment trial, partial treatment acceptance, intermittent treatment adoption, premature discontinuation following treatment adoption, and adherent. Early intervention goes hand-in-hand with early detection. Once treatment is determined to be clinically appropriate, providers can take specific steps to increase the chances of successful treatment initiation such as demonstrated in the study of ADHD (Coletti et al. 2012). Nonetheless, over the course of treatment, there will inevitably be challenges to adherence.

Case Vignette 10.1.3 Conclusion

You see Lono every month and carefully titrate his medication to a tolerated therapeutic dose. He experiences some nausea and appetite suppression at the onset of treatment and with dose increases that last a couple of days and improves by having him eat breakfast before taking the medication. Despite having occasional days during the week when he forgets to take the medication, his grades at school improve from mostly D's to a B average by the end of the school year. His teachers continue to praise him for his progress, attentiveness to classwork, and turning in assignments more consistently and on time. Lono tells you that his mother was so proud of his progress that she finally agreed to let him play football. He plans on starting training over the summer and agrees that wearing the appropriate safety equipment will be important to decreasing injuries.

The next time you see Lono he is 14 years old and just started his second quarter of ninth grade. He is playing high school football. His grades have dropped back down to C's and two D's. When you ask about his absence from the clinic and academic decline, he explains that he stopped taking medication because he thought he "got better" and no longer needed medicine. His mother wants him to take the medication at school because this would be better supervised and more consistent since no adults are at home when Lono leaves for school in the mornings. She admits that she was reluctant to stop medication treatment, but she agreed to try off medication when extended family members found out he was taking medication and pressed to stop "Western medicine." When his mother steps out of the room, Lono discloses that he started using cannabis because his older cousin on the football team told him it helped him to focus and not be so hyper. He notices that he is more relaxed, yet his short-term memory seems worse.

You offer education on how heavy cannabis use during development has been associated with lower intelligence quotient (IQ), short-term memory loss, and brain volume loss (e.g., smaller hippocampal volume compared to non-users). Lono agrees to refrain from cannabis use and resume ADHD medication treatment. He adds that he also had an incident during preseason football practice when he sustained a hard hit and felt dazed and "saw stars" for a couple minutes. He felt dizzy when he got home from practice and took a 90-min nap. The next day he awoke in the morning with a headache. He did not tell anyone about this incident because he thought he would be cut from the team.

Your office gets a call 2 months later. The nurse updates you that the patient cancelled his future monthly appointments. You call the family back, and the mother tells you that they stopped giving the medication because her son "almost had a heart attack" when he was on a church youth trip. With further investigation, you find out that he only got 3 h of sleep because he stayed up late with friends. In the morning, he drank a proprietary caffeinated energy drink on an empty stomach and took a double dose of his regular stimulant medication to help him stay awake and pay attention better. He was taken to the emergency department (ED) by the youth pastor.

You later review the ER notes, which reveal an unremarkable cardiac work up. His urine drug screen was only positive for the prescribed medication. The final ER diagnosis was panic attack. You again call the family to help reengage them in treatment. The mother thanks you for your concern and diligent care. She informs you that they are receiving counseling support through their church, and Lono has actually been getting mostly C's and occasional B's in school. She proudly adds that his football team made it to the state championships, and his father is returning from American Samoa permanently in the summer.

This case vignette helps to illustrate that treatment adherence is indeed dynamic across time. When nonadherence is conceptualized as a clinical problem, a biopsychosocial formulation can be constructed with consideration of predisposing, precipitating, perpetuating, and positive factors that modify adherence. Once these factors are identified and understood, then specific interventions can be implemented as part of the overall comprehensive treatment plan.

Common reasons for nonadherence are shown in Table 10.1:

Please take this opportunity to construct a biopsychosocial formulation. Keep in mind potential targets for treatment and corresponding biopsychosocial treatments. Studies have been conducted to better understand strategies to increase both medication (Osterberg and Blaschke 2005) and psychosocial (Gearing et al. 2012)

Table 10.1 Risk factors for nonadherence. (Adapted from Gearing and Mian 2005)

Factors associated with decreased treatment adherence in children and adolescents		
Diagnosed with major psychiatric disorders		
Medication side effects	Lack of insight	Poor family adhesiveness
Subtherapeutic dosage of medication	Cultural beliefs	Poor family support/involvement in treatment
Oral (rather than depot) medication	Religious beliefs	Family rejection
Older (rather than newer) medications	Poor memory	Family attitude toward illness and treatment
Complicated dosing schedules	Feelings of helplessness	Family criticism/expressed emotion
Comorbid conditions (specifically, substance abuse, behaviour problems, and double depression)	Feelings of hopelessness	Less social support
Severity of symptoms (e.g., delusions, suspiciousness)	Stress (real/perceived)	Lack of appropriate follow-up
Persistence of symptoms	Low self-esteem	Missing follow-up appointments
Harder to treat symptoms		Poor therapeutic alliance with treating health-care professionals
Poorer prognosis		Limited financial resources
Genetics		Cost of treatment
		Loss or change in discharge accommodations

treatment adherence. Zullig et al. (2013) have advocated for addressing four main ingredients to improve adherence—patient knowledge, counseling and accountability, self-monitoring, and costs. Although more research is needed, both high-tech and low-tech interventions have been demonstrated to be effective in boosting adherence. For example, telephone-administered cognitive behavioral therapy (CBT) was shown to improve adherence when compared to more traditional face-to-face CBT (Mohr et al. 2012).

10.1 Additional Topics of Interest

- Role of interdisciplinary collaboration and coordination of care in promoting adherence.
- Cultural and spiritual factors that influence treatment adherence.
- Adherence in the context of working with families and systems of care.
- Impact of nonadherence across development.
- Use of technology (e.g., smartphone apps, biometric monitors, smart blister packaging, social media, etc.) in medication adherence.
- Family/social disruption and the influence on child and adolescent mental health.

10.2 Review Questions

1. About what percentage of medications that are prescribed for chronic health conditions are taken as prescribed?

    a. 25%
    b. 50%
    c. 75%
    d. 100%

2. Adherence is dynamic throughout the course of treatment.

    a. True
    b. False

3. What factor will increase adherence?

    a. Limiting patient knowledge
    b. Counseling and accountability
    c. Reduced self-monitoring
    d. High medication costs

4. Psychosocial factors influence medication treatment adherence.

    a. True
    b. False

5. Which of the following is most true when considering treatment nonadherence?

    a. Patients who do not follow treatment plans must have cluster B personality traits.
    b. Families always support the treatment plan ordered by the doctor.
    c. A healthy therapeutic alliance with healthcare providers enhances adherence.
    d. Therapy over the telephone is inferior to face-to-face therapy.

Appendix A: Tables with Possible Answers to the Vignettes

Case Vignette 10.1: Presenting Situation Lono

Learning Issue Table 10.1

Facts	Hypotheses	Information needed	Learning issues
Lono is a 13-year-old Hawai'ian and Samoan male eighth grader from Oahu, Hawai'i who has come to your pediatric clinic for a school physical exam and with parental concerns that he has not been focusing well in school	ADHD	Comprehensive psychiatric and medical evaluation	At the very first visit, clinicians should assess factors that would promote treatment adherence
Vitals—height in the 90th percentile and a weight greater than the 98th percentile	Specific learning disorder	Physical and neurological exam	How does the physician integrate previous successful treatment interventions in the current treatment plan?
Lono has a history of mild asthma that improved over the years	Medical illness	Vital signs	You consider the family's experiences and nonadherence with previous treatment and wonder if the family's concerns were explored to an appropriate degree or if ample education about ADHD and its treatment were provided in a nonjudgmental and supportive manner?
Family history was significant for diabetes, hypertension, nicotine use disorder, and stroke in the mother, obesity and alcohol use disorder in the father, a paternal uncle with amphetamine use disorder and legal problems, and possible ADHD in two other siblings	Substance use disorder	Baseline labs, EKG	Based upon the initial labs and additional history about diet and exercise habits, you make recommendations about cutting back on simple carbohydrates and eating more fiber-rich alternatives
Mother smoked cigarettes throughout her pregnancy and occasionally consumed alcohol in the first trimester before finding out she was pregnant	Head trauma, sports-related injury	Records from his PCP	How does parent education address Lono's mother's worries that her son was labelled as "lazy" and does not want him to be on medications that will turn him into a "zombie" or make him addicted

Facts	Hypotheses	Information needed	Learning issues
Lono was born 2 weeks early with no significant delays in development requiring clinical attention, his milestones were met on time, however, he struggled throughout school especially in reading	Significant family and developmental history	Records from and communication with school	You discuss the latest evidence and recommendations for omega-3 in treating ADHD in children and adolescents
Lono's mother asks about natural supplements or other diet changes that could be tried	Consider the influences of cultural values and previous treatment experiences with adherence with the current treatment plans	You review the ER notes, which reveal an unremarkable cardiac work up. Urine drug screen was only positive for the prescribed medication, and the final ER diagnosis was panic attack	You explain how treatment is associated with decreased risk for ADHD patients developing substance use disorders and legal troubles into adulthood
The next time you see Lono he is 14 years old and just started his second quarter of ninth grade	Treatment adherence can be understood as a dynamic process that is subject to modification across a continuum		You again call the family to help reengage them in treatment, and mother thanks you for your concern and diligent care
Mother admits to stopping the medication when extended family members found out he was taking medication and pressed to stop "Western medicine"	Consider resources available to the family		She informs you that they are receiving counseling support through their church
Lono discloses that he started using cannabis and sustained a head injury during a preseason football practice and did not tell anyone			
You speak to Lono's mother by phone 2 months later, she reports the medication was stopped when he was taken to the ED while at a church youth trip where he had little sleep, drank a proprietary caffeinated energy drink on an empty stomach and took a double dose of his medication			

ADHD attention-deficit/hyperactivity disorder, *EKG* electrocardiogram, *PCP* primary care physician, *ED* emergency department

Appendix B: Answers to Review Questions

Answers 1. b, 2. a, 3. b, 4. a, 5. c

References

American Psychiatric Association. (2013). *Diagnostic and statistical manual of mental disorders* (5th ed.). Washington D.C.: American Psychiatric Publishing.

Bloch, M. H., & Qawasmi, A. (2011). Omega-3 fatty acid supplementation for the treatment of children with attention-deficit/hyperactivity disorder symptomatology: Systematic review and meta-analysis. *Journal of the American Academy of Child and Adolescent Psychiatry, 50*(10), 991–1000.

Charach, A. (2008). Stimulant medication adherence-theoretical perspectives. *Child Adolescent Psychopharmacology News, 13*(1), 1–5.

Coletti, D. J., Pappadopulos, E., Katsiotas, N. J., Berest, A., Jensen, P. S., & Kafantaris, V. (2012). Parent perspectives on the decision to initiate medication treatment of attention-deficit/hyperactivity disorder. *Journal of Child Adolescent Psychopharmacology*, 22(3):226–237.

Gearing, R. E., & Mian, I. A. (2005). An approach to maximizing treatment adherence of children and adolescents with psychotic disorders and major mood disorders. *The Canadian Child Adolescent Psychiatry Review, 14*(4), 106–113.

Gearing, R. E., Townsend, L., MacKenzie, M., & Charach, A. (2011). Reconceptualizing medication adherence: Six phases of dynamic adherence. *Harvard Review of Psychiatry, 19,* 177–189.

Gearing, R. E., Schwalbe, C. S., & Short, K. D. (2012). Adolescent adherence to psychosocial treatment: Mental health clinicians' perspectives on barriers and promoters. *Psychotherapy Research, 22*(3), 317–326.

Lichtenstein, P., Halldner, L., Zetterqvist, J., Sjölander, A., Serlachius, E., Fazel, S., et al. (2012). Medication for attention deficit-hyperactivity disorder and criminality. *The New England Journal of Medicine, 367*(21), 2006–2014.

Mohr, D. C., Ho, J., Duffecy, J., Reifler, D., Sokol, L., Burns, M. N., et al. (2012). Effect of telephone-administered vs face-to-face cognitive behavioral therapy on adherence to therapy and depression outcomes among primary care patients. *JAMA: The Journal of the American Medical Association, 307*(21), 2278–2285.

NEHI. (2011). Improving patient medication adherence: A $290 billion opportunity. Retrieved from http://www.nehi.net/bendthecurve/sup/documents/Medication_Adherence_Brief.pdf. Accessed Dec 2014.

Osterberg, L., & Blaschke, T. (2005). Adherence to medication. *The New England Journal of Medicine, 353*(5), 487–497.

Zullig, L. C., Peterson, E. D., & Bosworth, H. B. (2013). Ingredients of successful interventions to improve medication adherence. *JAMA: The Journal of the American Medical Association, 310*(24), 2611–2612.

Chapter 11
Stress and Health

Lisa A. Calvo and Alex A. Morrison

In most cases stress is the root cause of death; illneses are just the wrap-up
Yordan Yordanov

Acute stress, aiding in the flight-or-fight response, is inherently beneficial to humans and aids in primitive survival techniques. However, persistent activation of the stress response—chronic stress—has many negative effects. Chronic stress, which can often go unidentified or underappreciated, can have a profound impact on the overall mental and physical health of patients. Health-care providers, regardless of their degree or level of training, can learn to effectively work with their patients to use the tools to identify stress, discuss the importance of stress management, and formulate appropriate and patient-specific stress management plans. Gaining an appreciation of the harmful effects of stress, and ensuring that your patient understands and appreciates these effects as well, have been shown to lead to improvements in specific diseases that are particularly affected by stress, as well as improvements in overall quality of life.

At the end of this chapter, the reader will be able to:

1. Describe the physiology of the stress response
2. Explain the effects, both harmful and helpful, of acute and chronic stress and give examples of each
3. Recognize patients at risk and identify validated screening tools for stress
4. Demonstrate ways to increase patient appreciation of the importance of stress on their health
5. List proven stress management techniques and develop a treatment plan appropriate for a particular patient

A. A. Morrison (✉) · L. A. Calvo
University of Nevada School of Medicine, 1531 Delucchi Ln, Unit F, Reno, NV 89502, USA
e-mail: amorrison@medicine.nevada.edu

D. Alicata et al. (eds.), *Problem-based Behavioral Science and Psychiatry*,
DOI 10.1007/978-3-319-23669-8_11

Vignette 11.1: Mrs. Spears

As a third-year medical student rotating in the gastroenterology clinic, you review the chart on the next patient of the day: Mrs. Spears, a 32-year-old woman with a history of severe Crohn's Disease, with multiple flares and complications who is being seen on follow up 2 weeks after a recent hospitalization for a flare. Your preceptor asks you if there is an association between stress level and severity of symptoms (Buckley et al. 2014) and asks you to discuss stress with the patient. Upon entering the room, you see a thin woman dressed in a business suit, sitting on the exam table looking anxious but otherwise comfortable. On discussing her symptoms, Mrs. Spears reports that she is eating well and having normal bowel movements, however she is still having ongoing moderate abdominal pain that gets slightly worse after meals. She also claims that her morning 6-mile runs aggravate her pain and make it hard to "start the day on a good note." She expresses frustration with being hospitalized "it seems like every month!" despite her compliance with the medications and recommended diet. You ask her if she thinks that stress may be playing a role. She responds, "Why are you asking me about stress? Do you think my disease is just in my head and that I'm bringing this upon myself?"

Please proceed with the problem-based approach using the worksheet located in the appendix of Chap. 1!

FACTS	HYPOTHESES	INFORMATION NEEDED	LEARNING ISSUES

You respond, "Not at all. The reason I am asking is because stress levels have been shown aggravate inflammatory bowel diseases, including Crohn's Disease. If there is stress in your life that you think may be playing a role and we can address it, we may be able to better manage your symptoms and avoid hospitalizations."

Upon hearing your explanation, the patient relaxes a bit.

Mrs. Spears: "Being in the hospital makes me fall behind at work and miss activities like my little sister's plays, which makes me sometimes get upset and tearful, but I had never perceived it as stress. Now that you mention it, when I am upset about missing work, my abdominal pain and bleeding do seem to get worse. Even coming to this appointment today forced me to miss an important meeting. But I don't feel stressed. And how big of a deal can stress be, anyway?"

Please proceed with the problem-based approach using the worksheet located in the appendix of Chap. 1!

FACTS	HYPOTHESES	INFORMATION NEEDED	LEARNING ISSUES

11.1 Learning Issues

11.1.1 Physiology of Stress

In medicine, the term *stress* refers to the "pattern of responses a person makes to stimulus events that disturb his or her equilibrium and tax or exceed his or her ability to cope" (DSM-5, APA 2013, p. 829). It is a person's response to a *stressor,* which is "any emotional, physical, social, economic, or other factor that disrupts the normal physiological, cognitive, emotional, or behavioral balance of an individual" (DSM-5, APA 2013, p. 829). Stress is often a complex interplay between fear, an emotional response to a real or perceived imminent threat, and anxiety, an anticipation of a future threat (DSM-5, APA 2013). When an individual begins to perceive stress, several adaptive mechanisms in the body, also known as the *stress response,* are activated to maintain a state of equilibrium in the organism. This equilibrium, or homeostasis, is essential for survival and, if disrupted too severely or too often, can lead to profound health effects. Though many homeostatic processes in the body are altered during the stress response, two of the most marked are the autonomic nervous system (ANS) and the hypothalamic–pituitary–adrenal axis (HPA).

The ANS is made up of two opposing divisions: the sympathetic, or "fight-or-flight" division, and the parasympathetic, or "rest-and-digest" division. When physical or mental stress excites the nervous system, the sympathetic division overrides the parasympathetic division to provide extra activation of the body, making it stronger, faster, and more alert. Fear tends to provide surges of autonomic arousal necessary for fight or flight, and anxiety prepares the body with muscle tension and vigilance for future danger. Blood flow increases to muscles and decreases to organs such as the gastrointestinal (GI) tract and kidneys, muscle strength increases, blood glucose concentration rises via increased glycolysis, mental activity is heightened, and heart rate, respiratory rate, and arterial pressure all increase. Even if the initial stressor is psychological (running late for a meeting) instead of physical (running away from a tiger), the response remains the same.

Just as physical and mental stress cause an immediate response by the nervous system, it activates just as marked of a reaction by the HPA axis of the endocrine system. Almost immediately, the anterior pituitary gland releases increased amounts of adrenocorticotropic hormone (ACTH), followed within minutes by adrenocortical secretion of cortisol. Increased levels of cortisol have a wide range of effects on the body. Glucocorticoids such as cortisol cause rapid mobilization of amino acids and fat from their cellular stores, making them available for energy. Cortisol also acts as an anti-inflammatory, helping to dampen the body's inflammatory response to injury or allergic reactions (Silverman and Sternberg 2012). Overall, it helps to relieve the damaging effects of the stress response so the body can more quickly return to homeostasis.

11.1.2 When Stress Is Good (Acute) and When It Can Go Bad (Chronic)

It is clear that the stress response is a highly complex and adaptive way for the body to survive and thrive under conditions of emotional or physical pressure. The acute stress response gives individuals energy and resources to persist through demanding situations. However, this *acute* response is meant to be transient. When stress is ongoing, chronic activation of the body's sympathetic nervous system and high levels of circulating cortisol can take its toll. Though cortisol is a potent anti-inflammatory, it also decreases immunity and causes patients to be more prone to infection (Silverman and Sternberg 2012). Excess glucocorticoids from chronic stress can also impair the body's ability to respond to insulin, leading to increased glucose and fat in the blood stream, both which increase a person's risk for Type 2 diabetes and heart disease. In addition, it acts on the hypothalamus to inhibit release of reproductive hormones luteinizing hormone (LH) and follicle-stimulating hormone (FSH), leading to reduced fertility (Gore et al. 2006). Acute stress is essential for activating the sympathetic nervous system to increase blood pressure and heart rate and divert blood flow from the stomach and kidneys to the brain and muscles, but over time, stress-induced chronic arterial constriction can lead to atherosclerosis or myocardial ischemia (Lazzarino et al. 2013). Disorders that are associated with chronic stress and HPA dysfunction range everywhere from gastrointestinal (irritable bowel syndrome; IBS, esophageal reflux, Crohn's), to respiratory (asthma), to dermatologic (eczema, acne), and, of course, psychiatric (substance abuse, anxiety disorders; Silverman and Sternberg 2012).

Vignette 11.1.3: Continuation

After completing the Perceived Stress Scale (Cohen et al. 1988), Mrs. Spears scores a 23. You review her score with her, which indicates a higher than normal level of stress.

Mrs. Spears: "Wow, I didn't realize that I was under so much stress. What can I do to decrease my stress level? I'll do anything that is going to keep me out of the hospital!"

Please proceed with the problem-based approach using the worksheet located in the appendix of Chap. 1!

FACTS	HYPOTHESES	INFORMATION NEEDED	LEARNING ISSUES

After discussing options for stress management techniques, Mrs. Spears decides on a regimen of meditation and slightly less high-impact forms of exercise, such as Pilates and yoga at the studio near her condo. She is optimistic about adding stress management techniques to her treatment regimen for her Crohn's Disease.

Upon seeing you a month later in clinic for a follow-up appointment, she reported that she is still eating well, having normal bowel movements and has noticed an improvement in her abdominal pain. She adds "what's more, I haven't had to miss any time with my family to go the Emergency Department for pain and bleeding since my last appointment!"

Vignette 11.2: Tristan

Tristan, one of your regular patients in your primary care clinic, is a 20-year-old college student who comes to your office with a complaint of worsening asthma symptoms. He says that in the past 6 weeks his asthma has gotten considerably worse, to the point now where he is using his inhaler almost twice as often as previously despite compliance with his full treatment regimen.

STOP

Please proceed with the problem-based approach using the worksheet located in the appendix of Chap. 1!

FACTS	HYPOTHESES	INFORMATION NEEDED	LEARNING ISSUES

Noticing that Tristan appears anxious, you ask him how things have been going in his life for the past 6 weeks. He says that he recently broke up with his girlfriend of 8 months and got a new job as a kids' soccer coach to supplement the money he gets from his soccer scholarship. He also recently moved out of his parents' house for the first time, which is another reason he needs the extra money. You ask him if he feels like he has been under an increased amount of stress than usual, to which he replies, "I guess a little bit, but isn't some stress a good thing?"

STOP

Please proceed with the problem-based approach using the worksheet located in the appendix of Chap. 1!

FACTS	HYPOTHESES	INFORMATION NEEDED	LEARNING ISSUES

You suggest to Tristan that chronic stress can worsen his asthma symptoms, even during times when he does not feel acutely stressed. Tristan thinks about it more and says "Compared to the people around me, I don't think I'm stressed at all. Any stress I might have is nothing compared to my dad's, and his blood pressure is through the roof and he seems to have aged twenty years since starting his new job six months ago. Could stress be doing that, too?"

STOP — Please proceed with the problem-based approach using the worksheet located in the appendix of Chap. 1!

FACTS	HYPOTHESES	INFORMATION NEEDED	LEARNING ISSUES

11.2 Learning Issues

11.2.1 How a Clinician Can Help

Who Is at Risk No age group, gender, socioeconomic group, or culture is immune to illness. In the same way, stress can be found in people of all different ages, lifestyles, and backgrounds. There have been several studies looking at groups who are at higher risk for reporting significant stress. Traditionally, higher-risk groups include female workers who balance professional and family demands, workers who report a low degree of job control, higher educated workers (especially those overqualified for their jobs), shift workers, and those with long commutes (Marinaccio et al. 2013). Screening is typically focused on recent or current stressors. However, research has shown that significant stress experienced as a child can disrupt some aspects of pivotal brain development, leading to a lower threshold for stress management as an adult (National Scientific Council on the Developing Child 2005). Therefore, asking about overall childhood experiences may be useful.

A myriad of stressful life events can both directly and indirectly contribute to illness. In addition, each person responds differently to life stressors, depending on factors such as previous coping skills and cultural background (Taylor et al. 2007). Since these life events may not always come up spontaneously during history-taking, it is important to ask detailed questions about social and developmental histories to get an estimate of the amount of stress the patient may be under. A few of the top stressors that are often linked to future illness include death of a spouse or close family member, divorce, personal injury or illness, illness in a family member, marriage, pregnancy, retirement, change in financial state, or being fired from work (Holmes and Rahe 1967). If any of these risk factors may appear during history-taking, it may be helpful to use screening tools to better identify the magnitude of the patients' stress levels so you can help them implement changes to minimize the toll that their stress may have on their health.

Despite the known risk factors for increased stress and its associated affect on health, it is important to note that what matters most is not the stressors themselves but rather the patient's perceived level of stress. For example, an event that may not traditionally be recognized as a significant stressor may in fact be causing a high level of stress in an individual patient. Therefore, if a patient reports increased stress, it is important to address it and discuss management tools (Posen 2013).

How to Screen The ability to identify and treat stress is an essential skill for providers, regardless of their specialty. Although patients are more likely to see their physician for stress or stress-related symptoms rather than a mental health professional, physicians rarely address stress (Beth Israel Deaconess Medical Center 2012). For initial stress screening, there are several validated tools which have been shown to correlate with pathological stress effects and higher risk of stress-related illness. These include the Holmes-Rahe Stress Inventory (Holmes and Rahe 1967), the Perceived Stress Scale (Cohen et al. 1988), and the Life Experiences Survey (Sarason et al. 1978), all of which have shown an association with adverse health outcomes ranging from increased health resources utilization to poorer control of diabetes (Al Kalaldeh and Abu Shosha 2012). Regardless of the tool used, the goal is to aid in recognition of an individual's stress for the overall purpose of addressing any increased level of stress that may be negatively impacting their health. Scores on the assessment tools may help a provider identify patients who may not otherwise mention specific stressful life events but who are in fact struggling with significant psychological stress. Asking a patient to complete one of the assessment tools may highlight an additional treatment option for stress-related illnesses and to improve overall health. Once stress has been identified, either by history alone or by using screening tools such as those referenced above, it is important to partner with your patient to formulate a treatment plan for management of their stress as a key part of the management of their chronic disease (Lorig et al. 2001).

Vignette 11.2.4 Continuation

You explain to Tristan that his dad may be feeling the effects of stress but that you want to focus on addressing how stress may be affecting him. Despite multiple significant life stressors that Tristan just mentioned, he remains insistent that he is not actually feeling stressed. You explain to him that you suspect his asthma symptoms are related to the effects of stress and it should be addressed, but he remains hesitant.

Please proceed with the problem-based approach using the worksheet located in the appendix of Chap. 1!

FACTS	HYPOTHESES	INFORMATION NEEDED	LEARNING ISSUES

Tristan skeptically agrees to do deep breathing mediation exercises once a day for 10 min. He also says that he will "call up a few buddies that I haven't seen in a while," since while with his girlfriend, he withdrew much of his other social support.

During his follow-up visit 4 weeks later, he said that he enjoys the deep breathing practice because it forces him to have times to "chill and relax." He has also been spending more time with his friends, which has made him happier and "not as worried about the future since we are all in the same boat." He also reports that his asthma symptoms are relatively well controlled, and that he does not need his rescue inhaler as often.

11.3 Learning Issues

11.3.1 How a Clinician Can Help (Continuation)

Helping the Patient Understand Why Stress Is Important In formulating a treatment plan, it is important that the patient understand the significant correlation between stress and their overall health. Providing the patient with information, including handouts (see Appendix C), may be helpful. Patients may initially be resistant to the possibility of stress playing a role and even more resistant to taking the time to address it. One effective method for increasing patient understanding, and ultimately adherence, is the *teach-back* method, in which the patient is asked to state back in their own words what they understand about their illness/diagnosis. Applying this to stress identification and management, a clinician asks the patient to explain his or her level of stress and how it is affecting overall health and/or disease. As with suggestions for other lifestyle changes, once the patient recognizes that they are under stress and is motivated to make life changes, they are more likely to buy-in to the treatment plan (Dunbar-Jacob 2000).

Table 11.1 Common stress management techniques

Healthy	Unhealthy
Relaxation (meditation, yoga, etc.)	Alcohol
Exercise	Drugs
Social Support (family, church, support groups, etc.)	Overeating
Formal stress management programs (such as Stanford Self-Management Program)	Avoidance

Stress Management Techniques Several evidence-based stress management techniques have been developed, and the approach to stress management varies with each patient (Ahn et al. 2013). There are several healthy ways in which to manage stress and perhaps just as many unhealthy ways. Some examples are listed in Table 11.1.

If a patient is practicing healthy stress management techniques, such as those listed above, it may be helpful to provide positive reinforcement for the goal of promoting that behavior. If the patient admits to what are generally unhealthy stress management techniques, you could use that as an opportunity to intervene and offer alternative therapies to try.

Relaxation exercises, such as yoga and meditation, have been quite extensively studied and have been shown to significantly offset the adverse clinical effects of stress in conditions such as hypertension and anxiety, at least partially through the potential induction of telomerases, which interestingly also slow the process of aging (Bhasin et al. 2013). For those patients who could benefit from or who would rather increase their physical activity, regular exercise has many proven benefits, including release of endorphins, which are known to increase mood, enhance immunity, and offset some of the psychological affects of stress (Salmon 2001).

Another studied intervention is small-group interventions teaching self-management skills, such as the Stanford Chronic Disease Self-Management Program (Lorig et al. 1999). Patients enrolled in these types of programs have shown statistically significant improvements in healthy behaviors and health status, using markers such decreased cortisol levels, improved cognitive symptom management and lower glycosylated hemoglobin levels, indicative of better control of blood sugar in diabetics (Lorig et al. 2001; Kramer et al. 2000). These effects persist, even up to 6 months following completion of the programs (Hammerfald et al. 2006).

Discussing a menu of potential treatment options, and allowing the patient to decide what modality to try, may increase their adherence to a particular program and therefore lead to more significant benefits. As with other treatment plans, readdressing patient compliance and response to intervention at regular intervals is important, so that any changes, if necessary, may be implemented.

11.4 Conclusion

Although acute stress is evolutionarily beneficial to humans, chronic activation of the stress response leads to multiple negative effects. Life stress is ubiquitous; many people can identify significant current stressors in their lives, however it is the provider's responsibility to recognize the role that stress may be playing in their patients' overall health, as well as the status of specific diseases known to be directly affected by chronic stress. A provider that is able to apply the skills outlined in this chapter to identify and manage stress can have a profound positive impact on their patients' overall quality of life.

11.5 Review Questions

1. In which of the following would a stress response be beneficial?
   a. A long and unpredictable work commute, with a boss who does not tolerate tardiness
   b. Fighting with a spouse almost daily for several months
   c. Working on a busy obstetrical service during overnight call
   d. Daily financial concerns about the ability to pay rent
2. Based on the chapter reading, which patient is at the greatest risk for an elevated perceived stress level?
   a. A small business owner, who solely owns and runs her own successful flower shop
   b. A waitress who is also is a part-time student
   c. An athlete training during the off-season
   d. An office manager who was a victim of child abuse and raised in foster care
3. Your patient is an overworked executive who comes to see you in clinic complaining of stress, which has caused him to increase his nightly alcohol use and fast food visits, causing unwanted weight gain. Explain your approach to stress management in this patient, including which stress management techniques you would recommend and why.
4. Which are the following statements is true?
   a. The parasympathetic system is responsible for increased physical and mental activation during the stress response.
   b. Stress activates the HPA axis, ultimately leading to elevated cortisol levels.
   c. A chronic stress response is beneficial for survival.
   d. Chronic stress has been shown to have beneficial effects on several diseases, including diabetes and hypertension.

Appendix A: Possible Answers to Vignettes

Vignette 11.1: Mrs. Spears

Table 11.1.1

Facts	Hypotheses	Information needed	Learning issues
32-year-old woman with Crohn's disease	Stress may be contributing to her disease	Does the patient identify that she is stressed?	How can stress cause worsening IBD symptoms?
Patient has severe IBD with multiple flares		Could stress be playing a role?	
Stress leads to worsening control of IBD symptoms			

IBD inflammatory bowel disease

Table 11.1.2

Facts	Hypotheses	Information needed	Learning issues
Patient does endorse stress in her life	If her stress is managed, her disease may be better managed	Does the patient realize that stress really does adversely affect her?	How much of a role can stress play in disease flares and management?
Patient does notice a relationship between stress and her symptoms			How can you tell the impact stress may be having on an individual patient?
Patient will allow the provider to discuss stress effects			

Table 11.1.3

Facts	Hypotheses	Information needed	Learning issues
Patient has a high level of stress	Stress management skills will improve her disease	How does the patient decrease stress?	How to work with a patient to device a stress management plan?
Patient is open to discussing stress reduction techniques	She is motivated and will be compliant with stress management techniques	How does the decrease in stress affect her disease?	What are the proven stress reduction techniques?
			How effective is stress reduction in disease management?

Vignette 11.2: Tristan

Table 11.2.1

Facts	Hypotheses	Information needed	Learning issues
20-year-old male with asthma	Factors in his life may be playing a role in his illness	Has the stress in his life increased in the past 6 weeks?	How can you discern if a patient is under an increased amount of stress?
Patient has had more frequent asthma attacks in the past 6 weeks			

Table 11.2.2

Facts	Hypotheses	Information needed	Learning issues
Patient reports significant stressors	His stress is playing a role in his illness	How can he decrease his stress?	When does stress become harmful?
Patient does not recognize that he is stressed			

Table 11.2.3

Facts	Hypotheses	Information needed	Learning issues
Patient's dad may also be stressed	His dad's stress is affecting his health	Can stress affect blood pressure and aging	What conditions are affected by stress?

Table 11.2.4

Facts	Hypotheses	Information needed	Learning issues
Patient remains hesitant to accept that he is stressed	He needs to acknowledge his stress to be open to treating it	Does he realize that he is stressed?	What are some ways to get patients to recognize that stress may be hurting them?
	If he treats it, his asthma will likely improve	Is he open to treatment?	

Appendix B: Answers to Review Questions

1. c. Working on a busy obstetrical service during overnight call
   The acute stress response is beneficial, as it leads to increased physical and mental alertness. This response would be beneficial in an acute setting when the increased vigilance portends better performance. However, chronic stress, which one would expect to be present in the other scenarios, has detrimental physical and mental effects, as described in the chapter.
2. d. An office manager who was a victim of child abuse and raised in foster care
   As discussed in the chapter, certain patient groups are at higher risk of perceived stress, including those with financial difficulties, low level of job control, and those with traumatic childhood experiences,
3. There are multiple effective stress management techniques that can be discussed with this patient. Given his lifestyle of obesity, poor diet, and alcohol use, counseling him on healthy diet choices and limiting alcohol use would be beneficial. Since he is complaining of weight gain, it would also be good to suggest the addition of exercise, as part of both stress and weight management. He may also benefit from relaxation techniques, such as yoga or meditation, since he is described as "overworked," and allowing sometime to slow down may help decrease his stress level. Regardless of the method chosen to discuss with this patient, the most important aspect is that he must be open to the suggested treatment.

Of note, this patient already recognizes that they are under stress, which makes screening for stress a bit less important but may still be beneficial for some patients to develop a true understanding of their degree of stress.

4. b. Stress activates the HPA axis, ultimately leading to elevated cortisol levels. The stress response has many effects on the body, including leading to elevated cortisol levels through the activation of the HPA axis. Chronic stress has been shown to have detrimental effects on several diseases, including diabetes and hypertension. The sympathetic response is responsible for increased physical and mental activation during the stress response. An acute stress response is beneficial for survival.

Appendix C: Information on Stress

Holmes-Rahe Stress Inventory (http://www.dartmouth.edu/~eap/library/lifechangestresstest.pdf)

Perceived Stress Scale (http://www.mindgarden.com/docs/PerceivedStressScale.pdf)

Life Experiences Survey (www.psych.uw.edu/research/sarason/files/lifeexperiencessurvey.pdf)

Stanford Self-Management Program (http://patienteducation.stanford.edu/programs/cdsmp.html)

References

Ahn, S., Basu, R., Smith, M.L. Jiang, L., Lorig, K., Whitelaw, N., et al. (2013). The impact of chronic disease self-management programs: Healthcare savings through a community-based intervention. *BMC Public Health, 13,* 1141.

Al Kaladeh, M. T., & Abu Shosha, G. M. (2012). Application of the Perceived Stress Scale in health care studies, an analysis of the literature. *International Journal of Academic Research, 4*(4), 45–50.

American Psychiatric Association. (2013). *Diagnostic and statistical manual of mental disorders* (5th ed.). Arlington: American Psychiatric Publishing.

Beth Israel Deaconess Medical Center. (2012). Stress management counseling in the primary care setting is rare. ScienceDaily.

Bhasin, M. K., Dusek, J. A., Chang, B-H., Joseph, M. G., Denninger, J. W., Fricchione, G. L., et al. (2013). Relaxation response induces temporal transcriptome changes in energy metabolism, insulin secretion and inflammatory pathways. *PLoS ONE*. doi:10.1371/journal.pone.0062817.

Buckley, M. M., et al. (2014). Convergence of neuro-endocrine-immune pathways in the pathophysiology of irritable bowel syndrome. *World Journal of Gastroenterology, 20*(27), 8846–8858.

Chen, E., & Miller, G. E. (2007). Stress and inflammation in exacerbations of asthma. *Brain, Behavior, and Immunity, 21*(8), 993–999.

Cohen, S., Spacapan, S., & Oskamp, S. (1988). Perceived stress in a probability sample of the United States. The social psychology of health (pp. 31–67). The Claremont Symposium on Applied Social Psychology.

Dunbar-Jacob, J., et al. (2000). Adherence in chronic disease. *Annual Review of Nursing Research, 18,* 48–90.

Gore, A. C., Attardi, B., & DeFranco, D.B. (2006). Glucocorticoid repression of the reproductive axis: Effects on GnRH and gonadotropin subunit mRNA levels. *Molecular and Cellular Endocrinology, 256*(1–2), 40–48.

Hammerfald, K., Eberle, C., Grau, M., Kinsperger, A., Zimmermann, A., Ehlert, U., et al. (2006). Persistent effects of cognitive-behavioral stress management on cortisol responses to acute stress in healthy subjects—a randomized control trial. Clinical Psychology and Psychotherapy, Institute of Psychology, University of Zurich, 43, CH-8044.

Holmes, T. H., & Rahe, R. H. (1967). The social readjustment rating scale. *Journal of Psychosomatic Research, 11*(2), 213–218.

Kramer, J. R., Ledolter, J., Manos, G. N., & Bayless, M. L. (2000). Stress and metabolic control in diabetes mellitus: Methodological issues and illustrative analysis. *Annals of Behavioral Medicine, 22*(1), 17–28.

Lazzarino, A. I., Hamer, M., & Steptoe, A. (2013). The association between cortisol response to mental stress and high-sensitivity caridac troponin T plasma concentration in healthy adults. *Journal of the American College of Cardiology, 62*(10), 1694–1701.

Lorig, K. R., Ritter, P., Stewart, A. L., Sobel, D. S., Brown, B. W., Bandura, A., et al. (2001, November/December). Effect of self-management program on patients with chronic disease. Effective Clinical Practice.

Lorig, K. R., Sobel, D. S., Stewart, A. L, Brown, B. W., Bandura, A., Ritter, P., et al. (1999). Evidence suggesting that a chronic disease self-management program can improve health status while reducing hospitalization: A randomized trial. *Medical Care, 37*(1), 5–14.

Marinaccio, A., Ferrante, P, & Iavicoli, S. (2013). The relevance of socio-demographic and occupational variables for the assessment of work-related stress risk. *BMC Public Health, 13,* 1157.

National Scientific Council on the Developing Child. (2005, cited 2007 April 9). Excessive stress disrupts the architecture of the developing brain. Working Paper No. 3. Cambridge: The Council.

Posen, D. (2013). *Always change a losing game* (4th Ed.). Oakville: Firefly Books.

Salmon, P. (2001). Effects of physical exercise on anxiety, depression, and sensitivity to stress: A unifying theory. *Clinical Psychology Review, 21,* 33.

Sarason, I., Johnson, J., & Siegel, J. (1978). Assessing the impact of life changes: Development of the Life Experiences Survey. *Journal of Consulting and Clinical Psychology, 46*(5), 932–946.

Silverman, M. N., & Sternberg E. M. (2012). Glucocorticoid regulation of inflammation and its behavioral and metabolic correlates: From HPA axis to glucocorticoid receptor dysfunction. *Annals of the New York Academy of Sciences, 1261,* 55–63.

Taylor, S. E., Welch, W. T., Kim, H. S., & Sherman, D. K. (2007). Cultural difference in the impact of social support on psychological and biological stress responses. *Psychological Science, 18*(9), 831–837.

Chapter 12
Health Care 101 and Systems-Based Practice

Paula Yoshioka and Michael H. Fukuda

12.1 Introduction

In 2010, the delivery of health care in America was dramatically and extensively changed by the Patient Protection and Affordable Health Care Act (ACA,; H.R. 3590) and the Health Care and Education Reconciliation Act (H.R. 4872). Both laws set forth insurance market reforms with the goals of achieving the *triple aim*: improving the individual patient care in terms of satisfaction and quality, improving the health of the population, and reducing and controlling the cost of care. This chapter will provide a broad overview of the ACA and its impact on the patient, health-care workforce, and health-care provider systems.

12.2 Objectives

After the completion of this chapter, students will be able to:

1. Discuss the major reform initiatives that were mandated by the ACA
2. Articulate how the ACA proposes to transform current access, quality, and cost issues, and

---

After a century of striving, after a year of debate, after a historic vote, health care reform is no longer an unmet promise. It is the law of the land.
Barack Obama

P. Yoshioka (✉)
The Queen's Health Systems, 1301 Punchbowl Street, Honolulu, HI 96813, USA
e-mail: pyoshioka@queens.org

M. H. Fukuda
Department of Psychiatry, University of Hawai'i John A. Burns School of Medicine, 1356 Lusitana Street, University Tower 4th Floor, Honolulu, HI 96813, USA
e-mail: fukudam@dop.hawaii.edu

D. Alicata et al. (eds.), *Problem-based Behavioral Science and Psychiatry*,
DOI 10.1007/978-3-319-23669-8_12

3. Describe the short- and long-term impacts of the ACA on the patient and health-care provider community

Health-care access in the USA can be complex, with a mix of public and private services which often overlap. To gain a better understanding of the complexities of the ACA, we introduce the Baker family, whose health issues range from simple to complex. We will illustrate how the ACA affects family access and ability to pay for health care.

Mrs. Betty Johnson: a 54-year-old self-employed graphic artist living in Hawai'i.

Mr. Bob Baker: a 62-year-old owner of a small auto parts company in Detroit, MI.

Mr. Brian Baker: Bob's son, a 19-year-old sophomore college student with an undeclared major. He is enjoying his early college years and does not have health insurance.

Ms. Bridget McGladrey: a 22-year-old who is healthy and has a 5-year-old child.

Based on the information above and your knowledge of health insurance options in the USA, consider the potential impacts on the characters as they face the ACA, which provides:

Expanded health-care access

Individual American citizen mandate to purchase insurance

State health exchanges where insurance could be purchased

Eligibility and cost containment consumer safe guards

Primary prevention and wellness for betterment of populational health and

Opportunities for states to increase quality and foster change to address rising health-care cost

12.3 Overview of the ACA

The intent of the ACA legislation was to expand health-care coverage to an estimated 32 million uninsured Americans. Provisions of the law provide for expanding access to insurance, improving quality in health-care settings, increasing the workforce, and addressing the rising health-care costs. With an estimated cost of $938 billion over a 10-year period (2010–2020), various complex provisions of the 900+ page law provided significant policy changes in the way health care was and now is provided in America. More specifically, the ACA expanded health-care access, instituted an individual mandate for American citizens to purchase insurance, provided for state-based exchanges through which insurance could be purchased, safeguarded consumers through eligibility and cost containment protections, emphasized prevention and wellness as a means to attain population health, provided opportunities for states to increase quality, and fostered change to address the rising cost of health care (AHA 2010). Let us now address how the ACA secured each of these policy changes.

12.3.1 *Increased Access to Health-Care Services*

Before the ACA, there were approximately 32 million uninsured people in America. Under an individual mandate provision, all citizens and legal residents must have obtained health insurance by January 2, 2014. Qualifying insurance coverage can be provided through private and public sources including Medicare, Medicaid, TRICARE, the Veteran's Health Care Program, employer-sponsored plans, and market place exchanges. The federal government imposed a phased-in tax penalty for those eligible who did not obtain or maintain a minimum prescribed essential coverage benefits. Under the individual (personal responsibility) mandate, individuals who elect not to purchase health insurance can be initially fined a tax penalty of $95 per year up to a maximum penalty of $2085 per year for a household or a flat fee of 1 % of taxable income in 2014. By 2016, the tax penalty for an individual would rise to $695 or 2.5 % of taxable income. The last increases will occur in 2016, when the penalty will increase by the consumer price index (CPI). Limited exemptions from the individual mandate are available based on a number of criteria, including, but not limited to, religious objections, tax incomes below the tax filing thresholds, and hardship.

In order to increase insurance enrollment for the eligible populations covered by Medicaid (a joint federal and state program that assists individuals and families with costs associated with long-term medical and custodial care) and Medicare (a federal insurance program that assists persons aged 65 and over as well as for certain disabled individuals under the age of 65), states could apply to expand their Medicaid Program to non-elderly individuals (parents, children, and adults up to 133 % of the Federal Poverty Level). States that chose to expand were provided federal assistance to pay for the cost of coverage for eligible childless adults up to 133 % of the federal poverty level. This ACA provision was effective from January 2014.

Vignette 12.1: Mr. Brian Baker

Brian just returned home from his first year in college and has learned that his parents cannot pay for his university health insurance. He decides to forgo health insurance for the year, and thinks he can afford the individual tax penalty. However, during his vacation he gets into a bicycle accident and is taken to the emergency room.

Brian complains of fatigue, frequent thirst, and unintentional weight loss. He believes the fatigue caused him to lose balance and fall off the bicycle. He does not have any serious injury; however, a routine basic metabolic panel shows a blood glucose level above 200 mg/dL. The emergency room discharges Brian and recommends follow-up with his primary-care physician for the elevated blood glucose level.

Later at home, Brian wonders how he is going to pay the $3000 emergency room visit, and now questions his choice to forgo health insurance.

Please proceed with the problem-based approach using the worksheet located in the appendix of Chap. 1!

Please fill in the facts, your hypotheses, further information needed, and learning issues for learning issue Table 12.1.

Learning issue Table 12.1.

FACTS	HYPOTHESES	INFORMATION NEEDED	LEARNING ISSUES

12.4 Overview of the US Health-Care System

How one pays for health care in the USA occurs through a variety of mechanisms: one may pay directly for services, obtain insurance through their employer, or (if a veteran) receive care from the federal government. Government funded programs also cover Americans through Medicare and—for the impoverished, for the disabled, for pregnant women in need, and for children—the state managed Medicaid program (U.S. DHHS. CMS 2014).

12.4.1 Employers

In determining health insurance requirements for employers, the ACA made a separation between small and large employers. Small employers are those with less than 50 employees, medium employers are those with 50–100 employees, and large employers are those with more than 100 employees. For small employers, there are no new requirements and additional insurance choices are offered through exchanges. Additionally, tax credits are available depending on the size and average age of the employee. Medium employers are subject to financial penalties ranging from 2000 to $3000 per employee if their employees purchase coverage through the exchanges. Large employers are largely not impacted as most of them continue to provide coverage. Financial penalties apply to large employers as they do to medium-sized employers.

Vignette 12.2: Mr. Bob Baker

Bob owns a company with 40 employees and is interested in how the ACA will affect his finances. He has coverage for some of his employees; however, a few have hypertension and diabetes. They were denied coverage by his insurer. Bob also was denied coverage due to his hypertension and history of a transient ischemic attack (TIA). He has not seen his internist in 2 years and wonders what are the consequences of not seeking treatment and if the new ACA will help him.

STOP

Please proceed with the problem-based approach using the worksheet located in the appendix of Chap. 1!

Please fill in the facts, your hypotheses, further information needed, and learning issues for learning issue Table 12.2.

Learning issue Table 12.2.

FACTS	HYPOTHESES	INFORMATION NEEDED	LEARNING ISSUES

Vignette 12.3: Mrs. Betty Johnson

Mrs. Johnson (Bob's sister) becomes faint and passes out while working on an art project in a client's business. Her client calls 911. In the emergency room, an electrocardiogram reveals atrial fibrillation, and she is admitted to the hospital. She discusses her condition with her cardiologist, and they decide that electrical cardioversion is her best option. Betty undergoes successful cardioversion and is discharged with a beta-blocker.

Betty decides that she needs health insurance, and she calls several health plans at her location. All of the health plans turn her down and refer her to the health exchange. Betty does not believe she is poor and wonders why the insurers have turned her down. She has an income of about $1000 a month from her business.

STOP

Please proceed with the problem-based approach using the worksheet located in the appendix of Chap. 1!

Please fill in the facts, your hypotheses, further information needed, and learning issues for Learning issue Table 12.3.

Learning issue Table 12.3.

FACTS	HYPOTHESES	INFORMATION NEEDED	LEARNING ISSUES

12.4.2 State-Based Health Insurance Exchanges

As discussed earlier in this chapter, the federal government also provided that states could establish insurance marketplaces or *exchanges* where employers or consumers could buy insurance based on a selection of offered plans. By January 2014, states were required to establish these exchanges and offer defined essential benefits to include a full range of services (inpatient/outpatient, rehabilitation, emergency, prescription drug, maternity and newborn, pediatric, chronic disease management, and prevention/wellness). States are allowed to establish more than one exchange within a state as long as geographic areas are served. Other arrangements are allowed, such as establishing exchanges between states and establishing an exchange to assist small qualified employers.

Exchanges are also required to provide information on offered health benefits and plan choices; to manage eligibility determinations; to enroll individuals in Medicaid, Children's Health Insurance Program (CHP), or other public programs; and to communicate information in a culturally and linguistically sensitive manner.

12.4.3 Consumer Protections

The ACA made several changes to the insurance market to protect consumers. Most notably, insurers can no longer rescind coverage if a covered individual becomes ill, impose lifetime benefit limits and unreasonable annual limits on the dollar value of these benefits, impose exclusions for preexisting conditions for children under age

19 years, or exclude preventive services. Additionally, health coverage increased the age of a covered dependent to 26 years and provided for an appeals process related to coverage and claims.

The ACA provided access to health-care insurance for those who had been previously denied because of preexisting conditions or because they were nearing retirement. Temporary high-risk and reinsurance programs were established for this population.

Vignette 12.1: Mr. Brian Baker Conclusion

Brian arranges a follow-up appointment with his parent's internist. He presents to the office and lets the registrar know he does not have insurance. She asks him to complete an office questionnaire, which asks for his previous health insurer. After completing the form, the registrar informs him that he may still be eligible for insurance under his parents. Brian agrees to contact the insurer.

Brian meets with the internist, who suspects he has type 2 diabetes. He recommends that Brian obtain a fasting plasma glucose test. Brian agrees and schedules a follow-up appointment with the internist. He also calls his former insurance plan and learns he is eligible; he therefore enrolls under his parents plan.

The follow-up appointment confirms the type 2 diabetes diagnosis. Brian goes over a plan with his internist and agrees with the recommendation on diet, exercise, and oral medication. Subsequent visits show Brian's diabetes is well controlled and he reports no problems with fatigue or weight loss.

Vignette 12.2: Mr. Bob Baker Conclusion

With the help of the state health exchange, Bob is able to find affordable coverage for his employees. He is quite pleased to learn that his previous existing health problems do not exclude him from coverage, and he now sees his internist on a regular basis. His hypertension is under control and is on antiplatelet medicine to prevent another transient ischemic attack (TIA).

Vignette 12.3: Mrs. Betty Johnson Conclusion

Betty signs on to the Hawai‘i Health Connector (the state health exchange) and determines she is eligible for Medicaid through the ACA expansion of Medicaid eligibility. She is pleased to find an internist at her community health center and is able to get ongoing treatment plus medication at one location (Federal Registry Notice 2014).

Vignette 12.4: Ms. Bridgette Baker-McGladrey

Ms. Baker-McGladrey is planning to enroll her 5-year-old daughter in health care and contacts her former employer to purchase a plan for both herself and her daughter. The employer is not able to enroll the child in their health-care plan and refers Ms. Baker-McGladrey to a health exchange.

Ms. Baker-McGladrey purchases a plan through the exchange, and has her first appointment with a family medicine doctor and pediatrician. During the exam, she wonders why both doctors ask so many questions? Her family medicine doctor inquires about depression and domestic violence. The pediatrician administers screening forms that ask if the child is sad, prefers to stay home, or is "clingy" when presented with new situations.

STOP

Please proceed with the problem-based approach using the worksheet located in the appendix of Chap. 1!

Please fill in the facts, your hypotheses, further information needed, and learning issues for learning issue Table 12.4.

Learning issue Table 12.4.

FACTS	HYPOTHESES	INFORMATION NEEDED	LEARNING ISSUES

12.4.4 Wellness and Prevention

One of the main foci for ACA is to improve the health of the population. In this regard, the ACA required that health insurers and group health plans cover certain prevention services as recommended by the US Preventive Services Task Force and immunizations as required by the Centers for Disease Control and Prevention. Women's health, a major focus, gained significant attention with the establishment of the Office on Women's Health within the Federal Health and Human Services (HHS) agency. A Prevention and Public Health Fund was also created to provide funding through HHS for expanded and sustained programming in prevention and public health and education and outreach to allow public awareness around life span health improvement. School-based health centers are supported through grant funding that provides preference to underserved areas of low-income children.

Specific to Medicare, beneficiaries are provided with annual wellness visits to include a health risk assessment, prevention services for conditions that require follow-up and referrals for health services.

With the goal of promoting healthy communities, the federal government instituted Community Transformation Grants for evidence-based preventive health, healthy aging grants for early detection of complications of aging, programs to increase health-care access for those with disabilities, and programs to improve immunization rates. See Chap. 3 for a thorough discussion of the impact of early prevention and intervention programs on lifelong health. Such programs are critical to the success of any future health-care system.

Vignette 12.4: Ms. Bridgette Baker-McGladrey Conclusion

Bridgette's physician explains that social, developmental, and behavioral health questions are standard protocol and not meant to embarrass her. The ACA focus on wellness and prevention takes a proactive role in finding and preventing both biological and behavioral health issues. If any of these issues are identified early, a plan can be developed to mitigate adverse effects and ensure long-term wellness. Bridgette is relieved and glad that her physicians take the time to emphasize health and wellness.

12.4.5 Quality

Transparency in costs and an emphasis on quality care have required hospitals to fund data infrastructure to be able to share medical records with physicians and report on patient outcomes. The ACA established Hospital Value-Based Purchasing (VBP) to reimburse hospitals for their individual performance on defined quality measures. These measures required hospitals to set up reporting systems—also known as Health Care Assessment Hospital Provider Services (HCAHPS)—to include reporting for patient satisfaction; surgical outcomes; and outcomes of care delivered for heart attack, heart failure, and pneumonia. Hospitals not meeting quality measure performance as compared to peer hospitals are penalized in the form of reduced Medicare reimbursements.

Hospitals are fined decreased Medicare payments based on higher than expected within-30-day readmission measures for heart failure, heart attack, and pneumonia. Based on a formula based on Medicare-expected readmission rates, the largest reduction for any particular hospital could be 1 % in 2013, 2 % in 2014, and 3 % for all other future years along with a potential expansion to other conditions.

In order to incentivize providers, accountable care organizations (ACOs) were authorized to be formed beginning in January 2012. Members of ACOs could include physician practices, hospital-employed physicians, joint ventures, and other non-MD clinicians. ACOs were required to have a legal structure and governance, processes to ensure evidence-based medicine, care coordination, and mechanisms to report patient satisfaction and quality. In return, members of the ACO could earn incentive payments based on meeting prescribed quality thresholds.

12.4.6 Graduate Medical Education

With the expansion of the insured population, the ACA recognized that resources to teaching hospitals would need to be increased in order to expand teaching capacity. In 2009, Medicare provided most of the funding for graduate medical education. An amount of $9.5 billion was allocated to support approximately 100,000 residents in America's teaching hospitals. While there is a significant recognition that supporting primary care is a key strategy for successful ACA implementation, medical students' interest in primary-care careers continues to decrease, with only 16–18% choosing general internal medicine.

Among other innovations in supporting America's health-care workforce, the ACA provided for redistribution of unused residency training positions: 70% to hospitals in states where the resident to population served ratios are in the lowest quartile and 30% to hospitals in rural and HPSA-identified areas.

12.4.7 Financing the ACA

When the ACA was passed, the federal government estimated that it would cost $1080 billion to finance health-care reform. In broad categories, the chart below depicts how this $938 billion was to be covered:

Category	Impact (billion $)
Medicare reductions	416.5
Medicare tax increases on high-income taxpayers	210
Insurer and medical producer fees	107
Medicaid reductions	45
"Cadillac" health plan excise taxes	32
Employer and individual penalty payments	69
Other revenue	149
Other spending reductions	52

12.5 Conclusion

The ACA policy is dynamic and ever changing; it will continue to significantly impact access and health-care delivery across the country. It is foreseeable that Congress will continue to shape this law as population health needs change over time.

12.6 Review Questions

1. What are the aims identified as outcomes of the Affordable Health Care Act (ACA)?
    a. Improving the patient experience in quality and satisfaction
    b. Improving the health of the population
    c. Reducing and controlling the cost of care
    d. All of the above
2. Approximately what percent of non-elderly insured Americans receive their insurance through an employer-sponsored plan?
    a. 10 %
    b. 30 %
    c. 60 %
    d. 90 %
3. Approximately what percent of the US gross national product (GNP) is spent on health care?
    a. 6 %
    b. 16 %
    c. 32 %
    d. 66 %
4. Match the type of insurance coverage with the most appropriate description.
    a. Medicare
    b. Medicaid
    c. Private Insurance

1. Federally funded and designed to cover the elderly and people with certain long-term disabilities
2. Federally and State funded, designed to cover primarily the poor
3. Primarily employer-based, *fee for service* and *health maintenance organization (HMO)* models exist

Appendix A: Tables with Possible Answers to the Vignettes

Vignette 12.1: Mr. Brian Baker

Learning issue Table 12.1

Facts	Hypotheses	Information needed	Learning issues
19-year-old unemployed college student evaluated in the emergency room after a bicycle accident Medical history reveals fatigue, frequent thirst, and unintentional weight loss No serious injury; however, basic metabolic panel shows a blood glucose level above 200 mg/dL He is discharged with the recommendation to follow-up with his PCP for the elevated blood glucose level Brian wonders how he is going to pay the $3000 emergency room visit	Student health plan availability and coverage, parental coverage of college-enrolled kids	Has he investigated potential sources of coverage: individual insurance, employer-sponsored (mother's or father's), self-pay	How has the ACA impacted Brian's options? What are Brian's options to receive primary care?

PCP primary-care physician, *ACA*

Vignette 12.2: Mr. Bob Baker

Learning issue Table 12.2

Facts	Hypotheses	Information needed	Learning issues
62-year-old owner of a small auto parts company	Potential source of coverage: employer-sponsored, self-pay	What is the existing coverage plan for Bob and his employees?	How would the ACA help Bob and his employees obtain health insurance?
History of HTN and TIA	Existing employee coverage has limitations		
He has not seen his internist in 2 years	Bob and employees are denied coverage for preexisting illness		How would expanding coverage to Bob and his employees control health-care cost?
	Bob considers the consequences of not seeking treatment, and whether the new ACA will help him		What are the financial benefits to small business to cover employee health care?

ACA, *HTN* hypertension, *TIA* transient ischemic attack

Vignette 12.3: Mrs. Betty Johnson

Learning issue Table 12.3

Facts	Hypotheses	Information needed	Learning issues
54-year-old self-employed, uninsured graphic artist experiences syncope while working and is evaluated in the Emergency Department (ED)	Denied coverage by health plan and was referred to Medicaid		What are Betty's options to receive care?
ECG reveals Afib, and she is admitted to the hospital			How has the health-care system impacted Betty's options?
Betty undergoes successful cardioversion and is discharged with a beta-blocker			How would the health exchange help Betty obtain insurance?
			Why was Betty referred to Medicaid?
			How will Betty decide which plan best meets her financial situation?

ECG electrocardiogram, *Afib* atrial fibrillation

Vignette 12.4-Ms. Bridgette Baker-McGladrey

Learning issue Table 12.4

Facts	Hypotheses	Information needed	Learning issues
A 22-year-old who is healthy, unemployed, and has a 5-year-old child	Potential source of coverage—Medicaid or SCHIP, self-pay	Income level, Medicaid requirements (especially concerning pregnancy)	Why did the family physician ask about depression?
			Why would the family physician ask about domestic violence?
			Why did the pediatrician ask about how the child responds to new situations?

SCHIP State Children's Health Insurance Program

Appendix B: Answers to Review Questions

Answers

1. d
2. c
3. b

4. a-1
   b-2
   c-3

References

American Hospital Association. Legislative Advisory. (2010). Summary of 2010 Health Care Reform Legislation. The Patient Protection and Affordable Care Act (H.R. 3590) and Health Care and Education Reconciliation Act (H.R. 4872).

U.S. Department of Health and Human Services. (2014) Center for Medicare and Medicaid Services "What's Medicare". www.medicare.gov/Pubs/PDF/11306. Accessed 11 Dec 2014.

Chapter 13
Stigma and Medicine

Barbara Kohlenberg

Archbishop Tutu: I think, I mean, that we have very gravely underestimated the damage that apartheid inflicted on all of us. You know, the damage to our psyches, the damage that has made—I mean, it shocked me. I went to Nigeria when I was working for the World Council of Churches, and I was due to fly to Jos. And so I go to Lagos airport and I get onto the plane and the two pilots in the cockpit are both black. And whee, I just grew inches. You know, it was fantastic because we had been told that blacks can't do this.
Ms. Tippett: Right.
Archbishop Tutu: And we have a smooth takeoff and then we hit the mother and father of turbulence. I mean, it was quite awful, scary. Do you know, I can't believe it but the first thought that came to my mind was, "Hey, there's no white men in that cockpit. Are those blacks going to be able to make it?" And of course, they obviously made it—here I am. But the thing is, I had not known that I was damaged to the extent of thinking that somehow actually what those white people who had kept drumming into us in South Africa about our being inferior, about our being incapable, it had lodged somewhere in me.
From On Being, with Krista Tippett (www.onbeing.org)

13.1 Introduction

As illustrated in the above quotation, human beings can have very clear values which are inconsistent with other thoughts and feelings that may arise. As noted, Desmond Tutu, while clearly standing for the equality of black people in South Africa, describes, during a turbulent airplane flight, having the thought "Hey, there's no white men in that cockpit. Are those blacks going to be able to make it?" He discusses a sense of almost being infected with the social norms that gave rise to that thought, despite his values and hard work promoting the equality of black people. Tutu describes a very normal human phenomenon, in which consciously held values may have very little to do with thoughts that feel automatic, and may not be subject to conscious control. He also demonstrates that he holds these troubling

B. Kohlenberg (✉)
Reno, NV, USA
e-mail: bkohlenberg@medicine.nevada.edu

D. Alicata et al. (eds.), *Problem-based Behavioral Science and Psychiatry*,
DOI 10.1007/978-3-319-23669-8_13

thoughts lightly, with a sense of playfulness, in his public telling of the story. He is clearly not hiding these thoughts, suppressing them, or avoiding them.

Turning to medicine, it is clear that the values embedded in the Hippocratic Oath involve practicing medicine with honor, competency, and respect. Yet, despite these core values, medical students and physicians still may have thoughts and feelings that are the opposite of these cherished values. These thoughts and feelings may emerge with respect to patient care, and notably, may also involve the care provided for themselves and for their colleagues. For example, with respect to patient care, one may feel that people who are obese are entitled to excellent care and can live a life of worth and integrity, while at the same time, also struggle with thoughts and feelings about that person being a "a slob, weak willed…they did this to themselves…," and thus, back away from providing effective, compassionate medical care. With respect to physician and medical student self care, one may truly believe that physicians are human and can experience depression and that professional help may be useful, while at the same time, one may also have thoughts about weakness and shame and thus avoid seeking or recommending care.

No one likes having thoughts and feelings that are not consistent with who we want to be or who we believe ourselves to be. And a natural, human, understandable response to being in this predicament would be to try to not feel that way. However, efforts to not feel undesired feelings, as we shall see, can result in actually intensifying those very feelings (Wegner 1994). One normal solution to intensely troubling thoughts and feelings would be to distance oneself from the people or circumstances that provoke such feelings. But this, as we shall see, can be set up for dehumanization and stigma.

Stigma in medicine is important because, when acted upon, believing or avoiding one's stigmatizing thoughts can result in restricted opportunities and thus poor outcomes when applied to oneself or to the patient's under one's care.

This chapter will explore the kinds of stigma relevant for health-care providers and for patients. This chapter will also focus, specifically, on stigma surrounding obesity as well as on some of the unique features of depression and suicidality in physicians and medical students. Methods of reducing the adverse impact that stigma of all kinds can have on the provision of health care will also be discussed.

In this chapter, a slightly different approach will be applied to problem-based learning (PBL). Cases will be presented that target personal, emotional, and cognitive responses from the reader, and the reader is invited to consider those responses as the cases unfold. In addition, the PBL tables have a different format from most chapters in this book. The tables invite further exploration of the reader's thoughts, feelings, and behaviors.

Objectives By the end of this chapter, the reader will be able to:

1. Define enacted stigma and describe how this may impact the provision of heath care.
2. Discuss the effects of self stigma, or "shame," on seeking and receiving health care.
3. Describe specific aspects of obesity-related stigma.
4. Describe specific aspects of medical student and physician self stigma as it relates to depression and suicidality.
5. Discuss how physicians and medical students might reduce the effects of stigma in health care.

Clinical Vignette 13.1.1 Presenting Situation: Betty

Betty is a 32-year-old, morbidly obese woman who is pregnant with her first child. She presents to the emergency department at approximately 27-week gestation, weighing 425 pounds. She is unsure about her last menstrual period; therefore, the gestational age of the fetus is estimated by an ultrasound performed at her last visit to the emergency department. Betty is dressed in sweatpants and a t-shirt. She is carrying a large purse, and you see soda and candy wrappers sticking out. She has a bad odor about her, resulting perhaps from poor hygiene.

Betty has been experiencing lower back pain for approximately 2 days. The pain comes and goes. She reports good fetal movement. There is no vaginal bleeding or discharge.

You are the emergency room (ER) physician assigned to Betty you have been working long hours and you are halfway through a 14-h shift.

Please proceed with the problem-based approach using the worksheet located in the appendix of Chap. 1!

Visualize this patient and notice what emotional reactions come up in you. Be honest and write down what first comes to mind without censoring your responses. Please proceed with the problem-based approach. In this case, your thoughts, feelings, and behavior will be explored. The following table is modified from Chiles and Strohsahl (2004; Fig. 13.1)

	My response	**How I feel about my own response?**
What is your primary *positive* emotional response?		
What is your primary *negative* emotional response?		
What aspects of this person's situation and behavior elicit the most *negative* or *judgmental* response from you?		
What aspects of this person's situation and behavior elicit the most *positive* or *compassionate* response from you?		
What is the biggest barrier you would encounter continuing to interact with this person?		

Fig. 13.1 Betty

Case Vignette 13.1.2: Continuation
During her previous visits to the county hospital, ER employees became frustrated with Betty. She missed follow-up prenatal appointments and continued to use the emergency department for routine care. She reported concern that the pregnancy clinic staff "won't take me seriously."

Betty approaches the admission staff, who know her by name from her visit 3 weeks prior. You hear the staff say reprovingly: "You will have to wait your turn, Betty. Did you even see your obstetrician at the clinic, are you even concerned about your baby?"

While you are experiencing emotional negative, judgmental feelings about Betty, you are also aware that people with obesity are stigmatized in a very severe way, as the stigma of being overweight cannot be concealed and is seen as a controllable condition (Crocker et al. 1993).

13.2 Learning Issue: Stigma

The general term "stigma" refers to a process that has both high social/political and personal implications. Stigma refers to a process of judging a particular category of people based upon group membership. So a blond woman might be viewed as *flakey* or *fun*, an obese person might be viewed as *lazy* or *weak willed*, an addict might be viewed as *hopeless* and to *be feared*, a depressed medical student might be viewed as *incapable* and *weak*. Physical disability, mental illness, medical status, addiction, race, ethnicity, religion, and gender are a few examples of stigmatized groups.

While stigma takes many forms, the *process of stigma* may be understood as a process of attempting to avoid or suppress people, thoughts, or situations that give rise to discomfort. This process would be the same whether one is stigmatizing or avoiding another person or group (enacted stigma), or whether one is avoiding a feeling or cognition about oneself (self stigma).

Enacted Stigma Enacted stigma, or how we stigmatize others, is part of a process that, throughout history and continuing today, has given rise to the extermination of large groups of people defined ethnically, geographically, and religiously. With respect to this case, enacted stigma refers to judging and dehumanizing Betty, the obese pregnant patient, because of her obesity.

Self Stigma Self stigma refers to feelings of shame and negative thoughts about oneself because of one's membership in a particular stigmatized group. Feelings such as "why try, I'm such a loser…I'm obese, I'll never get that job…Doctor's never take me seriously, because I am so slovenly…" are all examples of statements reflecting self stigma.

13.3 Learning Issue: Weight Stigma

Overweight and obese people are pervasively stigmatized, including in employment settings, health-care settings, and romantic relationships. It is thought to be one of the last socially acceptable forms of discrimination (Vartanian et al. 2014). Literature suggests that while other conditions such as physical disability or being a member of a disadvantaged ethnic group can elicit empathy and sympathy, obese people do not receive that advantage (Chen and Brown 2005). Obesity is a dangerous epidemic, associated with many chronic disease conditions (e.g., US Department of Health and Human Services 2001). Medical professionals are known to have negative feelings about obese patients (Puhl and Heuer 2009). In fact, the Social Security Administration (http://www.disability-benefits-help.org/disabling-conditions/obesity-and-social-security-disability) does not list morbid obesity as a disabling condition. Furthermore, it is typical for insurance plans to exclude obesity treatment from coverage (Puhl and Brownell 2001). Such negative and judgmental feelings can lead to enacted stigma, that is, behavior that minimizes, marginalizes, and restricts opportunities to those with the stigmatized condition.

STOP

Please proceed with the problem-based approach using the worksheet located in the appendix of Chap. 1!

Now, imagine how Betty may feel and experience her interaction with health-care providers. Imagine *her* responses when filling out the table below (Fig. 13.2):

	Betty's response	**How Betty feels about her response?**
What is your primary *positive* emotional response to your health care providers?		
What is your primary *negative* emotional response to your health care providers?		
What is the biggest barrier you would encounter continuing to receive health care from these providers?		

Fig. 13.2 Betty's responses. (Adapted from Chiles and Stohsahl 2004)

13.4 Case 13.1.3 Continued

Betty leaves the ER in tears. You, as her health-care provider, are full of mixed feelings. Your peers share your feelings of discouragement and support your tendency to blame Betty for this difficult interaction. You feel justified and also feel worried about her likelihood of returning for the needed follow-up. You are worried about her unborn baby and also wish that the interaction had gone better. You are very glad to be off work after your shift, and you hope that if she returns, she will not be your patient.

Betty likely felt shamed and stigmatized as a result of her interactions with the health-care system (Puhl and Heuer 2009). Like many other patients with obesity, she may avoid health care, in order to avoid feeling so shamed and stigmatized (Vartanian et al. 2014). This kind of stigma, stigma that is internalized, is called felt stigma, and results in avoidance of situations that would bring about such feelings. How can this situation be improved, that is, how can the providers reduce enacted stigma and the patients reduce self stigma?

13.5 Learning Issue: Reducing the Impact of Enacted and Self Stigma

In every patient encounter, the physician brings biases about certain groups or categories of people based on their own experience. For example, a physician might negatively stigmatize a patient seeking pain medication if the physician him or herself has a history of a substance use disorder. In such an example, the patient might be inappropriately categorized as an addict, user, or drug seeker and denied treatment for pain. At the other end of the continuum, physicians may have a positive feeling about a patient, who may then not receive the care appropriate for their illness. For example, physicians are likely to assume adherence to medical regimens in patients with whom they are well acquainted, an assumption that may be false (Wailoo 2006).They may think, "I know this patient really well, and I'm sure they are taking their medications." The provider may not fully engage with the evaluation of the patient. Often, clinical judgments are based on outward features of a patient, previous actions, or membership in a certain group. This bias may result in suboptimal care because the details of the patient's medical problems are not assessed. At both ends of the continuum, enacted and self stigmatization describe how a physician judges a person and how that person responds, all leading to a distance between the patient's needs and their treatment.

Betty is a person who is among the most stigmatized in our society, due to her obesity. Her condition can give rise to enacted and self stigma, a process resulting in social isolation and rejection (Lazare 1997) and clearly impacting health care. In Betty's case, the physician might engage in negative enacted stigma, which might result in the following behaviors:

1. Failure to elicit Betty's concerns.
2. Inadequate time spent educating and treating her because of her past failure and her predicted failure to follow through in the future.
3. Blame toward Betty for her poor health.
4. Rationalization for not optimally engaging with this patient, followed by feelings of guilt, defeat, and burnout.

Betty may feel a great deal of shame about her present situation. She may, in fact, have avoided health care just because of her own shame around her condition (Lazare 1997). She may be afraid about pregnancy and being morbidly obese, and her avoidance of health care may be related to her attempts to not think about her own precarious health. After all, if she does not see a doctor, perhaps she can forget that she is, in fact, so overweight. Perhaps she can ignore her pregnancy and the addition of new responsibilities. In addition, she may be accurately afraid of coming in for help from past experiences of being stigmatized by health-care providers. In this situation, both enacted stigma and felt stigma are interacting to produce a very poor health-care outcome.

13.6 Learning Issue: How Might the Physician Improve This Situation?

First, it is important to note that it is not possible to completely eliminate judgmental thoughts and feelings from one's mind. Indeed, we are trained on many levels to make judgments of our patients in an attempt to evaluate and help them. These judgments include features of personality and risk factors for poor compliance and prognosis. When these judgments cause us to under-evaluate a patient, to treat them condescendingly or harshly, or to withhold our best intentions, then we begin the downward spiral of stigma. It is not possible to be without judgment but it is possible to decide not to allow one's actions toward patients to reflect these judgments. Physicians may strive to provide excellent health care even when their thoughts and feelings are inviting them to take short cuts that do not serve the patient's health-care needs.

To be more effective, think about how you might engage less with the judgmental thoughts and feelings you identified with this case, and focus on how to provide respectful, effective health care. In daily life, there are many examples where we behave effectively even when our thoughts and feelings dictate otherwise, such as going to work even when tired or depressed. It is possible to provide effective health care even when you feel discouraged and defeated by the patients themselves. These sensibilities are aspects of Acceptance and Commitment Therapy (Hayes et al. 1999).

13.7 Learning Issue: Avoiding Stigmatization

Here is an example of how one doctor might avoid stigmatizing Betty or another patient:

> Physician: "It is great you came in. I am glad you are here. You look really tired. Was it hard to get here?"
> Patient: "I'm so tired. The buses were all late and I had to borrow money for the fare. I'm not feeling good at all and I am worried about my baby…"
> Physician: "I'm glad you care so much. We want to help. I notice this is your fourth visit to the ER. It must be hard, but did you have chance to make it to your obstetrician appointment since we last saw you? Is there something that can be done to help make it easier for you to attend your outpatient appointments? I wonder if there is a way to get you some bus passes … would that help?"

In caring for a patient with felt stigma and shame, it could help to be empathic and to invite the patient to share what she may feel and to discuss how important it is to seek health care anyway. Much the way you have to learn to behave as a competent physician in spite of judgmental feelings, the patient must also take care of her body even when she is feeling ashamed (Fig. 13.3). For example:

> Physician: "Betty, I know how hard it must be to come in here. I know that many times, people who have had problems like this feel embarrassed and feel some shame. I am so glad that you are in here today; even though it is hard, and I am going to try really hard to have this visit go well for you."

How might you, as her physician, elicit the most *positive* and cooperative responses from Betty?	

How might you, as her physician, feel positive and engaged with Betty and proud of your medical care for her and her unborn child?	

Fig. 13.3 Strategies to improve physician and patient responses in Vignette 13.1

Vignette 13.1.4: Conclusion

Betty returns to the ER a few weeks later, just as a follow-up. You, her physician, notice your negative reactions, and also greet her warmly and thank her for returning. You notice that Betty is teary, and you ask her to tell you about what is wrong. She tells you that she is worried that her overweight might negatively impact her baby, and also tells you (while seeming very embarrassed) that she is trying to diet while pregnant. You lean toward her and discuss candidly her concerns, focusing on her commitment to her unborn child and on her desire to do what recommended for the duration of the pregnancy. You both leave that interaction feeling that effective, compassionate, care has been provided and has been received. You feel that you have done good work in this case, and are quite open to seeing Betty again.

Vignette 13.2.1 Presenting Situation: Mary

Mary is a 25-year-old medical student who is currently a clerk on your internal medicine service. You have worked with her for a few weeks, and saw her as bright and engaged. Of late, you notice that she seems tearful and withdrawn. She has been late, distracted, unprepared, and seems very fatigued. You notice bandages on her wrists. You ask her into your office to see if you can give her feedback about her sudden drop in performance.

Mary begins to cry, she notes she is not sleeping, has lost about 10 pounds in the last few weeks, her boyfriend broke up with her, and she feels totally unprepared for boards. She confides that her brother was recently diagnosed with cancer. She states she has been using alcohol for sleep, unsuccessfully. You ask her if she is receiving support from her peers or if she is in counseling or taking any psychiatric medication. She states "yeah, right, who has time for that...." You want to help her further, but she gets up and thanks you for your attention, assures you she is doing just fine, promises to do better, and rushes out of your office.

Please think about your reactions to Mary as her attending physician and work through the table below (Fig. 13.4):

	Please proceed with the problem-based approach using the worksheet located in the appendix of Chap. 1!

You are uncomfortable about Mary's behavior, as you want to believe in this talented medical student, and you do not want to negatively impact her training. You remember being a medical student, and you remember struggling with depression, and even using alcohol inappropriately, and how important it felt to hide it in order

	My response	**How I feel about my own response. Include both positive and negative feelings.**
What is your primary *positive* emotional response?		
What is your primary *negative* emotional response?		
What aspects of this person's situation and behavior elicit the most *negative* or *judgmental* response from you?		
What aspects of this person's situation and behavior elicit the most *positive* or *compassionate* response from you?		
What is the biggest barrier you would encounter continuing to interact with this person?		

Fig. 13.4 Responses to Mary

to not lose the confidence of your peers and teachers. The bandages on her wrists are very troubling to you, you want to ask her about them but do not want to embarrass her and also are unsure of what to do if she, in fact, has been engaging in suicidal behavior.

You are also aware that medical students have higher rates of depression, burnout, and mental illness than the general population, and that these issues tend to get worse as training continues (Schwenk et al. 2010). You are also aware that physicians commit suicide more than twice as often as nonphysicians, and that female physicians are particularly vulnerable. And you know that rates of suicidal thoughts occur in just under 10% of fourth-year medical students and residents (Goebert et al. 2009).

Now imagine how it might feel to be Mary, experiencing emotional struggles, and then being called in to her attending physician's office (Fig. 13.5).

Medical students experience significant enacted and felt stigma around their emotional struggles, depression, and suicidal ideation (Schwenk et al. 2010). That is, they are not only subject to significant stress and emotional struggle, but also feel that seeking help and revealing their struggles will negatively impact their careers. They also experience significant felt stigma, that is, they feel shame around admitting their vulnerability in a culture where appearing strong, independent, and competent is so highly valued (Fig. 13.6).

Mary is falling into the category of possibly having depression and may be abusing alcohol. You are not sure. She is also possibly cutting her wrists. These problems are very difficult for anyone, including physicians, to deal with. These

	Mary's response	Positive and negative effects on Mary
What might she have felt in her attending physicians office that felt positive to her? What might she have felt felt negative to her? What is her primary *positive* emotional response?		
What is her primary *negative* emotional response?		
What aspects of this situation and staff behavior elicit the most *negative* or *judgmental* response from her?		
What aspects of this situation and staff behavior elicit the most *positive* or *compassionate* response from her?		
What is the biggest barrier she would encounter in continuing to try to receive help?		

Fig. 13.5 Mary's feelings in Vignette 13.2

How might you encourage Mary to talk about her struggles and to be open to getting help and support?	

Fig. 13.6 Strategies to elicit the most positive and cooperative responses in Vignette 13.2

types of mental health issues are highly stigmatized in our culture. People with mental illness are often severely judged, feared, and given suboptimal health care (Corrigan 2005). Mary's dysfunctional behavior may be particularly difficult to accept because she is a medical student and may evoke particular responses on the part of the physician. In the area of substance abuse, enacted stigma is particularly severe, as it tends to evoke even greater negative social attitudes (Crisp et al. 2000).

Vignette 13.2.2 Conclusion
Mary is distraught during rounds later that day. You approach her again and offer to talk. She does not want to tell the attending physician that she is feeling hopeless because her boyfriend broke up with her and is feeling suicidal.

She fears he will not take her seriously as a student. The attending's pager beeps.

"I have some really acute patients to take care of Mary. What do you need right now?"

Mary cannot pinpoint what she needs. She does know that she feels intense anxiety about her relationship and her studies. She is suddenly unsure that she can trust the attending to maintain confidentiality.

"Nothing! I have nothing. I need nothing! I'll go home deal with it"

STOP — Please proceed with the problem-based approach using the worksheet located in the appendix of Chap. 1!

When physician judgments result in enacted stigma, the following may occur:

1. Referral to psychiatry immediately, without any discussion with Mary.
2. Minimization of the problems because of her medical student status, for example, "You will feel better after finals…"
3. Blame toward the patient for their poor health. "You didn't take your meds…"
4. Temporary feelings of justification in not having engaged with this patient; followed by feelings of defeat and burnout.

When physician judgments do not lead to enacted stigma, the following might occur:

1. Quality time spent with the student; genuine engagement with her and understanding of her problems; development of a thoughtful, collaborative referral if indicated.
2. Connection with her medical student status; empathy, and encouragement to take care of herself.
3. Assessment of her problems with adherence to medications, including an assessment of side effects, costs and benefits, and alternative treatment regimens.
4. Consultation from trusted colleagues about your own feelings about treating someone who is so distressed and yet may share a profession with you.

In this case, it is likely that Mary feels tremendous felt stigma or shame. Seeking treatment from the same people who teach and evaluate her is likely very difficult. She may, in fact, have avoided seeking help earlier due to her own shame about her condition. In addition, statistically, her suicide risk is high.

To be more effective with Mary, think about how you might engage less with your judgmental thoughts and feelings and focus more on the provision of respectful, effective health care. It is possible to provide effective health care even when you feel judgmental and defeated. Learning these skills will help you teach them to

Mary. Empathize with how she may be feeling under these conditions and reinforce her willingness to seek help when needed. Connect with Mary's value of taking care of herself and thus succeeding in her medical career.

13.8 Learning Issue: Avoiding Stigmatization

Please consider the following as one possible way to avoid stigmatizing Mary or another patient:

> Physician: "Mary, I understand you may feel uncomfortable because we know each other and I am your teacher. You have opened up to me a little, which I know is awkward, and I feel strongly that your courage is very admirable and a good step in taking care of yourself. I will do my best to keep what we discuss here between the two of us."
> Mary: "Thank you. I'm so upset. My boyfriend just broke up with me. I'm scared. I'm scared to be alone. And exams are coming. I can't focus or concentrate. I can't do what I need to do."
> Physician: "It's hard to focus when you are trying to sort out feelings. I am wondering if you are having feelings about harming yourself."
> Mary: "I've had those thoughts. That's probably what scares me the most. I have been cutting … see my wrists? It takes away the pain for a while and then it becomes unbearable all over again."
> Physician: "It must be hard for you to share this with me. You sound worried about your thoughts and feelings. I am concerned about you and want to make sure that you get the help you need. What is important is that you get help when you need it so that you can pursue your goals and stay healthy."

13.9 Conclusion

Avoiding the effects of stigma may well be the most difficult aspect of providing equal health care to all people. This may be the case because doing so requires the disciplined efforts of all health-care personnel to monitor their feelings and thoughts and to control their actions. Within groups, one person has the power to promote a culture of tolerance and compassion. Consider an internal medicine resident asking the staff psychiatrist to help him understand a patient with borderline personality disorder: "She has brought me to my wit's end … I can't stand her … I feel terrible." For a minute, the psychiatrist sits with the resident, validates his feelings, commends him for recognizing the problem in himself, and then states simply that this patient's emotional progress became retarded ever since she was raped at home as a teenager. "And so she still sees the world as a young teenager in many ways, even though she is well educated and physically very capable." The resident and the patient will benefit because the resident sought help to manage his feelings of frustration and burn out, and a senior colleague took time to think the problem through.

13.10 Discussion Questions

1. Why do you think enacted stigma causes others to feel shame? What kind of verbal and nonverbal signals have you seen people use to send this demeaning signal to others?
2. Why should a patient's self-imposed stigma burden a physician who is adequately treating the patient otherwise?
3. What specific personal goals can you make to reduce the demoralizing and debilitating effects of stigma of your working environment?
4. When is shame a positive emotion? When is shame a negative emotion? When have you felt stigma in your life? How can you ward off the ill effects of this stigma?

References

Chen, E. Y., & Brown, M. (2005). Obesity stigma in sexual relationships. *Obesity, 13*(8), 1393–1397.

Chiles, J., & Strosahl, K. (2004). *Clinical manual for assessment and treatment of suicidal behavior*. Washington D.C.: American Psychiatric Publishing.

Corrigan, P. W. (2005). *On the stigma of mental illness: Practical strategies for research and social change*. Washington, D.C.: APA. http://dx.doi.org/10.1037/10887–000.

Crisp, A. H., Gelder, M. G., Rix, S., Meltzer, H. I., & Rowlands, O. J. (2000). Stigmatisation of people with mental illnesses. *British Journal of Psychiatry, 177*, 4–7.

Crocker, J., Cornwell, B., & Major, B. (1993). The stigma of overweight: Affective consequences of attributional ambiguity. *Journal of Personality and Social Psychology, 64*(1), 60–70.

Goebert, D., Thompson, D., Takeshita, J., Beach, C., Bryson, P., Ephgrave, K., et al. (2009). Depressive symptoms in medical students and residents: A multischool study. *Academic Medicine, I*, 236–241. doi:10.1097/ACM.0b013e31819391bb.

Hayes, S. C., Strosahl, K., & Wilson, K. G. (1999). *Acceptance and commitment therapy: An experiential approach to behavior change*. New York: Guilford Press.

Lazare, A. (1997). Shame, humiliation, and stigma in the medical interview. In M. Lansky & A. Morrison (Ed.), *The widening scope of shame* (pp. 383–396). NJ: Analytic Press.

Puhl, R. M., & Brownell, K. D. (2001). Bias, discrimination and obesity. *Obesity Research, 9*(12), 788–805.

Puel, R., & Heuer, C. A. (2009). The stigma of obesity: A review and update. *Obesity, 17*, 941–964.

Schwenk, T., Davis, L., & Wimsatt, L. (2010Depression, stigma, and suicidal ideation in medical students. I, Sep 15;304(11):1181–90. doi: 10.1001/jama.2010.1300. Washington, DC, APA, http://dx.doi.org.

US Dept of Health and Human Services. (2001). *The surgeon general's call to action to prevent and decrease overweight and obesity*. Rockville: U.S. Department of Health and Human Services.

Vartanian, L. R., Pinkus, R. T., & Smyth, J. M. (2014). The phenomenology of weight stigma in everyday life. *Journal of Contextual Behavioral Science, 3*(3), 196–202.

Wegner, D. M. (1994). Ironic processes of mental control. *Psychological Review, 101*, 34–52.

Wailoo, K. (2006). Stigma, race, and disease in 20th century America. *Lancet, 367*, 531–533.

Chapter 14
Culture, Ethnicity, and Medicine

Anthony P. S. Guerrero and Asad Ghiasuddin

Culture is a part of who we are and how we manage our health and illnesses. During training, most physicians are confronted with people who represent cultures and values that are remarkably different from their own background. This chapter offers information on approaching cultural differences.

At the end of this chapter, the readers will be able to:

1. Discuss the definitions of culture and culturally competent care
2. Discuss ethnic factors that can impact the epidemiology and presentation of common medical illnesses
3. Approach situations in which culture may impact help-seeking behavior and treatment adherence
4. Be familiar with DSM-5 section on cultural formulation

Case Vignette 14.1.1 Pinky

"Pinky" is a 7-year-old female brought by her mother to the pediatrician for symptoms of acute gastroenteritis. The mother recently immigrated to the USA, and speaks English as a second language. While the physician and patient share the same ethnic background, the physician was born and raised in the USA.

Mother: So what does my daughter have?

Physician: It seems that your daughter may have a stomach flu, and that's why she's having the stomachaches and diarrhea.

Mother: What medicine does she need?

A. P. S. Guerrero (✉) · A. Ghiasuddin
Department of Psychiatry, John A. Burns School of Medicine, University of Hawai'i,
1356 Lusitana Street, University Tower 4th Floor, Honolulu, HI 96813, USA
e-mail: GuerreroA@dop.hawaii.edu

A. Ghiasuddin
e-mail: ghiasuddina@dop.hawaii.edu

D. Alicata et al. (eds.), *Problem-based Behavioral Science and Psychiatry*,
DOI 10.1007/978-3-319-23669-8_14

Physician: Actually, she doesn't need medicine at this time. Because it's a virus, there's no antibiotic that can treat this. She needs to drink a lot of fluids, though.

Mother: Is she normal, then?

Physician: Not necessarily "normal," but certainly, this is "common."

Mother: So she just needs to drink more? (almost crying)

Physician: I think that's what would help her the most.

Mother: (silence, definitely crying at this point)

Physician: I'm sorry to see that you're crying. Can you tell me what you're thinking?

Mother: Nothing, really…

Please proceed with the problem-based approach using the worksheet located in the appendix of Chap. 1!

Please fill in the facts, your hypotheses, further information needed, and learning issues for Learning Issue Table 14.1.1.

Learning Issue Table 14.1.1

FACTS	HYPOTHESES	INFORMATION NEEDED	LEARNING ISSUES

Basic Principles and Definitions Whether or not we believe that a patient is from a "culture" different from our own, it is important to recognize that in every patient encounter, we bring with us a set of assumptions and styles of communication that undoubtedly affect the care the patient receives. In the above case, in which the parent seems confused and upset over what would ordinarily be a routine explanation for a benign acute illness, any of the following may have occurred:

- Physician's failure to elicit (or recognize the need to elicit) what the parent is most worried about and/or what the parent feels the child needs most at this time (e.g., medication)
- A language barrier, in which terms such as "virus" and "not normal but common" do not necessarily provide the intended reassurance
- Physician's assumption that asking directly "what are you thinking" is the most effective way to elicit concerns or questions
- Parent's fear that they will not be able to satisfactorily explain the child's illness to the decision-maker or authoritative figure in the family (who was unable to make this visit)

Case Vignette 14.1.2
Concerned and perplexed, you consult with your front office receptionist, who is able to speak in the native language with the mother. As it turns out, Pinky's mother is concerned that her own mother (child's grandmother) will be upset if the child does not go home with a medication. The mother seemed relieved as further explanation was given while the grandmother was on the telephone.

Traditionally, culture has been defined along the lines of values, beliefs, and/or practices shared by populations of people. Obviously, culture is not the same as "ethnicity" or "race," as there can be many different types of "culture" (e.g., the medical culture) that have nothing to do with race—which is not even universally accepted as a valid concept.

Lewis-Fernandez and Kleinman (1995) have defined culture as the *"processes* that emerge out of the patterns of everyday social life—taken-for-granted common sense, historically determined ways of being and doing, preferred forms of ordinary interpersonal interaction, socially elaborated bodily states." We will use this definition for the purposes of this chapter.

The DSM-5 provides a revised outline for cultural formulation to systematically assess:

1. The cultural identity of the individual, including race, ethnicity, immigrant status, and language abilities
2. Cultural conceptualization of distress, including cultural syndromes and coping/help seeking behaviors
3. Psychosocial stressors and cultural features of vulnerability and resilience, including the role of family, religion, and social networks
4. Cultural features of the relationship between the individual and the clinician
5. Overall cultural assessment, summarizing the implications of the above factors on diagnosis and treatment.

Adaptiveness of Diversity We believe that culture—like anything else for which "differences" among people exist—is best understood as something that must have been adaptive. In order to provide optimal care for a diverse patient group, this principle is important to consider, in terms of both medical/biological issues and social/cultural issues.

Case Vignette 14.2.1: Presenting Situations—Junior, John-boy, and Lisa
You are a busy pediatrician at a community health center in a large west-coast city. The following are vignettes from your practice:

Junior, a 3-day old Filipino-Caucasian male infant, comes to your office for a routine post-hospitalization check. He is feeding both breast milk and formula. He is jaundiced to the mid-trunk. Mother is O+, and baby is also O+, Coombs' negative. You wonder how much you should be concerned about the jaundice, since it does not appear that there are obvious risk factors.

John-boy, a 7-year-old Pacific Islander boy, comes in with a stuffy nose, headache, fever, and a history of ill contacts. His throat was mildly sore in the beginning but not now. On exam, his throat is minimally red, no exudates or adenopathy. You wonder whether you should obtain other studies. Although this is not a well-child check (and therefore only his weight is measured and not his height or body mass index (BMI)), you notice that he is significantly overweight.

Lisa, a 17-year-old Japanese female, comes in with nausea, vomiting, and headaches. She was recently started on escitalopram by her psychiatrist, who was concerned that there may be other causes of her physical symptoms, since the starting dose given of the medication was very small.

Please proceed with the problem-based approach using the worksheet located in the appendix of Chap. 1!

Please fill in the facts, your hypotheses, further information needed, and learning issues for Learning Issue Table 14.2.1.

Learning Issue Table 14.2.1

FACTS	HYPOTHESES	INFORMATION NEEDED	LEARNING ISSUES

Culturally competent care implies not only integrating awareness of cultural dynamics (as illustrated in the first case) into the patient care encounter, but also considering biologically mediated differences—whether they correspond to ethnicity, gender, or other classification—that may impact medical care. While it is likely true that there is little biological reality behind the entire concept of "race," it is undeniably true that there are populational differences (even within "races") in disease prevalence, drug metabolism, and dietary practices. Similar to how "cultural" differences must have had an adaptive function, such biological differences are also likely a product of evolution and adaptation to environment. Some examples are summarized in Table 14.1.

Table 14.1 Potential adaptiveness of certain genotypes associated with certain illnesses and other conditions

Phenotype	Higher prevalence in	*Possible* evolutionary adaptive role of associated genotype
Cystic fibrosis	Caucasians	Protection against cholera (Bertranpetit and Calafell 1996)
Thalassemia	Southeast Asians, Mediterranean peoples	Protection against malaria (Kwiatkowski 2005)
Glucose-6-phosphate dehydrogenase deficiency	Southeast Asians, Mediterranean, and African peoples	Protection against malaria (Kwiatkowski 2005)
Obesity, diabetes mellitus, metabolic syndrome, in the context of Western diets	Pacific Islanders, other indigenous peoples	Energy conservation during prolonged periods of limited food access (Chukwuma and Tuomilehto 1998)
Lactose *tolerance* (rather than intolerance)	Caucasians	Ability to have dairy products as part of diet
Aldehyde dehydrogenase *non*-deficiency	Non-Asians	Ability to have fermented drinks as part of diet

Table 14.1 (continued)

Rheumatic fever	Polynesians (Kurahara et al. 2002)	Immunogenetic factors that otherwise may confer protection against other rheumatological illnesses and possibly infections
Cytochrome P450 2C19 ultra-metabolizer	North Africans, Middle Easterners (de Leon et al. 2006)	Role in detoxification

Case Vignette 14.2.2

Regarding Junior, your newborn patient, you astutely ask further details about the infant's ethnicity and learn that the mother identifies herself as pure Filipino. You also inquire about any family history of any blood problems or dietary restrictions, and you learn that there is a maternal male cousin who was jaundiced as an infant and who needed to avoid certain foods and medications. You therefore order (in addition to your usual tests) a test for glucose-6-phosphate dehydrogenase and monitor the child very carefully over the next few days.

Regarding John-boy, the 7-year-old boy, you appropriately query whether or not existing practice guidelines for the evaluation of possible streptococcal pharyngitis are truly applicable to your population. You decide to obtain a throat culture, which proves to be positive for group A beta-hemolytic streptococcus. You also provide the patient and parent counseling on diet and activity, attempting to be sensitive to: the family's indigenous dietary preferences, the role of other family members in the child's care, and other realities (e.g., expense of healthier meals, access to safe recreational areas, etc.) related to their socioeconomic status. Finally, given the prevalence of childhood obesity in your practice, you decide to implement new clinic protocols to adequately screen for and manage obesity (also refer to Chap. 27).

Regarding Lisa, your 17-year-old patient, you conduct a history and physical examination and conclude that an adverse reaction to the escitalopram is the most likely cause of her symptoms. You research the drug metabolism of escitalopram and discover that it is metabolized by cytochrome P450 2C19 and that 10–25% of East Asians are, in fact, cytochrome P450 2C19 poor metabolizers (de Leon et al. 2006). You communicate with her psychiatrist, who eventually is able to successfully treat her using an alternate medication.

While a discussion of all diseases that vary in prevalence by ethnicity is beyond the scope of this textbook, we advocate that culturally competent physicians should be of the mindset that certain conditions may affect certain ethnic groups more than others presumably because of evolutionary adaptation and not because any ethnic group is inferior or superior to the other.

Reducing Health Disparities We also advocate that culturally competent physicians should consider social and environmental factors that may lead to health disparities among cultural and ethnic groups.

Case Vignette 14.3.1: Presenting Situation—Sammy
You are a family physician who is seeing Sammy, a 25-year-old Pacific Islander male with a history of a seizure disorder. He is intermittently homeless in urban Honolulu and receives inconsistent primary medical care. The record indicates a long history of "noncompliance" and subtherapeutic levels of his anticonvulsant medications. Before you enter the room, your more senior colleagues tell you that he only comes back for appointments whenever he needs bus pass form signed. You begin to wonder how you will address issues of compliance in this patient.

STOP

Please proceed with the problem-based approach using the worksheet located in the appendix of Chap. 1!

Please fill in the facts, your hypotheses, further information needed, and learning issues for Learning Issue Table 14.3.1.

Learning Issue Table 14.3.1

FACTS	HYPOTHESES	INFORMATION NEEDED	LEARNING ISSUES

As suggested in Chap. 10, apparent "noncompliance" should be viewed as a clinical finding that has its own set of differential possibilities. The above case illustrates possible causes for "noncompliance" that should be considered by the culturally competent clinician, in particular:

- Is the regimen too costly for the patient?
- Does the patient metabolize a medication in an unexpected way (leading to too many side effects or inadequate response)?
- Does the patient have alternative beliefs about the illness, including etiology and treatment?
- Does the patient have adequate social support or access to resources?
- Does the patient have an interfering psychiatric illness, the symptoms of which are underreported because of the stigma of mental illness?
- Are there language barriers that prevent adequate explanations from being given?
- Did the clinician fail to involve key family members who are important in the patient's care?

Case Vignette 14.3.2

Sammy insists, with a somewhat bland affect, that he has been taking the medications. He is able to repeat (again with a bland affect) that he has a "seizure problem" and that the medications are "for the seizures."

He denies any other medical or psychiatric illnesses, including substance abuse. A review of records indicates that neuroimaging done several years ago was negative and that he has had several missed appointments with the neurologist. Although he denies any history of depression, he admits to not being quite as talkative as he used to be. He denies any use of herbal medications or visits to a traditional healer for his condition.

When he is not on the streets, he lives with a few of his girlfriend's extended family. He is a migrant to Hawai'i. English is a second language for him; however, he is able to converse fluently and appears to understand most of the explanations given. He denies that there is anyone else who is significantly involved in making decisions about his treatment or in implementing treatment recommendations. He does, however, often rely on his girlfriend for transportation, as he does not feel comfortable driving given the history of his seizure disorder. He is on government-supported health insurance, which completely covers the cost of his medications. He denies any unusual stressors in his life other than his illness.

Please proceed with the problem-based approach using the worksheet located in the appendix of Chap. 1!

Please fill in the facts, your hypotheses, further information needed, and learning issues for Learning Issue Table 14.3.2.

Learning Issue Table 14.3.2

FACTS	HYPOTHESES	INFORMATION NEEDED	LEARNING ISSUES

There are numerous examples of health disparities in medicine, which are likely explained by complex interactions between biological, social, and environmental factors. Prominent examples, according to the Centers for Disease Control and Prevention (CDC), are summarized in Table 14.2 (CDC 2009).

Table 14.2 Disparities in prevalence of illness by ethnicity

Condition	Higher in
Infant mortality	African Americans, Native Americans, Puerto Ricans
Mortality from cervical cancer	African Americans
Mortality from breast cancer	Caucasian Americans
Death from cardiovascular disease	African Americans
Diabetes mellitus	Native Americans and Alaska Natives
AIDS	African Americans and Hispanics
Underimmunization for influenza and pneumococcus in the elderly	Hispanics and African Americans
Depression and substance abuse	Native Americans and Alaska Natives
Hepatitis B	Asians and Pacific Islanders
Syphilis	African Americans
Tuberculosis	Asians and Pacific Islanders

It is also important to minimize cultural barriers and stigma (see Chap. 13) that may occur on the individual clinician level. Use of the DSM-5 cultural formulation interview, a set of 16 questions used to assess cultural factors in the clinical encounter, may aid in this regard. It uses a person-centered approach to assess each individual's interpretation of his or her illness and help seeking, and is designed to avoid stereotyping by culture (American Psychiatric Association 2013).

Case Vignette 14.3.3
You refer Sammy to a psychiatrist, who happens to be co-located in the clinic, for possible depression. Because of subtle cognitive findings and the history of neurological disorder, the psychiatrist suggests a follow-up neuroimaging study, which actually shows a localized infection in an anatomic location that fully explains the seizures experienced by the patient, as well as the blunted affect and potentially poor judgment. Following medical treatment of the brain infection, his affect appears to brighten, and he no longer has issues of non-compliance. He is able to sustain employment and reasonably stable housing.

In summary, when approaching the issue of health disparities, the culturally competent clinician should be mindful that (1) a patient may be at risk for certain illnesses as a consequence of living in a biological/psychological/social environment different from what they may be initially adapted to (e.g., a dark-skinned person being at risk for vitamin D deficiency in a polar latitude, or a light-skinned person being at risk for skin cancer in an equatorial latitude), and (2) cultural differences between the clinician and the patient may prevent optimal diagnosis and treatment of illness (as illustrated in Vignette 14.1). We close with the following case:

Case Vignette 14.4.1: Presenting Situation—Julius
You are a supervising physician in a pediatric clinic. Your resident raises the concern that Julius, a mixed Asian/Pacific Islander toddler, seen for a well-child check, has on his back several marks that might suggest abuse. Your resident states, "This almost feels like a board review question… where they're sort of checking our so-called cultural competence. I thought about coining and cupping as indigenous healing practices, but these marks don't look like they come from coins or cups. I also thought about Mongolian spots, and these definitely don't look like them. I really think these were inflicted by a hand. I hate to stereotype, but I've heard from other families that corporal punishment is standard discipline in certain cultures."

Please proceed with the problem-based approach using the worksheet located in the appendix of Chap. 1!

Please fill in the facts, your hypotheses, further information needed, and learning issues for Learning Issue Table 14.4.1.

Learning Issue Table 14.4.1

FACTS	HYPOTHESES	INFORMATION NEEDED	LEARNING ISSUES

You and the resident examine the patient together, and you confirm that this likely is a case of child abuse, probably inflicted by the stepfather. You inform the mother, who becomes tearful, that you will need to involve child protective services.

You commend the resident for identifying a case of child abuse, which is likely under-identified in primary care practice (see Chap. 7). You encourage the resident to critically appraise the notion that child abuse could ever be a culturally acceptable or adaptively advantageous practice. You discuss the principle of “acculturative stress,” and help the resident to elicit the further history that this child’s family, in immigrating to the USA lost the strong extended family and community network that they otherwise would have had in their native countries, experienced significant financial stress, and became exposed to substances of abuse that would have been relatively absent in their traditional culture. Your resident is grateful for your instruction and plans to integrate knowledge of these issues into a comprehensive, “bio-psycho-social-cultural-spiritual” (see Chap. 1) treatment plan to prevent child further child abuse, should this child ever return to the mother’s care.

14.1 Review Question

1. Which of the following could be called “effective habits” of the culturally competent clinician:

   a. Evaluating one’s own style of communication with patients
   b. Asking patients how they understand their condition and its treatment

   c. Knowledge about ethnic differences in risk for certain conditions and response to treatment
   d. Advocacy for improving access to care and reducing health disparities
   e. All of the above

2. Culture can be defined as:

   a. "*Processes* that emerge out of the patterns of everyday social life—taken-for-granted common sense, historically determined ways of being and doing, preferred forms of ordinary interpersonal interaction, socially elaborated bodily states"
   b. Something that is synonymous with race or ethnicity
   c. Something that is not important when it comes to health care

3. Which of the following are elements of the DSM-5 outline for cultural formulation?

   a. Cultural identity of the individual
   b. Cultural conceptualization of distress
   c. Psychosocial stressors and cultural features of vulnerability and resilience
   d. Cultural features of the relationship between the individual and the clinician
   e. Overall cultural assessment
   f. All of the above

4. Nervios in Latin America, Nerva among Greeks in North America, Nierbi among Sicilian in North America, and Nerves among whites in Appalachia and Newfoundland are related ________________

   a. Idioms of distress
   b. Classic DSM-5 psychiatric disorders
   c. Discredited syndromes

5. The ________________ is a 16-item semistructured interview for systematically assessing cultural factors in the clinical encounter that may be used with any individual. It is a person-centered approach that is designed to avoid stereotyping

   a. Minnesota Multiphasic Personality Inventory
   b. Cultural Formulation Interview
   c. Vineland Adaptive Behavior Scale

Appendix A: Tables with Possible Answers to the Vignettes

Case Vignette 14.1: Presenting Situation—Pinky

Case 1: Basic Principles and Definitions

Learning Issue Table 14.1.1

Facts	Hypotheses	Information needed	Learning issues
7-year-old child with acute gastroenteritis, and mother	Mother does not understand diagnosis?	More info needed on cultural and familial context of this situation	Define culture, race, and ethnicity
Recent immigrants	Mother does not believe diagnosis?		Be familiar with the DSM-5 Outline for Cultural Formulation
ESL	Mother is worried about another possible cause of child's illness?		
Mother crying when told of child's diagnosis	Mother feels inadequate or has her own mental health issues?		
	Language barrier?		
	Are there other people involved in the child's care?		

Case Vignette 14.2: Presenting Situations—Junior, John-boy, and Lisa
Case 2: Adaptiveness of Diversity
Learning Issue Table 14.2.1

Facts	Hypotheses	Need to know	Learning issues
Filipino-Caucasian newborn with jaundice	Physiologic jaundice since no obvious risk factors? Or something more to consider?	Does ethnicity or family history put this child at risk for jaundice?	Culturally competent clinicians should be aware that certain conditions may affect certain ethnic groups more than others
7-year-old Pacific Islander (PI) boy, overweight, with stuffy nose, headache, fever	Need for a throat culture? How to address obesity?	Do current treatment guidelines for strep throat apply to this patient?	
17-year-old Japanese female with nausea, vomiting, and headache, recently started in escitalopram	Is this a drug reaction or is there another cause for her symptoms?	What role do culture and family play in managing this child's obesity?	
		How is escitalopram metabolized?	
		Does Patient's (pts) ethnicity put her at higher risk for a possible drug reaction?	

Case Vignette 14.3: Presenting Situation—Sammy
Case 3: Reducing Health Disparities
Learning Issue Table 14.3.1

Facts	Hypotheses	Information needed	Learning issues
25-year-old PI male	Possible contributors to "noncompliance"	Patient's cultural context	Be aware that cultural factors may place certain groups at risk for certain illnesses
Seizures	Cost of medication	What is a useful tool for evaluating cultural factors in a clinical encounter?	Cultural differences between clinician and patient may pose a barrier at times
Intermittently homeless	Unexpected metabolism of medication	What is patient's health insurance?	Be familiar with the DSM-5 Cultural Formulation Interview
Inconsistent primary medical care	Language barrier		
Needs bus pass form to be completed	Inadequate support network		
	No transportation		
"Noncompliance"			

Case Vignette 14.4: Presenting Situation—Julius
Case 4: Cultural Concepts of Distress
Learning Issue Table 14.4.1

Facts	Hypotheses	Information needed	Learning issues
Mixed Asian/PI toddler with bruises	Child abuse?	Cultural context of child and family, including traditional healing methods	Culturally competent physician needs to be aware of DSM-5 Cultural Concepts of Distress, including:
	Occult medical illness?	Thorough medical examination	1. Cultural syndromes
	Cultural healing practice? (Cupping?)		2. Cultural idioms of distress
			3. Cultural explanations or perceived causes
			As well as traditional healing practices

Appendix B: Answers to Review Questions

1. e
2. a
3. e
4. a
5. b

References

American Psychiatric Association. (2013). Cultural formulation. In American Psychiatric Association (Ed.), *Diagnostic and statistical manual of mental disorders* (5th ed.).

Bertranpetit, J., & Calafell, F. (1996). Genetic and geographical variability in cystic fibrosis: Evolutionary considerations. *Ciba Found Symposium, 197,* 97–114 (discussion 114–118).

CDC Office of Minority Health. (2009). Eliminating racial & ethnic health disparities. http://www.cdc.gov/omhd/About/disparities.htm. Accessed 20 Nov 2015.

Chukwuma, C. Sr., & Tuomilehto, J. (1998). The 'thrifty' hypotheses: Clinical and epidemiological significance for non-insulin-dependent diabetes mellitus and cardiovascular disease risk factors. *Journal of Cardiovascular Risk, 5*(1), 11–23.

de Leon, J., Armstrong, S. C., & Cozza, K. L. (2006). Clinical guidelines for psychiatrists for the use of pharmacogenetic testing for CYP450 2D6 and CYP450 2C19. *Psychosomatics, 47,* 75–85.

Kurahara, D., Tokuda, A., Grandinetti, A., Najita, J., Ho, C., Yamamoto, K., Reddy, D. V., Macpherson, K., Iwamuro, M., & Yamaga, K. (2002). Ethnic differences in risk for pediatric rheumatic illness in a culturally diverse population. *Journal of Rheumatology, 29*(2), 379–383.

Kwiatkowski, D. P. (2005). How malaria has affected the human genome and what human genetics can teach us about malaria. *American Journal of Human Genetics, 77*(2), 171–192.

Lewis-Fernandez, R., & Kleinman, A. (1995). Cultural psychiatry. Theoretical, clinical, and research issues. *Psychiatrics Clinics of North America, 18*(3), 433–448. (Review).

Chapter 15
Quantitative Measures in Health Care

M. Anand Samtani, Earl S. Hishinuma and Deborah A. Goebert

Medical students often ask themselves, "Why should I learn statistics for my future medical practice?" Statistical techniques are used in just about every discipline and profession as tools to organize and analyze data. In medicine, it is essential to have a basic understanding of statistics to:

1. Critically understand and interpret studies in the medical literature
2. Properly conduct well-designed studies on human participants
3. Make informed and sound decisions about existing and new medications and treatments for one's clinical practice (source: Appleton (1990, p. 1013))

At the end of this chapter, the reader will be able to:

1. Discuss fundamental concepts of statistical measurement
2. Discuss fundamental concepts of study design
3. Describe fundamental concepts of hypothesis testing and statistical inference
4. Interpret the medical literature with basic statistical concepts

The primary goal of this chapter is to provide the students with a fundamental knowledge of the statistical tools relevant to clinical practice and clinical research. This chapter assumes some basic knowledge of quantitative measurements.

M. A. Samtani (✉)
Department of Commerce and Consumer Affairs, Public Utilities Commission, Research Section, 465 South King Street, #103, Honolulu, HI 96813, USA
e-mail: mohan.a.samtani@hawaii.gov

E. S. Hishinuma · D. A. Goebert
Department of Psychiatry, University of Hawai'i John A. Burns School of Medicine, 1356 Lusitana Street, University Tower 4th Floor, Honolulu, HI 96813, USA
e-mail: hishinumae@dop.hawaii.edu

D. A. Goebert
e-mail: goebertd@dop.hawaii.edu

D. Alicata et al. (eds.), *Problem-based Behavioral Science and Psychiatry*,
DOI 10.1007/978-3-319-23669-8_15

Case Vignette 15.1.1 Melinda

Melinda, a fourth-year medical student, presents a patient at the state mental hospital at the weekly case conference. This patient had been diagnosed with bipolar disorder with psychotic features, has been on a certain atypical antipsychotic (with supposedly fewer extrapyramidal side effects) for several years, and is now exhibiting Parkinson-like symptoms. After discussion at morning report, Melinda is asked to present an article on drug-related movement disorders.

One week later, Melinda presents an article titled "Predicting the incidence of antipsychotic-induced movement disorders in long-stay patients," published in *Epidemiology and Psychiatric Services* (Bakker et al. 2013). She recounts the case she presented the previous week. She discusses the link between long-term use of antipsychotic drugs and movement disorders commonly found in Parkinsonism. Following her presentation, the attending psychiatrist (who is well known for successfully mentoring students and residents in clinical research) proposes that she should investigate the topic further by conducting her own research project on movement disorders in patients treated with this particular antipsychotic at their facility.

The attending psychiatrist explains that before Melinda can embark on her project, she has to consider several key elements in selecting a study design and analyzing the collected data.

Please proceed with the problem-based approach using the worksheet located in the appendix of Chap. 1!

Please fill in the facts, your hypotheses, further information needed, and learning issues in the Learning Issue Table 15.1.

Learning Issue Table 15.1

FACTS	HYPOTHESES	INFORMATION NEEDED	LEARNING ISSUES

Table 15.1 Study designs

Type of study	Experimental/ observational	Analytical/ descriptive	Retrospective/ prospective	Description/ examples	Advantages	Disadvantages
Case-control	Observational	Analytical	Retrospective	A study design that compares two existing groups that differ on an outcome (e.g., disease)	Economical	More difficulty making causal statements because of confounding variables
				Often used to study rare diseases	Data can be analyzed relatively quickly (Kuzma 1992)	
				Examines the outcome to determine the possible risk factors		
				Case group: participants with disease		
				Control group: participants without the disease		
				Odds ratio often used in analysis		

Table 15.1 (continued)

Type of study	Experimental/ observational	Analytical/ descriptive	Retrospective/ prospective	Description/ examples	Advantages	Disadvantages
Cohort	Observational	Analytical	Prospective; it can also be retrospective	As a prospective study: data are collected over a determined period of time	Better control over sample selection and data collected	More costly and time-intensive
				The influence of the selected risk factors on the outcome is examined in the group exposed to vs. the group not exposed to the risk factors	Prospective study design reduces bias	
Cross-sectional	Observational	Descriptive	Retrospective/ prospective	Examines relationship of variables at a specific point in time. It is a snapshot view of what is happening	Requires fewer resources and time than longitudinal designs	More difficulty making causal statements because of lack of longitudinal data and confounding variables
				Often used to assess prevalence		
				Example: a political poll		

Table 15.1 (continued)

Type of study	Experimental/ observational	Analytical/ descriptive	Retrospective/ prospective	Description/ examples	Advantages	Disadvantages
Case series	Observational	Descriptive	Retrospective/ prospective	A descriptive study of a group with common attributes, experiences, etc.	Relatively straightforward without a comparison group	More difficulty making causal statements because of confounding variables and lack of comparison group
				Also used to determine the association between exposure to a particular factor and outcome	Less costly	
				Data may include personal background and diagnoses		
Community surveys	Observational	Descriptive	Prospective	A study designed (e.g., questionnaires and surveys) to provide a basic understanding of a selected community (e.g., demographic, concerns, opinions)	Provides the opportunity to obtain more community-based data and information	Accuracy of community-based information dependent upon the representativeness of the data

Table 15.1 (continued)

Type of study	Experimental/ observational	Analytical/ descriptive	Retrospective/ prospective	Description/ examples	Advantages	Disadvantages
Longitudinal studies	Observational	Analytical	Retrospective/ prospective	A study where a sample is tracked and measured at multiple time points	Ability to detect individual changes	More costly and time-consuming
					Eliminates confounding of studies that rely on the recall of the participants	Requires larger sample sizes for data analysis and representativeness
					Potential to make temporal and perhaps causal statements	Possible high attrition rate across longer durations

Table 15.1 (continued)

Type of study	Experimental/ observational	Analytical/ descriptive	Retrospective/ prospective	Description/ examples	Advantages	Disadvantages
Clinical trials	Experimental	Analytical	Prospective	Apply intervention (e.g., therapy, new drugs, procedure) to one of the groups studied to determine its effects against a control group (receiving a placebo intervention or the standard treatment)	Offers more robust data (reduces bias) and is considered the "gold standard" in research	More time and capital-intensive
				Often single- or double-blinded measures (in which either the patient or both the patient and the administrator do not know whether what is being administered is a placebo or active treatment)		
				Example: testing whether a new drug is more effective than the current drug for a particular disease		

Table 15.1 (continued)

Type of study	Experimental/observational	Analytical/descriptive	Retrospective/prospective	Description/examples	Advantages	Disadvantages
Community intervention trials	Experimental	Analytical	Prospective	Experiments are done at the community rather than the individual level (as with clinical trials)	May increase external validity, i.e., the generalizability of the results to the community members	Requires significant coordination with community leaders (e.g., community advocates and tribal and religious leaders)

15.1 Learning Issues

In this section, we break down Melinda's project into 15 discrete steps. Her chances of success are significantly increased if she is able to think through each of the 15 steps and get help with the research design and data analysis *before* she starts her project.

1. Identify the research question:
    a. What is the primary research question of your study?
    b. Write down your research hypothesis (i.e., your proposed theory to answer your research question).
    c. Identify other goals/objectives of your study.
2. Conduct a literature review:
    a. Are there similar studies that have been conducted?
    b. What new idea or information can you contribute?
3. Select the appropriate study design:
    a. Decide on the type of study.

After the research question has been defined, selecting the right type of study design is essential to the success of the project. The aim and research question(s) of your study must fit the study design.

There are many ways to categorize study designs. Here, studies are classified into two main groups: observational and experimental. Experimental studies involve indirect and/or direct intervention by the investigator(s) during the data collection process, whereas observational studies require no intervention in the collection process. Many experimental studies require informed consent from the participants.

In general, experimental studies are considered more rigorous than other studies because these studies are prospective in nature (i.e., current and future data are collected vs. past data in a retrospective study) and there is more control over the participants and treatment(s). However, experimental studies usually require more protocols, institutional review board (IRB) oversight, and expenses. Table 15.1 describes the types of studies:

1. Observational studies: These studies involve no intervention with the participants/patients and treatments used in the study. Many study designs fall under this category. They include cohort, case-control, cross-sectional, case series, and community surveys.
2. Experimental studies: These studies involve intervention (e.g., treatment) on the part of the investigator(s). Studies under this category include clinical trials and community intervention trials.
   Refer to Table 15.1 for a summary of the different study designs.

4. Select tools for measurement (scales, types of measurement)

Table 15.2 Scales of measurement

Type of data	Examples	Discrete/ continuous	Characteristics	Type of statistical test
Nominal	Gender, ethnicities, religion	Discrete	Membership May be assigned numeric value; however, these values have no true meaning	Nonparametric
Ordinal	Educational level (e.g., elementary, graduate to professional education), Likert scale (agreement scale)	Discrete/ continuous[a]	Membership Values are in some rank order Spacing between values are *not* equivalent	Nonparametric
Interval	Temperature (i.e., Celsius and Fahrenheit)	Continuous	Membership Values are in some rank order Equivalent intervals Arbitrary zero point	Parametric
Ratio	Age, length, weight, height, screening tests (e.g., prostate-specific antigen (PSA) levels)	Continuous	Membership Values are in some rank order Equivalent Intervals Absolute zero	Parametric

[a] As a general rule, ordinal data may be treated as continuous data if there are many ranks (similar to an interval scale). Nonetheless, some researchers disagree with this rule, arguing that ordinal data are only discrete (or categorical)

It is important to know what type of data you have before selecting a statistical test for analysis. Data can be categorized into four levels, known as scales or types of measurement (see Table 15.2). The type of measurement will determine the statistical test employed. Since nominal and ordinal data are considered discrete (or categorical) data, nonparametric tests would be needed to analyze the data. This is because nonparametric tests do not assume a normal distribution. For interval and ratio scale data, parametric tests may be used for analysis.

Parametric statistical tests assume that the outcome data approximate a normal distribution (interval and ratio data), whereas nonparametric tests are less restrictive, assuming no particular distribution of the data (nominal and ordinal). With multiple data types in an analysis (i.e., discrete and continuous), nonparametric tests are applied. However, when possible, parametric tests should be employed as they have more explanatory power.

5. Instruments and diagnostic tests

How consistent and accurate are your instruments? You should assess the reliability and validity of your instruments (e.g., surveys). These two concepts and how to test for them are discussed in the next case. If your study requires the use of a screening test for a particular disease, testing the accuracy of the results is crucial. Relatively simple calculations are used to produce the sensitivity and specificity of these tests.

Sensitivity refers to the probability that a positive result on a screening test truly indicates that the patient does have a certain disease or condition for which he or she is tested. It is the probability of a true positive.

On the other hand, *Specificity* refers to the probability that a negative result on a screening test truly indicates that the patient does not have a certain disease or condition for which he or she is tested. It is the probability of a true negative. Providing accurate results is important as lack of treatment (if the result is a false negative result) could result in harm to the patient's health.

Tables 15.3, 15.4, and 15.5 apply this to an example: detecting Parkinson's disease.

For predictive values, if the test is negative, the negative predictive value is TN/(FN+TN). It is the probability that a negative test result is a true negative. If the test is positive, the positive predictive value is TP/(TP+FP). It is the probability that a positive test result is a true positive (Table 15.5).

The false positive rate (also referred to as α = alpha) is the relative frequency of a positive test result of a certain disease when in fact the patient does not have the dis-

Table 15.3 Sensitivity and specificity

	Parkinson's disease		Total
	Present	Absent	
Test Positive	(TP) 85	(FP) 7100	(TP+FP) 7185
Test Negative	(FN) 15	(TN) 92,800	(FN+TN) 92,815
Total	(TP+FN) 100	(FP+TN) 99,900	(TP+FP+FN+TN) 100,000

TP true positive, *FP* false positive, *FN* false negative, *TN* true negative

Table 15.4 Sensitivity and specificity

Sensitivity	Specificity
TP/(TP+FN)	TN/(FP+TN)
85/100=85%	92,800/99,900=93%

TP true positive, *FP* false positive, *FN* false negative, *TN* true negative

Table 15.5 Predictive values

Positive predictive value	Negative predictive value
TP/(TP+FP)	TN/(FN+TN)
85/7185=1.18%	92,800/92,815=99.98%

TP true positive, *FP* false positive, *FN* false negative, *TN* true negative

ease (i.e., healthy people incorrectly identified as being sick). Using Table 15.3, the calculation is FP/(FP + TN) = 7100/99,900 = 7 % (or 1 − specificity). False negative rate (also referred to as β = beta) is the relative frequency of a negative test result when in fact the patient does have the disease (i.e., sick people incorrectly identified as being healthy). The calculation for this rate is FN/(TP + FN) = 15/100 = 15 % (or 1 − sensitivity).

6. Sampling

Selecting an appropriate and feasible sampling technique and sample size is essential for providing data for a more robust analysis with minimal bias (good representation of the population being studied). *Simple random sampling* is when a sample of the population is randomly selected, making sure each observation has an equal chance of being picked. *Stratified sampling* is when there are several different groups within the population and each one needs to be represented equally. For each group, the simple random sampling technique is applied to generate the sample. *Self-selection sampling* is when the sample is based on convenience of data collection or some other factor determined by the investigator (e.g., selection of a set of schools or programs in which consent could be easily obtained). This technique could result in bias in the data. *Systematic sampling* or *assignment* is when a list of the population is available, the first observation is randomly selected, and then every *n*th observation (decided by the investigator) is selected until the determined sample size has been reached.

7. Significance level and statistical errors

In the simplest case, the *null hypothesis* typically states that there is no relationship between two variables, whereas the *alternative hypothesis* typically states that there is a relationship between two variables.

Hypothesis testing involves comparing empirically observed sample findings with theoretically expected findings—expected if the null hypothesis (H_0) is true. This comparison allows one to compute the probability that the observed outcome could have been due to chance or random error.

Significance level is the *alpha* or significance level that is set by the researcher, generally at 5 %. It is the level at which the test results are determined to be statistically significant. The significance level is also:

- The probability at which the null hypothesis (H_0) would be rejected
- The level or probability selected by the researcher that determines the probability of committing a type I error (see Table 15.6 below)

Table 15.6 Type I and type II errors

	Reject the null hypothesis	Do not reject null hypothesis
Null hypothesis is true	*Type I error* Alpha	Correctly determining there is no difference 1 − alpha
Null hypothesis is false	*Power* Correctly determining that there is a difference 1 − beta	*Type II error* Beta

Type I error is rejecting a true null hypothesis. A researcher can mistakenly reject the null hypothesis when in reality it is true (not false). It gives "false affirmation" to the results of a study (Vogt and Johnson 2011). This, in turn, generates a false positive. The objective of minimizing type I error is to have a small probability claiming something is true when in reality it is not true (e.g., statistically significant difference between two drugs, when there is no difference). It is inversely related to a type II error.

Type II error is failing to reject a false null hypothesis (accepting a false null hypothesis). It is failing to reject (mistakenly accepting) the null hypothesis when in reality it is false. It is giving "false denial" (Vogt and Johnson 2011) to the results of a study (e.g., no significant difference between two drugs, when there is a difference). This, in turn, generates a false negative.

Statistical power is the probability of rejecting a truly false null hypothesis. In other words, it is the probability that statistically significant differences will be found in a study. It is the inverse of the probability of a type II error (e.g., if power = 80 %, then the probability of a type II error = 20 %). A general rule is that statistical power of 80 % or higher is acceptable.

8. Establish protocols for the study (the actual steps necessary on how you conduct your study):
    a. Determine how your participants will be selected.
    b. Are signed adult consent and/or youth assent forms needed? If yes, develop a plan to collect and store the confidential data.
    c. Train the project members/administrators on collecting data (e.g., interviews, IQ tests).
9. Run the study on a test group (i.e., a pilot study).
10. Develop a codebook of all variables and possible values collected.
11. Conduct the study (collect primary data).
12. Clean/recode the data (making appropriate notes in the codebook).
13. Analyze the data:
    a. Revisit the hypothesis stated.
    b. Descriptive and inferential analyses:
        1. Run basic frequencies, means, and correlations of the study variables.

A correlation *(r)* is the statistical relationship between two variables. This numerical relationship is often referred to as a bivariate association. It tests whether or not there is an association between the variables. The r values range from −1 to +1. A value of −1 indicates a perfect negative or inverse relationship. A value of +1 indicates a perfect positive or direct relationship. A value of 0 indicates no relationship, except in the case of a curvilinear relationship. For the latter, other techniques need to be employed to determine the association.

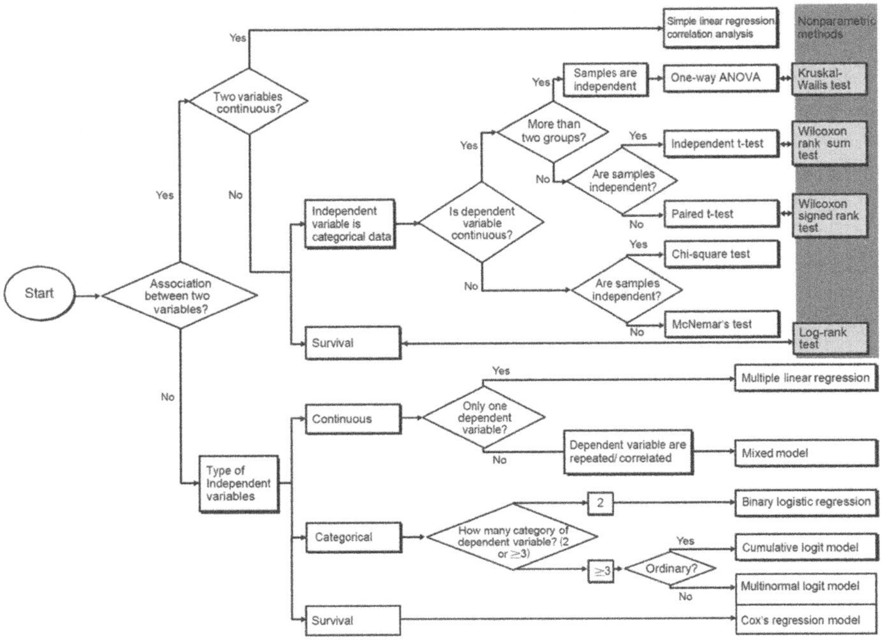

Fig. 15.1 Flowchart on the appropriate statistical tests to use as a function of the types of independent and dependent variables (from Nam and Chung 2012, p. 579)

There are many ways to calculate the correlation coefficient depending on the type of variables being used (i.e., ordinal, interval, and ratio). The most common and widely used correlation coefficient is Pearson's product–moment *r*. Pearson's *r* carries certain assumptions and distribution requirements. It is this statistic that measures the degree of the linear relationship (i.e., strength and direction of the association) between variables. If the scale of measurement for the variables is ordinal (i.e., a ranking order with no uniform intervals or absolute zero), then Spearman's rho or Kendall's tau may be applied.

2. Choose the appropriate statistical test (see Fig. 15.1). The more basic and common tests are those that involve two variables and are parametric (i.e., upper half of Fig. 15.1; e.g., simple linear regression correlation analysis or Pearson's correlation).
3. Review results: Is there a statistically significant difference to reject the null hypothesis?

14. Write your paper.
15. Submit the paper for presentation and publication.

Case Vignette 15.1.2 Conclusion

Following considerable thought to her study design options, Melinda selects a case-control study to evaluate the relationship between long-term use of antipsychotic drugs and movement disorders commonly found in Parkinsonism. A randomized clinical trial with case and control groups would be ideal. However, that option requires a significant amount of time and capital.

After receiving permission from the hospital, she conducts 100 chart reviews (retrospective data) of patients with and without the Parkinsonism symptoms. The correlation was applied to test for an association. The result was 0.7, confirming a reportable and direct relationship. The next step is to apply a randomized controlled trial to determine whether or not a significant causal relationship exists. Melinda noted that this study may provide useful insight into further studies (i.e., experimental) and assist in successfully applying for grants that would provide the funding for more involved data collection.

Case Vignette 15.2.1 Shyla Sing

Shyla Sing is a 12-year-old girl who was brought to the primary care clinic by her mother. Mrs. Sing explains to the medical psychologist and the first-year resident who is shadowing that day that though Shyla appears to be physically fine, she is worried about her child's mental development. Some of Mrs. Sing's concerns include Shyla's difficulty in interacting with her peers. Also, Shyla is extremely shy and refuses to separate from her mother.

Please proceed with the problem-based approach using the worksheet located in the appendix of Chap. 1!

Please fill in the facts, your hypotheses, further information needed, and learning issues in Learning Issue Table 15.2.1.

Learning Issue Table 15.2.1

Case Vignette 15.2.2 Continuation

Shyla's physical examination revealed no abnormalities and suggested that she is a normal 12-year-old girl. Furthermore, the results of standard laboratory tests did not reveal any medical problems.

Mrs. Sing explains that for the past 2 years, Shyla has had "erratic behavior." Examples include simple dialogue resulting in major tantrums. Mrs. Sing may ask for a spoon from the kitchen drawer, and Shyla would suddenly start to cry. When Mrs. Sing approaches her, Shyla would often yell out, "Get away from me. You don't care whether I live or die!" At times, she would escalate the situation by throwing utensils and/or hitting her mother. This type of behavior usually occurs when she is alone with her mother.

Furthermore, Shyla's academic performance has shown a decline over the past 2 years. Her parents have met with the school principal on three occasions during the time period to discuss her failing to near-failing grades in her classes. After meeting with the principal, the parents, mainly the mother, would talk with the Shyla about improving her grades. Sometimes it would result in a "shouting match." Usually, within a month, Shyla's grades would show a steady improvement. This would last for 3–4 months and then decline again.

Since there is an array of possible diagnoses related to the patient's behavior, the behavioral health consultant suggests conducting a structured interview with the patient. The Diagnostic Interview Schedule for Children (DISC) was brought up as a possibility. The resident was not very familiar with this instrument. Therefore, he decides to investigate its application for this particular case.

Please proceed with the problem-based approach using the worksheet located in the appendix of Chap. 1!

Please fill in the facts, your hypotheses, further information needed, and learning issues in Learning Issue Table 15.2.2.

Learning Issue Table 15.2.2

FACTS	HYPOTHESES	INFORMATION NEEDED	LEARNING ISSUES

15.2 Learning Issues

There are advantages of employing the DISC scoring algorithms for mental health diagnoses. It has been reviewed and approved by the National Institute of Mental Health (NIMH; e.g., Shaffer et al., 2000). In addition, since the DISC is a highly structured interview, the administration of the computerized version requires no clinical and little hands-on training.

In terms of the instrument's *reliability* and *validity,* the DISC has been widely used since 1983. Since that time, there have been many inquiries and reviews as to its reliability. Although there may be some detractors, the DISC appears to have a history of reliable and valid results.

Reliability is concerned with the consistency of a measurement or instrument over multiple applications. With a survey or questionnaire, it is the consistency of the results over time with the same individual or the consistency within a set of items administered at the same time. While reliability is focused on the consistency of the instrument, *validity* is concerned with its accuracy. Does the instrument measure what it is expected to measure? A test could be reliable or consistent over time; however, it might not be an accurate or valid measure.

A common metaphor used to describe the relation between the two concepts of reliability and validity is a dartboard or target. The objective is to hit the center (i.e., the bull's eye) of the board. One possibility may involve a tight grouping of darts on the periphery of the board. This result would be considered very reliable but not valid or accurate (i.e., totally missing the center). The ideal case is for all the darts to hit the bull's eye. This result would be both reliable and valid.

There are many types of reliabilities. In this chapter, three types are discussed: *internal reliability* (or internal consistency), *test–retest reliability* (or stability), and *inter-rater reliability.* Internal reliability assesses the consistency of the responses in measuring the same construct (such as depression). Test–retest reliability assesses the degree to which the same construct is measured across a certain time period. Inter-rater reliability assesses the consistency of the raters' or observers' assessment of the same event.

One popular measure of internal reliability is Cronbach's alpha. It is a reliability coefficient, ranging from 0 to 1 (values close to 1 are considered to reflect a high reliability). Values of 0.7–0.8 are regarded as satisfactory; however, clinical applications require higher values (Bland and Altman 1997).[1]

A common indicator of test–retest reliability is the correlation between Time 1 and Time 2 scores. The correlation can range from −1 to +1. In general, the shorter the test–retest duration, the higher the positive correlation would be expected.

[1] For the calculations of Cronbach's alpha, see Campbell and Machin (1999, pp. 174–175).

A way to gauge for inter-rater reliability is *Cohen's kappa.* Its values range from 0 to 1. Values less than 0.4 are considered to be "poor," 0.4–0.6 are "moderate," 0.6–0.8 are "substantial," and above 0.8 are "almost perfect."[2]

Test *validity* refers to the accuracy of the test. If a test purports to measure depression, and it ends up doing so, then it is a valid test. Note that in order for a test to be valid, it must be reliable. However, a reliable test may not be valid. There is some movement away from listing the different types of validity and definitions to understanding the overall logical arguments for making a case of test validity (e.g., American Educational Research Association, American Psychological Association and National Council on Measurement in Education 1999). However, using more traditional lists may be instructive in providing a brief summary of several of the more basic types of test validity. Table 15.7 presents these different types of basic test validity.

Validity can also be conceptualized regarding the results of a research study. *Internal validity* is the extent to which the observed results demonstrate a causal relationship between the variables (dependent and independent) examined. In other words, to what extent do the studied independent or explanatory variables cause a variation (one way or another) in the dependent or outcome variable? This is the degree to which valid conclusions can be drawn about the causal effects of one variable on another (Vogt and Johnson 2011). *External validity* is the ability to apply the results outside the study or generalize them to another group.

Case Vignette 15.2.3 Conclusion

Before committing to the DISC as a diagnostic tool, the resident further examines its reliability and validity. For internal consistency, the calculated Cronbach's alpha was 0.89. This is more than satisfactory. For inter-rater reliability, the calculated Cohen's kappa was 0.72, considered substantial.

Finally, for validity, the resident gains permission to review past medical charts from different clinics where the DISC was used. He then compares DISC results with physicians' diagnoses. For the most part, the outcomes were consistent. The resident continued to evaluate its validity by comparing a small group of at-risk patients (potential for suicidal thoughts or actions based on DISC results) with their follow-up appointments. His investigation validates the DISC results as many of these patients later admit to have had suicidal thoughts and some have attempted to act on it.

In the end, the resident decides to administer the structured interview with the patient. After running the computerized version and reviewing the results

[2] For the calculations of Cohen's kappa, see Campbell and Machin (1999, p. 175).

with the Diagnostic and Statistical Manual of Mental Disorders, Fifth edition (DSM-5), the resident felt better equipped to diagnose the patient. Shyla was diagnosed with depression and anxiety disorder. Six months later with the behavioral treatment and medication, she showed significant and consistent improvement in her behavior.

Case Vignette 15.3.1 Michael

Michael, a third-year medical student, is doing a rotation at the outpatient anxiety specialty clinic. During one of the team meetings, he realizes that the many different types of anxiety disorders are associated with different levels of impairment and the prognosis can also be a function of the type of anxiety disorder. Upon inquiring about this during the team meeting, he is directed to look into this by briefly reviewing the scientific literature on the subject. He is warned, however, that the relationship between anxiety disorders and impairment can be complex and may involve advanced research and statistical designs, including structural equation model (SEM).

Please proceed with the problem-based approach using the worksheet located in the appendix of Chap. 1!

Please fill in the facts, your hypotheses, further information needed, and learning issues in Learning Issue Table 15.3.1.

Learning Issue Table 15.3.1

FACTS	HYPOTHESES	INFORMATION NEEDED	LEARNING ISSUES

Table 15.7 Test validity

Validity type	Description	Example of depression construct
Face	Experts agree that the items of the test reflect the construct purported to be measured	"I feel sad" as one of the items
Content	Experts agree that the items of the test are representative of the various elements of the construct	"I feel sad," "My sleep pattern has changed," "My eating habits have changed," etc.
Concurrent	Test scores correlate strongly with another established indicator that purports to measure the same or very similar construct	Correlates strongly with Beck Depression Inventory scores
Convergent	Test scores correlate moderately to strongly with an indicator that is theoretically related	Correlates strongly with anxiety scores
Divergent	Test scores correlate weakly or not at all with an indicator that is theoretically not related	Correlates weakly with an indicator of conscientiousness
Discriminant	Test scores differentiate between two or more different types of people	High scores differentiate people who have attempted suicide, and low scores differentiate people who have not attempted suicide
Predictive	Test scores strongly predict in the future another related indicator	Strongly predicts Beck Depression Inventory scores or a suicide attempt 1 month later
Construct	Test scores perform as expected if the test measures the purported construct	Experimental group who receives a depression intervention scores lower on the depression test than control group that does not receive the depression invention. (Note: Construct validity can be conceptualized as a more general type of validity for which all other types of validity contribute.)

15.3 Learning Issues

SEM is a relatively new method of analyzing more complex data. SEMs "… provide estimates of the strength of all the hypothetical relationships between variables in a theoretical model" (Murayama 1998, p. 4). Although SEM can entail observable variables (i.e., path analysis; Hoyle 1995) and exploratory models (e.g., Schumacker and Lomax 2004), it is typically employed with confirmation models that may include latent (unobserved) variables (Murayama 1998). There are many advantages of using SEM for the analysis of complex data: (1) able to "confirm" theory-driven models, (2) able to test moderating and mediating-intervening effects of variables, (3) when working with longitudinal data, better able to make temporal and causal inferences (e.g., McArdle et al. 2014; Hishinuma et al. 2012), (4) able to incorporate latent (non-observable) variables (e.g., Hoyle 1995; Loehlin 2004), and (5) able to address missing or incomplete data with current powerful software packages (e.g., *Mplus*; Muthén and Muthén 2012).

Case Vignette 15.3.2 Conclusion

After conducting a brief review of the literature, one of the articles is directly related to the topic of interest: "A longitudinal examination of psychosocial impairment across the anxiety disorders," by Naragon-Gainey et al. (2014), published in the journal *Psychological Medicine.* In glancing through article, you find the following structural equation modeling figure and description (Fig. 15.2).

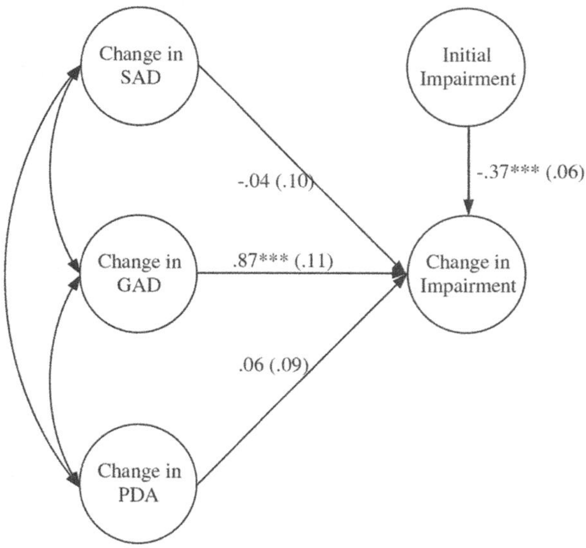

Fig. 15.2 Change in disorder constructs as unique predictors of change in impairment, controlling for initial levels of impairment. Parameter estimates are standardized and standard errors are shown in parentheses. $n = 606$. Model fit: $\chi^2_{902}=2054.75$ ($p<0.001$), comparative fit index = 0.94, Tucker–Lewis index = 0.93, root mean square error of approximation = 0.05, standardized root-mean-square residual = 0.06. Model $R^2 = 0.92$. Initial level of impairment is the impairment intercept from the latent growth model, whereas change values are slopes from the latent growth models. *SAD* social anxiety disorder, *GAD* generalized anxiety disorder, *PDA* panic with or without agoraphobia. *$p < 0.05$, **$p < 0.01$, ***$p < 0.001$ (Naragon-Gainey et al. 2014, p. 1696)

After carefully reviewing the entire article, Michael realizes that the "fit" of the model was good, resulting in the conclusion, "Because change in GAD was most specifically related to change in impairment, treatment for those with multiple anxiety disorders could focus on treating GAD symptoms first or treating transdiagnostic processes" (p. 1691).

Michael also realizes that before drawing any definitive conclusions, he will need to review more articles from the literature search. However, the strengths of this article, with its longitudinal design and structural equation modeling analysis, will serve as a valuable foundation to incorporate other articles.

Case Vignette 15.4.1 Nate

As an assignment for his next journal club, Nate, a second-year medical student, was asked to present on the essential elements in critically understanding a journal article. He selected an article from a reputable, peer-reviewed journal that conducted a meta-analysis on an existing oral hypoglycemic medication (Drug X) that has been on the market for 10 years.[3]

In his presentation, Nate notes that the authors of the study applied a meta-analysis to examine retrospective data from 40 of 104 relevant studies in which Drug X was used. They proposed that Drug X is potentially harmful because it increases the incidence of cardiac events (i.e., myocardial infarction). Literature searches were conducted using various public and private databases. Inclusion criteria for the meta-analysis included studies that had a randomized control group not receiving Drug X, studies that were conducted for at least a period of 20 weeks, and studies with outcome data for cardiovascular events.

The average age of the participants was approximately 53 years. Of 13,100 patients on Drug X, 95 experienced a cardiovascular event. Of 12,700 patients not on Drug X, 70 experienced a cardiovascular event. When comparing the treatment group to the control group, the odds ratio for a cardiovascular event was 1.32 (at the 95% confidence interval (CI), 1.04–1.85, $p=0.04$). The authors concluded that Drug X is associated with a significant increase in the risk of a cardiovascular event.

[3] This fictitious case is loosely based on facts and findings from an article published in the *New England Journal of Medicine* (Nissen and Wolski 2007).

Please proceed with the problem-based approach using the worksheet located in the appendix of Chap. 1!

Please fill in the facts, your hypotheses, further information needed, and learning issues in Learning Issue Table 15.4.1.

Learning Issue Table 15.4.1

FACTS	HYPOTHESES	INFORMATION NEEDED	LEARNING ISSUES

It is important that consumers of the research literature be critical of the methods, analyses, and results of any study. Most journal articles offer current and relevant information on research topics of interest. It is the responsibility of health-care professionals to be informed and to properly evaluate and interpret published studies in order to provide the best clinical care for their patients.

Case Vignette 15.4.2 Continuation

After reading the article a few times, Nate made a list of questions to critically examine the methods and results of the published study.

The list includes:

1. Have you critically examined the methods to determine the validity of the study? How was the sample selected (e.g., simple random sample, stratified sampling)?
2. Pretend that you were conducting the study yourself (see the previous case for the checklist of designing a study). Would you do it differently? If yes, how would you change it? Would your changes significantly impact the results of the published study?
3. What do the results mean?
4. Can the findings be applied in a practical sense (e.g., in my practice)? If yes, how can I apply them?

Additional questions for meta-analysis include:

5. When dealing with multiple studies, you have to deal with multiple study designs, sampling methods, data collection techniques, and protocols. Were the values from different studies placed on a standard or common scale?

6. How were the data combined into one data set? Do you have access to the original data sets? Did any of the studies in the meta-analysis use the same data set (partial or complete)? This would entail double-counting.
7. Were the studies with opposing or negative results reported?

STOP

Please proceed with the problem-based approach using the worksheet located in the appendix of Chap. 1!

Please fill in the facts, your hypotheses, further information needed, and learning issues in Learning Issue Table 15.4.2.

Learning Issue Table 15.4.2

FACTS	HYPOTHESES	INFORMATION NEEDED	LEARNING ISSUES

15.4 Learning Issues

A *meta-analysis* is conducted by gathering data from multiple journal articles to increase its sample size. The data, from various secondary sources, are compiled and considered as one large data set in the analysis. Each study included in the meta-analysis is considered a unit of measurement.

15.4.1 Criteria for an Acceptable Meta-analysis

1. The study objectives were clearly identified.
2. Inclusion criteria of articles in general and specific data to be accepted were established before selection.
3. An active effort was made to find and include all relevant articles.
4. An assessment of "publication bias" was made, that is, the bias that articles with statistically significant results are more likely to be published in journals.
5. Specific data used were identified.

Table 15.8 Example of relative risk

		Liver disease		
		Present	Absent	Totals
Exposure to alcohol	Yes (50 or more)	*(a)* 70	*(b)* 150	*(a + b)* 220
	No (1–8)	*(c)* 250	*(d)* 950	*(c + d)* 1200

The relative risk is calculated by the following formula:

$$\frac{a/(a+b)}{c/(c+d)} \rightarrow \frac{70/(70+150)}{250/(250+950)} \rightarrow \frac{0.318}{0.208} \rightarrow 1.53$$

The odds ratio is calculated by the following formula:

$$\frac{a/c}{b/d} \rightarrow \frac{70/250}{150/950} \rightarrow \frac{0.280}{0.158} \rightarrow 1.77$$

6. Assessment of article comparability (e.g., controls, circumstances) was made.
7. The meta-analysis was reported in enough detail to allow replication.

Source: Riffenburgh (2006, p. 163).

Individual studies, as well as meta-analyses, can involve relative risk of odds ratios.

Relative risk is a risk ratio comparing the probability of developing a disease in two groups: the incidence of those exposed to a specific risk factor (e.g., smoking and alcohol consumption) and the incidence of those not exposed to the risk factor. It is often applied in prospective data analysis (e.g., cohort studies and clinical trials), where the two groups are selected at the beginning of the study. Consequently, this ratio is not used in case-control studies (retrospective data analysis with a focus on the outcome first). The following example of relative risk examines the influence of alcohol on liver disease (see Table 15.8). The exposure group included men who drank the alcohol equivalent of 50 or more beers a week. The group not exposed to significant alcohol consumption drank the alcohol equivalent of 1–8 beers a week (social drinking).

Based on the calculated relative risk, a man who drank heavily was approximately 1.5 times more likely to develop a liver disease than a man who drank socially.

The *odds ratio* is the ratio of two probabilities: the probability that an event will occur (a/c for simplicity, the data in Table 15.8 are used) and the probability that an event will not occur (b/d). It is often used in the analysis of retrospective cases (e.g., case-control studies of rare diseases).

While the odds ratio is often used as an estimate for relative risk, we can see by applying the same example from Table 15.8 that the odds ratio is different from the relative risk. A man who drank heavily was approximately 1.8 times more likely to develop a liver disease than a man who drank socially. As the ratios move away from 1, the difference becomes more apparent. (Note: Odds ratios can be less than 1.0. Odds ratios less than 1.0 simply mean that the ratio of the numerator is less than that of the denominator. In these instances, to convert the odds ratios to the greater-than-1.0 odds-ratio equivalents, simply take the reciprocal of the less-than-1.0 odds ratios (i.e., 1 divided by the less-than-1.0 odds ratio). For example, an odds ratio of 0.5 would convert to an odds ratio of 1 divided 0.5 = 2.0.)

Case Vignette 15.4.3 Conclusion
Nate applies the critical questions to examine the validity of the authors' claims. Based on the data, methods, and analysis, it is difficult to say with confidence that the association between Drug X and cardiac events is truly noteworthy. Specific reasons include:

1. Methods: The retrospective data come from other multiple sources. Moreover, the authors did not have access to the original source data. This is a considerable limitation.
2. Methods: It appears that most of these studies were not designed to study cardiac outcomes.
3. Analysis: The actual number of cases with cardiac outcomes was relatively small, given the sample size. For participants on Drug X, 95 of 13,100 patients experienced a cardiovascular event. For participants not on Drug X, 70 of 12,700 patients experienced a cardiovascular event.
4. Analysis: Although statistically significant ($p=0.04$), the odds ratio of 1.32 appears to be low. Nonetheless, to test whether this ratio is relatively high or low, a comparative analysis with other similar drug(s) should be conducted.

Ideally, a randomized clinical trial (prospective analysis) should be conducted to properly examine whether a significant causal relationship exists. In the end, it is up to an informed practitioner to decide how to interpret and apply the findings of this article and other journal articles in his/her practice.

15.5 Review Questions

1. Study designs:
   A group of clinician researchers hypothesized that household crowding may be an important risk factor for pediatric obsessive–compulsive disorder (via increased risk for streptococcal pharyngitis). The researchers chose to analyze a database that was derived from a one-time survey of youth attending community high schools who agreed to participate in the study. The surveys included questions on the number of people in the household and structured interview questions to assess for symptoms of obsessive–compulsive disorder. While all students at the high schools were approached for potential participation in the surveys, the only students included in the study were those for whom there were

both youth assent and parental permission. Which of the following statements pertaining to the study design is *false?*

a. The study would involve retrospective data analysis.
b. This is a cohort study design.
c. This is a cross-sectional study design.
d. Self-selection sampling was done.
e. None of the above.

2. Sensitivity, specificity, positive predictive value, negative predictive value:
Suppose the prevalence of coronary heart disease (CHD) among older adults is 25 %. Angiography can test for CHD, and it has a sensitivity of 60 % and a specificity of 80 %. What are the positive predictive value and negative predictive value, respectively? It may be helpful to use a total *N* of 100.

a. 25 %; 14 %
b. 50 %; 86 %
c. 60 %; 80 %
d. 80 %; 50 %

3. Correlations:
One study finds a Pearson's correlation coefficient of +0.85 between depression and anxiety, and another study finds a Pearson's correlation coefficient of −0.20 between depression and anxiety. Which correlation is statistically significant (alpha $< .05$)?

a. −0.20
b. +0.85
c. Depends on *N* (i.e., degrees of freedom)
d. Cannot determine from the information given

Appendix A: Tables with Possible Answers to the Vignettes

Case Vignette 15.1

What are the facts?	What are your hypotheses?	What do you want to know next?	What specific information would you like to learn about?
There appears to be a link between long-term use of antipsychotic drugs and movement disorders commonly found in Parkinsonism	There is a relationship between long-term use of this particular atypical antipsychotic drug and movement disorders commonly found in Parkinsonism	Have observational or experimental studies been conducted on this topic?	How to select and conduct a study?
			Study designs
			Scales of measurement for data collection
			Types of sampling techniques
	A significant portion of the variation in occurrence of this movement disorder can be explained by the long-term use of this drug		Sensitivity and specificity tests
			How to analyze data (e.g., basic statistical tests used to analyze data)?

Case Vignette 15.2

What are the facts?	What are your hypotheses?	What do you want to know next?	What specific information would you like to learn about?
12-year-old girl	Possible anxiety disorder	Physical appearance (e.g., any bruises and residual marks)	What are the normal developmental milestones at this age?
			Other ways to approach and communicate with this girl
Mother worried about mental development	Normal separation anxiety of temperamental variation		Available diagnostic tools/instruments
	Depression	Cognitive awareness of environment	
	Child abuse	Home environment	
	Post-traumatic stress disorder	School performance	
		Parents' disposition (temperament)	
		Possible substance use	Reliability
	Nutritional deficiency		
	Possible endocrine disorder (hypothyroidism)		

What are the facts?	What are your hypotheses?	What do you want to know next?	What specific information would you like to learn about?
Difficulty interacting with peers	Mother is overly concerned	Possible parental substance use	Validity
Shy			
Refuses to separate from mother			

Case Vignette 15.3

What are the facts?	What are your hypotheses?	What do you want to know next?	What specific information would you like to learn about?
There may be a relationship between different types of anxiety disorders and impairment	Different anxiety disorders will have different associations with impairment	What does the scientific literature reveal?	Relationship between anxiety disorders and impairment
More advanced research designs and statistical methods may be used	Structural equation modeling might be involved	What else needs to be known before making a conclusion?	Structural equation modeling

Case Vignette 15.4

What are the facts?	What are your hypotheses?	What do you want to know next?	What specific information would you like to learn about?
The journal article purports that through the use of meta-analysis, Drug X is associated with a significant increase in the risk of a cardiovascular event	The study has many limitations and should be treated with cautious reception	Of the 64 relevant studies not selected, how many claimed no significant relationship between Drug X and cardiac events?	Meta-analysis
			Relative risk
			Odds ratio

Appendix B: Answers to Review Questions

Answers

1. Study designs:
   Answer: (b).
2. Sensitivity, specificity, positive predicative value, negative predictive value:
   Answer: (b).

Disease		
	Present	Absent
Test Positive	TP	FP
Test Negative	FN	TN

TP true positive, *FN* false negative, *FP* false positive, *TN* true negative

Sensitivity=TP/(TP+FN)	Specificity=TN/(FP+TN)
Positive Predictive Value=TP/(TP+FP)	Negative Predictive Value=TN/(FN+TN)

Explanation: The prevalence of CHD is 25 %. Assume a sample of 100 and put 25 people in the CHD-present column and 75 people in the CHD-absent column. The sensitivity of the test is 60 %; therefore, 60 % of the 25 people with CHD (or 15 people) will test positive and the other 10 will test negative. The specificity is 80 %; therefore, 80 % of the 75 CHD-absent people (or 60 people) will test negative and the other 15 will test positive. Thus, 15 + 15 = 30 people will test positive, and 15 of them will really have CHD; therefore, the positive predictive value is 15/30 or 50 %. A total of 10 + 60 = 70 people will test negative, and 60 of them really will not have CHD; therefore, the negative predictive value is 60/70 or 86 %.

3. Correlations:
   Answer: (c).

Although the Pearson *r* or correlation coefficient of +0.85 is very high, if the sample size was very small, the correlation may not be statistically significant. Although the other correlation of −0.20 is much lower, the sample size could be much larger and the correlation could be statistically significant. Therefore, because the statistical significance is dependent on both the size of the correlation and the number of participants, we do not know which of the two correlations is statistically significant. We would need to know the *N* size for each to determine whether each is statistically significant or not.

References

American Educational Research Association, American Psychological Association, & National Council on Measurement in Education. (1999). *Standards for educational and psychological testing*. Washington, DC: American Psychological Association.

Appleton, D. R. (1990). What statistics should we teach medical undergraduates and graduates? *Statistics in Medicine, 9,* 1013–1021.

Bakker, P. R., de Groot, I. W., van Os, J., & van Harten, P. N. (2013). Predicting the incidence of antipsychotic-induced movement disorders in long-stay patients: A prospective study. *Epidemiology and Psychiatric Services, 22*(4), 375–379.

Bland, J. M., & Altman, D. G. (1997). Cronbach's alpha. *British Medical Journal, 314,* 572.

Campbell, M. J., & Machin, D. (1999). *Medical statistics: A commonsense approach* (3rd ed.). West Sussex: Wiley.

Hishinuma, E. S., Chang, J. Y., McArdle, J. J., & Hamagami, F. (2012). Potential causal relationship between depressive symptoms and academic achievement in the Hawai'ian High Schools Health Survey using contemporary longitudinal latent variable change models. *Developmental Psychology, 48*(5), 1327–1342. doi:10.1037/a0026978.

Hoyle, R. H. (1995). The structural equation modeling approach. In R. H. Hoyle (Ed.), *Structural equation modeling: Concepts, issues, and applications* (pp. 1–15). Thousand Oaks: Sage.

Kuzma, J. W. (1992). *Basic statistics for the health sciences.* Mountain View: Mayfield.

Loehlin, J. C. (2004). *Latent variable models: An introduction to factor, path, and structural equation analysis* (4th ed.). Mahwah: Lawrence Erlbaum.

McArdle, J. J., Hamagami, F., Chang, J. Y., & Hishinuma, E. S. (2014). Longitudinal dynamic analyses of depression and academic achievement in the Hawai'ian High Schools Health Survey using contemporary latent variable change models. *Structural Equation Modeling: A Multidisciplinary Journal, 21,* 1–22. doi:10.1080/10705511.2014.919824. (Online version).

Murayama, G. M. (1998). *Basics of structural equation modeling.* Thousand Oaks: Sage.

Muthén, L. K., & Muthén, B. O. (2012). *Mplus: Statistical analysis with latent variables: User's guide*. Los Angeles: Muthén & Muthén.

Nam, C. M., & Chung, S. Y. (2012). Statistical methods for medical students. *Journal of the Korean Medical Association, 55*(6), 573–581.

Naragon-Gainey, K., Gallagher, M. W., & Brown, T. A. (2014). A longitudinal examination of psychosocial impairment across the anxiety disorders. *Psychological Medicine, 44,* 1691–1700.

Nissen, S. E., & Wolski, K. (2007). Effect of rosiglitazone on the risk of myocardial infarction and death from cardiovascular causes. *New England Journal of Medicine, 356,* 2457–2471. http://content.nejm.org/cgi/content/full/NEJMoa072761. Accessed 13 Oct 2007.

Riffenburgh, R. H. (2006). *Statistics in medicine*. Burlington: Elsevier.

Schumacker, R. E., & Lomax, R. G. (2004). *A beginner's guide to structural equation modeling* (2nd ed.). Mahwah: Lawrence Erlbaum.

Shaffer, D., Fisher, P., Lucas, C. P., Dulcan, M. K., & Schwab-Stone, M. E. (2000). NIMH Diagnostic Interview Schedule for Children Version IV (NIMH DISC-IV): Description, differences from previous versions, and reliability of some common diagnoses. *Journal of the American Academy of Child and Adolescent Psychiatry, 39*(1), 28–38.

Vogt, W. P., & Johnson, R. B. (2011). *Dictionary of statistics and methodology: A nontechnical guide for the social sciences* (4th ed.). Thousand Oaks: Sage.

Chapter 16
Death, Dying, and End-of-Life Care

Lori Murayama-Sung and Iqbal Ahmed

All physicians face end-of-life issues during their training and many continue to work in specialties where life and death are part of their daily duties. This chapter addresses a key challenge for physicians who work with older and critically ill patients.

At the end of this chapter, the reader will be able to:

1. Understand psychological issues surrounding the end of life, including stages of grief, psychiatric illness, and psychosocial/spiritual needs.
2. Understand what the standard of care is with regard to euthanasia and physician-assisted suicide (PAS).
3. Discuss sensitive issues with patients including diagnosing death, organ donation, and how to address families at the time of death.
4. Understand what palliative care is and when to refer someone to hospice.

Case Vignette 16.1.1

Mr. Kim is a 63-year-old Chinese man who is admitted for pleuritic chest pain and dyspnea. He has no known medical or psychiatric history except for an 80-pack-year smoking history. He had not sought medical treatment in years but finally decided to seek treatment at the urging of his second wife.

After you perform a full workup, you gently break the bad news to him that he has end-stage lung cancer. You explain to him that his prognosis is poor and that the recommended treatment at this time would be palliative chemotherapy.

L. Murayama-Sung (✉)
2756 K Pali Highway, Honolulu, HI 96817, USA
e-mail: murayamalori@yahoo.com

I. Ahmed
Department of Behavioral Health, Tripler Army Medical Center, 1 Jarrett White Road, Tripler AMC, Honolulu, HI 96859, USA
e-mail: ahmedi96822@gmail.com

D. Alicata et al. (eds.), *Problem-based Behavioral Science and Psychiatry*,
DOI 10.1007/978-3-319-23669-8_16

Mr. Kim barely says a word during this discussion, but you brush this off because he seems "all right" at the time. Later, however, you become concerned that he may be suffering from depression because the nursing staff has witnessed him crying frequently in his room. He also has been barely touching his food.

You decide to address these issues; however, before you do, you try to recall the recent grand rounds on "stages of grief." You also think about how you will need to differentiate between depression that needs treatment and an adjustment reaction that will dissipate with time.

Please proceed with the problem-based approach using the worksheet located in the appendix of Chap. 1!

Please fill in the facts, your hypotheses, further information needed, and learning issues in Learning Issue Table 16.1.1.

Learning Issue Table 16.1.1

FACTS	HYPOTHESES	INFORMATION NEEDED	LEARNING ISSUES

Kubler-Ross's stages of grief provide a model for the different emotional and cognitive stages that people experience when they are faced with loss (Kubler-Ross 1996). Not everyone progresses through these stages in this particular order and some people skip stages. Table 16.1 describes the stages and offers examples for each of them.

In addition to recognizing stages of grief, you need to determine if Mr. Kim meets criteria for a normal grief reaction (preparatory grief) versus a major depressive episode. While people can have symptoms similar to those seen in depression, during acute grief, the intensity and duration of symptoms appear less (Widera 2012). Grief also does not typically have symptoms of extreme guilt or suicidal thoughts. Please see Chap. 8, "The Physician–Patient Relationship" for information on breaking bad news (Table 16.2).

Table 16.1 Stages of grief (Kubler-Ross 1969)

Stage	Example
Denial	Mr. Kim is in disbelief that he has lung cancer
Anger	Mr. Kim gets angry with himself or his physicians for not recognizing his illness earlier. He also gets angry with God because he feels his situation is unjust
Bargaining	Mr. Kim tries to make deals with God or with himself such as "If my cancer remits, I promise I won't smoke anymore."
Depression	Mr. Kim starts to feel sad or despondent
Acceptance	Mr. Kim realizes that he has cancer, starts to cope with the realities of having cancer, and starts to focus on treatment and his day-to-day relationships

Table 16.2 Distinguishing characteristics of grief and depression in terminally Ill patients (Widera and Block 2012)

Characteristic	Normal grief	Depression
Nature of response	Adaptive	Maladaptive
Focus of distress	Distress is in response to a particular loss and does not affect all aspects of life	Distress is pervasive and affects all aspects of life
Symptom fluctuations	Comes in waves but generally improves with time	Constant
Mood	Sadness and dysphoria	Protracted and constant depression or flat affect
Interests/capacity for pleasure	Interests and capacity for pleasure intact, although engagement in activities may be diminished because of functional decline	Anhedonia with markedly diminished interest or pleasure in all activities
Hope	Episodic and focal loss of hope; hopes may change over time, giving persons positive orientation toward the future	Hopelessness is persistent and pervasive
Self-worth	Maintained self-worth, although feelings of helplessness are common	Worthlessness with feeling that one's life has no value
Guilt	Regrets and guilt over specific events	Excessive feelings of guilt
Suicidal ideation	Passive and fleeting desire for hastened death	Preoccupation with a desire to die

Case Vignette 16.1.2

Mr. Kim tells you that for months he knew that something was "not right" with his body but delayed seeking treatment because of concerns that it could be something bad. He explains that when you initially told him he had end-stage cancer, he felt numb and was in disbelief. However, after a few days, his situation started to sink in.

Mr. Kim admits to feeling sad and anxious with regard to his cancer. He denies actual thoughts of wanting to hurt himself at this time. He also denies any feelings of hopelessness or worthlessness. He does admit to recent weight loss, decreased energy, and some difficulty sleeping due to lower back pain secondary to compression fractures from bony metastasis.

Please proceed with the problem-based approach using the worksheet located in the appendix of Chap. 1!

Please fill in the facts, your hypotheses, further information needed, and learning issues in Learning Issue Table 16.1.2.

Learning Issue Table 16.1.2

FACTS	HYPOTHESES	INFORMATION NEEDED	LEARNING ISSUES

At this point, it seems most likely that Mr. Kim may be suffering from a grief reaction. However, in addition to assessing for grief and depression, it is also important to assess for other psychiatric conditions such as anxiety disorders, mood and anxiety disorders secondary to another medical condition, and delirium.

Case Vignette 16.1.3

When discussing his medical issues, Mr. Kim describes his fear about what will happen to his body and his ability to function as he approaches death. He remembers watching his father die from gastric cancer and is worried that he will experience the same amount of pain. He states that if the pain became unbearable, he would want you to put him out of his misery like those people in the television special he saw on Dr. Jack Kevorkian. Mr. Kim tells you how important it is for him to have a dignified death. You pause to think about what other goals patients may have at the end of life.

Please proceed with the problem-based approach using the worksheet located in the appendix of Chap. 1!

Please fill in the facts, your hypotheses, further information needed, and learning issues in Learning Issue Table 16.1.3.

Learning Issue Table 16.1.3

FACTS	HYPOTHESES	INFORMATION NEEDED	LEARNING ISSUES

Although Mr. Kim brings up end-of-life issues on his own, for many patients, these discussions are often avoided for various reasons including (Bernacki and Block 2014) the following:

- Patient barriers: the patient may be scared, confused, unaware of the seriousness, or too embarrassed to approach topic. Cultural or family factors may impede discussions as well.
- Physician barriers: the physician may feel too nervous to deliver bad news or may not feel adequately trained in delivering this type of news.
- Systems barriers: with multiple physicians treating the patient, it may be unclear who is responsible for bringing up this discussion.

In order to improve these end-of-life discussions, Balaban (2000) created a four-step approach described below:

- Initiate end-of-life discussion
  - Provide a supportive/sympathetic environment for the patient and their family by listening and encouraging open discussions
  - Designate a durable power of attorney (DPOA) or surrogate decision-maker
  - Elicit the patient's general ideas about end-of-life care
- Clarify prognosis
  - Be frank yet compassionate about their prognosis
  - It may be necessary to repeat explanations
  - Clarify the patient's understanding
  - Avoid medical jargon
- Identify goals at the end of life
  - See table below
  - Discuss goals in terms of medical care
- Create a treatment plan
  - Help patient understand their medical options including where they will receive their care and about pain management

Table 16.3 Common treatment goals at the end of life (Block 2000; Larson and Tobin 2000)

Goals	Ways to approach these topics
1. Maintain sense of identity and operate as independently as possible within the limits of illness and prognosis	"What barriers prevent you from feeling comfortable and in control as you deal with your illness?"
	"How would you like your loved ones to remember you?"
	End-of-life discussions including treatment options can provide sense of control
2. To avoid/limit pain and suffering	"Is pain or the possibility of pain/suffering a concern for you?"
	Do not say: "There is not much that can be done for you."
	Instead say: "I believe there is much that can be done to manage your pain, provide you comfort, and assist you in living every day to its fullest."
3. Maintain/enhance important relationships and resolve conflicts with others	"Are there people in your life you want to get closer to or make up with?"
	"How do you want to tell your loved ones good bye?"
	Encourage families to share emotions and memories, and collect memorabilia
4. Pursue remaining dreams and setting goals	"When you think about your future, what is of greatest importance to you?"
	"Are there unresolved issues that you need to take care of and bring closure to?"
	Help patient come up with goals such as attending their son's wedding or going to a grandchild's graduation
5. Finding meaning in life and death	Patients often question what type of legacy they have left behind. Allowing patients to share memories, words of wisdom
6. Preparation for death: being able to hand over control to family and loved ones	"In what ways can you help your family prepare for and cope with your death?"
	Organize end-of-life plans (living wills and funeral arrangements)
	Having a frank conversation with the patient about their prognosis and what happens as they are about to die can be helpful
	Telling the patient that you will be there until the end can be reassuring to patients

- Provide treatment recommendations
- Identify the patient's preferences with regard to resuscitation
- Discuss palliative care if appropriate

During this case, Mr. Kim brought up his goal of having a "good death." End-of-life conversations should include finding out from patients what their goals are even if faced with a terminal illness. Here are some common goals that people have at the end of life and ways to phrase these conversations (Table 16.3).

16.1 Pain Management in Palliative Care

Another issue that Mr. Kim was trying to ask is "will my pain be addressed?" This is an important concern for many end-of-life patients that often is incompletely addressed as evident by the SUPPORT study (The SUPPORT Principal Investigators 1995).

When evaluating pain for palliative care patients, the physician must assess etiology, quality, severity, timing, and relieving/exacerbating factors. Principles for pain management (particularly with cancer patients) include the following (DeSandre and Quest 2010):

- Mild-to-moderate pain→nonopioid analgesics (NSAIDs, aspirin, acetaminophen) +/– adjunctive agents.
- Moderate-to-severe pain→addition of opioid analgesics, to provide additive analgesic effects.
  - Moderate pain→opioids such as codeine or hydrocodone.
  - Moderate-to-severe pain→use higher potency opioids such as morphine, methadone (long half-life), or fentanyl (short half-life).
- When prescribing for patients with chronic pain, it is better to have scheduled, rather than pro re nata (PRN) analgesics to decrease breakthrough pain.
- Other adjunctive agents can be use for various types of pain. Medications such as tricyclic antidepressants or gabapentin can be used in neuropathic pain.
- Behavioral techniques such as relaxation techniques, biofeedback, or cognitive restructuring can be used as well.
- Physical methods, such as heat/cold and acupuncture may be tried.
- Treat comorbid psychiatric conditions, which can increase the patient's subjective experience of pain.

16.2 Physician-Assisted Suicide and Euthanasia

Euthanasia is when the physician actively participates with intentionally ending a patient's life. It is illegal and considered a criminal act in all states but some countries such as the Netherlands have had regulated systems for its practice (Steck et al. 2013).

By contrast, PAS is when the physician provides the patient with medications, interventions, or information that the patient will use to commit suicide. While this is currently legal in certain states, many medical organizations such as the American Medical Association have made statements against these practices (American Medical Association 2005; Weinberger 2014).

Many Americans support euthanasia and PAS for those in severe pain (Emanuel 2002). Pain, however, does not appear to be the main reason why people request these interventions. Psychosocial and existential factors appear to play more of a role. According to a systematic review performed by Hudson et al. (2006), depression/hopelessness, burdening others, loss of autonomy, physical symptoms, anxiety about the future, and existential worries were common themes behind these requests.

If Mr. Kim were to bring up the topic of PAS/euthanasia, it would be important to consider the following:

- How serious is the request?→Was Mr. Kim just reacting to his current situation or was he actually seeking information or assistance?
- What is the underlying reason for wanting PAS/euthanasia?→Mr. Kim discussed his concerns about unaddressed pain.
- Do not assume that a decision is final. Studies have shown that depression and hopelessness have been strongly associated with requests for euthanasia or PAS and that such requests can dissipate with time (Chochinov et al. 1995; Monforte-Royo 2011).
- Assess for psychiatric symptoms and even consider a psychiatric consultation→Is depression contributing to Mr. Kim's request?
- Find out about the patient's support system.
- Educate the patient that alternatives such as treatment withdrawal, aggressive management of pain (even if it may shorten the patient's life), and withholding fluids or nutrition are legal and not considered PAS.

Case Vignette 16.1.4

Mr. Kim appears to have accepted his prognosis. You initiate a discussion about his end-of-life goals. He reflects on all the things he would still like to accomplish, especially since he has only been married to his wife for 2 years. He describes the plans they had to travel to Europe when he retired at age 65. He also tells you that he has not spoken to his three adult children for several years after a bitter divorce from their mother and how he would like to reconcile with them. He worries about his wife, who also has multiple medical problems, and asks you if his death could possibly impact her health. You ask Mr. Kim whether faith or religion is an important part of his life. He says that he has not attended church in years but would like to speak with the hospital chaplain.

STOP

Please proceed with the problem-based approach using the worksheet located in the appendix of Chap. 1!

Please fill in the facts, your hypotheses, further information needed, and learning issues in Learning Issue Table 16.1.4.

Learning Issue Table 16.1.4

FACTS	HYPOTHESES	INFORMATION NEEDED	LEARNING ISSUES

16.3 Impact of Death on the Surviving Spouse

Studies have shown that the loss of a spouse can significantly impact the physical and psychological health of the survivor. Rates of hospitalizations and mortality are increased with higher rates from accidental, alcohol-related causes, and violent means and moderate increases from lung cancer and ischemic heart disease (Moon 2011).

16.4 Spirituality and Religion at the End of Life

Physicians are often uncomfortable asking about faith, but as Mr. Kim has shown, spirituality can play an important role for the terminally ill. Research has shown that only 10 % of physicians discuss spirituality with their patients despite 65–95 % of patients wanting this addressed (Puchalski 2002). Thus, simply asking, "Is your faith important to you in this illness?" can open up the discussion (Larson and Tobin 2000).

Religion or spirituality can be the way that people explore the meaning of their death and cope with their dying process. Studies have shown that positive religious coping is significantly associated with fewer symptoms of depression in old age (Bjorklof et al. 2013). It can also be a protective factor against despair experienced at the end of life (Puchalski 2002).

Discussions about faith are important because many religions have certain beliefs about end-of-life care. Finding out the patient's religious background and specific needs during the dying process can show commitment to caring for the patient as a whole. For example, some religions want their religious leaders present at the time of death (Roman Catholics have last rites) or have special requests for the care of the body before and after the patient's death. Certain religions such as Islam and Judaism also have traditions that can impact autopsy or organ donation (Oliver et al. 2011).

Case Vignette 16.1.5
Mr. Kim then asks you about hospice and about the process of organ donation because the social worker came in earlier asking if he would like more information. As you glance over his electronic record, you notice that his code status has not been updated; therefore, you ask him about his resuscitation wishes. After reviewing hospital policies and Internet resources (e.g., at http://www.polst.org/), you complete an updated Physicians Orders for Life Sustaining Treatment (POLST) form.

Hospice/Palliative Care
Mr. Kim asks you about hospice, but before this topic can be discussed further, the general principle of palliative care should be discussed. The goals of palliative care are to enhance quality of life and relieve pain and suffering for patients with advanced disease (Morrison and Meier 2004; American Family Physician 2014). A multidisciplinary approach addresses psychosocial as well as spiritual issues and offers support to patients and families. Palliative care may be offered alongside other medical treatments. It aims to neither quicken nor delay death.

In order to qualify for hospice, a patient must be deemed to be terminally ill with a life expectancy of 6 months or less (Morrison and Meier 2004). The patient and their family's goals must be directed at symptom relief rather than curative treatments aimed at prolonging life.

Organ Donation
In this vignette, Mr. Kim asks about the process of organ donation and the criteria for it. Most organ transplantations are the result of donations from deceased donors (Institute of Medicine 2006).

Previously, the criteria for organ donation were strict with potential donors being under 50 years with limited comorbid conditions. Today, there is no national standard in terms of absolute or relative contraindications. Transplant centers each have their own criteria, often on a case-by-case basis, because of the few absolute contraindications. Patients and their families may need to understand the concept of brain death and the process of organ donation in order to decide what is best for them.

Case Vignette 16.1.6
After discussing his code status with you, Mr. Kim decides that he does not want life-sustaining measures if there is no hope for recovery or if he is unable to interact with his family. He names his wife as his DPOA in case he becomes incapacitated and is unable to make medical decisions for himself.

Several days later, Mr. Kim's respiratory function rapidly deteriorates. He becomes increasingly hypoxic and less responsive. Sensing the gravity of his situation, you gather his family members, including his estranged children.

Because of his previously stated wishes, you prepare to deliver comfort care to minimize his feelings of dyspnea as well as his bony pain. There is conflict, however, among the newly arrived family members. They are pushing for intubation despite the patient's wishes. You are frustrated by Mr. Kim's children who demand aggressive treatment against his stated wishes.

16.5 End-of-Life Discussions with Family Members

The conflict between Mr. Kim's and his family's wishes is a common theme seen in the hospital. Here are some ways to address this issue (Balaban 2000; Weissman 2004):

- Understand that acceptance of the patient's prognosis occurs differently for different people. Often times, it is more difficult for families to accept the patient's impending death than it is for the patient.
- Go over clinical information with the patient and their family in a manner that is simple and jargon free.
- Allow the patient and their family time to express their feelings and ask questions.
- Sometimes families want "everything done" despite the patient having a poor prognosis. In these cases, it is important to uncover the underlying motivation. Assessing the family dynamics can provide insight into unresolved issues or conflicts. Occasionally, families may not realize the futility of treatment; therefore, prognosis should be discussed.
- If these discussions are unable to progress, the ethics committee or legal counsel can help.

Case Vignette 16.1.7
You arrange a family meeting to ascertain the family's understanding of Mr. Kim's condition and overall prognosis. His children repeatedly ask, "Why can't we use machines to help him breathe so we can keep him alive until he recovers?" They also ask why he is unresponsive and whether he is brain-dead. You explain to them the difference between coma and brain death.

Diagnosing Death
Mr. Kim's family brings up a topic that can often be confusing for families. Below is a table that helps to distinguish between persistent vegetative state (PVS), coma, and brain death. While there are differences in opinion regarding what to do with patients in a PVS, if a patient is diagnosed as brain-dead, they are considered legally dead. However, there is a great deal of variability from state to state regarding the definition and declaration of brain death. Since many states offer little guidance in diagnosing brain death, it is up to individual hospitals to develop policies for addressing brain death and organ donation. It is important that the patient is

Table 16.4 Differentiating between various states of conscious. (Multi-Society Task Force on PVS 1994)

Persistent vegetative state (PVS)	Coma	Brain death
The patient is awake and has sleep/wake cycles but is unaware of themselves and their surroundings	Sustained unconsciousness can progress to consciousness, PVS, or death	Irreversibly comatose legally dead; therefore, life support is futile
Hypothalamic and brain-stem autonomic functioning is intact but there are no purposeful responses to stimuli	Due to dysfunction in the ascending reticular activating system (which can be damaged at the site of the brain stem or both cerebral hemispheres). The patient is unable to be aroused, and this status lasts longer than 1 h	Absence of all brain functions including the brain stem, reflexes, and cranial nerves

pronounced brain-dead as per the policy used at a given hospital. Once a person is considered legally dead, organ donation can commence and life support can be disconnected (Table 16.4).

Case Vignette 16.1.8

Soon after the family meeting, there is a call from Mr. Kim's nurse saying that he is increasingly tachycardic and tachypneic. Family members at the bedside are distressed by his breathing pattern and are asking for measures to make him comfortable. "He looks like he's drowning. Can't you do something?" After you give him morphine to make him feel better, he eventually becomes more hypoxic with agonal breathing, progressing to complete unresponsiveness and asystole.

As you are performing the "death pronouncement," you can hear the family sobbing at the bedside. You then turn to them and say, "I'm very sorry. When you are ready, we can meet in the family room where we can talk and I can answer any questions you may have."

	Please proceed with the problem-based approach using the worksheet located in the appendix of Chap. 1!

Please fill in the facts, your hypotheses, further information needed, and learning issues in Learning Issue Table 16.1.5–16.1.8.

Learning Issue Table 16.1.5–16.1.8

FACTS	HYPOTHESES	INFORMATION NEEDED	LEARNING ISSUES

16.6 How to Address the Family at the Time of Death (Jurkovich et al. 2000; Williams et al. 2000)

Addressing Mr. Kim's death with his family is difficult, but here are some ways to improve these conversations with families:

- Meet the family in a private area. Identify their relationships with the deceased.
- Families like to be told in a sympathetic and unrushed manner what happened. Use the patient's name rather than "the patient." Advise them if an autopsy is required.
- Allow family to ask questions and express their feelings.
- Allow them time to view the deceased and prepare them if there are any medical devices left or if the body has been altered physically.
- Assist family with what to do next (e.g., how to make funeral arrangements, when they can go home).
- Offer to request a visit from a pastoral counselor.
- Give handouts about the grieving process.

16.7 Review Questions

1. Which of the following is more likely a sign of depression rather than attributable to a grief reaction?

    a. Difficulty sleeping for several days
    b. Minor guilt
    c. Feelings of worthlessness

2. What are the stages of grief?

    - A. Denial
    - B. Anger
    - C. Bargaining

- D. Depression
- E. Acceptance
- F. All of the above

3. True/False:

   a. Euthanasia is legal in the USA.
   b. PAS is illegal in all states.

Appendix A: Tables with Possible Answers to the Vignettes

Case Vignette 16.1: Mr. Kim

Learning Issue Table 16.1.1

Facts	Hypotheses	Information needed	Learning issues
63-year-old Chinese man	Normal grief reaction	Does he meet DSM-5 criteria for major depression?	What are the stages of grief?
80 pack-year smoking history	Major depressive episode		
Had not sought medical treatment in years	Adjustment reaction		
Has end-stage lung cancer			
Recommended treatment would be palliative chemotherapy			
Barely says a word during this discussion			
Nursing staff has witnessed him crying frequently in his room, barely touching his food			

Learning Issue Table 16.1.2

Facts	Hypotheses	Information needed	Learning issues
Delayed seeking treatment because of concerns that it could be something bad	Grief reaction	Monitor for other mental status changes	How does the clinician differentiate grief and depression?

Felt numb and was in disbelief	Rule out anxiety disorders, mood and anxiety disorders secondary to another medical condition, and delirium	What else is he worried about?	
Sad and anxious, denies actual thoughts of wanting to hurt himself		How much pain does he have and how well is it controlled?	
Denies any feelings of hopelessness or worthlessness			
Recent weight loss, decreased energy, some difficulty sleeping due to lower back pain			

Learning Issue Table 16.1.3

Facts	Hypotheses	Information needed	Learning issues
Afraid of what will happen to his body and his ability to function as he approaches death	Afraid of pain	What other goals may he have at the end of life?	What are common treatment goals at the end of life?
Saw his father die (with pain) from gastric cancer			What is the AMA Code of Medical Ethics, Opinion 2.211, position on PAS?
Saw a television special on Dr. Jack Kevorkian			
Important to have a dignified death			

Learning Issue Table 16.1.4

Facts	Hypotheses	Information needed	Learning issues
Appears to have accepted his prognosis			What is the impact on the surviving spouse?

Been married to his wife for 2 years			How can the physician determine whether spirituality and religion are relevant for the patient?
They had plans to travel to Europe when he retired at age 65			
He has not spoken to his three adult children for several years after a bitter divorce from their mother and would like to reconcile with them			
He worries about his wife, who also has multiple medical problems			
He has not attended church in years but would like to speak with the hospital chaplain			

Learning Issue Table 16.1.5–16.1.8

Facts	Hypotheses	Information needed	Learning issues
Increasingly tachycardic and tachypneic	Family may have grief issues	What questions do the family members have?	How does the clinician engage family members in end-of-life discussions?
Family members at the bedside are distressed			How does the physician address the family at the time of death?
"He looks like he's drowning. Can't you do something?"			
Morphine given to make him feel better			
Progresses to complete unresponsiveness and asystole			
Family sobbing at the bedside			

Appendix B: Answers to Review Questions

Answers: 1. C, 2. F, 3. a—False. b—False

References

American Family Physician. (2014). End of life care. (Last update: 06/17/2014). http://www.aafp.org/afp/topicModules/viewTopicModule.htm?topicModuleId=57#0. Accessed 27 Feb 2015.

American Medical Association. (2005). E-2.211 Physician-assisted suicide. (Last updated 2005). http://www.ama-assn.org/ama/pub/physician-resources/medical-ethics/code-medical-ethics/opinion2211.page?. Accessed 3 Sept 2015.

Balaban, R. B. (2000). A physician's guide to talking about end-of-life care. *Journal of General Internal Medicine, 3,* 195–200.

Bernacki, R. E., & Block, S. D. (2014). American college of physicians high value care task force: Communication about serious illness care goals: A review and synthesis of best practices. *JAMA Internal Medicine, 174*(12), 1994–2003.

Block, S. D. (2000). Assessing and managing depression in the terminally ill patient. *Annals of Internal Medicine, 132,* 209–218.

Block, S. D. (2001). Psychological considerations, growth, and transcendence at the end of life. *Journal of the American Medical Association, 285*(22), 2898–2905.

Bjorklof, G. H., Engedal, K., Selbaek, G., Kouwenhoven, S. E., & Helvik, A. S. (2013). Coping and depression in old age: A literature review. *Dementia Geriatrics Cognitive Disorders, 35,* 121–154.

Chochinov, H. M., Wilson, K. G., Enns, M., Mowchun, N., Lander, S., Levitt, M., & Clinch, J. J. (1995). Desire for death in the terminally ill. *American Journal of Psychiatry, 152,* 1185–1191.

Da Silva, I., & Frontera, J. A. (2015). Worldwide barriers to organ donation. *JAMA Neurology, 72*(1), 112–118.

Desandre, P. L., & Quest, T. E. (2010). Management of cancer-related pain. *Hematology/Oncology Clinics of North America, 24*(3), 643–658.

Dirckx, J. H. (Ed.). (1987). Stedman's concise medical dictionary for health professions (1st ed., p. 408). Williams & Wilkins.

Emanuel, E. J. (2002). Euthanasia and physician-assisted suicide. *Archives of Internal Medicine, 162,* 142–152.

Goy, E., & Ganzini, L. (2003). End-of-life care in geriatric psychiatry. *Clinics in Geriatric Medicine,* 19(4), 841–856.

Hudson, P. L., Kristjanson, L. J., Ashby, M., Kelly, B., Schofield, P., Hudson, R., Aranda, S., O'Connor, M., & Street, A. (2006). Desire for hastened death in patients with advanced disease and the evidence based of clinical guidelines: A systematic review. *Palliative Medicine, 20,* 693–701.

Institute of Medicine. (2006). *Committee on increasing organ donation: Organ donation: Opportunities for action* (1st ed.). Washington: National Academy of Sciences.

Jurkovich, G. J., Pierce, B., Pananen, L., & Rivara, F. P. (2000). Giving bad news: The family perspective. *The Journal of Trauma: Injury, Infection, and Critical Care, 48,* 865–870.

Kahn, M. J., Lazarus, C. J., & Owens, D. P. (2003). Allowing patients to die: Practical, ethical, and religious concerns. *Journal of Clinical Oncology, 21*(15), 3000–3002.

Kelly, B., Mc Clement, S., & Chochinov, H. M. (2006). Measurement of psychological distress in palliative care. *Palliative Medicine, 20,* 779–789.

Koenig, H. G., Cohen, H. J., Blazer, D. G., Kudler, H. S., Krishnan, K. R., & Sibert, T. E. (1995). Religious coping and cognitive symptoms of depression in elderly medical patients. *Psychosomatics, 36*(4), 369–375.

Kubler-Ross, E. (1969). *On death and dying*. New York: MacMillan.
Levy, M. H. (1996). Pharmacological treatment of cancer pain. *New England Journal of Medicine, 335*(15), 1124–1132.
Monforte-Royo, C., Villavicencio-Chávez, C., Tomás-Sábado, J., & Balaguer, A. (2011). The wish to hasten death: A review of clinical studies. *Psychooncology, 20*(8), 795–804.
Moon, J. R., Kondo, N., Glymour, M. M., & Subramanian, S.V. (2011). Widowhood and mortality: A meta-analysis. *PLoS ONE, 6*(8), e23465.
Morrison, R. S., & Meier, E. D. (2004). Palliative care. *New England Journal of Medicine, 350*(25), 2582–2590.
Multi-Society Task Force on PVS. (1994). Medical aspects of the persistent vegetative state—first of two parts. *New England Journal of Medicine, 330,* 1499–1508.
Oliver, M., Woywodt, A., Ahmed, A., & Saif, I. (2011). Organ donation, transplantation and religion. *Nephrology Dialysis Transplantation, 26,* 437–444.
Periyakoil, V. S., & Hallenbeck, J. (2002). Identifying and managing preparatory grief and depression at the end of life. *American Family Physician, 65*(5), 883–90.
Puchalski, C. M. (2002). Spirituality and end-of-life care: A time for listening and caring. *Journal of Palliative Medicine, 5*(2), 289–294.
Siminoff, L. A., Arnold, R. M., Caplan, A. L., Virnig, B. A., & Seltzer, D. L. (1995). Public policy governing organ and tissue procurement in the United States. *Annals of Internal Medicine, 123*(1), 10–17.
Steck, N., Egger, M., Maessen, M., Reisch, T., & Zwahlen, M. (2013). Euthanasia and assisted suicide in selected European countries and US states: Systematic literature review. *Medical Care, 51*(10), 938–944.
Sullivan, A. D., Hedberg, K., Feming, D. W. (2000). Legalized physician-assisted suicide in Oregon—the second year. *New England Journal of Medicine, 342*(8), 598–604.
The SUPPORT Principal Investigators. (1995). A controlled trial to improve care for seriously ill hospitalized patients. The study to understand prognoses and preferences for outcomes and risks of treatments (SUPPORT). *Journal of the American Medical Association, 274*(2), 1591–1598.
Weinberger, L. E., Sreenivasan, S., & Garrick, T. (2014). End-of-life mental health assessments for older aged, medically ill persons with expressed desire to die. *Journal of the American Academy of Psychiatry and the Law, 42*(3), 350–361.
Weissman, D. E. (2004). Decision making at a time of crisis near the end of life. *Journal of the American Medical Association, 292*(14), 1738–1743.
Widera, E. W., & Block, S. D. (2012). Managing grief and depression at the end of life. *American Family Physician, 86*(3), 259–264.
Williams, G., O'Brien, D. L., Laughton, K. J., & Jelin, G. A. (2000). Improving services to bereaved relatives in the emergency department: Making healthcare more human. *Medical Journal of Australia, 173,* 480–483.

Chapter 17
Basic Principles of Evaluation: Interviewing, Mental Status Examination, Differential Diagnosis, and Treatment Planning

Anthony P. S. Guerrero and Daniel A. Alicata*

This chapter helps bring everything you are learning full circle as we discuss the actual patient encounter. We compare and contrast the psychiatric evaluation to that of general medicine and describe what is expected in your psychiatric clerkship as you examine, diagnose, and develop a treatment plan. This provides the context for applying the principles of psychiatry.

17.1 Objectives

At the end of this chapter, the reader will be able to:

1. Discuss the basic structural components of a psychiatric interview, including history and mental status examination (MSE).
2. Discuss the basic principles to guide the process of an effective interview, including establishing and maintaining rapport, prioritizing safety, and efficiently gathering data sufficient to yield a differential diagnosis.
3. Discuss the process of differential diagnosis according to the Diagnostic and Statistical Manual of Mental Disorders, 5th Edition (DSM-5).
4. Discuss the process of biopsychosocial–cultural formulation and treatment planning.

* Co-first editor of the book.

A. P. S. Guerrero (✉) · D. A. Alicata
Department of Psychiatry, John A. Burns School of Medicine, University of Hawai'i,
1356 Lusitana Street, University Tower 4th Floor, Honolulu, HI 96813, USA
e-mail: GuerreroA@dop.hawaii.edu

D. A. Alicata
e-mail: alicatad@dop.hawaii.edu

D. Alicata et al. (eds.), *Problem-based Behavioral Science and Psychiatry*,
DOI 10.1007/978-3-319-23669-8_17

Case Vignette 17.1.1 Dan, Tony, and Melissa
Dan, Tony, and Melissa are second-year medical students who are starting their "brain and behavior" clinical skills preceptorship. They are quite apprehensive about performing their first interview because they believe that "everything is totally different when it comes to psych."

Students often worry that the basic history and examination skills they learned on other clinical services will not work in psychiatric settings. In reality, the entire assessment and treatment planning process learned in other parts of medicine are completely relevant to psychiatry, with a few relevant adaptations, as shown in Table 17.1.

Table 17.1 Components of the psychiatric assessment

Traditional "medical exam" component	Psychiatric assessment component
Identifying data	Same
Source and reliability	Same
Chief complaint	Same
History of the present illness, with attention to "pertinent positives" and "pertinent negatives"	Same—with attention to the psychiatric review of systems and the different psychiatric and another medical conditions that should be "ruled in" and "ruled out"
Past medical history	Same *plus* a specific past psychiatric history
Family history	Same—with attention to psychiatric conditions
Social history	Same—often more lengthy because of the role of social factors in psychiatric illness
Review of systems	Same—because another medical conditions (detectable in the review of systems) can often explain psychiatric symptoms
Physical examination	Same—with more emphasis on the neurological exam and the MSE as a detailed branch step of the physical examination
	MSE (described further below)
Problem list and assessment of each problem	Psychiatric formulation and differential diagnosis, based on the DSM-5
Plan, with additional information/diagnostic testing, specific treatments, and patient education	Same

MSE mental status examination, *DSM-5* Diagnostic and Statistical Manual of Mental Disorders, 5th Edition

Case Vignette 17.1.2 Continued

The three students feel less anxious, knowing that they can apply the skills that they have already learned. They successfully met the requirements of the preceptorship.

The three students are now third-year medical students new to the psychiatry clerkship. They each are about to do their first patient interview for the clerkship. Dan, who received positive recognition in his previous clerkships for his patience and his excellent bedside manner, states: "All I need to do is listen, and I think the patient will tell me what I need to know in 30 min (which is the time allotted to the interview)." Tony, who was recognized in his previous clerkships for his high exam scores, states: "I think I have everything figured out: all I need to do is ask the patient everything in this master template that I made, and everything will be fine." Finally, Melissa, who was recognized in her previous clerkships for her overall stellar performance, states: "I've never had a problem interviewing patients. I just need to get Honors in this clerkship because I want to go into a competitive specialty."

Following their first interview, the three students are flustered. In a debriefing meeting with their clerkship director, Dr. Nicole, Dan states: "I couldn't get a word in during the interview. All I was able to find out was that this patient is married and that he is a Christian. I was totally lost during the rest of the interview, and I didn't want to interrupt him because it seemed like he would get mad." Tony states: "Even though I kept telling the patient how important it was to answer all of my questions, all he could do was give one-word answers, look quickly from one side of the room to the next, and then ask to go back to his room …which he did anyway after only 15 min. I ran out of time and we didn't even get to why he overdosed." Melissa states: "Because my patient kept crying so much, I didn't get a chance to test all of that important stuff for psychiatry, like ask about rolling stones gathering no moss and what to do with a stamped envelope."

Dr. Nicole, hoping to help their subsequent interviews with these patients to go smoother, encourages them to think of the interview as an opportunity to apply the problem-based approach. "What do you mean?" they ask. Dr. Nicole encourages them to proceed with a modification of the familiar problem-based approach.

Although this is not the typical problem-based learning (PBL) scenario, use of a modified PBL issue table may be helpful in guiding the process of the interview, as shown in Learning Issue Table 17.1.1–17.1.2.

Learning Issue Table 17.1.1–17.1.2

What are the observations about the process of the interview?	What are the hypotheses about why the interview is going this way?	What might I need to ask about and/or do next?
(For Dan) Difficult to interrupt patient “I’m lost”	Bipolar mania	Summarize, ask clarifying questions
	Schizophrenia	Do one’s best to elicit relevant history
	Methamphetamine intoxication	
(For Tony) One-word answers Looking quickly from one side of the room to the next Wants to go back to room	Suspicion about the interview process	Ask about and try to optimize patient’s comfort
	Irritability from depression	Reorient patient to purpose and context of interview
		Do one’s best to elicit relevant history
(For Melissa) Crying so much	Depression	Recognize patient’s emotions and provide empathic comments as appropriate
	Grief	

While the structural elements of the psychiatric interview are essentially identical to elements of the general medical interview, a distinguishing characteristic of psychiatric interviewing is the likelihood that the very illness that one is trying to assess (such as the primary mood or psychotic disorder that Dan’s patient above likely was demonstrating symptoms of) may impact the very *process* of the interview. Whenever something unexpected happens in an interview (ranging from intense tearfulness, to a request to leave the interview early, to an unusual question being asked of the interviewer), the most appropriate next step is often to use this occurrence as an opportunity to gather more information about what might be happening. For example, “I notice that you’re really wanting to go back to your room … We’ll be done in a few minutes, but I wonder if you could tell me what you’re thinking right now or if there’s anything we could do to help you feel more comfortable right now.”

Even though it is easy to remember what the structural elements of an interview should be, students often feel challenged in getting through a “complete interview” in a time-limited period—which often needs to be done in real-life situations. We suggest that, during a time-limited interview, students should establish the following priorities:

1. *Attempt to establish and maintain rapport through:*
   - Unconditional positive regard for the patient and attentiveness to patient comfort. This can be conveyed through a friendly demeanor and supportive and empathic statements (“That must have been a tough time for you.”)
   - Adequate preparation for the interview (explaining the context)
   - Appropriate use of open-ended (yet context-appropriate) questions, such as “What happened that led to your hospitalization?” or “Could you tell me more about that?” or “What’s your understanding of what the medications are being prescribed for?”

- Responsiveness to the patient's emotions and other potential barriers to effective rapport. For example, Tony felt irritation in his interview, and Melissa felt overwhelmingly sad during her patient interview but neither responded to the patient's mood state. Failure to address such barriers may interfere with subsequent data gathering and may be more time consuming in the long run.

2. *Assess safety, specifically:*

   - Suicidality and thoughts of violence towards others: current ideations as well as previous dangerousness, command hallucinations, acute stressors, mood symptoms, and (if a recent attempt had been made) degree of premeditation (including suicide notes and other preparatory acts), method of discovery, perception of lethality, and what the patient perceives as having changed since the attempt. (Apparently, Tony did not prioritize this in his interview)
   - Abuse and being victimized (particularly for minors and dependent adults)
   - Serious psychotic symptoms that impair reality testing and would interfere with a patient's ability to meet basic needs
   - Other serious medical conditions
   - Substance intoxication and/or withdrawal (which could be life threatening)

3. *Attempt to elicit history and examination findings to at least establish a differential diagnosis* (not necessarily the definitive diagnosis, which may be unrealistic to determine in a short period of time):

   - Pertinent positives and pertinent negatives, based on criteria from the Diagnostic and Statistical Manual of Mental Disorders, currently in its 5th edition, text (DSM-5)
   - To the degree possible, review of the key areas of history and psychiatric review of systems

Another distinguishing characteristic of the psychiatric interview is the need to thoughtfully perform an MSE. While it may initially seem (as it probably did to Melissa) that the MSE is an academic exercise with little relevance to the rest of medicine, each of the elements have practical clinical relevance and represent an indirect assessment of neurological functions. Detailed descriptions of observations are more clinically relevant than clinical jargon. A good MSE will "paint a picture" of the patient at the time of the exam. The components of the MSE are summarized in Table 17.2.

Following the psychiatric interview and MSE is the biopsychosocial–cultural–spiritual formulation (discussed in Chap. 1) and a differential diagnosis with diagnostic classification made according to the DSM-5 (American Psychiatric Association 2013; Sadock et al. 2015, p. 214).

It may sometimes seem that the checklist approach used by DSM-5 for diagnosing psychiatric disorders seems like "cookbook" medicine because there is no "gold standard" along the lines of a definitive blood test or histopathological finding. However, it should be noted that other medical conditions, such as rheumatologic disorders and disorders affecting multiple systems, are diagnosed and very effectively treated through a similar approach.

Table 17.2 Components of the mental status examination

Mental status examination component	How assessed	Sample descriptive terms	Part(s) of the brain being tested	Examples of practical clinical relevance
General appearance	Observation	Well developed, well nourished, thin, overweight, good/poor hygiene, no obvious deformities, etc.	Multiple	Patients whose illness affects ability to care for self may have significant findings on general appearance
Eye contact	Observation	Good, adequate, fair, poor, etc.	Multiple	May be decreased as a result of depression or distraction from hallucinations, etc.
Cooperation with interview	Observation	Cooperative with interview, guarded, etc.	Multiple	Several conditions can impact upon rapport
Motor activity	Observation; sometimes formal testing for abnormal motor movements, tremor, and/or rigidity	Psychomotor agitation or retardation (or none), abnormal motor movements (or none), tremor, and/or rigidity present (or not)	Basal ganglia, motor cortex, other areas	Major depression may cause psychomotor retardation, while mania may cause psychomotor agitation. Antipsychotic medications may cause abnormal motor movements, tremor, and/or rigidity
Speech	Observation	Normal or increased or decreased rate and/or volume and/or amount; normal (or not) clarity	Multiple areas, including speech centers	Mood disorders and/or substance intoxication may affect the rate, volume, and/or amount of speech. Neurological conditions (that may also cause psychiatric symptoms) may affect clarity of speech

Table 17.2 (continued)

Mental status examination component	How assessed	Sample descriptive terms	Part(s) of the brain being tested	Examples of practical clinical relevance
Mood—expressed emotional state	Direct questioning about how the patient has been feeling; rate mood from 1 to 10, 10 = best possible	Euthymic, depressed, anxious, expansive, irritable	Hypothalamus, limbic system, other parts	Mood disorders and/or substances may affect patient's reported mood and observed affect
Affect—observed emotional state	Observation	Mood-congruency (mood-congruent, mood-incongruent)		
		Range (broad, restricted, flat)		
		Lability (labile or not)		
		Overall quality (neutral, depressed, anxious, euphoric, irritable)		
Thought process	Observation	Linear (remains on topic) and goal directed, circumstantial (goes off topic but eventually returns to the original topic), tangential (goes off topic without ever returning to the original topic), flight of ideas (without production of a coherent thought), word salad (in which even the individual words may not coherently link together)	Inappropriate mesolimbic dopamine release, poor cortical filtering; other areas	Primary psychotic disorders such as schizophrenia and/or substances may affect thought processes
Thought content	Observation, some direct questions	Delusions (present or not, with specific examples), paranoid ideations (present or not, with specific examples), future-orientation, etc.		Primary psychotic disorders such as schizophrenia and/or substances may affect result in delusions;depression with suicidal ideations may lead to a patient not having a future-orientation

Table 17.2 (continued)

Mental status examination component	How assessed	Sample descriptive terms	Part(s) of the brain being tested	Examples of practical clinical relevance
Perceptions	Direct questions, with some observation for distractibility of other evidence of response to internal stimuli	Auditory and visual hallucinations (present or not), appearance (or not) of seeming to respond to hallucinations, other hallucinations (e.g., tactile, olfactory, etc.) also important to note if present	See above, relevant sensory cortices (auditory, visual, etc.)	Primary psychotic disorders such as schizophrenia, substances, and/or delirium may result in hallucinations
Alertness	Observation	Alert, drowsy, stuporous, comatose	Reticular activating system	Delirium may cause fluctuations in level of alertness
Orientation	Direct questions, with some observation	Oriented (or not) to person, place, time (date, month, year), situation	Often depends on alertness and memory	Delirium may cause disorientation. Other memory-impairing conditions such as dementia may cause disorientation
Concentration	Direct questions, with some observation	Able (or not) to perform serial 7s (“take the number 100, subtract 7, and then keep subtracting 7 from your answer until I tell you to stop…”)	Reticular activating system	Delirium primarily affects alertness and concentration
		Able (or not) to spell 5-letter words such as “world” or “ocean” backwards. (Usually, one of these tests will suffice)		

Table 17.2 (continued)

Mental status examination component	How assessed	Sample descriptive terms	Part(s) of the brain being tested	Examples of practical clinical relevance
Memory	Direct questions	Ability to immediately recall three unrelated words that are not objects in the room (e.g., "umbrella," "car," "happiness") and to recall these words approximately 5 min later (if not spontaneously recalled, prompting or giving hints may suggest more impairment of memory retrieval than memory storage)	Hippocampus (memory encoding), other parts of the cerebral cortex	Dementia results in memory impairment along with other cognitive findings. Cortical dementias are associated with memory storage difficulties, while subcortical dementias are associated with memory retrieval difficulties
		Longer term memory may be assessed by asking the last five presidents, etc.		
Abstraction	Direct questions	Ability (or not) to state similarities (e.g., apple and orange are both fruits, table and chair are both furniture, newspaper and radio both tell the news, opera and a painting are both works of art) or accurately interpret proverbs (though proverbs often test more than just abstraction)	Frontal lobe	Schizophrenia often is associated with frontal lobe maldevelopment
Judgment	Observation, possibly direct questions	Ability (or not) to exercise good judgment with regards self-care, behaving appropriately	Frontal lobe	As above
Insight	Observation, possibly direct questions	Insight into illness, need for treatment	Frontal lobe	As above
Suicidality, homicidality, violence	Direct questions	Presence or absence: ideations and/or intentions	Multiple areas	Important to explicitly cover, in the interests of safety

Table 17.3 Treatment planning template

	Biological	Psychological	Social/cultural
Additional information	Old records (e.g., to look at previous diagnoses and medication efficacy)	Additional interviews	Talk to family, others if patient gives consent
		Speak with previous therapists, etc.	
	Ensure a recent physical exam	Psychological testing, for example, intelligence testing, personality testing, projective testing (to evaluate for psychotic processes)	
	Relevant labs, for example:		
	Chemistry profile		
	Complete blood count		
	Thyroid function tests		
	Tests to rule out infection (e.g., syphilis, HIV)		
	Toxicology screen		
	Neuroimaging		
Treatment	Continue effective medications, usually	Individual psychotherapy to build rapport	Family psychotherapy, if appropriate
	Abstinence from substances	Groups, for example, anger management, Alcoholics/Narcotics Anonymous	Social services, stable living
			Structured setting,for example, to remain safe, substance free, etc.
			Other resources
Patient education (often covered above)	Education on benefits and side effects of medications	Psychoeducation on need for compliance, crisis resources, etc.	Family psychoeducation as appropriate

HIV human immunodeficiency virus

Other medical conditions and substance-induced conditions, while often overlooked, are important to include in the differential diagnosis of many psychiatric conditions.

The final step of the psychiatric assessment is to develop a treatment plan that adequately considers the formulation and differential diagnosis. Please refer to Chap. 1 for a diagrammatic illustration of how a successful plan addresses the various components of a biopsychosocial–cultural–spiritual formulation. Table 17.3 shown below helps to develop a comprehensive plan.

We close, in Appendix 17.C, with a sample write-up of a fictitious patient (with gratitude to George Lucas, creator of the Star Wars series (Disney and Lucasfilm Ltd.), where many of the fictitious names came from).

17.2 Review Questions

1. You are interviewing a patient, who suddenly becomes very quiet and possibly tearful when the topic of her childhood is discussed. The next most appropriate thing to do is to:
   a. Switch the topic to something less sensitive
   b. Immediately perform a cognitive examination
   c. Recognize the change in affect and empathically acknowledge the likely difficulty in discussing such a topic
   d. Immediately terminate the interview and postpone any further attempts at interview until the patient can regain composure
   e. Reassure the patient that you know exactly how he or she feels, and that it is perfectly okay to cry
2. During the course of a diagnostic interview, your patient asks, for a second time, "Doctor, how old are you, anyway?" Which of the following is the best response:
   a. "Once again, this interview is about you, not about me, so let's talk about something else."
   b. "I'm old enough to be a physician and old enough to be interviewing you."
   c. "I'm very uncomfortable talking about my personal life with patients."
   d. "I notice that you're really interested in how old I am. I wonder what your thoughts are behind wanting to know."
   e. "I'm somewhere between 20 and 60."
3. All of the following statements are correct *except:*
   a. Affect describes one's observation of the patient's emotions during the interview.
   b. Mood describes what the patient's emotional state has generally been.
   c. Mood can be elicited through direct questioning of how the patient has been feeling.
   d. Tangential thoughts never return to the original topic or question.
   e. Circumstantiality is pathognomonic for a psychotic disorder.
4. Which of the following statements best describes the role of testing "serial 7's"
   a. Difficulties with this test may indicate delirium.
   b. This test is intended to primarily test mathematical abilities.
   c. Difficulties with this test always reflect dysfunction of the reticular activating system.
   d. Psychotic individuals invariably have difficulty with this test.
   e. This test must always be done in combination with asking the patient to spell "world" forwards and backwards and recall digit spans.

5. Which of the following statements about psychiatric assessment are correct:
   a. A biopsychosocial–cultural–spiritual formulation, because of its inherent inclusion of "psychiatric jargon" terms, is rarely useful for patients or other health professionals involved in patient care.
   b. Effective rapport is the foundation for all patient interviews, whether in psychiatry or in any other specialty of medicine.
   c. Psychiatrists should never perform physical examinations or order laboratory studies.
   d. Assessment of safety is merely an assessment of current suicidal or homicidal ideations.
   e. Learning disorders and pervasive developmental disorders are noted on Axis II.

Appendix A: Tables with Possible Answers to the Vignettes

Case Vignette 17.1: Dan, Tony, and Melissa

Appendix B: Answers to Review Questions

Answers

1. c
2. d
3. e
4. a
5. b

Appendix C: Sample Write-up

Name: Luke Skywalker, MS3
Attending psychiatrist: Master Yoda, M.D.
Date: 05/01/2014

Identifying Data Princess Leia is a 34-year-old cosmopolitan female, divorced, employed as a secretary.

Reason for Examination Psychiatric consultation for patient on the general medical ward; medical student write-up #1

Referring Physician Obi-Wan Kenobi, M.D. (internal medicine)

Source and Reliability Patient, who appears fairly reliable. Chart also reviewed.

Chief Complaint Acetaminophen overdose

History of the Present Illness

> Summarize information relevant for eventual formulation and differential diagnosis

Ms. Leia is a 34-year-old female admitted last night for an acetaminophen, acetaminophen/oxycodone, and ibuprofen overdose. This overdose occurred late yesterday afternoon (Saturday) at her apartment. She ingested several extra strength acetaminophen tablets, a few acetaminophen/oxycodone tablets, and a few ibuprofen tablets following an argument with her boyfriend over his recent infidelity. This argument started on Friday night and caused her to essentially not sleep the whole night. Immediately following the ingestion, she called her boyfriend, who then brought her to the emergency room, from where she was subsequently admitted because of an acetaminophen level in the toxic range.

> Assess safety

Ms. Leia states that she thought that she would die as a result of the ingestion but denies that she had been premeditating the act prior to yesterday's argument. She denies having left a suicide note and denies any history of giving away possessions in preparation for death. She says that what she did was "the dumbest thing I've ever done" and that she is "grateful to be alive." She cannot really say what has changed in their relationship, but says, "no matter what happens, it's not worth dying for."

Ms. Leia denies any past history of suicide attempts, command hallucinations telling her to commit suicide, or any intoxication at the time of the overdose. She notes that, for the past 4 months, she has had, more days than not, a depressed mood related to relationship difficulties, associated with: decreased enjoyment of usually pleasurable activities (e.g., going out with her friends, playing with her 6-year-old son at the beach, etc.), terminal insomnia (e.g., waking up at 3 a.m. and not being able to go back to sleep), increased appetite with an unintentional 5-pound weight gain, decreased energy level, feelings of worthlessness, and difficulty concentrating in her job. She admits to some degree of sensitivity to perceived rejection, for example, crying when her friends go somewhere without her or when her boyfriend is unable to make it for a planned date.

Past Psychiatric History Ms. Leia reports that when she was around 28 years old, she experienced similar symptoms during the ending of her 5-year marriage to her ex-husband. In retrospect, she believes that her symptoms started within about 1 month following the birth of her son. She saw a psychiatrist (Dr. Qui-Gon Jinn) and took fluoxetine for around 9 months. She reports that the fluoxetine was helpful and stopped this medication because she felt she no longer needed it.

She denies any history of manic symptoms (e.g., sustained abnormally elevated mood, racing thoughts, decreased need for sleep, rapid speech, psychomotor agitation, grandiosity, impulsive spending).

She admits to sometimes feeling, especially in the past 4 months, a fast heartbeat and light-headedness associated with feeling "stressed and overwhelmed with everything that's going on." These feelings would last less than a minute and would occur no more frequently than every few weeks. She denies any history of feeling any impending sense of doom during these instances, and she denies any worry about feeling these symptoms again in between these instances. She denies any history of repetitive, intrusive thoughts or behaviors. She also denies any history of anxiety in places where she may be under public scrutiny. In terms of any exposure to trauma, she reports having been involved in a car accident when she was 8 years old. Her mother's car was rear-ended on the freeway by a large truck, resulting in her mother needing to be hospitalized overnight. She says she coped reasonably well with this incident, and she denies any nightmares, flashbacks, or other reexperiencing phenomena related to this incident. She denies any past experience of physical or sexual abuse, and she denies any physical abuse in her current relationship.

She admits to drinking socially since age 18 or 19. The last time she had anything to drink was last week, with her friends. She reports only having one or two drinks each time. She denies any history of alcoholic blackouts, hallucinations related to drinking, or withdrawal seizures. She responded negatively to all components of the "CAGE" questionnaire. She denies any other history of substance use.

She denies any history of binging (e.g., eating large quantities of food in one sitting, feeling a lack of control over eating) or purging behavior.

Past Medical History Ms. Leia is otherwise healthy, without any chronic health problems. She denies any past history of seizures, major head trauma, or loss of consciousness. However, she notes that she had her wisdom teeth extracted 5 days ago and is still experiencing a significant amount of discomfort.

Ms. Leia has been pregnant only once, with her 6-year-old son. She reports a history of irritability and sadness before and during her menstrual periods. She has just started her menstrual period and denies any possibility of current pregnancy.

Current medications: acetaminophen/oxycodone

Allergies: Allergic to penicillin, which causes hives

Family History Ms. Leia believes that her father (65 years old) may have developed depression following a heart attack. He was prescribed an antidepressant, which he took for about 1 year. Her brother also had a history of school difficulties and marijuana abuse as a teenager. She denies any other known family history of depression, completed suicides, other psychiatric disorders, or substance abuse. She has a maternal aunt with a history of hypothyroidism, for which she takes thyroid replacement on an ongoing basis.

(*Optional* graphic depiction)

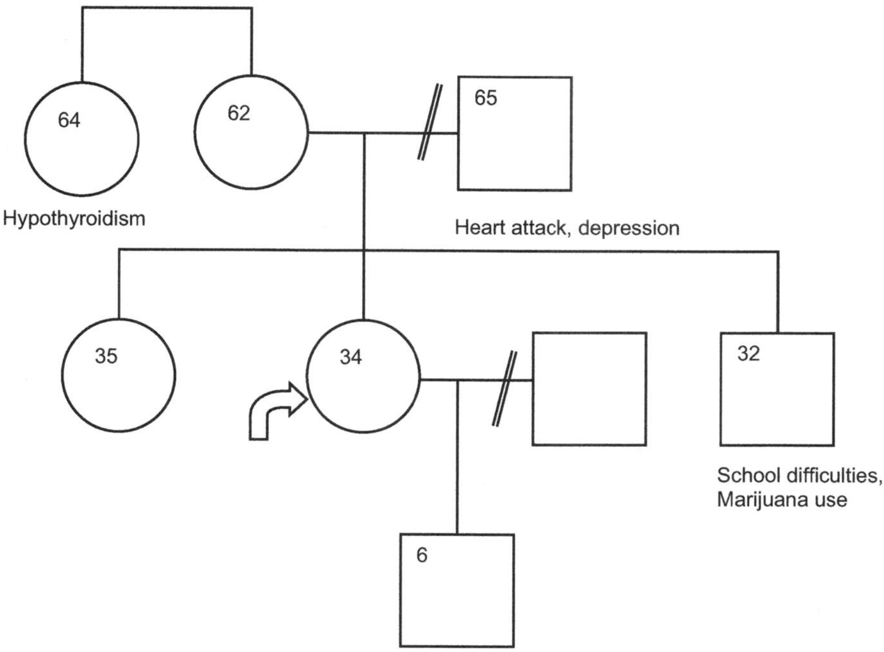

Developmental and Social History Ms. Leia grew up in Honolulu. Her parents divorced when she was 3 years of age. She denies that there was any domestic violence around the divorce, only arguing. She recalls being sad when her parents divorced but admits that she does not really remember details. Her mother raised her. While growing up, she had infrequent contact with her father, who remarried. She reports that she did not get along well with her mother because her mother was "too strict."

Ms. Leia reports having had difficulties in school, especially in math. She reports having been in special education for a few years. She denies any particular difficulty with concentrating/paying attention in school. She dropped out of 11th grade because she was "sick of school" and wanted to be with her boyfriend at the time. She completed her general equivalency diploma (GED) at the age of 18. She would like to return to school sometime and obtain a college degree, perhaps in education or psychology. She has held various jobs: as a cashier, food service provider, and office secretary. Most recently, she has worked as a secretary for a research company for the past 3 years.

Ms. Leia had been married to the father of her 6-year-old son for 5 years. Prior to that, she had only been in one long-term serious relationship (from high school). She reports that the marriage ended "mostly because he started getting more and more into drinking and I couldn't count on him to be around anymore." There had not been any domestic violence. She has been with her current boyfriend for the past 2 years. She reports that they had been arguing more especially in the past 5 or 6 months, generally over his ongoing friendship with ex-girlfriends.

Ms. Leia lives with her 6-year-old son. Her sister and brother help to provide childcare while she is at work. Her son stays with his father (who shares legal custody) during the weekends and was not with her during the time of the ingestion. She states that she misses her son when he is at his father's place. Her ex-husband pays child support but still notes that it is "hard to make ends meet" especially now that her son has started private school at their local church. She currently sees her mother at least once per week and talks to her father around once every few months. She feels close to her older sister and sees her frequently during the week. Her sister has come to visit her in the hospital and has been supportive.

Ms. Leia is active in church and reports that her friends from church are also very supportive. When she stopped seeing Dr. Qui-Gon Jinn, she had hoped she could stay emotionally well if she prayed and talked regularly to her pastor.

Ms. Leia denies having any access to firearms or other weapons.

Review of Systems Constitutional: History of weight gain, decreased energy level.

Eyes: Negative.

Ear, Nose, and Throat (ENT): History of recent extraction of wisdom teeth.

Cardiovascular (CV): For the past 4 months, occasional fast heartbeat and lightheadedness when she is anxious. No history of any chest pain, shortness of breath, or other cardiac symptoms.

Respiratory: Negative.

Gastrointestinal (GI): Some nausea following overdose; otherwise negative.

Genitourinary (GU): Regular urinary pattern, no discharge. Recently started menses.

Musculoskeletal: Negative.

Skin: Negative.

Neuro: Negative. No headaches, speech/gait abnormalities, weakness, numbness, paresthesias.

Psych: Depressed mood, suicidal ideation (see history of present illness, HPI).

Endocrine: No known history of thyroid disease. Endorses some history of feeling cold easily, even when others feel warm.

All others: Negative.

Physical Examination Constitutional: Well developed, well nourished, no acute distress. Normal body habitus, no obvious deformities. Adequate groom, dressed in hospital gown. Vital signs: Temperature 98.6 F, Pulse 72/min, blood pressure (BP) 110/70, respiratory rate (RR) 18, oxygen saturation (SaO_2) 100 % in room air (RA).

Eyes: Pupils 3 mm, reactive.

Musculoskeletal: No abnormal movements, rigidity, or tremor. Appears to have normal use of all extremities.

Skin: Warm and dry, no diaphoresis.

Mental Status Examination Eye contact: Good. Cooperation with interview: Cooperated well.

Motor activity: No psychomotor agitation or retardation.

Speech: Normal rate, volume, clarity, and amount.

Mood: "Sad and depressed, not my usual self."

Affect: Congruent, depressed, and tearful at appropriate points of the interview (e.g., discussing recent relationship difficulties, discussing how she feels when her son is not there). Affect brightened somewhat upon discussing her son's achievements in school.

Thought process: Linear, goal directed.

Thought content: No delusions or paranoid ideations. Conveys future-orientation: return to work, see her son as soon as she is able.

Perceptions: Denies any auditory or visual hallucinations. Does not appear to be responding to hallucinations.

Orientation: Oriented to person, place, time, and situation.

Attention/concentration: Attended well to the interview and was able to spell "world" forwards and backwards without difficulty.

Memory: Able to register 3/3 unrelated words without difficulty and to remember 3/3 after 5 min. Able to name the past five US presidents in reverse chronological order.

Knowledge: Good fund.

Abstractions: Able to note similarities (apple/orange, table/chair, opera/painting) appropriately.

Judgment: Fair. She states that, if she were ever feeling suicidal again, she would call her sister or someone else who was able to assist her.

Insight: Fair. Able to recognize that her suicidal thoughts may be related to a recurrence of depression and that she may benefit from psychiatric care once again.

Suicidal ideations: Denies, even with repeated questioning. Verbally agrees not to do anything to harm herself in the hospital and agrees to inform staff if she were to feel distressed again.

Homicidal ideations: Denies.

Laboratory Studies (on Admission) Urine toxicology: Positive for opiates, otherwise negative.

Electrocardiogram: Normal sinus rhythm, normal electrocardiogram (EKG).

Acetaminophen level: Borderline toxic range.

Acetylsalicylic acid level: Negative.

Complete blood count (CBC) with differential: All values within normal range.

Comprehensive metabolic profile: All values within normal range, including liver function tests (LFTs).

Prothrombin time/partial thromboplastin time (PT/PTT): Within normal range.

Serum human chorionic gonadotropin (HCG): Negative.

Formulation In summary, Ms. Leia is a 36-year-old female admitted to the hospital for a potentially toxic intentional acetaminophen overdose and a history of depression.

Relevant biological factors include a possible genetic predisposition to depression (family history), recent physical discomfort (status-post tooth extraction, sleep deprivation) just prior to the suicide attempt, and possible hormonal influences (history of postpartum onset of depression, history of mood changes before and during menses, which she is currently having). Other, less prominent (though possibly still relevant) factors include current use of a pain medication that could affect mood (oxycodone) and infrequent use of alcohol (none in the past few days).

Relevant psychological factors include the recent argument with her boyfriend and possibly the fact that her son was not with her at the time of the suicide attempt (as the more recent, precipitating factors); a past history of losses and transitions, including her parents' divorce, a less-than-optimal relationship with the parent who raised her, and the breakup of a previous marriage; other factors (e.g., school difficulties) that could have led to a loss of self-esteem and predisposed her to depression; and what she describes as an increased sensitivity to perceived rejection. Also, she is at a stage in life where she may be hoping for more stability in her relationship/family life and financial situation than she currently has, and this may be an additional factor contributing to depression.

Relevant social/cultural/spiritual factors include ongoing financial stress and working in the single parent role. She describes receiving emotional and other support from siblings and friends. She has maintained a stable job for the past few years. Her beliefs about the nature and treatment of depression may be influenced by her religious orientation. Her religious involvement is positive influence in her life.

Depicted graphically (with treatment interventions enclosed in ovals)—*also optional:*

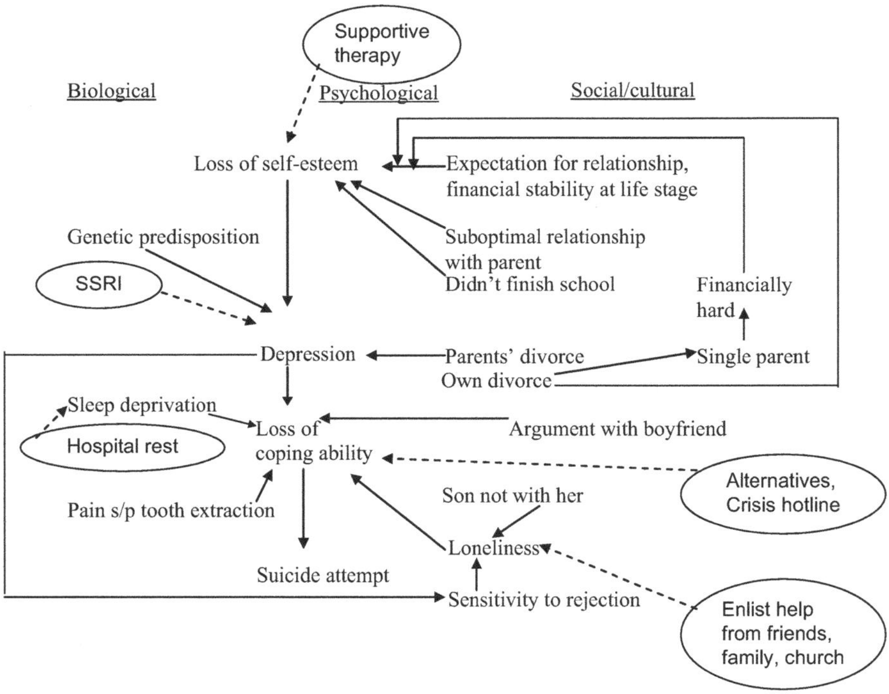

Differential Diagnoses

1. Major depressive disorder, moderate, recurrent episode: Patient meets DSM-5 criteria for this diagnosis. She also may meet the criteria for atypical features.
2. Bipolar II disorder: A consideration given the history of recurrent major depressive episodes; however, no definite history of manic symptoms endorsed in this interview.
3. Adjustment disorder with depressed mood: With the stressors being the relationship difficulties; however, because she meets the criteria for a major depressive disorder, the latter diagnosis would supersede.
4. Panic disorder: Patient describes a history of fast heartbeat and light-headedness; however, does not meet full criteria for panic attacks, and these symptoms occurred only in the context of what appears to be a major depressive episode.
5. Alcohol use disorder and substance-induced depressive disorder: based on the history provided, would not meet criteria for a substance use disorder; collateral information would be helpful in ruling out this possibility.
6. Premenstrual dysphoric disorder: Patient describes some symptoms around menses that may be consistent with this condition; however, it is unclear that they were absent following menses and not merely an exacerbation of what is likely a major depressive disorder.
7. Depressive disorder due to another medical condition (with depressive features): Thyroid disorder (given family history) and primary heart condition (with anxiety symptoms) should be considered.
8. Specific learning disorder (with impairment in mathematics) or other specific learning disorder: given history of school difficulties and special education.
9. Borderline personality disorder—trait specified: with sensitivity to abandonment; however, it is not clear that her history is necessarily characterized by "a pattern of unstable and intense relationships…." or "recurrent" suicidal behavior.
10. Dependent personality disorder—trait specified: With discomfort of being alone; however, it is also not clear that criteria are met for this personality disorder.
11. Status-post overdose (acetaminophen, hydrocodone, ibuprofen)
12. Status-post tooth extraction
13. *Penicillin allergy (important to recall, though not necessarily directly relevant to current psychiatric status)*
14. Possible thyroid disorder: family history of thyroid disorder, history of cold intolerance.
15. Possible cardiac arrhythmia: Given history of fast heartbeat, light-headedness; however, the timing of these symptoms seemed to coincide with the episode of depression, and the EKG done on admission was negative.

Working diagnoses:

Major depressive disorder, moderate, recurrent episode
Specific learning disorder (with impairment in mathematics—provisional)
Status-post overdose
Status-post tooth extraction with pain

Treatment Plan Treatment setting: Ms. Leia should remain in the hospital because she needs general medical treatment for the overdose. A standard hospital suicide risk assessment form has been completed, and orders have been written appropriate to her level of suicide risk, with removal of potentially injurious objects and frequent nursing checks.

Other specific interventions are as follows:

	Biological/medical	Psychological	Social
Additional information	1. Review past records from previous treating psychiatrist, with attention to medication issues	1. Meet again with patient to clarify diagnostic issues as noted above	1. With patient's permission, speak with family members for collateral information
	2. Consider checking a TSH	2. Review past records from treating psychiatrist	2. Assess whether son (minor) is under appropriate care currently
		3. Consider rating scales for depression and other mood disorders	
Treatment	1. Medical treatment of overdose as per general medical team	1. Individual supportive psychotherapy to be provided during medical hospitalization, with focus on psychoeducation about depression and discussion of feelings about current and past stressors	1. Enlist support from family members and friends where appropriate
	2. Patient may be a candidate for restarting of SSRI, such as fluoxetine, which had been helpful in the past. Consider monitoring response using standard rating scales for depression		2. Disposition (e.g., discharge to outpatient care vs. psychiatric hospitalization) to be determined during follow-up visits
	3. Encourage adequate rest while in the hospital	2. In the longer term, may be a candidate for cognitive-behavioral psychotherapy (e.g., to address feelings of worthlessness, rejection) or interpersonal psychotherapy (e.g., to address role transitions, losses)	

	Biological/medical	Psychological	Social
Patient education	1. Education about the alternatives to and potential benefits/risks of treatment with SSRI	1. Provide information on crisis phone numbers	With patient's permission, enlist family's help in insuring safety in the environment (e.g., no large bottles of dangerous medications) and in encouraging patient make use of available resources
	2. Advise patient to avoid drinking alcohol at this time, as it may impair judgment and render her more vulnerable to self-destructive acts	2. Provide information on the importance of depression treatment, including ongoing medical follow-up	

TSH thyroid-stimulating hormone, *SSRI* selective serotonin reuptake inhibitor

Prognosis: Ms. Leia's prognosis at this point would seem to be fair to good. One important risk factor is current relationship instability. However, from the standpoint of completed suicide risk, she has a fairly favorable demographic profile (young, female, employed), no past history of suicide attempts, and no apparent substance abuse problem. From the standpoint of major depression, she has a history of good response to selective serotonin reuptake inhibitor (SSRI) treatment in the past. Her social supports and church involvement may also be factors that weigh in her favor.

Further Readings

American Psychiatric Association. (2013). *Diagnostic and statistical manual of mental disorders DSM-5* (5th ed.).

Guerrero, A. P. S., Hishinuma, E. S., Serrano, A. C., & Ahmed, I. (2003). Use of the "Mechanistic Case Diagramming" technique to teach the biopsychosocial–cultural formulation to psychiatric clerks. *Academic Psychiatry, 27,* 88–92.

Guerrero, A. P. S., Ling, C. Y. L., Ahmed, I., Takeshita, J., & Bell, C. K. (2007). Development of a structured module to teach psychiatric interviewing competencies to medical students. *Focus on Health Professional Education: A Multidisciplinary Journal, 9*(3), 65–75.

Sadock, B. J., Sadock, V. A., & Ruiz, P. (2015). *Mood disorders. Kaplan and Sadock's synopsis of psychiatry: Behavioral sciences/clinical psychiatry* (11th ed., pp. 347–386). Philadelphia: Wolters Kluwer.

Chapter 18
Disorders of Childhood

Erika Ryst and Jeremy Matuszak

Childhood is a time of great vulnerability to psychiatric illness. According to the World Health Organization, around 20 % of the world's children and adolescents have mental disorders or problems. This chapter will introduce three cases that will highlight some of the most common disorders and treatments.

At the end of the chapter, the reader will be able to:

1. Describe the *fundamental* differences between a child and an adult psychiatric evaluation
2. Differentiate between the diagnostic criteria for adult and childhood psychiatric illnesses
3. Describe the epidemiology, phenomenology, etiology, and treatment for six childhood psychiatric diagnoses.

Vignette 18.1.1 Presenting Situation: Sam

A mother brings in Sam, her 7-year-old boy in second grade, to you for a child psychiatric evaluation. She tells you she is here at the insistence of the boy's classroom teacher, who notices an inability to sit still, decreased academic performance compared to his age-mates, and generally disruptive classroom behavior. These concerns have been going on for 2 months since the beginning of the school year. The mother seems a bit irritated that the school is requesting your evaluation. Sam is a cute, brown-haired boy with normal-

"The foundation for good mental health is laid in the early years of childhood and adolescence." Mental Health Promotion in Young People—an Investment for the Future: World Health Organization, 2010.

J. Matuszak (✉)
Willow Springs Center, 690 Edison Way, Reno, NV 89502, USA
e-mail: jeremymatuszak@gmail.com

E. Ryst
Department of Psychiatry, School of Medicine, University of Nevada, Reno, NV, USA

D. Alicata et al. (eds.), *Problem-based Behavioral Science and Psychiatry*,
DOI 10.1007/978-3-319-23669-8_18

appearing features. He gets up frequently from his seat but tends to hover in the immediate vicinity of his mother.

Please proceed with the problem-based approach using the worksheet located in the appendix of Chap. 1!

Table 18.1.1

FACTS	HYPOTHESES	INFORMATION NEEDED	LEARNING ISSUES

The psychiatric evaluation of a child differs from that of an adult in a number of fundamental ways. To start, children rarely present to your office with a chief complaint or treatment agenda. Rather, it is the parents or caregivers who will provide the reason for referral and evaluation. The process of evaluating a child or adolescent necessitates taking histories from not only the child, but the caregiver and school environments as well. When interviewing the child, it is important to communicate in a way that is appropriate to developmental level. The child may not be able to say in words what is wrong, but observation of his behavior may give clues as to the diagnosis. A thorough chronological history including conception, childbirth, physical development and medical history, school functioning, and emotional development help clinicians develop differential diagnoses and treatment plans. Special attention must be paid to any history of trauma (emotional, physical, or sexual) that may have precipitated the child's symptoms. Generating a differential diagnosis requires both time and caution, as symptoms of different disorders may present in the same way. For example, irritability could reflect a biological mood disorder or an environmental stressor such as child abuse. Therefore, the Diagnostic and Statistical Manual of Mental Disorders, Fifth Edition (DSM-5; APA 2013), while a useful diagnostic guide, may not be as applicable to children as it is to adults.

The differential diagnosis for Sam at this point is broad and includes attention deficit hyperactivity disorder (ADHD), autism spectrum disorder (ASD), intellectual disability (ID) or learning disorder, mood or anxiety disorder, environmental causes (e.g., being bullied at school), and oppositional defiant disorder (ODD).

18.1 Continuation

Sam's school sends evaluation results from testing by the school psychologist as part of an Individualized Education Plan (IEP). He has a high IQ with academic performance in the expected range for age. However, on the Weschler Intelligence Scale for Children (WISC), the working memory and attention scales show current impairment. A WISC performed 1 year ago showed a slightly higher IQ with attention and memory in the average range. During your classroom observation, you observe that Sam is highly distractible, particularly in high-stimulation situations. He jumps at loud noises and then has trouble returning to his schoolwork. At times, he gazes out the window and seems to be lost in his own world. You are able to speak with Sam's first-grade teacher and she indicates that none of the current behavioral and cognitive problems existed 1 year ago.

Please proceed with the problem-based approach using the worksheet located in the appendix of Chap. 1!

Table 18.1.2

FACTS	HYPOTHESES	INFORMATION NEEDED	LEARNING ISSUES

This new information should now narrow the differential diagnosis. ADHD has now moved lower in the differential as these symptoms have not persisted for at least 6 months. Additionally, it is now evident that the changes in attention and cognition are of a more recent onset (i.e., <6 months), thus placing an ASD lower on the differential as well. Normal IQ and onset outside of early development effectively rules out an ID. Note that a diagnosis of ID relies heavily on adaptive functioning deficits and does not directly correlate to IQ scores. IQ testing, nonetheless, yields important information about intellectual capacity, strengths, and deficits. Some degree of intellectual impairment is needed for a diagnosis of an ID. At this time, a mood disorder, anxiety disorder, or an environmental cause to these behaviors are still possibilities.

Although ADHD is lower on our differential, it is an important diagnosis in child psychiatry. DSM-5 (APA 2013) requires a pattern of either inattentive symptoms or hyperactivity-impulsivity lasting at least 6 months. These symptoms must be both maladaptive and inappropriate for developmental age. To make a formal diagnosis, some of these symptoms must have been present before age 12. Additionally, there must be evidence of impairment in social, academic, or occupational function in two or more settings. Again, taking a comprehensive school, home, and individual history is needed to make an informed diagnosis.

The prevalence of ADHD likely falls between 3 and 7% in school-age children. Twin studies have shown the heritability of this disorder to be as high as 80%. Likewise, if a parent meets criteria for ADHD, there is a 50% chance that the child will as well (Faraone et al. 2005). In searching for the genetic basis for ADHD, it is evident that there are disruptions in both the norepinephrine and dopamine neurotransmitter systems. Among these systems, irregularities in the cingulate gyrus, caudate, and cerebellum (each with a corresponding dopamine pathway) have been implicated (Abbeduto et al. 2014).

Psychostimulants, which effect both norepinephrine and dopamine pathways, are the mainstay for treatment of ADHD. Medications that work on norepinephrine alone (e.g., atomoxetine), while more effective than placebo, do not appear to be quite as effective. The Multimodal Treatment Study of ADHD (MTA) study (Arnold et al. 1997) showed that these pharmacological treatments have been so effective that approximately 75% of subjects receiving *a first trial* of stimulants show academic *and* behavioral improvement compared to 0–25% receiving placebo. Up to 90% of children with ADHD respond if a second trial of medication is tried or medication dosage is altered. It is important to mention here that the risk of dependence on low-dose oral stimulants is remarkably low (Arnold et al. 1997).

The MTA established a strong evidence base for the medication treatment of ADHD in children. This rigorous large-scale, NIMH-sponsored study was originally designed to test whether medications alone, psychosocial treatments alone, or a combination of the two best treated the symptoms of ADHD. The study found that while medication was the best treatment for the core symptoms of ADHD, combined treatment was superior to the other groups in addressing some of the associated problems of ADHD such as poor social skills and disrupted family relations. Helpful adjunctive psychosocial treatments include psychoeducation, parent training in behavior management skills, school advocacy, and social skills training (Arnold et al 1997).

While it used to be felt that the majority of children would "grow out of" their ADHD symptoms, recent studies indicate that ADHD continues at least into early adolescence in the majority of cases (Arnold et al 1997). Due to a paucity of data regarding adult outcomes, as well as methodological differences between the few existing studies, it is not clear at this time how frequently ADHD persists into adulthood. However, there is some evidence that many adults continue to suffer from some, if not all, of the symptoms of ADHD (APA 2013). Persistent ADHD is also associated with significant comorbidity including lower educational achievement, conduct disorder and antisocial personality disorder, major depression, car accidents, and cigarette smoking (APA 2013).

18.2 Conclusion

You speak with the pediatrician, who has known Sam since birth and who is very happy that Sam is now under psychiatric care. His parents separated when he was 3 months of age, and Sam's mother has always given the impression of being a sensitive and caring parent. However, the pediatrician has noticed a change in the mother's overall demeanor over the last year, which has coincided with the entry of a new boyfriend into the home. Since then, the pediatrician has felt that Sam's mother has seemed more distant and closed. On one occasion, the boyfriend accompanied the family to an appointment, and the pediatrician thought he may have smelled alcohol on his breath. Just last week, the pediatrician had been able to speak separately with the mother, who admitted, after initially denying any problems, that her boyfriend, when intoxicated, would become physically abusive towards her and verbally belittling towards Sam. He reported this information to Child Protective Services (CPS) and is scheduled to see Sam in follow-up.

Please proceed with the problem-based approach using the worksheet located in the appendix of Chap. 1!

Table 18.1.3

FACTS	HYPOTHESES	INFORMATION NEEDED	LEARNING ISSUES

When child abuse is suspected, the first and foremost concern is the child's ongoing safety. As a physician, you are legally mandated to report the child (even if only suspected and not confirmed) to CPS. If needed, the police can be called, or the child can be admitted to the hospital to protect them while awaiting a CPS evaluation. Failure to report could result in further injury or even the child's death (Cheng and Myers 2005). Of the 3.4 million referrals alleging maltreatment to CPS in 2012, there were 686,000 true cases identified which included 1640 child fatalities (U.S. Department of Health and Human Services 2012). Child abuse leads to approximately 1100 deaths a year in the USA alone. Please refer to Chap. 7 for a further discussion of child abuse. Given the high prevalence, child abuse needs to be considered in the differential diagnosis for any behavioral disorder in a child.

A victim of child abuse may display a number of changes including anxiety, depression, aggression, or posttraumatic stress disorder (PTSD). One study demonstrated that as high as 60% of children who experience sexual abuse and 42% of children who have been physically abused go on to develop PTSD (Dubner et al 1999). Children understandably respond to trauma differently than adults, and therefore diagnostic criteria of PTSD in children are somewhat different than for adults (see Chap. 22 for a full discussion of PTSD). In fact, there is a different set of diagnostic criteria for PTSD in children aged 6 and younger. Children may experience trauma through witnessing, personally experiencing, or learning of a traumatic event that happened to a caregiver. They may reexperience their trauma through post-traumatic play, play reenactment of the event, nightmares, flashbacks/dissociations and distress at reminders of the event. Avoidance in children may be evidenced by constricted play, social withdrawal, restricted range of affect, *and* loss of previously acquired developmental skills. Alterations in arousal (Criterion D) may present with irritability, problems with concentration, and sleep disturbances (APA, 2013).

Once safety issues are addressed, there are a number of psychotherapeutic and biologic treatments available. Psychotherapeutic treatments should facilitate the child feeling safe and being able to recall the traumatic events without feeling powerless. There are a number of evidence-based psychotherapeutic treatments for childhood PTSD including trauma-focused cognitive-behavioral therapy (Deblinger et al. 1999). Medication options include treatment with selective serotonin reuptake inhibitors (SSRIs) or alpha-2-agonists (clonidine or guanfacine), which can attenuate impulsive behaviors arising from the event and limit arousal symptoms (Lewis 2002). As noted in Chap. 22, SSRI use in adolescents and children is controversial.

18.3 Case 18.2.1 Presenting Situation: Teddy

Teddy is a 9-year-old boy who presents to his pediatrician with a 4-month history of bowel incontinence. These episodes only occur while awake and never during sleep. Teddy had been previously bowel trained at the age of 4, though his mother recalls that toilet training had been a struggle. Since he was a young child, Teddy has suffered from intermittent constipation, which has required medical intervention including hospitalization for bowel clean-out. However, except during episodes of severe constipation, when he has had some leaking, he has been able to stay clean. His mother is now concerned because over the last few months she has noticed significant fecal staining of Teddy's underwear, which includes formed stools as well as leaking.

STOP

Please proceed with the problem-based approach using the worksheet located in the appendix of Chap. 1!

Table 18.2.1

FACTS	HYPOTHESES	INFORMATION NEEDED	LEARNING ISSUES

The DSM-5 (APA 2013) defines encopresis as repeated (at least once per month for at least 3 months) passage of feces into inappropriate places (e.g., clothing or floor) in a child who is 4 years or older. This should not be exclusively the result of a substance, medication, or general medical condition except through a mechanism involving constipation. There are two subtypes for encopresis: with (retentive) and without (nonretentive) constipation and overflow incontinence. If a patient has never achieved continence, the diagnosis is primary encopresis. On the other hand, as in Teddy's case, if there has been a period of continence with subsequent bowel incontinence, the condition is secondary encopresis. Several studies cite the prevalence of encopresis as 4 % in 4–5 year olds and 1.5 % in 11–12 year olds. It is more common in males (Katz et and DeMaso 2011).

The differential diagnosis of encopresis at this time includes spinal cord injury (leading to dysregulation of the anal sphincter), Hirschsprung disease, anal stenosis, imperforate anus with fistula, or psychological factors.

The etiology of encopresis can be physiologic, psychological, or a combination of both (Har and Croffie 2010). In physiologic encopresis, chronic constipation leads to a vicious cycle of ongoing bowel problems and incontinence. For example, the child avoids making bowel movements because they are hard and painful; more and more fluid gets reabsorbed from the bowel, and the retained feces becomes harder and harder. Over time the child becomes obstructed, and liquid waste leaks around the retained feces causing soiling. In psychologically mediated encopresis, unresolved psychological issues get played out in the realm of bowel movements. For example, a child with a strong need for control (who perhaps is in conflict with a controlling parent) exasperates the parent by willfully defecating at inopportune times and inappropriate places. Finally, physiological and psychological processes often go hand in hand. Encopresis may start out as a willful behavior on the part of the child but develop into a problem of chronic constipation as a result of the child's habit of holding in feces.

18.3.1 Continuation

Physical examination, including rectal examination, is unremarkable. A plain film of the abdomen fails to reveal any evidence of constipation, obstruction, or impaction. There is neither recent nor remote history of trauma. Teddy's film of the abdomen fails to reveal any evidence of constipation, obstruction, or impaction. Teddy's mother relates to you that she and Teddy's father were divorced shortly before these problems began. Since their separation, Teddy has had little contact with his father.

Please proceed with the problem-based approach using the worksheet located in the appendix of Chap. 1!

Table 18.2.2

FACTS	HYPOTHESES	INFORMATION NEEDED	LEARNING ISSUES

Although the initial history is consistent with retentive encopresis, Teddy's presentation is now somewhat different. There is no mention of bouts of constipation consistent with retentive constipation. Furthermore, physical examination is unremarkable. Given this, a biologic cause is lower on the differential, and one must look closely for psychological contributors to this problem.

The treatment of encopresis in children is multipronged. The use of laxatives (either short or long term) may relieve the constipation that frequently causes pain in this disorder. A behavioral approach is also commonly employed, included a structured bowel training program (using the restroom at set intervals) and a program of biofeedback which teaches the child to relax the external anal sphincter successfully. Psychological treatment, such as play therapy to allow the child to work out unresolved conflicts, may also be appropriate if there are significant psychological factors involved (Reid and Bahar 2006).

It is important to effectively rule out any potential medical cause for encopresis before concluding that it is psychologically based. When it is psychologically based, however, the underlying motivator is frequently control. Children are dependent on caregivers in nearly every aspect of their lives—food, clothing, shelter, when to wake up, when to go to bed. One thing a child *does* have control over is his or her bowels. By holding in feces or soiling themselves, children may employ the little autonomy they do have in a very tangible way. For this reason, encopresis often reflects a child's attempt to regain control over feelings of helplessness (such as when a child is being hurt or abused). Alternatively, it may embody the dynamics of a control struggle between child and parent. Psychological treatment allows further exploration of these issues and identification of the unique meaning of the encopretic symptom for the child and his or her family. If unconscious conflicts driving this symptom are uncovered, the symptom itself resolves (Drake 2005). Please see Chap. 27 on eating disorders for related topics.

Vignette 18.3.1 Presenting Situation: Michael

You are a pediatrician and have been treating Michael, a 3-year-old boy, since his birth. Michael's mom is a first-time parent, and you have perceived her as relatively anxious and insecure about her parenting experience. She is bringing Michael to you for his 3-year-old check-up. At this visit, when reviewing normal developmental milestones, it becomes clear that Michael's language is significantly delayed. He has a few words, such as "baba" for milk, which his mother is able to understand but is unintelligible to others. He has trouble getting his needs met because he does not point or gesture for what he wants.

Please proceed with the problem-based approach using the worksheet located in the appendix of Chap. 1!

Table 18.3.1

FACTS	HYPOTHESES	INFORMATION NEEDED	LEARNING ISSUES

At this point, a differential diagnosis could include language delay, ID, ASD, and various general medical causes of the latter two diagnoses. The investigation should therefore include a comprehensive assessment (Volkmar et al. 2014) that includes:

- Birth history (e.g., problems with pregnancy, prenatal exposures, anoxia at birth).
- Previous development (e.g., regression in milestones vs. earlier hints of developmental delay, development in other areas).
- Temperament as an infant (e.g., colicky, responsive/nonresponsive/cuddly).
- Social development and interaction between mother and infant (e.g., was there give-and-take or social reciprocity between mother and child? Was there a social smile at 2 months, peek-a-boo play at 5–6 months, back-and-forth play with parent at 9–11 months, and pointing to indicate interests at 12–18 months?).
- Language milestones (e.g., vocalizations as an infant, one-word utterances at 1 year, two-word phrases at 2 years?).
- Medical assessment: seizure history; sensory deficits (hearing/vision); signs/symptoms of specific genetic disorders such as Fragile X, audiometry, and visual exam; routine lead screening.
- Physical examination with attention to growth, developmental status, and facial features looking for dysmorphology.
- Laboratory tests in the presence of global developmental delay:
  - Chromosomal microarray genetic testing
  - Fragile X testing
  - Neuroimaging
- Other laboratory tests, selected based on physical findings
  - Wood's lamp testing (tuberous sclerosis)
  - Urinary amino acids (metabolic disorder)
  - Blood organic acids (metabolic disorder)
  - Biochemical tests for any suspected inborn errors of metabolism
  - Electroencephalogram (EEG; seizure disorder)

- Psychological testing
  - Occupational therapy/physical therapy assessment
  - Speech and Language testing (vocabulary, syntax/grammar, articulation/oral-motor skills, pragmatic skills)
  - Intelligence testing
  - Adaptive testing (e.g., Vineland Adaptive Scales)

18.3.2 Continuation

Michael's workup reveals the following results. All laboratory tests are within normal limits. There is no evidence of dysmorphology on physical examination, and genetic testing reveals no abnormalities. Speech and language testing shows significant language delay—currently at the 12-month level (2 years language delayed). Adaptive skills testing shows both fine motor and gross motor delays, though not as severe as the language and social developmental delays.

Michael's mother reports normal pregnancy and delivery but has always felt that "something is wrong with my child." As a newborn, he was not as "cuddly" as other babies. He slept a lot and appeared to get overstimulated very easily. His mother does not recall playing "peek-a-boo" or other types of give-and-take games. Michael does not use gestures to communicate or indicate interest. Upon direct observation, he is minimally interactive, even with his mother. He maintains minimal eye contact and does not appear to be curious about toys in the office. Michael plays repetitively with cars and lines them up in sequence over and over. His mother reports that he does this at home, too, for hours at a time. Additionally, there is no use of fantasy play, and he is very inflexible. For example, he gets upset if the examiner tries to engage him in playing with the car. The examiner also notices that the child seems to self-stimulate himself by twisting and turning his body.

Please proceed with the problem-based approach using the worksheet located in the appendix of Chap. 1!

Table 18.3.2

FACTS	HYPOTHESES	INFORMATION NEEDED	LEARNING ISSUES

At this point, Michael's social developmental and communication delays point to autistic spectrum disorder. Also, because of what appear to be global developmental delays, he may eventually meet the criteria for ID.

The cardinal features of ASD as defined by the DSM-5 (APA 2013), include persistent deficits in social communication and social interaction across multiple contexts and restricted, repetitive patterns of behavior, interests, or activities. Deficits in social communication are manifested by a lack of social-emotional reciprocity (such as the back and forth of normal conversation), poor use of nonverbal communication such as eye contact, and trouble developing, maintaining, and understanding social relationships. Children with ASD can have stereotyped or repetitive motor movements such as lining up toys or objects, inflexible insistence on sameness, abnormally intense, restricted, unusual interests, and under or over-reactivity to sensory stimuli. Of note, language delay is not enough in itself to make a diagnosis of autism; most important is the demonstration of specific deficits in social communicative interaction. While ASD often co-occurs with ID, it requires the presence of social communication deficits that are below those expected for the child. The DSM-5 (APA 2013) also includes a new diagnosis, social (pragmatic) communication disorder, which reflects deficits in the social use of verbal and nonverbal communication without the restricted, perseverative interests and stereotyped motor movements that are characteristic of autism. The American Academy of Pediatrics recommends that all children be administered the Modified Checklist for Autism in Toddlers, Revised (M-CHAT-Revised), at 18 and 24 months (Robins et al. 2014). The M-CHAT is a screening tool administered by pediatricians; a child unable to pass the M-CHAT requires further assessment for autism. The gold-standard assessment tool for autism is the Autism Diagnostic Observation Schedule (ADOS; Lord et al. 2003).

According to the Center for Disease Control (2010), the most recent estimated prevalence of ASD in the USA is 1 in 68 children. ASD is almost five times more common in boys than girls. The etiology of ASD is, at this time, unknown. Current hypotheses suggest both a genetic and environmental contribution to this disorder (CDC 2010).

Evidence supporting a genetic etiology includes robust data on concordance between identical twins, which indicates a heritability of 80% or greater (Ronald and Hoekstra 2011). Parents who have a child with ASD have an 18.7% chance of having another child with autism. However, despite the strong genetic heritability of autism spectrum disorder, no single genetic etiology accounts for more than 1–2% of cases (Abbeduto et al. 2014). There is also growing evidence in regard to underlying brain differences between autistic and normal children. Specifically, neuroimaging studies show volume abnormalities in both gray and white matter and that such volume abnormalities are associated with atypical functional and structural connectivity in the brain (Stigler et al. 2011).

From an environmental perspective, intrauterine infections have been suggested to predispose a child to autism, as have other risk factors such as prematurity, low birth weight, and parental age. A lingering controversy has been whether or not childhood vaccinations lead to an increased risk of autism, but research has failed to suggest such a link (Abbeduto et al. 2014).

There is no specific treatment for the core features of autism, but intervention is focused on improvement of function, which includes a multimodal treatment plan such as social skills training, speech and language services, occupational therapy, applied behavioral analysis, educational interventions, advocacy, and sometimes medication to treat associated symptoms such as anxiety or aggression (Gabbard 2014). Recently, several exciting studies suggest that some medication treatments (such as risperidone) help not only with reducing aggression and agitation associated with autism but may in fact also promote small developmental gains (Williams 2006). Currently, aripiprazole and risperidone are the only two FDA-approved medications for the treatment of irritability and aggression associated with autism (Baribeau and Anagnostou 2014).

While children who are identified and helped early (before ages 3–4) have the best prognosis, intervention at any age can promote developmental gains and improve functioning (Council on Children with Disabilities 2006). The key to successful intervention is to employ as many modalities as possible to promote the child's development. A child with autism spectrum disorder requires a comprehensive assessment to identify areas of deficit, which should then inform a targeted and multifaceted treatment plan.

The DSM-5 (APA 2013) defines ID as a disorder with onset during the developmental period that includes both intellectual and adaptive functioning deficits in conceptual, social, and practical domains. Deficits in intellectual function (that include reasoning, problem solving, planning, abstract thinking, judgment, academic learning, and learning from experience) must be confirmed by both clinical assessment and individualized, standardized intelligence testing. Of particular importance is the presence of adaptive functioning deficits that result in failure to meet developmental and sociocultural standards for personal independence and social responsibility. Because of both standardized intelligence testing is unreliable during the early childhood years and the fact that children's developmental capacities can substantially change as a result of learning experiences and early intervention, most clinicians avoid labeling a child as having an ID until school age (Molfese and Acheson 1997).

Severity levels for ID range from mild, moderate, severe to profound, which correspond to progressively limited adaptive functioning in the conceptual, social, and practical domains, as indicated in Table 18.1.

18.4 Conclusion

The diagnostic breadth of childhood psychiatric illness is as broad as (if not broader) that of adult disorders. In addition to a number of disorders unique to those persons under the age of 18 (Table 18.2), there are diagnoses common to both age groups, but they may have different presentations in childhood (Table 18.3). It is important to understand the fundamental differences in presentation and diagnostic criteria of these disorders.

Table 18.1 Categories of intellectual disability and areas of impairment

Severity	Conceptual domain	Practical domain	Social domain
Mild	Difficulties in learning academic skills, applying abstract skills, and executive functioning	Need some support with complex daily living tasks. Judgment may require support to make health-care, financial, or occupational decisions	Immature in social interactions. Concrete communications, difficulties in recognizing social cues
Moderate	Academic skills lag behind age-matched peers throughout the developmental cycle. For adults, academic ability does not exceed elementary level	Need considerable support for employment and attending to normal activities of daily living. With support, they can function relatively well, however	Communication is basic and primarily verbal. Social limitations are significant and require support
Severe	Little understanding of written language or numerical concepts. Caretakers must provide extensive support for problem solving	Requires support for all activities of daily living (ADLs). Cannot make responsible decisions for their own well-being. They can acquire skills but require long-term teaching and ongoing support. Some maladaptive behaviors, including self-injurious behavior, present in a significant minority	Spoken language is limited in grammar and vocabulary. Speech is single word or phrases and is focused on the here and now. Relationships are primarily with immediate family
Profound	Conceptual skills involve the physical, tangible world. Difficulties understanding symbolic processes. May use objects in a goal-directed fashion. Motor and sensory problems are prevalent and prevent functional use of objects	Dependent on others for all aspects of care and need high levels of support. Simple actions with objects may be the way to participate in any sort of vocation	Very limited understanding of symbolic communication and gestures. May understand some simple instructions or gestures. Expresses desires through nonverbal, nonsymbolic communications. Connects only with those that are very well known to them

Table 18.2 Other diagnoses specific to children and adolescents

	Diagnostic features	Special features
Disruptive behavioral disorders of childhood		
Oppositional defiant disorder	A pattern of hostile, irritable, and defiant behavior	Must be more oppositional than developmental peers
Conduct disorder	Aggressive, destructive, delinquent (criminal) behaviors	Precursor to antisocial personality disorder in adults
Depressive disorders		
Disruptive mood dysregulation disorder	Severe, recurrent (at least three times per week) temper outbursts grossly out of proportion in intensity or duration	Diagnosis to be made between the ages of 6 and 18 years; a new DSM-5 diagnosis meant to capture chronically irritable and aggressive children who lack cardinal symptoms of depression or mania
Anxiety disorders		
Separation anxiety disorder	Developmentally inappropriate and excessive fear regarding separation from attachment figures	Must last at least 4 weeks in children and adolescents and more than 6 months in adults
Selective mutism	Persistent failure to speak in social situations despite speaking in other situations	Often a precursor to social anxiety disorder in adulthood
Trauma-related disorders		
Reactive attachment disorder	Pathogenic care-giving history associated with a consistent pattern of inhibited, socially withdrawn behavior	Associated with internalizing disorders
Disinhibited social engagement disorder	Pathogenic care-giving history associated with a consistent pattern of actively approaching and interacting with unfamiliar adults in an overly familiar and indiscriminate way	Associated with externalizing disorders
Learning, motor disorders, and language disorders		
Specific learning disorder	Difficulties learning and using academic skills for at least 6 months despite receiving targeted interventions for the difficulties	Specific subtypes include: with impairment in reading, with impairment in written expression, with impairment in mathematics
Developmental coordination disorder	Low levels of coordination/motor performance	Possible delays in developmental milestones
Language disorder	Limited vocabulary	Not attributable to hearing impairment, medical, or neurological condition or intellectual disability
	Errors in grammar	
	Difficulty understanding words	

Table 18.2 (continued)

	Diagnostic features	Special features
Speech sound disorder	Difficulties in speech sound production	
Childhood-onset fluency disorder (stuttering)	Disturbances in the normal fluency and timing of speech	
Stereotypic movement disorder	Repetitive, seemingly driven, and apparently purposeless motor behavior	May be associated with a known medical or genetic condition (e.g., Lesch–Nyhan syndrome), neurodevelopmental disorder, or environmental factor
Tic disorders	Consist of sudden, rapid, recurrent, nonrhythmic motor movement or vocalizations	Onset before age 18 If > 1 year: Persistent (chronic) motor tic Persistent (chronic) vocal tic Tourettent (chronic) vocal tics and vocal tics If < 1 year: Provisional tic disorder

Table 18.3 Adult disorders that may present in childhood

Disorder	Diagnostic features	Special features in children
Major depression	Same as adults	Mood may be irritable instead of sad; failure to make expected weight gains
Persistent depressive disorder (dysthymia)	1-year duration	Mood may be irritable
Bipolar disorder	Same as adults	Controversial in children
Specific phobia	Minimum duration 6 months; anxiety may be expressed by crying, tantrums, or freezing	May not recognize fear as unreasonable; animal and natural environment phobias usually are childhood onset
Generalized anxiety disorder	One symptom of anxiety in children for at least 6 months	"Overanxious Disorder of Childhood"
Social anxiety disorder (social phobia)	Minimum duration 6 months; anxiety may be expressed by crying, tantrums, or freezing	May not recognize fear as unreasonable; anxiety in peer and adult settings
Obsessive compulsive disorder	Same as adults	May not recognize obsessions or compulsions as unreasonable; association with strep infections
Personality disorders	Same as adults	Usually not diagnosed in children due to developmental variations and evolving nature of personality that is not fixed until adulthood
Schizophrenia	Same as adults	Rare
Gender dysphoria	Incongruence between experienced gender and assigned gender of more than 6 months duration	Onset usually in childhood

Review Questions

1. The psychiatric evaluation and diagnosis of a child
   (a) Is primarily obtained from observation of the child.
   (b) Must always conform to DSM-5 criteria.
   (c) Must include at least three settings of problematic behavior to diagnose ADHD.
   (d) Should include a thorough history including school functioning, developmental milestones, and conception.
   (e) Two of the above.

2. Which of the following statements is true about treatment of ADHD?
   (a) Atomoxetine (Strattera) exerts its main effects on the serotonin neurotransmitter system.
   (b) It is especially controversial because of a lack of large-scale, non-pharmaceutical industry sponsored studies.
   (c) Methylphenidate should be avoided because of its addictive properties.
   (d) Should focus exclusively on the dopamine neurotransmitter system.
   (e) None of the above.

3. Which of the following statements is true regarding child abuse?
   (a) Abuse can result in symptoms of play reenactment of the event, restricted affect, night walking, and avoidance.
   (b) CPS should be notified only if suspicion for abuse is high because they have a responsibility to always separate the child from suspected perpetrators.
   (c) If the family admits to one isolated case of abuse, you can delay notifying CPS in order to maintain the therapeutic alliance which must be maintained for successful intervention and treatment.
   (d) More than half of all CPS-reported cases are confirmed as real.
   (e) Studies show that child abuse is considerably more common in low socioeconomic class, minority communities.

4. Which of the following diagnoses may present after the age of 18 years?
   (a) Conduct disorder
   (b) Autism spectrum disorder
   (c) Schizophrenia
   (d) Disruptive mood dysregulation disorder
   (e) Tourette's disorder

Appendix A: Tables with Possible Answers to the Vignettes

Vignette 18.1: Sam

Table 18.1.1

Facts	Hypotheses	Information needed	Learning issues
Referral was initiated by the school	Attention deficit hyperactivity disorder (ADHD)	Collateral information including history from teacher, direct observation of the child in the classroom, input from the child's pediatrician	Elements of a comprehensive child psychiatry evaluation and how it differs from an adult evaluation
Poor school performance, hyperactivity, and behavior problems at school	Autism spectrum disorder	A more detailed history including (1) In what environment(s) do these behaviors occur in?, (2) Are there other symptoms that might narrow the differential including sleep disturbances, change in appetite, loss of interests in activities, moodiness, tearfulness, anxiety, etc.?, (3) Are these new or old behaviors?, (4) What is the child's level of function in different areas (e.g., home, school, and with friends), (5) social/environmental details, and (6) family history	Differential diagnosis of childhood attentional and learning problems
Mother seems irritated that an evaluation has been requested	Intellectual disability (ID)	An individualized education program (IEP) evaluation to assess IQ and academic functioning	Recognition of important aspects of the child mental status exam including the parent–child relationship
	Specific learning disorder		
	Mood or anxiety disorder		
	Environmental causes (e.g., being bullied at school)		
	Oppositional defiant disorder (ODD)		

Table 18.1.2

Facts	Hypotheses	Information needed	Learning issues
High IQ, no impairment in academic performance	ADHD, autism spectrum disorder, and intellectual disability are less likely	More thorough social history	Synthesis of data to develop working hypothesis
Deficits in working memory and attention scales as demonstrated by the WISC	Still on the differential are: Mood disorder Anxiety disorder Environmental cause		Prevalence and treatment of ADHD
Child is highly distractible			Recognition of posttraumatic stress disorder as a potential cause of acute attentional problems
Hypervigilant to loud noises			
Symptoms have started within the last year; previous school functioning was normal			

WISC Weschler intelligence scale for children, *ADHD* attention deficit hyperactivity disorder

Table 18.1.3

Facts	Hypotheses	Information needed	Learning issues
Pediatrician's impression of the mother is overall favorable	Child abuse	Is there physical evidence of child abuse? For example, multiple bruises in different stages of healing, fractures not consistent with normal injury	The importance of considering abuse and trauma as potential causes of changes in child mental status
The patient's mother has become more withdrawn since a new boyfriend has moved into her home	Witness to domestic violence		Appreciation of the role of the health provider as a mandated reporter of child abuse
Pediatrician believes he smelled alcohol on the boyfriend's breath during an in-office visit			

Vignette 18.2: Teddy

Table 18.2.1

Facts	Hypotheses	Information needed	Learning issues
Previously bowel trained	Spinal cord injury	Physical examination	Differential diagnosis of encopresis to include possible physiological and psychological causes
History of intermittent constipation requiring medical intervention	Hirschsprung disease	Plain film of the abdomen	
Encopresis does not occur at night	Anal stenosis	Anorectal manometry sometimes useful	
	Imperforate anus with fistula	History of trauma suggesting spinal cord injury	
	Psychogenic origin	Detailed social history	

Table 18.2.2

Facts	Hypotheses	Information needed	Learning issues
Physical examination is unremarkable	Retentive encopresis less likely	Family patterns of interaction around issues of control	Common physical manifestations of psychological conflicts in childhood
Onset of problems coincided with the divorce of Teddy's parents	Psychological etiology more likely		

Vignette 18.3: Michael

Table 18.3.1

Facts	Hypotheses	Information needed	Learning issues
Language delay	Language delay	Birth history	Diagnostic assessment procedures for developmental delay
No pointing or gestures	Intellectual disability	Developmental history	
	Autism spectrum disorder	Infant temperament	
		Social development and parent–child interaction	
		Language milestones	
		Medical assessment	
		Physical exam	
		Laboratory tests	
		Psychological testing	

Table 18.3.2

Facts	Hypotheses	Information needed	Learning issues
Labs normal	Autism spectrum disorder	Detailed information about child's strengths and weaknesses to help inform treatment plan	Diagnostic criteria for autism spectrum disorder
Normal facial features	Possible intellectual disability		
Genetics normal			
2 years language delayed			
Fine/gross motor delays			
No social reciprocity			
No communicative intent			
No nonverbal gestures			
Poor social interaction			
Perseverative motor behaviors			
Limited interests			
Inflexible			
No fantasy play			

Appendix B: Answers to Review Questions

1. d
2. e
3. a
4. c

References

Abbeduto, L., Ozonoff, S., Thurman, A. J., McDuffie, A., & Schweitzer, J. (2014). Neurodevelopmental disorders. In R. E. Hales, S. C. Yudofsky, & L. W. Roberts (Eds.), *The American psychiatric publishing textbook of psychiatry* (6th ed., pp. 229–272). Arlington: American Psychiatric Publishing.

American Psychiatric Association. (2013). *Diagnostic and statistical manual of mental disorders* (5th ed.). Arlington: American Psychiatric Publishing.

Arnold, L. E., Abikoff, H. B., Cantwell, D. P., Conners, C. K., Elliott, G., Greenhill, L. L., Hechtman, L., Hinshaw, S. P., Hoza, B., Jensen. P. S., Kraemer, H. C., March, J. S., Newcorn, J. H., Pelham, W. E., Richters, J. E., Schiller, E., Severe, J. B., Swanson, J. M., Vereen, D., & Wells, K. C. (1997). National Institute of Mental Health Collaborative Multimodal Treatment Study of Children with ADHD (the MTA). Design challenges and choices. *Archives of General Psychiatry, 54*(9), 865–870.

Baribeau, D. A., & Anagnostou, E. (2014). An update on medication management of behavioral disorders in autism. *Current Psychiatry Reports, 16*(3), 437–450.

CDC Morbidity and Mortality Weekly Report. (2010). Prevalence of autism spectrum disorder among children aged 8 years-autism and developmental disabilities monitoring network, 11 sites, United States. *Surveillance Summaries, 63*(SS02), 1–21.
Cheng, K., & Myers, K. M. (2005). *Child and adolescent psychiatry: The essentials*. Philadelphia: Lippincott Williams & Wilkins.
Council on Children with Disabilities, Section on Developmental Behavioral Pediatrics, Bright Futures Steering Committee, Medical Home Initiatives for Children with Special Needs Project Advisory Committee. (2006). Identifying infants and young children with Developmental disorders in the medical home: An algorithm for developmental surveillance and screening. *Pediatrics, 118*(1), 405–420.
Deblinger, E., Steer, R. A., & Lippmann, J. (1999). Two-year follow-up study of cognitive behavioral therapy for sexually abused children suffering post-traumatic stress symptoms. *Child Abuse and Neglect, 23*(12), 1371–1378.
Drake, D. (2005). Understanding play in the treatment of an encopretic boy. *Child and Adolescent Social Work Journal, 22*(2), 229–242.
Dubner, A. E., & Motta, R. W. (1999). Sexually and physically abused foster care children and posttraumatic stress disorder. *Journal of Consulting Clinical Psychology, 67*(3), 367–373.
Faraone, S. V., Perlis, R. H., Doyle, A. E., Smoller, J. W., Goralnick, J. J., Holmgren, M. A., et al. (2005). Molecular genetics of attention-deficit/hyperactivity disorder. *Biological Psychiatry, 57*(11), 1313–1323.
Gabbard, G. O. (2014). Autism spectrum disorder. In *Gabbard's treatments of psychiatric disorders* (5th ed.). Arlington: American Psychiatric Publishing.
Har, A. F., & Croffie, J. M. (2010). Encopresis. *Pediatrics in Review, 31*(9), 368–374.
Katz, E. R., & DeMaso, D. R. (2011). Encopresis. In R. M. Kliegman, B. F. Stanton, J. W. St. Geme, N. F. Schor & R. E. Behrman (Eds.), *Nelson textbook of pediatrics* (pp. 70–75). Philadelphia: Elsevier.
Lewis, M. (2002). *Child and adolescent psychiatry: A comprehensive textbook* (3rd ed.). Philadelphia: Lippincott Williams & Wilkins.
Lord, C., Rutter, M., & DiLavore, P. (2003). *Autism diagnostic observation schedule*. Los Angeles: Western Psychological Services.
Molfese, V. G., & Acheson, S. (1997). Infant and preschool mental and verbal abilities: How are infant scores related to preschool scores? *International Journal of Behavioral Development, 20*(4), 595–607.
Reid, H., & Bahar, R. J. (2006). Treatment of encopresis and chronic constipation in young children: Clinical results from interactive parent-child guidance. *Clinical Pediatrics, 452,* 157–164.
Robins, D. L., Casagrande, K., Barton, M., Chen, C. M., Dumont-Mathieu, T., Fein, D., Chen, C. M., Dumont-Mathieu, T., & Fein, D. (2014). Validation of the Modified Checklist for Autism in Toddlers, Revised with Follow-up (M-CHAT-R/F). *Pediatrics, 133*(1), 37–45.
Ronald, A., & Hoekstra, R. A. (2011). Autism spectrum disorders and autistic traits: A decade of new twin studies. *The American Journal of Medical Genetics, 156,* 255–274.
Stigler, K. A., McDonald, B. C., Anand, A., Saykin, A. J., & McDougle, C. J. (2011). Structural and functional magnetic resonance imaging of autism spectrum disorders. *Brain Research, 1380,* 146–161.
U.S. Department of Health and Human Services, Administration for Children and Families, Administration on Children, Youth and Families, Children Administration for Child maltreatment. (2012). Resource document. http://www.acf.hhs.gov/programs/cb/research-data-technology/statistics-research/child-maltreatment. Accessed 13 March 2015.
Volkmar, F., Siegel, M., Woodbury-Smith, M., King, B., McCracken, J., State, M., & The American Academy of Child and Adolescent Psychiatry (AACAP) Committee on Quality Issues (CQI). (2014). Practice parameter for the assessment and treatment of children and adolescents with autism spectrum disorder. *Journal of the American Academy of Child and Adolescent Psychiatry, 53*(2), 237–257.
Williams, S. K. (2006). Risperidone and adaptive behavior in children with autism. *Journal of the American Academy of Child and Adolescent Psychiatry, 45*(4), 431–439.

Chapter 19
Substance-Related and Addictive Disorders

William F. Haning and Anthony P. S. Guerrero

Multiple illnesses comprise the substance use disorder spectrum. The management of any illness within the spectrum relies heavily on the availability of diagnostic and treatment resources and upon the level of participation by the patient. The two cases in this chapter demonstrate different problems and approaches to these challenging disorders.

At the end of this chapter, the reader will be able to:

1. Discuss the epidemiology, mechanisms, clinical presentation, clinical evaluation, differential diagnosis, treatment, and prevention of substance-related disorders, with particular attention to alcohol, tobacco, cannabis, opioids, and stimulants.
2. Describe medical comorbidities and counter-transference issues that need to be considered when caring for patients with substance use disorders.

Vignette 19.1.1: Benton Bentham

Benton Bentham is a 50-year-old male admitted to the orthopedic service yesterday after jumping off of a four-story building. He sustained a significant leg fracture and multiple bruises and contusions. A psychiatric consultation was ordered for evaluation of suicidal behavior. In the emergency room, Mr. Bentham was noted to smell of alcohol and to have "track marks" on his arms. His blood alcohol level was 0.31 mg/dL and his urine toxicology screen was positive for alcohol, cocaine, and opiates. Before you enter the room, the attending orthopedic surgeon, who appears quite worried, informs you that the patient is threatening to leave the hospital, and has even tried to climb out of his bed.

W. F. Haning (✉) · A. P. S. Guerrero
Department of Psychiatry, University of Hawaiʻi John A. Burns School of Medicine,
1356 Lusitana Street, University Tower 4th Floor, Honolulu, HI 96813, USA
e-mail: haning@hawaii.edu

A. P. S. Guerrero
e-mail: GuerreroA@dop.hawaii.edu

D. Alicata et al. (eds.), *Problem-based Behavioral Science and Psychiatry*,
DOI 10.1007/978-3-319-23669-8_19

Mr. Bentham is superficially cooperative and gives only minimal answers. He appears diaphoretic and seems to have difficulty focusing on your questions. He says blandly that he wants to leave the hospital because he is tired and wants to rest. He gives the same answer when the same question is repeated and cannot state what may happen to him if he were to refuse the recommended care. He states that he jumped off the ledge of his apartment building because he was "just fed up with it all … but I guess I learned my lesson now."

Please proceed with the problem-based approach using the worksheet located in the appendix of Chap. 1!

Please fill in the facts, your hypotheses, further information needed, and learning issues for Learning Issue Table 19.1.1.

Learning Issue Table 19.1.1

FACTS	HYPOTHESES	INFORMATION NEEDED	LEARNING ISSUES

Epidemiology

Substance use and addiction is common in the USA. Consider these facts:

- According to the Centers for Disease Control and Prevention (CDC 2013), approximately 9 % of persons in the USA aged 12 years or older have used any illicit drug in the past month.
- Approximately 7 % of persons in the USA aged 12 years or older have used marijuana in the past month.
- 2.6 % of persons in the USA aged 12 years or older have made nonmedical use of a psychotherapeutic drug in the past month.
- With regard to substances that are currently legal, tobacco smoking prevalence varies from approximately 10–33 % across the USA and territories.
- In the USA, over 50 % of the adult population drank alcohol in the past 30 days; over 6 % of the total population drank heavily; and over 15 % of the population binge drank (defined as more than four drinks).

The morbidity and mortality related to legal and illegal drug use in the USA is also significant. For example:

- Annually in the USA, cigarette smoking results in serious illnesses in approximately 8.6 million people and death in 440,000 people. It is the most preventable cause of premature death in the USA.
- In 2013, there were approximately 88,000 deaths in the USA attributable to excessive alcohol use, which is the third leading lifestyle-related cause of death in the USA. This extrapolated to 2.5 million years of potential life lost (YPLL), 2006–2010.
- According to the Office of National Drug Control Policy (2004a, 2004b, 2015), the economic cost of drug abuse is around $193 billion, which represents the cost of health consequences ($11 billion), the criminal consequences ($61 billion), and loss of productivity from death and inability to work ($120 billion) (see summary below).
- In 2004, poisoning was second only to motor vehicle crashes as a cause of death from unintentional injury in the USA. Nearly all of these deaths were from drugs.
- Costs of substance abuse:
  - Social/health cost to US society: ½ trillion/year
  - Illicit drugs: $193 billion/year
  - Tobacco: $168 billion/year
  - Alcohol: $185 billion/year
  - Diabetes: $132 billion/year
  - Cancer: $210 billion/year

Mechanisms, Clinical Manifestations, and Acute Treatment
Substance abuse and its medical sequelae are common in general medical settings, as illustrated in the case of Mr. Bentham. While his urine toxicology was positive for alcohol, opiates, and cocaine, it is important to identify which of these substances—in intoxication or withdrawal—may be producing his symptoms. It is also critical to identify the intoxication or withdrawal syndrome that is the most life-threatening and requires the most urgent treatment. Table 19.1 provides a summary of mechanisms and key clinical findings associated with intoxication and withdrawal of the major substances of abuse.

Mr. Bentham presents with apparent confusion, which could be explained by several of the intoxication or withdrawal symptoms listed above, and certainly by alcohol withdrawal delirium, which may be life-threatening. The consulting physician needs to ask Mr. Bentham about his pattern of substance use and past medical history, with attention to comorbid general medical conditions that could increase his risk of complications from intoxication and/or withdrawal. Mr. Bentham's physicians also need to monitor his vital signs and to note any other symptoms of intoxication and withdrawal on his physical examination. They will also obtain laboratory studies to screen for comorbidities.

Table 19.1 Mechanisms and clinical manifestations of the major substances of abuse

Substance	Mechanism	Clinical manifestations in intoxication	Clinical manifestations in withdrawal
Alcohol and sedative/hypnotic-anxiolytics, including benzodiazepines and barbiturates	Facilitation of GABA binding to its receptor	Respiratory depression, slurring of speech, lateral nystagmus, sedation, disinhibition, nausea/vomiting	Alcohol withdrawal delirium ("delirium tremens"), seizures, hypertension, tachycardia, diaphoresis, tremors *(withdrawal risk higher with chronic heavy use and sudden cessation as well as with concurrent illness or trauma)*
Cocaine, methamphetamine, and "stimulants"	Increased release of catecholamines and/or blockage of catecholamine reuptake	Cardiac arrhythmias, hypertension, vasospasm, agitation, mydriasis	Depression, sedation, lethargy
Ecstasy or methylene-dioxymethamphetamine (MDMA)	Release of catecholamines and serotonin	As above (with stimulants), and dehydration	Withdrawal uncommon; some characteristics associated with stimulants, when present
Gamma-hydroxy-butyrate (GHB)	GABA and dopamine receptor agonism	Seizures, coma (synergistically with alcohol)	Uncommon, but resembles benzodiazepine withdrawal when present
Inhalants	Cell membrane disruption	Cardiac arrhythmias, encephalopathy,	Lethargy, anhedonia, irritability
Hallucinogens, including lysergic acid diethylamide (LSD)	Serotonin receptor agonism	Agitation, delirium	No syndrome described
Marijuana	Cannabinoid receptors	Delirium uncommonly, not associated with coma or death; sedation, confusion	Irritability, insomnia, distractibility and inattention, anxiety
Opioids (including heroin)	Opioid receptor agonism	Respiratory depression/apnea, miosis, hypotension, constipation, sedation/coma	Autonomic hyperactivity, mydriasis, pain, diarrhea *(withdrawal risk higher with chronic heavy use and sudden cessation)*
Phencyclidine	N-methyl-D-aspartic acid (NMDA)	Agitation, fever, muscle rigidity	No syndrome described

GABA gamma-aminobutyric acid

Vignette 19.1.2 Continuation

Mr. Bentham says that he had been drinking "a lot" for the past "week or so," and that he has been a "good drinker" since he was "a boy." He denies any past history of withdrawal seizures. He admits to almost daily heroin use but says he only uses cocaine "once in a while." He says that he was on methadone maintenance therapy "about 5 years ago" but can't remember his dose, only that it was "high." He denies current use of other drugs, including barbiturates and prescription medications.

His past medical history is significant for cellulitides on his arms from injecting drugs. He takes no medications regularly. He smokes two packs per day of cigarettes. In the hospital, he receives Demerol (meperidine) p.r.n. for pain.

Physical exam:

Vital signs: Temperature 99.8 °F, Respirations 22/min, heart rate (HR) 112/min, blood pressure (BP) 146/92. He rates his pain as 5 on a 10-point scale.

General appearance/mental status: Mr. Bentham is disheveled, with poor eye contact. His speech is soft and minimally slurred and his mood is mildly irritable. His affect is anxious. Mr. Bentham denies any auditory or visual hallucinations or current suicidal or homicidal ideations. He appears to have a hard time following your questions. He is able to state his name, but he gives the wrong name of the hospital and is unable to give the date. He is unable to repeat more than 3 digits forward and 2 digits backward.

HEENT: Pupils 5 mm.

Neck: Supple.

Abdomen: Liver edge appreciated 2 fingerbreadths below the ribcage.

Neurologic: Tremors of outstretched hands. He has difficulty with finger-to-nose testing. Gait cannot be assessed due to the leg fracture.

Skin: "Track marks" are present. He is diaphoretic. There is no jaundice.

Review of labs and other studies:

Complete blood count (CBC): Mild anemia with a mildly elevated mean corpuscular volume

Chemistry panel: Elevated gamma glutamyl transferase and other liver function tests

Head computed tomography (CT) scan: Normal

Electrocardiograph (EKG): Normal except for sinus tachycardia

The psychiatric consultant contacts the admitting physician to discuss immediate recommendations, which include:

1. Patient should not be allowed to leave the hospital as he appears delirious and to lack decisional capacity.
2. A sitter at bedside.

3. Initiation of a benzodiazepine protocol to manage alcohol withdrawal.
4. Thiamine, vitamins, and folic acid.
5. Initiation of a patient-controlled analgesia (PCA) unit, with close monitoring of pain control and pupil size.
6. Close monitoring of vital signs and placement of a pulse oximeter.
7. Consideration of other laboratory tests, including HIV and hepatitis B/C.
8. Close attention to hydration, nutrition, and overall health.

Over the next few days, with intensive treatment, Mr. Bentham's mental status improves and his vital signs normalize. Although he still seems to have some difficulty with finger-to-nose testing, he is much less tremulous. He is able to remain alert and oriented, with an improved capacity to perform digit spans.

STOP

Please proceed with the problem-based approach using the worksheet located in the appendix of Chap. 1!

Please fill in the facts, your hypotheses, further information needed, and learning issues for Learning Issue Table 19.1.2.

Learning Issue Table 19.1.2

FACTS	HYPOTHESES	INFORMATION NEEDED	LEARNING ISSUES

The tachycardia, elevated BP, tremulousness, and confusion all are consistent with alcohol withdrawal delirium, in combination with opioid withdrawal and cocaine intoxication. At this point, it is important to review the treatment of intoxication and withdrawal of the major substances, summarized in Table 19.2.

While a discussion of the organ systems affected by alcohol is beyond the scope of this textbook, it is worth noting that Mr. Bentham likely had medical complications of alcohol use, including elevated liver function tests, macrocytic anemia, and cerebellar dysfunction. Because of the multi-organ effects of substances of abuse and the poor access to care that patients who abuse substances often experience, it is important to thoroughly evaluate such patients for medical complications of substance abuse. For Mr. Bentham, an electrocardiogram was obtained to rule out

Table 19.2 Treatment of intoxication with and withdrawal from the major substances of abuse

Substance	Treatment of intoxication	Treatment of withdrawal
Alcohol and sedative/hypnotics, including benzodiazepines (BZs) and barbiturates	Supportive care, including attention to airway, breathing, circulation; benzodiazepine antagonist (flumazenil) for BZs only	Thiamine, magnesium sulfate, anticonvulsants arguably, benzodiazepine-based protocols (for alcohol); BZs for BZ and other sedative–hypnotic dependence
Cocaine, methamphetamine, and "stimulants"	Benzodiazepines for agitation, appropriate cardiac antiarrhythmic medication	Under investigation, present recommendations off-label. In interim, support sleep (trazadone, antihistamines, sedatives circumspectly); feed/hydrate
Ecstasy/MDMA	As for stimulants	None generally required; as for stimulants, if syndrome present
Gamma-hydroxy-butyrate (GHB)	Respiratory support	None
Heroin and opioids	Nalloxone (Narcan) acutely	Opioid agonists (buprenorphine, methadone); clonidine, anitiemetics (promethazine)
Inhalants	Respiratory support	None
Hallucinogens, including lysergic acid diethylamide (LSD)	Antipsychotic medication (risperidone, haloperidol), benzodiazepines	None
Marijuana	Conservative	None
Phencyclidine	Antipsychotic medication (risperidone, haloperidol), benzodiazepines	None

MDMA 3,4-methylenedioxy-methamphetamine

cardiovascular sequelae of cocaine and alcohol use, and neuroimaging was obtained in order to rule out intracranial pathology (perhaps from unrecognized trauma) as a cause of the delirium. Finally, tests for hepatitis B/C and HIV were obtained because of the history of injection drug use.

In addition, without treatment with thiamine (to be given before any dextrose-containing solution) and effective management of the alcohol withdrawal, Mr. Bentham may be at risk for Korsakoff's syndrome (alcohol-induced major neurocognitive disorder, amnestic-confabulatory type), typically also associated with Wernicke's encephalopathy. The mechanisms and signs and symptoms associated with this condition are indicated in Fig. 19.1.

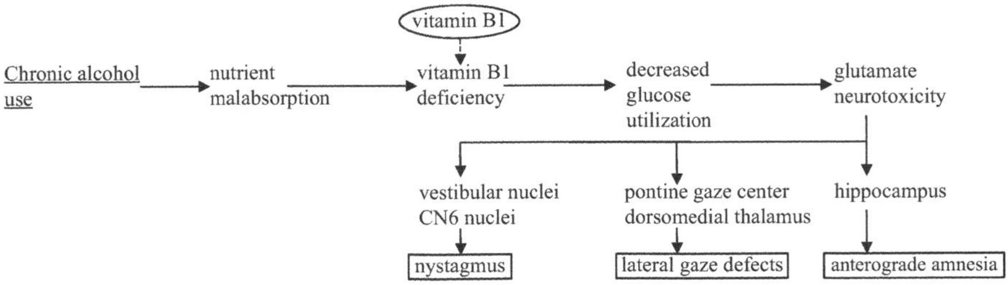

Fig. 19.1 Mechanisms, signs, and symptoms associated with Wernicke's encephalopathy and alcohol-induced persisting amnestic disorder

Beyond acute management, Mr. Bentham's physicians will gather further history about Mr. Bentham to formulate a comprehensive management plan.

Vignette 19.1.3 Continuation

Mr. Bentham reports that he has been feeling very depressed for the past week after losing a job that he had held for almost 1 year. He had been drinking more heavily than usual. He reports a history of regular drinking, mostly after work, usually six beers each evening, for the past 25 or so years. He went through an alcoholism rehabilitation program about 8 years ago and attended Alcoholics Anonymous (AA) for a few months afterwards. His longest period of sobriety from alcohol was 10 months, during and after the rehabilitation episode, but he continued to use other drugs "a little" during that period. He acknowledges one Driving Under the Influence (DUI) conviction and gives positive responses to all four "CAGE" items (need to *c*ut down, *a*nnoyance with criticism, *g*uilt about drinking, use of alcohol as an "*e*ye opener"; refer to Appendix C). Mr. Bentham gives further details about his heroin use: he had relapsed after having been on methadone for about 1 year and occasionally was involved in selling drugs to support his habit. He denies any other history of illegal activity or trouble with the law. He states that he snorted cocaine on the day of admission "…and maybe a few days before that," and that he only uses it every few months. He admits to having experimented with other drugs in the past, including hallucinogens during the 1970s: "You name it, I tried it." He acknowledges having friends who "are worse drug addicts than I am," from whom he buys drugs.

He denies any past history of psychiatric treatment, suicide attempts, or diagnosis of depression. He admits that he had been thinking of suicide the day prior to admission but says that he deeply regrets what he had done, especially now that he is sober. He denies any persistent depression or anhedonia lasting longer than 2 weeks prior to having lost his job. He denies any past history of manic symptoms unrelated to cocaine intoxication. He denies having experienced any hallucinations or delusions.

Mr. Bentham lives by himself in a small apartment in town. He had been homeless in the past. He has one half-brother in Hawai'i, with whom he has limited contact, but otherwise his family is on the mainland. His 7-year marriage ended 15 years ago, and he has limited contact with his previous wife and teenage son. He believes that several of his uncles had problems with alcoholism. He says: "I sure hope my son doesn't turn out like I do."

The order for a bedside sitter is discontinued.

As Mr. Bentham's medical status improves, he is switched from PCA morphine to a modest daily dose of methadone (given in liquid form in orange juice) and offered disulfiram, which he politely refuses now but says he will consider later. You also recommend the use of the medication acamprosate while awaiting improvement in his liver function studies and offer community resources for substance abuse treatment and general medical follow-up.

Mr. Bentham is visibly relieved to learn that his tests for HIV and hepatitis were negative. You discuss safe sex and HIV prevention guidelines, which he says he will follow ("I need to get my life together.") He asks you if and when he should have his HIV test repeated.

You also advise him on the importance of smoking cessation. Although he is not yet ready to set a quit date, he is open to hearing your advice regarding the "5 Rs": relevance of quitting smoking, risks of smoking, rewards of quitting smoking, perceived roadblocks to quitting smoking, and importance of repetition. He promises to discuss this issue at his medical follow-up visit. He also asks whether or not the nicotine patch or bupropion might be appropriate for him.

Differential Diagnoses

The Diagnostic and Statistical Manual for Mental Disorders, 5th edition (2013), or DSM-5, offers a categorical description of substance use disorders, summarized below in Table 19.3.

At the time of his admission, in addition to the acute intoxication and withdrawal syndromes discussed above, it is likely that Mr. Bentham meets criteria for alcohol and opioid use disorders, severe; tobacco use disorder, moderate to severe; and cocaine use disorder, mild.

The mechanisms to explain Mr. Bentham's current presentation are shown in Fig. 19.2.

Comprehensive Management and Prevention

As indicated in Fig. 19.2, long-term management will need to include a biopsychosocial approach, which is essential for the treatment of all substance use disorders. Table 19.4 summarizes the medication interventions that may be appropriate for each specific substance of abuse. The American Society of Addiction Medicine (ASAM) Criteria, 2013, provide detailed crosswalks matching the level of care to symptomatic expression during intoxication and withdrawal.

Table 19.3 Relevant categories of substance use disorders specified in the Diagnostic and Statistical Manual of Mental Disorders, 5th edition (DSM-5)

Disorder	Highlights
Substance use disorder	Problematic pattern
	Clinically significant impairment or distress
	At least two within a 12-month period
	Taken in larger amounts or over a longer period than intended
	Persistent desire or unsuccessful efforts to cut down or control use
	Significant time spent obtaining, using, recovering
	Craving or a strong desire to use
	Failure to fulfill major role obligations
	Continued use despite persistent/recurrent social/interpersonal problems caused or exacerbated by substance
	Important social, occupational, or recreational activities given up or reduced
	Recurrent use in situations where physically hazardous
	Continued use despite knowledge of having a persistent physical or psychological problem likely to have been caused or exacerbated by substance
	Tolerance
	Withdrawal
	Modifiers
	Early remission: >3 months, <12 months (no criteria other than craving/desire)
	Sustained remission: >12 months (no criteria other than craving/desire)
	Mild: 2–3 symptoms
	Moderate: 4–5 symptoms
	Severe: 6+ symptoms
Substance/medication withdrawal or intoxication delirium	Other criteria for delirium, namely disturbance of consciousness and attention; change in cognition (e.g., memory, orientation) or perceptual disturbances not better accounted for by dementia; acute onset with fluctuation in symptoms
	Temporally related to substance withdrawal or intoxication
Substance/medication-induced major or mild neurocognitive disorder	Significantly impairing memory impairment that represents a decline from previous functioning
	Not fully explained by delirium, dementia, or substance withdrawal
	Etiologically related to the persisting effects of substance use

For Mr. Bentham, methadone might address both opioid withdrawal and his need for pain management, given the recent injuries. The conscientious clinician in this case also made sure to address the tobacco use, which (in spite of its legality) is a serious health risk in the long term. The clinician can refer to treatment resources in US Public Health Service (2012).

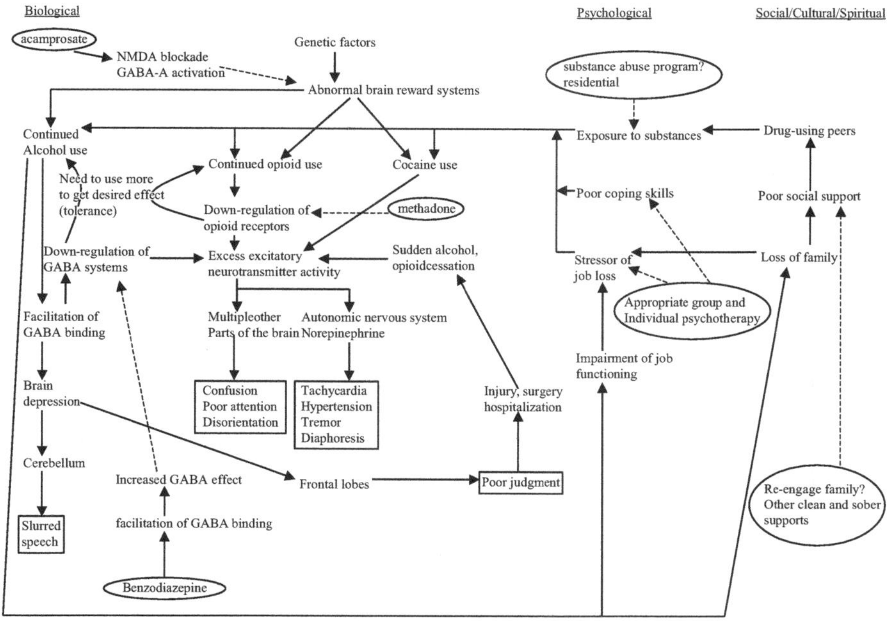

Fig. 19.2 Mechanisms to explain Mr. Bentham's current presentation

Prevention

Finally, Mr. Bentham raised the important issue of how to best prevent his son from having the same substance use problems that he had. As reviewed by the National Institute on Drug Abuse (2003), effective prevention principles include enhancement of protective factors (e.g., parental support), reduction of risk factors (e.g., psychosocial adversity and negative peer influences), and enhancement of academic and social competence through prevention-based curricula in the schools. From the clinician standpoint, it is important to detect substance abuse risk factors as well as substance abuse itself as early as possible in order to optimize outcome. The next case illustrates the importance of this principle.

In contrast to the previous case, the following is a description of an outpatient setting, where the "patient" is not the one recognizing the problem or seeking help.

Vignette 19.2.1: Dr. Caleb

You are the primary care physician for Dr. Caleb, a 55-year-old male physician with progressive impairment in multiple spheres in his life. He is famous in the medical community for once having successfully sued the major community hospital for restraint of trade issues centering on his medical staff privileges.

On a busy Friday, his wife, Dr. Jenny, drags her reluctant husband into your office during an overbooked calendar. She wants to talk to you about "his behavior," which may have something to do with drinking. She says, "I thought of bringing him in to see the local addiction specialist, but Dr. Caleb would be paranoid seeing a psychiatrist. He would be worried about what people might think: patients, other doctors."

On further questioning (constrained by Dr. Caleb's presence in the room), Dr. Jenny reports the following:

Home life: His behavior has been reclusive. He has taken to driving home and going directly to his study. On weekends, he no longer hikes. There are two teenage children who avoid him because he is unfriendly, judgmental, and sometimes punitive.

- Not reported: He has struck Jeremy, one son, in an argument over how he was speaking to the mother, Jenny.
- Not reported: His daughter, Carmen, has a friend who is Dr. Caleb's patient. Dr. Caleb fondled the friend during a recent physical examination. A Licensing Board complaint has been filed.

Professional life: Dr. Caleb is constantly paged at home, yet never seems to need to go to the hospital; he manages most of his practice by calling in medications.

- Not reported: He splits meds with his patients; he offers to "discard legally" unused pills and then diverts them to his own use ("diversion").
- Not reported: Self-prescribed zolpidem until several years ago, when it became a controlled substance.
- Health: He has gained weight. She thinks he has hypertension but he never sees a doctor; he tells her, "It's under control."

Behavior: He is angry when she asks about his drinking.

- Not reported: She is terrified of asking him.

"What is your concern or fear?" you ask. She answers that she is worried because Dr. Caleb's father was alcoholic.

You begin by having Dr. Caleb sign releases for communication with several key people: his wife, a colleague, the children, his primary physician. Regardless of how you originally met Dr. Caleb, your management of his problems follows a Change Model of intervention (please refer to Chap. 10: Adherence in Medicine).

You proceed with a comprehensive history and examination.

Table 19.4 Pharmacotherapy of addictions (limited list)

Class	Medication	Indication	Efficacy	Considerations
Agonist	Methadone	Opioid withdrawal/maintenance (controlled substance CII)	High	Dispensing restrictions beyond CII; overdose risk; lengthy withdrawal
	Buprenorphine, buprenorphine + naloxone	Opioid withdrawal/maintenance (controlled substance CIII)	High	Milder restrictions than with methadone; little risk of overdose. Risk of diversion diminishes with addition of naloxone
	Nicotine replacement therapy (NRT)—gum, patch, nasal insufflation. Vapor inhalation?	Nicotine dependence	Low-moderate	Best in conjunction with adjunctive therapy (bupropion, varenicline). Efficacy and safety of vapor inhalation ("e-cigarettes") not yet determined
	Benzodiazepines—diazepam, alprazolam, etc.	Alcohol or sedative-hypnotic withdrawal (GABA agonist)	High	Risk of overdose in outpatient setting
Antagonist	Naloxone	Opioid overdose	High	Abrupt withdrawal, profoundly dysphoric; IV only
	Naltrexone	Opioid dependence; some efficacy in alcohol dependence	Moderate	Blocks effects of self-administered opioids, useful in monitored abstinence. Oral and long-acting injection
	Flumazenil (Mazicon)	Benzodiazepine overdose	High	Abrupt withdrawal, dysphoric, seizure risk; short-acting so principally diagnostic; expensive
Aversive agents	Disulfiram (Antabuse)	Alcohol dependence	Moderate	Interrupts alcohol metabolism to create acetaldehyde accumulation; profoundly distressing: N/V, HA, hypotension, dysphoria when challenged with ethanol intake. Rare acute psychosis. Do not co-prescribe with other acetaldehyde dehydrogenase inhibitors (e.g., metronidazole)
Other (anticraving agents, satiety agents, others of unknown mechanism)	Naltrexone—Diminution of craving, early alcohol satiety (harm reduction strategy as well as abstinence enhancement)	Alcohol dependence	Moderate	Available as oral (Revia—daily); or injectable (Vivitrol—monthly), though latter is markedly costlier

Table 19.4 (continued)

Class	Medication	Indication	Efficacy	Considerations
	Acamprosate—NMDA blocker, GABA-A activation	Alcohol dependence	Low-Moderate	Low risk, some SEs (HA/N), best initiated in abstinence
	Bupropion—antidepressant with catecholaminergic and dopaminergic agonism, nicotinergic antagonism	Nicotine dependence,	Low-moderate	Reduces seizure threshold. With nicotine dependence, best employed with concomitant Nicotine replacement therapy
	Varenicline (Chantix)—nicotine receptor partial agonist	Nicotine dependence	Moderate	May be best employed with bupropion; use with NRTs increases side effect profile
	Clonidine—alpha-2 adrenergic agonist	Opioid withdrawal—symptom management without controlled substances	Moderate	Best employed with promethazine or ondansetron (anti-nauseants), anticonvulsants. Risk of suppression of vital signs in alcohol withdrawal delirium
	Anticonvulsants—divalproate/ Depakote, others	Alcohol and sedative-hypnotic withdrawal (where benzodiazepenes not indicated)	Moderate	Incomplete efficacy in controlling seizures; not indicated for delirium. Consider adjunctive use of other sedating agents (trazadone, promethazine) for sleep

GABA gamma-aminobutyric acid, *IV* intravenous drip, *NMDA* N-methyl-D-aspartic acid, *N/V* nausea/vomiting, *HA* headache

STOP — Please proceed with the problem-based approach using the worksheet located in the appendix of Chap. 1!

Please fill in the facts, your hypotheses, further information needed, and learning issues for Learning Issue Table 19.2.1.

Learning Issue Table 19.2.1

FACTS	HYPOTHESES	INFORMATION NEEDED	LEARNING ISSUES

From a primary care standpoint, useful resources for assessment of alcohol and other substance abuse are listed below:

- See Treatment Improvement Protocols, Center of Substance Abuse Treatment of Substance Abuse and Mental Health Services Administration: TIPs 24 and 34 http://www.kap.samhsa.gov/products/manuals/tips/index.htm
- CAGE Questionnaire (Appendix C)
- Michigan Alcohol Screening Test (MAST) (Appendix D)
- Structured Clinical Interview for DSM-IV TR (SCID) (SCID for DSM-5 not yet available 1/2015)
- Alcohol Use Disorders Identification Test (AUDIT) (Appendix E)

Vignette 19.2.2 Continuation

Dr. Caleb's first-person history is significant for the following:

- Raised to a Taiwanese mother and a German–Dutch father, Dr. Caleb had four siblings. Two survive. His father was a military officer whose social life centered on alcohol use; when he retired, it became the centrally organizing theme in his life.
- Dr. Caleb's mother lived with the father until his death; she remarried, to a Native American casino owner.
- Dr. Caleb resolved at an early age to never drink or smoke.
- He moved to Hawai'i for residency in family practice, married another doctor—she is a pathologist—and developed a demanding community and hospital practice in a large-group partnership.
- In 2008, he decided to go solo.

- He has suffered headaches most of his adult life. They are commonly disabling.
- For medical care, he used to see whoever of his partners was available; he has provided his own care to himself, since.
- In 2009, in a suit to get out of his previous practice agreement, he alleged misconduct against two of his colleagues. One, a recovering alcoholic, he accused of "…always being drunk." His contention was that he left because of increased joint liability. The suit was withdrawn when the partnership agreed to settle.

Salient Findings:

- Dr. Caleb acknowledges that his headaches have worsened and that they frequently do not respond to opioids.
  - Not reported: He has been ordering and using injectable Stadol/butorphanol through the mail.
- He agrees that he has given up most of his social and athletic interests. He indicates that this is because his practice is too busy.
  - Not reported: He spends as much time as always at work, 60 h. His productivity has fallen 20 % since 2008.
- He believes that his wife will leave him if he doesn't recover; he states that he wants the marriage to continue.
  - Not reported: He has always felt that Jenny was a superior physician and the more successful partner in the marriage. He sees this illness as yet another acknowledgment of his inferiority to her. He is actually ambivalent about the marriage.
- He thinks that he has an ulcer. He has been taking cimetidine (Tagamet).
  - Not reported: Hematemesis 2 weeks ago after a binge.
- He is short of breath on exertion, but ascribes this to cigarettes, 20+ pack-years.
  - Not reported: He has edema.

You perform a physical examination and appropriate laboratory studies and draw diagnostic conclusions. Your impression is: alcohol use disorder, severe; with opioid use disorder and sedative–hypnotic–anxiolytic use disorder, mild-moderate.

Dr. Caleb is willing to see an addiction specialist, who develops a treatment plan predicated on his level of readiness for change, using ASAM Criteria:

1. Inductive care (residential, day treatment, or outpatient as appropriate and available). Motivational interviewing (MI) strategies are employed to

reach a level of readiness for change. Psychotherapies in the treatment of addictions include: cognitive behavioral therapy, 12 step facilitation, and contingency management. Please refer to Chap. 4 on learning principles of human behavior for more information. These occur in the context of group psychosocial rehabilitation. A patient's required level of care can be identified using a level of care algorithm developed by ASAM.

2. Medication therapy
3. Community reinforcement (also known as network therapy) is a contractual management for behavioral monitoring, treatment adherence, and relapse prevention. (Gallanter)
4. Peer identification, such as physician support groups
5. Recovering community identification such as AA and Narcotics Anonymous
6. Family treatment (reflecting family unit disruption and "contagion," associated with substance use disorder)
7. Medical care (somatic consequences of substance use disorder) and psychiatric care (neuropsychological comorbid consequences of substance use disorder)

Situations such as Dr. Caleb's are clinically, ethically, and legally complex, yet not uncommon. Physicians in need of addiction treatment should be referred to an addiction specialist. The number of physicians involved in the care of a physician should be generous, and their communications with one another should be frequent. At least one objective of this is to prevent the colleague from resuming the role of self-physician.

Review Questions

1. Which of the following statements about the epidemiology of substance use disorders is *false*?

   a. Smoking prevalence varies from approximately 10–33 % across the 50 states, the District of Columbia, Guam, Puerto Rico, and the US Virgin Islands
   b. Excessive alcohol use is the third leading lifestyle-related cause of death in the USA
   c. Annually in the USA, cigarette smoking results in serious illnesses in approximately 8.6 million people and death in 440,000 people
   d. The percentage of persons in the USA aged 12 years or older who have used any illicit drug in the past month is approximately 3 %
   e. None of the above is false

2. A patient on the medical/surgical unit requests "something to take the edge off of my alcohol withdrawal." Following many years of heavy, regular drinking, he had his last drink 4 days prior to his admission for pneumonia. He has tachycardia, elevated BP, and difficulty sustaining attention. The most appropriate treatment(s) at this time is (are):

a. Thiamine, multivitamins, and benzodiazepines
b. Alpha-2-adrenergic agents such as clonidine or guanfacine
c. Therapeutic prescription for beer to be given with each meal
d. Either naltrexone or acamprosate to reduce cravings
e. All of the above

3. A 15-year-old patient uses cannabis nearly every day in order to "mellow myself out so that I can function." She describes significant anxiety symptoms, almost to the point of panic, if she is unable to have access to it. She obtains the cannabis mostly through trafficking it in her high school. She states that, for the past several months, she has used significantly more of the drug "because I can afford it now." Her academic record reflects an ability to "get straight As when I put my mind to it." She is often in trouble with her parents for staying out late with her drug-using peers. She denies any past psychiatric symptoms other than "hating her parents" prior to the age of 13, when she first began using cannabis. The most likely diagnosis is:

a. Attention deficit hyperactivity disorder
b. Cannabis use disorder, moderate
c. Panic disorder with self-medication
d. Antisocial personality disorder
e. None of the above

4. Which of the following is *not* a component of the CAGE questionnaire?

a. Cut down (use)
b. Anger (with discussion)
c. Anxiety (with cessation of drinking)
d. Guilt (over use)
e. Eye opener

5. A 23-year-old male is brought to the emergency room with combativeness, paranoia, and pressured speech. His HR and BP are elevated. Which of the following is (are) likely substance(s) to explain these findings:

a. Methamphetamine
b. Oxycodone
c. Volatile inhalants
d. Diazepam
e. a and b only

Appendix A: Tables with Possible Answers to the Vignettes

Vignette 19.1: Benton Bentham

Learning Issue Table 19.1

Facts	Hypotheses	Information needed	Learning issues
"Good drinker", daily heroin use	*Alcohol withdrawal, delirium likely*	Comprehensive medical and psychiatric evaluation	Which of these substances in intoxication or withdrawal may be producing his symptoms?
History of cellulitides from injecting drugs	Tobacco use disorder	Comprehensive physical and neurological examination	It is critical to identify the intoxication or withdrawal syndrome that is the most life-threatening and requires the most urgent treatment
Smokes cigarettes	Liver damage	Monitoring of pain control	It is important to review the treatment of intoxication and withdrawal of the major substances
Temperature 99.8 °	Some sort of encephalopathy	Monitoring of vital signs	It is important to review the treatment of intoxication and withdrawal of the major substances
HR 112/min BP 146/92	Anemia from nutritional deficiency?	Screen for HIV and hepatitis B and C	Is the patient at risk for Korsakoff's syndrome typically also associated with Wernicke's encephalopathy?
Hard time following questions, gives the wrong name of the hospital, unable to give the date, unable to repeat more than 3 digits forward and 2 digits backward		Electrocardiogram was obtained to rule out cardiovascular sequelae of cocaine and alcohol use; and neuroimaging was obtained in order to rule out intracranial pathology	Consider the biological, psychological, and social/cultural/spiritual elements of comprehensive treatment management
Liver edge appreciated 2 fingerbreadths below the ribcage\tremors of outstretched hands difficulty with finger-to-nose testing, diaphoretic			
Mild anemia with a mildly elevated mean corpuscular volume, elevated gamma glutamyl transferase and other liver function tests			

HR heart rate, *BP* blood pressure

Vignette 19.2: Dr. Caleb

Learning Issue Table 19.2

Facts	Hypotheses	Information needed	Learning issues
55-year-old male physician dragged into your office	Alcohol use disorder	Comprehensive history and examination	Consider the biological, psychological, and social/cultural/spiritual elements of comprehensive treatment management
Would be worried about what people think	Prescription medication use disorder	Appropriate laboratory studies	Physicians in need of addiction treatment should be referred to an addiction specialist
Reclusive, unfriendly, judgmental, and sometimes punitive	Other medical condition		
Licensing Board complaint	Suffered headaches most of his adult life		
Constantly paged; he manages most of his practice by calling in medications	Marital stressors		
Has gained weight			
Father was alcoholic			

Appendix B: Answers to Review Questions

1. d
2. a
3. b
4. c
5. a

Appendix C: CAGE Questionnaire (Ewing 1984)

(High sensitivity and specificity in most medical populations. Manner of questioning influences outcome, questioner should avoid leading the answer with affect. Recommended that more neutral risk screening be conducted first—e.g., diet/exercise/seat belts/smoking.)

Has the patient any of these responses, to the suggested questions?

*C*ut Down (or discontinued) Use

- Because symptoms worsened
- Because a doctor or therapist or advisor suggested

Angry when Using or Annoyed when Drug or Alcohol Use Discussed

- Anger or altercation during use
- Hostile defensiveness surrounding use

Guilt Surrounding Use

- Guilt or shame regarding behaviors while using
- Any suicidal gesture

*E*ye-Opener

- Effort to medicate withdrawal, e.g., alcohol or sedatives to suppress hangover symptoms or to permit function at work

Appendix D: Michigan Alcohol Screening Test (MAST)

A score of two or more positive responses suggests an alcohol use disorder corresponding to dependence (DSM4TR) (Buschbaum et al. 1991) and warrants re-screening with MAST (Michigan Alcohol Screening Test) or S-MAST (Short MAST), or full diagnostic review with the SCID (Structured Clinical Interview for DSM-4TR).

Appendix E: Short MAST (Seltzer et al. 1975)

Do you feel you are a normal drinker?	Yes	*No*
Do your spouse or parents worry or complain about your drinking?	*Yes*	No
Do you ever feel bad about your drinking?	*Yes*	No
Do friends or relatives think you are a normal drinker?	Yes	*No*
Are you always able to stop drinking when you want to?	Yes	*No*
Have you ever attended a meeting of Alcoholics Anonymous?	*Yes*	No
Has drinking ever created problems between you and your spouse?	*Yes*	No
Have you ever gotten into trouble at work because of drinking?	*Yes*	No
Have you ever neglected your obligations, your family, or your work for 2 or more days in a row because you were drinking?	*Yes*	No
Have you ever gone to anyone for help about your drinking?	*Yes*	No
Have you ever been in the hospital because of drinking?	*Yes*	No
Have you ever been arrested even for a few hours because of drinking?	*Yes*	No
Have you ever been arrested for drunk driving or driving after drinking?	*Yes*	No

Scoring:

1 point for each of answers in italics.
2 points = possible problem in use of alcohol
3 points = probable problem in use of alcohol

Appendix E: Alcohol Use Disorders Identification Test (AUDIT) Public Domain, http://pubs.niaaa.nih.gov/publications/arh28-2/78-79.htm

AUDIT

PATIENT: Because alcohol use can affect your health and can interfere with certain medications and treatments, it is important that we ask some questions about your use of alcohol. Your answers will remain confidential, so please be honest.

For each question in the chart below, place an X in one box that best describes your answer.

NOTE: In the U.S., a single drink serving contains about 14 grams of ethanol or "pure" alcohol. Although the drinks below are different sizes, each one contains the same amount of pure alcohol and counts as a single drink:

12 oz. of beer (about 5% alcohol) =

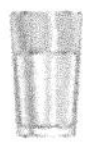

8-9 oz. of malt liquor (about 7% alcohol) =

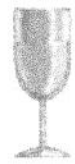

5 oz. of wine (about 12% alcohol) =

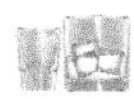

1.5 oz. of hard liquor (about 40% alcohol)

Questions	0	1	2	3	4	
1. How often do you have a drink containing alcohol?	Never	Monthly or less	2 to 4 times a month	2 to 3 times a week	4 or more times a week	
2. How many drinks containing alcohol do you have on a typical day when you are drinking?	1 or 2	3 or 4	5 or 6	7 to 9	10 or more	
3. How often do you have 5 or more drinks on one occasion?	Never	Less than monthly	Monthly	Weekly	Daily or almost daily	
4. How often during the last year have you found that you were not able to stop drinking once you had started?	Never	Less than monthly	Monthly	Weekly	Daily or almost daily	
5. How often during the last year have you failed to do what was normally expected of you because of drinking?	Never	Less than monthly	Monthly	Weekly	Daily or almost daily	
6. How often during the last year have you needed a first drink in the morning to get yourself going after a heavy drinking session?	Never	Less than monthly	Monthly	Weekly	Daily or almost daily	
7. How often during the last year have you had a feeling of guilt or remorse after drinking?	Never	Less than monthly	Monthly	Weekly	Daily or almost daily	
8. How often during the last year have you been unable to remember what happened the night before because of your drinking?	Never	Less than monthly	Monthly	Weekly	Daily or almost daily	
9. Have you or someone else been injured because of your drinking?	No		Yes, but not in the last year		Yes, during the last year	
10. Has a relative, friend, doctor, or other health care worker been concerned about your drinking or suggested you cut down?	No		Yes, but not in the last year		Yes, during the last year	
					Total	

Note: This questionnaire (the AUDIT) is reprinted with permission from the World Health Organization. To reflect drink serving sizes in the United States (14g of pure alcohol), the number of drinks in question 3 was changed from 6 to 5. A free AUDIT manual with guidelines for use in primary care settings is available online at *www.who.org*.

Excerpted from NIH Publication No. 07-3769 **National Institute on Alcohol and Alcoholism** ***www.niaaa.nih.gov/guide***

References

American Psychiatric Association. (2000). *Diagnostic and statistical manual for mental disorders IV-TR*. Arlington: American Psychiatric Press.

American Psychiatric Association. (2006). Work group on substance use disorders. Practice guideline for the treatment of patients with substance use disorders (2nd ed.). http://psychiatryonline.org/pb/assets/raw/sitewide/practice_guidelines/guidelines/substanceuse.pdf. Accessed 16 Feb 2015.

American Psychiatric Association. (2013). *Diagnostic and statistical manual of mental disorders DSM-5* (Fifth ed.). Arlington: American Psychiatric Press.

Buchsbaum, D. G., Buchanan, R. G., Centor, R. M., Schnoll, S. H., Lawton, M. J. (1991). Screening for alcohol abuse using CAGE scores and likelihood ratios. *Annals of Internal Medicine, 115,* 774–777.

Centers for Disease Control and Prevention. (2013). http://www.cdc.gov. Accessed 16 Feb 2015.

Ewing, J. A. (1984). Detecting alcoholism: The CAGE questionnaire. *JAMA, 252,* 1905–1907.

Mee-Lee D. (Ed.). (2013). ASAM Criteria (AKA "PPC-3"). PPC-2 openly accessible in TIP 51, SAMHSA. http://162.99.3.213/products/manuals/tips/pdf/TIP51.pdf. Accessed Jan 2015.

National Institute of Alcoholism and Alcohol Abuse (NIAAA)—AUDIT Questionnaire. (2008). http://pubs.niaaa.nih.gov/publications/arh28-2/78-79.htm.

National Institute on Drug Abuse. (2003). Preventing drug use among children and adolescents (2nd ed.). http://www.drugabuse.gov/pdf/prevention/RedBook.pdf. Accessed 16 Feb 2015.

Office of National Drug Control Policy. (2004a). The economic costs of drug abuse in the United States, 1992–2002. Washington, DC: Executive Office of the President (Publication No. 207303). http://www.whitehousedrugpolicy.gov/publications/economic_costs/economic_costs.pdf. Accessed Jan 2015.

Office of National Drug Control Policy. (2004b). (Publication No. 207303). 2004.; CDC. *MMWR, 54*(25), 625–628, July 1, 2005; Harwood, H. Lewin Group for the NIAAA, 2000.

Office of National Drug Control Policy. (2015). Fact sheets: http://www.whitehouse.gov/ondcp/ondcp-fact-sheets/how-illicit-drug-use-affects-business-and-the-economy. Accessed Jan 2015.

Seltzer, M. A., Vinokur, A., Van Rooijen, L. J. (1975). A self-administered short michigan alcohol screening test (SMAST). *Journal of Studies on Alcohol, 36,* 117–126.

Substance Abuse and Mental Health Services Administration (SAMHSA), Behavioral Health Barometers. (2014). This link provides access to PDF files, with both national and individual states' reports on behavioral health and substance use data. http://www.samhsa.gov/data/browse-report-document-type?tab=46. Accessed 16 Feb 2015.

U.S. Public Health Service, Hays, J. T., Treatment of Tobacco Dependence. (2012). http://www.cdc.gov/primarycare/materials/smokingcessation/docs/Smoking_Cessation_Teleconference_Speaker_Presentation_508_2012-04-25.pdf. Accessed Jan 2015.

Chapter 20
Schizophrenia Spectrum and Other Psychotic Disorders

Steven J. Zuchowski and Brian Kirkpatrick

Schizophrenia is arguably the worst disease affecting mankind (Editor, 1988).

Psychotic disorders are often devastating to patients and their families. The symptoms can be both terrifying and disabling. While delusions and hallucinations are the often the most obvious manifestation of a psychotic disorder, a wide range of more subtle symptoms may also be present. Current antipsychotic treatments, while they can be effective, do not impact all aspects of psychotic illness and frequently carry a significant side effect burden. This chapter will provide an overview of the psychotic disorders, touching on their clinical presentation, neurobiology, and treatment. In addition, some of the psychosocial and medical consequences of the psychotic disorders and their treatments will be discussed.

At the end of this chapter, the reader will be able to:

1. Recognize common symptoms and signs of the major psychotic disorders and discuss a differential diagnosis
2. Discuss the appropriate assessment, including necessary general medical workup, of a new onset of psychotic symptoms
3. Outline a biopsychosocial treatment plan for a patient with a chronic psychotic disorder such as schizophrenia

S. J. Zuchowski (✉)
Department of Psychiatry, University of Nevada School of Medicine,
Suite 215, 401 W. 2nd Street, Reno, NV 89503-0354, USA
e-mail: szuchowski@medicine.nevada.edu

B. Kirkpatrick
Department of Psychiatry and Behavioral Sciences, University of Nevada School of Medicine,
64 North Virginia St Mail Stop 0354, Reno, NV 89557-0354, USA
e-mail: bkirkpatrick@unr.edu

D. Alicata et al. (eds.), *Problem-based Behavioral Science and Psychiatry*,
DOI 10.1007/978-3-319-23669-8_20

Vignette 20.1.1 Presenting Situation: Christina Moreno
Christina Moreno is a 19-year-old college sophomore who was healthy and active until 6 months ago when she started to withdraw socially, staying in her dorm room and often missing classes. In spite of getting all "As" in high school, Christina struggled to pass her college classes last semester and was placed on academic probation. She presents to your office accompanied by her parents. They are worried that something is medically wrong with their daughter. She is at risk of losing her scholarship if she cannot turn her grades around this semester.

Her parents report that Christina was very popular and socially active in high school. At the beginning of the summer, Christina seemed happy to be home with her family. However, after about a week, she began spending extended periods of time alone in her room. She declined all invitations by friends to go out. She became irritable when her parents coaxed her to come out to dinner with them. By the end of the summer, she rarely left her room and had to be reminded to shower and brush her hair. In spite of her symptoms, Christina has returned to campus to begin her sophomore year.

STOP

Please proceed with the problem-based approach using the worksheet located in the appendix of Chap. 1!

A dramatic change in personality and behavior as described in this patient is a very serious finding that requires further evaluation. Although a primary psychiatric condition may seem likely, general medical causes must also be considered and ruled out. For example, general medical conditions that can present with psychiatric symptoms include infections, electrolyte disturbances, endocrine disorders, and seizures. A normal set of screening blood tests is reassuring but does not completely rule out a general medical condition. On the other hand, brain imaging is not routinely recommended unless there are other suspicious symptoms or signs that point to a neurological process such as a suspected seizure, unilateral weakness or numbness, hyperactive reflexes, or pupillary changes.

Substance abuse can also present with symptoms such as these and may be carefully concealed from parents and others, including medical professionals. While a negative urine drug screen is helpful information, it does not rule out illicit substances as a possible cause for symptoms as drug screens—of urine or blood—do not test for all possible substances of abuse. Also, some substances have short half-lives and may be undetectable within a few hours after use. Finally, some experienced drug users may successfully reduce the accuracy of urine drug screens through various methods.

Case 20.1.2: Continuation

On examination, Christina looks somewhat unkempt. She has poor eye contact and little spontaneous speech. She describes her mood as "fine," but she has little range of emotional expression on her face. She seems uncomfortable, and it is difficult to get any sort of conversation going with her. When asked for her perspective on what has been going on with her, she says, "I guess I'm not that interested in college after all." She denies using recreational drugs or drinking alcohol. She says that she is not feeling ill or experiencing any pain in her body. Christina also denies any history of feeling suicidal or violent. When asked if she is hearing, seeing, or experiencing anything unusual, she seems distracted momentarily and then answers, "No, nothing like that."

STOP

Please proceed with the problem-based approach using the worksheet located in the appendix of Chap. 1!

20.1 Psychotic Symptoms

20.1.1 Delusions

The most obvious and well-known manifestations of psychotic disorders are delusions and hallucinations. Delusions are fixed, false beliefs that are not shared by the person's subculture, frequently of a suspicious nature (Hales et al. 2014). Not all false beliefs are delusions. However, delusional beliefs are quite inflexible even in the face of strong evidence to the contrary. Although a caring attitude and offering reassurance is appropriate, argument or pointing out inconsistencies is unlikely to change her belief system in the moment. In fact, an overly aggressive stance against her delusional beliefs may result in a breakdown of trust between doctor and patient and potentially a missed opportunity for treatment. On the other hand, there is evidence for the efficacy of cognitive behavioral therapy in softening the impact of delusional beliefs, although this would generally not be considered in an acute presentation.

Delusional beliefs occur on a continuum between the ordinary and the bizarre. For example, a person may develop the delusional belief that his spouse is having an affair with a neighbor, which is plausible even if false in this instance. At the bizarre end of the spectrum, another patient may believe that extraterrestrials are controlling him by beaming radio waves to a microchip implanted in his brain.

20.1.2 Hallucinations

Hallucinations are false sensory *perceptions* in any of the five senses. The false perceptions can be vague or clear. Patients may hear auditory hallucinations in the form of one or more voices that talk to them or about them, or they may hear unformed noises. They are often distressing but not always. Not uncommonly, the voices are critical, insulting, profane, and/or threatening, or they may provide a running commentary on the person's behavior (Hales et al. 2014). Occasionally, patients may describe a voice as helpful or friendly.

Hallucinations may wax and wane throughout the day or may occur less frequently than each day. Persistent hallucinations may be contrasted with the fleeting misperceptions that most nonpsychotic people experience from time to time; these are referred to as illusions. For instance, you may briefly think that you hear your name being called or may see something strange out of the corner of your eye. Patients can be reassured that illusions are normal experiences that do not signal the onset of psychiatric illness.

Visual hallucinations can be of fully formed figures that appear exactly like—and may be mistaken for—real people or can be of vague shapes, colors, or shadows. In addition to auditory and visual hallucinations, psychotic misperceptions can occur in other sensory modalities such as the olfactory, gustatory, and tactile systems. An individual patient may experience a variety of hallucinations simultaneously. Auditory hallucinations are the most common type of hallucinations in chronic psychotic disorders.

Case 20.1.3 Conclusion

Christina's parents are politely asked to leave the room for the physical examination. As soon as her parents are out of the room and the door is closed, Christina whispers, "Those aren't my real parents. They're kidnappers. You should call the police." There is a moment when you think she may be joking, but you quickly realize that she is not only serious but also quite fearful. You offer reassurance but it seems to have little impact on her level of fear. You step out, leaving a medical assistant to stay with Christina. The labs you ordered have been completed, and all is within normal limits. Her urine drug screen is negative. Vitals signs are unremarkable, but you notice that her weight is down 20 lb since 3 months. Her parents, obviously very concerned, share an additional observation: over the summer, Christina was heard conversing with someone when alone and not on the telephone.

20.2 Risks Associated with Psychosis

Patients with psychotic disorders are at an increased risk for suicide attempts and suicide. Patients with schizophrenia have an estimated 5% risk of completed suicide in their lifetimes, and about one in five patients will attempt suicide at least once (Palmer et al. 2005).

In general, people with psychiatric illness are no more likely than the general population to commit acts of violence (Coid et al 2015). However, sometimes, people with psychiatric illness do act violently, and it is essential that clinicians consider violence risk and do what is possible to mitigate it, such as hospitalizing the patient when necessary. While most patients—even those with suspicious delusions—are not violent, the presence of this type of delusion is one factor that increases violence risk. Command auditory hallucinations that instruct or insist on a specific behavior of a violent nature are another risk factor. Although patients rarely, if ever, act like automatons in response to command hallucinations, they may feel some compulsion to obey a voice that persistently bosses them around or threatens harm if the commands are not carried out. For example, a patient heard auditory hallucinations that she thought were the voice of Satan telling her the only way to save her son's soul was to kill him.

Patients with psychotic disorders may also injure themselves unintentionally due to disorganized behavior or in reaction to delusions or hallucinations. Disorganized or highly distracted patients, especially when acutely ill, may be unable to care for themselves and meet their own basic needs for safety, shelter, or medical care. They may also be vulnerable to being victimized by other people. Every state has specific criteria for involuntary hospitalization for psychiatrically ill people who are a risk to themselves or others; clinicians should familiarize themselves with the laws and procedures in their state.

Patients suffering from chronic psychotic disorders are at higher than average risk for various comorbid medical conditions, including obesity, heart disease, stroke, and diabetes mellitus. Some of these comorbidities may be secondary to lifestyle factors such as increased rates of smoking and substance abuse, poor nutritional habits, and lack of access to medical care. Many antipsychotic medications are associated with higher rates of obesity and metabolic abnormalities such as diabetes mellitus and lipid dysregulation. There is also a growing body of research suggesting that individuals with chronic psychotic disorders such as schizophrenia are at increased risk for general medical conditions impacting various organ systems and that these risks are independent of lifestyle and medication (Fernandez-Egea et al. 2009, 2013). In addition to periodic mental status assessments, patients with psychotic disorders (especially those on antipsychotic medications) should be monitored medically, as summarized in Table 20.1.

Table 20.1 Recommended monitoring for patients on antipsychotics

Measure	Minimum frequency
Fasting lipids	Every 6 months
Fasting blood sugar	Every 6 months
Formal assessment for extrapyramidal movements	Every 6 months (for typical antipsychotics) and every 12 months (for atypical antipsychotics), using the Abnormal Involuntary Movement Scale (AIMS)
Eye examination	Every 6 months for quetiapine
Electrocardiogram	At baseline and as indicated for medications that may prolong the QT interval
Body mass index	At each visit for the first 6 months, then quarterly thereafter

Vignette 20.2.1 Presenting Situation: Kenneth Crabb

Mr. Crabb is a 44-year-old man who was admitted to the psychiatric inpatient service on a legal hold from the emergency department. He was brought in by his family and was described as having decreased need for sleep (1–2 hours per night), beliefs of being a god-like figure as well as jumbled thoughts for the past two weeks. His family explained that he stopped taking his regular medications (risperidone and divalproex) and simultaneously began using marijuana and alcohol again about a month ago after losing his job at the local humane society. On approach, Mr. Crabb has rapid speech and is hyperverbal. He is very difficult to interrupt, making an interview with him very challenging. He sarcastically answers each question you pose to him with the same question turned back on you. He is physically restless and hyperactive, walking around the examining room, looking at pictures while maintaining a stream of comments that are difficult to follow. He uses some unusual words that sound made up. When you attempt to redirect him with a bit more assertiveness, he abruptly becomes irritated, asking to see your supervisor and refusing to talk with you any further.

Please proceed with the problem-based approach using the worksheet located in the appendix of Chap. 1!

Vignette 20.2.2: Continuation

You step out and review his paperwork from the emergency department. His blood counts and metabolic profile appear within normal limits except for a mildly low serum protein level, an elevated mean corpuscular volume (MCV) value, and a mild anemia. Urinalysis reveals nothing of significance except very concentrated urine. Serum toxicology screen was positive for cannabinoids. Blood alcohol level was 0.01 % about 3 hours ago, and his valproic acid level was zero.

Mr. Crabb was allowed to settle in to his room for about an hour. He was given a snack of graham crackers and juice and then seemed less irritated. Upon approach the second time, you open with the question of "Mr. Crabb, is there something we might be able to help you with right now? Is there anything that you need?" Mr. Crabb becomes tearful and says that listening to everyone's prayers day and night has become intolerable. He cannot sleep or eat, and he fears he is going crazy. When asked if anything was helpful for this in the past, he acknowledges that risperidone was very helpful. He asks, "Do you have that here?"

Please proceed with the problem-based approach using the worksheet located in the appendix of Chap. 1!

Vignette 21.2.3: Conclusion

Mr. Crabb was admitted to the hospital, started back on risperidone, and he improved within a few days. He asked that his divalproex be restarted and it was, with lab monitoring of his blood level. He became less accelerated and less irritable. He said that the voices he was hearing were much quieter and less frequent. He was sleeping 6 hours per night. His thinking was easier to follow. However, he began spending more time alone in his room and refused group therapy. He did not want to participate in arts and crafts or in staff-led discussions on current events. He began to look flat and emotionless and to answer questions with one-word responses. He reported his mood was "all right; in the middle," and he denied side effects from his medications. On observation, you noticed no tremor or muscle rigidity, and his gait was normal. His family reported that he has had manic episodes several times before in his life but that between these more dramatic episodes, he continues to have some degree of impairment from delusions and hallucinations. In spite of this, he has been able to live independently in his own apartment.

20.3 Learning Issues

20.3.1 Other Types of Delusions

Delusional beliefs occur in a variety of different themes and are frequently of a mixed nature. Grandiose delusions are relatively common and consist of false beliefs of power, wealth, or talent. People with these types of delusions may believe they are powerful deities but may become angry when others do not treat them as such. A patient admitted to a psychiatric ward may believe that she is actually an undercover investigator and that she was admitted to expose abuses of patients. In this way, grandiose delusions may be entwined with paranoid beliefs.

Delusions involving a patient's body, organs, or health status are also relatively common and are referred to as somatic delusions. For example, a man believed that his natural organs were replaced with mechanical ones that could be manipulated by evil forces. It is important to distinguish between a somatic delusion and a somatic symptom disorder (see Chap. 23) because the treatment is very different. However, making this distinction can be difficult in patients with severe somatic symptom disorders.

20.3.2 Thought Process Disorders

A person's thought processes are typically relatively linear and easy for others to follow, although everyone occasionally goes off on an irrelevant tangent or takes longer than necessary to get to a point. However, in a case of a person with disordered thought processes, speech is typically difficult or even impossible to follow. A thought-disordered person may repeatedly go off on tangents and may lose track of the original point they were trying to make. This is termed tangential thinking. Circumstantial thinking is similar, but the speaker eventually realizes the digression and gets back to the point without redirection. A degree of tangential and circumstantial thinking is normal. Try paying attention to how others speak when they tell stories and converse; this will help you to calibrate what degree of nonlinearity of thought is normally seen.

Loose associations are an extreme form of tangential thinking. One idea is followed by another and another, and the listener cannot follow the connection between the various thoughts. For example, when a patient was asked how he was feeling, he answered, "I'm a non-participant; they are obese and re-obese; government intrusion with rumors of homosexuals; voices of poetic upbringing."

Manic patients (see Chap. 21 on mood disorders) may demonstrate a pattern of thinking and speech referred to as flight of ideas, which is closely related to and may include loose associations. Flight of ideas is a rapid succession of ideas that are at best only superficially connected. For example, when asked how he was feeling, a patient with rapid speech and flight of ideas answered, "Feeling fine, fine as the sunshine, getting my vitamin D and working on my tan, planning my next vacation, going to the beach or to Holland, I do love tulips and windmills, they produce energy and I love energy."

Patients with thought disorders sometimes use an idiosyncratic vocabulary, coining new words called neologisms. Occasionally, patients are so disorganized that their speech is completely unintelligible. This is sometimes referred to as a word salad.

20.3.3 Negative Symptoms

Hallucinations and delusions are often referred to as positive symptoms because something is added that is not normally present. Negative symptoms, on the other hand, refer to a reduction or absence of something that is normally present, such as emotional expression, motivation, or cognition. The range of someone's emotional expression is referred to as their affect. In the extreme, patients with chronic psychotic disorders such as schizophrenia may have a flat affect and may appear emotionless. The term flat affect should be reserved to describe the extreme end of a spectrum of blunted or diminished affect; it is, therefore, incorrect to describe a patient as having "a little flat affect." In addition to flat affect, a person's range of emotional expression is frequently described using such terms as full, appropriate, reduced, blunted, mood congruent, or incongruent. For example, a person who smiles and giggles while describing the death of their child would usually be described as demonstrating a mood-incongruent affect.

Some patients with chronic psychotic disorders demonstrate significant avolition. They may have difficulty with tasks requiring sustained attention, concentration, and motivation. Thus, they may be unable to sustain employment or success in school with subsequent socioeconomic implications. Some patients may qualify for disability payments such as may be available through the social security system. However, it is important to note that this is not true of all patients with chronic psychotic disorders. Patients who are successfully treated may hold gainful employment and may succeed academically and socially, although they typically have some residual impairment, even if it is subtle.

It is sometimes difficult to discern between negative symptoms inherent to the illness and side effects of medications used to treat the illness. Patients with prominent parkinsonian side effects from potent dopamine antagonist medication may display a mask-like face that is indistinguishable from blunted affect. Please refer to Table 20.2 below for a summary of antipsychotic side effects.

Medications can also be sedating and be associated with feelings of low motivation and cognitive slowing, which again mimic negative symptoms. It is important to consider whether a patient's medications may be contributing to his or her apparent negative symptoms and make adjustments if possible.

20.4 Neurobiology of Psychosis

20.4.1 Dopamine Overactivity Hypothesis

The hypothesis that the symptoms of schizophrenia are due to overactivity of the brain dopaminergic system was based on the observation that the early antipsychotic drugs such as chlorpromazine were dopamine antagonists. Sixty years after the advent of chlorpromazine, which was the first antipsychotic, all antipsychotic

Table 20.2 Major side effects of antipsychotic medications

Syndrome	Manifestations	Mechanism	Treatment
Neuroleptic malignant syndrome	Hyperthermia, muscle rigidity, autonomic instability, rhabdomyolysis, and renal failure	Functional denervation (from dopamine blockade) of the sympathetic nervous system from central control	Supportive care, dantrolene, bromocriptine
Acute dystonia	Acute muscle spasm; may involve the eye muscles (oculogyric crisis) and/or neck muscles	Relative excess of acetylcholine relative to dopamine effect in the basal ganglia	Anticholinergics (e.g., benztropine, trihexaphenadyl, diphenhydramine)
Akathisia	Significant motoric restlessness and discomfort		Beta-adrenergic blockers, benzodiazepines
Parkinsonism	Resting tremor, cogwheel rigidity, shuffling gait, blunted affect	Relative excess of acetylcholine relative to dopamine effect in the basal ganglia	Anticholinergics like benztropine
Tardive dyskinesia	Typically involves lip-smacking, chewing, or other orofacial movements	Possibly oxidative damage in the basal ganglia secondary to chronic dopamine blockade and unregulated excitatory neurotransmission	No strong evidence of effective treatment; prevention and early detection are key. Resuming antipsychotic treatment may suppress TD symptoms

TD tardive dyskinesia

drugs continue to have a significant action as a dopamine antagonist or partial agonist (which also has the effect of decreasing the dopaminergic signal in the brain). Please refer to Table 20.3 for an overview of antipsychotic mechanisms of action and side effects.

There are other observations that suggest psychotic symptoms are associated with dopaminergic dysfunction. Decreased dopaminergic signaling is a key pathophysiological feature of Parkinson's disease, and many antipsychotics cause pseudoparkinsonian symptoms. Amphetamines and methylphenidate increase psychotic symptoms in patients with schizophrenia and cause psychotic symptoms in people who do not have any history of a psychotic illness.

However, the mechanism of action of a group of medications may be an imperfect guide to the pathophysiology of a disease. After all, strep throat is not caused by a patient's penicillin deficiency. The relationship between dopamine and schizophrenia is not specific in a couple of senses. First, antipsychotics lack disease specificity: (a) they are superior to placebo in the treatment of psychotic symptoms in other disorders, for instance, in dementia and (b) they are effective in the treatment of disorders other than psychosis, such as nonpsychotic mania, and as adjuncts in the treatment of depression. Second, people with schizophrenia have, as a group, a number of other neuropsychiatric and metabolic problems

Table 20.3 Mechanisms of action and possible side effects of antipsychotics

Medication	Mechanisms	Possible side effects
Atypical antipsychotics (e.g., clozapine, risperidone, olanzapine, quetiapine, ziprasidone, aripiprazole, paliperidone)	Dopamine receptor blockade (there are several different dopamine receptors)	Extrapyramidal symptoms (described further below) via dopamine blockade in the nigrostriatal tract
		Weight gain and sedation (via histamine receptor blockade)
	Serotonin receptor blockade	Metabolic complications of weight gain (e.g., hyperglycemia, hyperlipidemia)
		Hyperprolactinemia (via dopamine blockade in the tuberoinfundibular tract)
		Potential drug–drug interactions
Typical antipsychotics (e.g., haloperidol)	Dopamine receptor blockade: higher in "higher potency" agents (e.g., haloperidol, fluphenazine) and lower in "lower potency" agents (e.g., thorazine)	More prominent in "higher potency" agents (because of dopamine receptor blockade):
		Extrapyramidal symptoms
		Hyperprolactinemia
		More prominent in "lower potency" agents (because of other receptor blockade):
		Anticholinergic side effects
		Sedation
		Hypotension (due to alpha-adrenergic antagonism)
		Cardiac rhythm disturbances (particularly QT prolongation)

other than psychosis, and dopaminergic medications do not treat these. Third, dopaminergic blockade can induce negative symptoms, including apathy, in some patients. Fourth, genetic studies have more frequently implicated genes related to glutamatergic function than those related to dopamine. As a group, people with schizophrenia appear to have excess dopaminergic signal in the brain, but the dopaminergic theory is a better theory of mechanism of action than a theory of etiology and pathophysiology.

20.4.2 Other Neurotransmitter Systems

Glutamate/N-methyl-D-aspartate (NMDA) Several observations suggest that the glutamatergic system plays a role in the pathophysiology of schizophrenia. Ketamine infusions increase the severity of psychotic symptoms, and a number of glutamatergic abnormalities have been found in the brains of people with schizophrenia. As noted above, genes related to glutamatergic signaling in the brain have been associated with risk of schizophrenia. Although there have been a number of treatment trials of drugs affecting glutamine, so far, none of these medications have been shown to be effective (Javitt et al 2012; Noetzel et al. 2012).

Serotonin Infusion of a serotonergic agonist increases the severity of psychotic symptoms in people with schizophrenia, and animal studies suggest that manipulation of the serotonergic system should work as an antipsychotic. One of the theories of the superior efficacy of clozapine compared to other antipsychotics is based on its strong interactions with serotonin receptors. However, other evidence leaves us uncertain as to the role of serotonin in the pathophysiology of psychotic symptoms (Remington 2008). Representative medications that have been developed for the psychotic disorders are summarized below. In most situations, atypical antipsychotics (other than clozapine) are the medications chosen for initial treatment of psychotic disorders. Refer to Table 20.4.

20.5 Schizophrenia

Schizophrenia is characterized by the presence of two or more of the following criteria A symptoms during a 1-month period (APA 2013):

Criteria A symptoms:

1. Delusions
2. Hallucinations
3. Disorganized speech
4. Grossly disorganized or catatonic behavior
5. Negative symptoms

For a person to meet the Diagnostic and Statistical Manual of Mental Disorders, Fifth Edition (DSM-5) diagnostic criteria for schizophrenia (APA 2013), at least one of the above symptoms must be delusions, hallucinations, or disorganized speech, and the individual's level of functioning is markedly impaired in one or more areas of life. Signs of the disturbance must be continuously present for at least 6 months, including any prodromal period, but note that the full criteria above must only be met for 1 month and can be even shorter if successful treatment is initiated. If significant mood episodes have occurred, they should be present for a minority of the total duration of illness if the diagnosis is to remain schizophrenia. For example, a patient with a 10-year life course of schizophrenia reports that she was depressed once for about a month in the past 10 years. Since 1 month represents only a minority of her overall life course, her diagnosis would remain schizophrenia. On the other hand, if a similar individual with apparent schizophrenic symptoms reported annual recurrences of depressive or manic episodes, a diagnosis of schizoaffective disorder would have to be considered.

Table 20.4 Representative antipsychotic medications

Medication	Available forms	Long-acting preparation	Special side effects	Other comments
Risperidone	Oral, rapidly disintegrating, liquid	Yes	Higher rate of extrapyramidal symptoms and hyperprolactinemia	Moderate weight gain
Paliperidone	Oral	Yes	Similar to risperidone	Moderate weight gain
Olanzapine	Oral, rapidly disintegrating, intramuscular	Yes	Higher rates of sedation and weight gain	Patients receiving long-acting preparation must be monitored for post-injection delirium/sedation syndrome
Quetiapine	Oral	No	Theoretical risk of corneal clouding	Moderate weight gain
Ziprasidone	Oral, intramuscular	No	Slightly higher risk (compared with the other atypical antipsychotics) of QT prolongation	Lower risk of weight gain and metabolic sequelae among the atypical antipsychotics
Aripiprazole	Oral	Yes	Agitation	Lower risk of weight gain and metabolic sequelae among the atypical antipsychotics
Asenapine	Sublinqual	No	Sedation	
Ilioperidone	Oral	No	Sedation	Orthostasis
Lurasidone	Oral	No	Sedation	Must be taken with food for maximal absorption
Clozapine	Oral	No	Higher rates of sedation and weight gain Agranulocytosis is a potentially life-threatening complication	Used in cases refractory to other atypical antipsychotics; initially requires weekly monitoring of neutrophil counts
Haloperidol	Oral, intramuscular, intravenous	Yes	Risks of typical antipsychotics as described above; IV administration carries an arrhythmia risk	Of the antipsychotics, haloperidol is the one with the most data for use in delirium (see Chap. 26)

20.5.1 Genetics and Environment

Although most individuals with schizophrenia have no family history of psychosis, there are genetic factors at play in determining risk for developing schizophrenia. Studies of identical twins yield a concordance rate of under 50 %. The exact mechanism for schizophrenia's pattern of inheritance remains uncertain, but it is clearly not a straightforward Mendelian pattern. There is likely to be a complex interaction of genes and nongenetic factors in most patients. Environmental factors posited to contribute to the risk of developing schizophrenia include, for example, low birth weight, summer birth, immigrant status, sexual abuse, marijuana use, and advanced paternal age (Hamlyn et al. 2013).

20.5.2 Schizoaffective Disorder

Schizoaffective disorder is essentially schizophrenia symptoms with superimposed mood symptoms (depressive or manic episodes) that are present for the majority of the total duration of the active and residual portions of the illness (APA 2013).

So, there must be periods of illness in which:

1. Major mood episodes occur concurrently with schizophrenic symptoms of hallucinations, delusions, disorganized speech, disorganized behavior, or negative symptoms and
2. Delusions or hallucinations have occurred for 2 or more weeks in the absence of major mood episodes

20.6 Substance/Medication-Induced Psychotic Disorder

Recreational substance use and prescribed medications are common causes of new-onset psychotic symptoms in the general hospital and emergency department settings. Most recreational substances are capable of inducing hallucinations and delusions in susceptible individuals. Psychotic symptoms can occur during acute intoxication or during withdrawal in dependent individuals, and the presentation may be indistinguishable from schizophrenia in the moment. However, resolution of symptoms within days or weeks following discontinuation of substance use suggests a substance-induced psychosis. Also, no history of hallucinations or delusions prior to substance use is suggestive, but this history is often unavailable or unreliable. Likewise, beginning antipsychotic treatment in an individual with a possible substance-induced psychosis complicates the question of why they improved quickly after admission to the hospital. It is important to keep in mind that many individuals with primary psychotic disorders like schizophrenia or schizoaffective disorder also utilize recreational substances, so the cause–effect relationship is rarely clear.

Psychostimulants such as amphetamine, cocaine, or methamphetamine are strongly associated with the development of psychotic symptoms (Bramness et al. 2012). Likewise, hallucinogens, true to their name, can induce a full-blown psychosis. In certain susceptible individuals, stimulants and marijuana can each trigger a sustained psychotic disorder that follows a course indistinguishable from schizophrenia (Radhakrishnan et al. 2014). With each drug, there is a complex relationship of genetic and nongenetic factors that renders certain individuals vulnerable to acute and chronic psychotic reactions.

Prescribed medications that are associated with the onset of psychotic symptoms include opiate analgesics and corticosteroids. Even antibiotics and gastrointestinal medications can have unintended effects on the brain. Medications with anticholinergic effects can induce hallucinations in susceptible patients. Finally, interactions between two or more prescription medications can induce psychotic symptoms.

20.7 Psychotic Disorder Due to Another Medical Condition

Delusions or hallucinations can occur that are attributed directly to the physiological effects of a general medical condition. General medical illness in a variety of body systems can lead to psychotic symptoms, but pathology that directly impacts the central nervous system (CNS) is a more likely candidate. Infections and metabolic disruptions can cause psychotic symptoms, although typically, there are others signs and symptoms that point to the underlying general medical cause, such as abnormal laboratory findings, neurological signs or symptoms, and alterations in vital signs. Seizures can manifest directly as hallucinations or psychotic symptoms can occur in the post-ictal period. CNS tumors only rarely present with psychotic symptoms.

Vignette 20.3.1 Presenting Situation: Sam Aloo

Mr. Sam Aloo presented to the dermatologist with concerns about "skin worms." He said that for the past several months, he has been developing open sores on his both of his forearms and ventral thighs. He states that the sores are extremely itchy and bothersome to him, and he admits to being unable to resist picking at them and scratching them frequently. They sometimes become frankly painful, and sometimes pus comes out of the sores. He has been reading about various types of parasitic worms that he may have picked up on a trip 6 months ago to sub-Saharan Africa.

A phone call between the dermatologist and the patient's primary care physician revealed that Mr. Aloo has a history of being extremely anxious about various somatic concerns. A year ago, he was convinced that he was suffering from vitamin deficiencies. Before that, he was focused on various chemical sensitivities. The primary care doctor confirmed that Mr. Aloo had received some traveler immunizations in preparation for his Africa trip (yellow fever, hepatitis A, and typhoid).

He makes fair eye contact and is conversant. His speech is normal in rate and articulation. His thinking in linear and goal-directed. Mr. Aloo's skin is normal other than the presence of two excoriations on the dorsal surface of each forearm and one on the ventral surface of each thigh. The lesion on the left thigh appears infected and is draining a small amount of purulent fluid.

Please proceed with the problem-based approach using the worksheet located in the appendix of Chap. 1!

Vignette 20.3.2: Continuation

After the examination of his skin, Mr. Aloo produces a small plastic baggie containing various fibrous-appearing threads, which he says he extracted from his skin lesions. He states they are dead parasites and that he can often feel them crawling just under his skin. At times, he can see movement in his skin lesions, and he sometimes has been able to "capture" one of the worms and place them in the baggie. Microscopic examination of the "worms" reveals fibrous tissue and nothing resembling any known parasite. Mr. Aloo is prescribed an oral antibiotic for his secondarily infected thigh lesion. He is gently told about the results of the microscopic examination and the dermatologist's conclusion that there is no parasitic infection present. He is given instructions on dressing the lesions and told not to pick at or scratch them. He is also prescribed hydroxyzine for itching and anxiety.

Please proceed with the problem-based approach using the worksheet located in the appendix of Chap. 1!

Vignette 20.3.3: Continuation

Mr. Aloo returns two weeks later with his lesions largely unchanged in appearance. He appears more anxious and produces another baggie full of fibrous tissue for the doctor to examine. After a gentle, but clear, explanation about the nature of his condition being "a trick of his mind," Mr. Aloo is prescribed risperidone, an atypical antipsychotic medication. He is also referred to a skilled psychotherapist. Mr. Aloo seems a bit confused by all of this but indicates his willingness to try whatever the doctor thinks will help.

Please proceed with the problem-based approach using the worksheet located in the appendix of Chap. 1!

Vignette 20.3.4: Conclusion
Mr. Aloo returns in a month and is considerably improved. His lesions are in various states of healing, and he reports that he has stopped picking and scratching them. His mood appears brighter, and he seems less anxious.

20.8 Learning Issues

The differential diagnosis in this case includes primary skin diseases including atopic dermatitis, scabies, or fungal infection, possibly with secondary bacterial infection. Skin picking disorder (or psychogenic excoriation) is also possible (see Chap. 22). Many dermatological disorders have psychiatric complications or co-morbidities. In this case, delusional disorder would have to be considered given the presentation. The possibility of skin infection cannot entirely be ruled out but is considerably less likely. Delusional disorder is characterized by the presence of one or more fixed, false beliefs without obvious bizarre thinking or behavior. Hallucinations are generally absent, but if present, they relate very closely with the delusional content. In this case, the patient describes a perception of a crawling sensation under his skin, a tactile hallucination closely related to his delusion about worm infestation. He even believed that he could see the movement of parasites under his skin.

A person with a delusional disorder usually presents without obvious psychiatric illness apart from their fixed, false belief. By definition, day-to-day functioning is not markedly impaired except to the degree that the delusion itself impacts behavior, which is not obviously bizarre or odd. Criteria A symptoms of schizophrenia cannot be present (i.e., hallucinations, disorganized speech or behavior, flattening of affect). Subtypes of delusional disorder include erotomanic, persecutory, somatic, grandiose, jealous, mixed, and unspecified (APA 2013). Please refer to Table 20.5 for an overview of several diagnoses that may present with psychotic or psychotic-like symptoms.

Mr. Aloo was open to considering antipsychotic medication after a tactful explanation of rationale. An atypical antipsychotic medication such as risperidone may help decrease distressing somatic preoccupation and may also help his sleep and mood. If clinically significant depressive or anxiety symptoms were present, consideration could be given to prescribing an antidepressant medication in addition to an antipsychotic. Topical creams could also help calm the inflammation and provide

Table 20.5 Several psychiatric diagnoses with psychotic or psychotic-like symptoms

Diagnosis	Key features	Would presence of delusions support this diagnosis?	Would hallucinations support this diagnosis?	Would disorganized thoughts, behavior, and/or significant impairment support this diagnosis?	Would prominent mood symptoms support this diagnosis?	Time course
Schizophrenia	Active symptoms must include at least two of the following: delusions, hallucinations, disorganized speech, grossly disorganized or catatonic behavior, negative symptoms (including flat affect)	Yes	Yes	Yes	No	At least 6 months, with at least 1 month of active symptoms
Schizophreniform disorder	Active symptoms of schizophrenia	Yes	Yes	Yes	No	At least 1 month but less than 6 months
Brief psychotic disorder	At least one of the following: delusions, hallucinations, disorganized speech, grossly disorganized or catatonic behavior	Yes	Yes	Yes	Usually not	At least 1 day but less than 1 month
Schizoaffective disorder	Active symptoms of schizophrenia plus either a major depressive, manic, or mixed episode (see Chap. 22)	Yes	Yes	Yes	Yes, however, there needs to be psychotic symptoms present for at least 2 weeks without any prominent mood symptoms	Major mood symptoms are present for the majority of the total duration of the illness.

Table 20.5 (continued)

Diagnosis	Key features	Would presence of delusions support this diagnosis?	Would hallucinations support this diagnosis?	Would disorganized thoughts, behavior, and/or significant impairment support this diagnosis?	Would prominent mood symptoms support this diagnosis?	Time course
Delusional disorder	Delusions for at least 1 month	Yes	No—except for hallucinations closely related to delusional theme	No	No	At least 1 month
Paranoid personality disorder	See Chap. 25	No—there is distrust and suspiciousness, without outright delusion	No	Usually not (though this disorder can be premorbid to schizophrenia)	No	Lifelong
Schizotypal personality disorder	See Chap. 25	No—there are only social/interpersonal deficits, perceptual distortions, and eccentricities	Illusions (though not frank hallucinations) are possible	Odd behavior and magical thinking are characteristic; can also be premorbid to schizophrenia	No	Lifelong

some relief from itching. A dermatologist or primary care physician may wish to consider comanagement of a patient like Mr. Aloo with a psychiatrist.

Denial of a psychiatric basis for illness is common in the psychotic disorders and can be difficult to overcome. This may be akin to anosognosia, seen in some neurological conditions like stroke or traumatic brain injury, in which patients fail to recognize their own severe deficits (Lehrer and Lorenz 2014). However, insight into psychiatric illness is a complex concept and occurs on a continuum. Patients may willingly accept treatment even while denying psychiatric symptoms. On the other hand, a lack of insight does increase the risk for treatment refusal or nonadherence.

Pharmacotherapy should not be considered the only available treatment modality for the psychotic disorders. Psychotherapy of a variety of kinds may also be useful in developing coping strategies, a stronger sense of self, and emotional resilience (Wykes 2014). For chronic psychotic disorders such as schizophrenia and schizoaffective disorder, psychosocial rehabilitation may be helpful in improving independence and quality of life. This comprehensive program of treatment targets improvements in social skills, the ability to live independently, and avoid repeated psychiatric hospitalizations. The overarching goal is to maximize the chances of patient success in whatever positive interpersonal, educational, and vocational endeavors that they choose for themselves. Psychotherapy that targets treatment adherence may also be helpful in reducing relapse and hospitalizations. For patients with residual hallucinations and delusions, cognitive behavioral therapy can be effective in reducing the impact of these symptoms.

20.9 Self-Assessment Questions

1. A 19-year-old man presents to the emergency department with 1 year of suspiciousness, auditory hallucinations in the form of commenting voices, and mild thought disorganization. Vitals signs are all normal. Drug abuse is denied, and a urine toxicology screen is negative. The most likely diagnosis is:

   a. Schizoaffective disorder
   b. Schizophrenia
   c. Delusional disorder
   d. Bipolar I disorder

2. A physical and neurological examination of the above patient reveals no abnormalities. Screening labs are normal. What is the best course of action?

   a. Psychiatric consultation
   b. Brain imaging
   c. Spinal tap
   d. Psychological testing

3. A 45-year-old woman has had a long history of mental illness, including auditory hallucinations and a mixture of suspicious and grandiose delusions. A chart review reveals at least five episodes of major depression as well as three manic episodes in her lifetime. Between mood episodes, she is chronically psychotic. She also intermittently drinks alcohol to excess and is often nonadherent to treatment. What is the most likely diagnosis?

   a. Schizophrenia
   b. Bipolar I disorder
   c. Alcohol-induced psychotic disorder
   d. Schizoaffective disorder

4. A 55-year-old truck driver presents for evaluation at the urging of his wife because he has become convinced that a local newscaster has fallen in love with him, despite the fact that they have never actually met. On exam, the patient is easily engaged in conversation, has good hygiene and grooming, and is fully oriented. He denies hallucinations, and his thinking is well organized. He has been functioning at work without difficulty. When his wife leaves the room, the patient describes that about a month ago, his favorite evening newscaster started wearing dresses in his favorite color and style, specifically to seduce him. He feels strongly that she is in love with him, although he acknowledges that this sounds "crazy." What is the most likely diagnosis?

   e. Schizophrenia
   f. Schizoaffective disorder
   g. Delusional disorder
   h. Bipolar I disorder

5. What evidence is supportive of the dopamine theory of schizophrenia?

   i. Proven antipsychotics all antagonize dopamine receptors to some degree
   j. Ketamine can induce psychotic symptoms
   k. One of the symptoms of Parkinson's disease is psychosis
   l. All of the above

6. A young woman with schizophrenia is well treated with risperidone, an atypical antipsychotic medication. She presents with tremor, blunted affect, shuffling gait, and cogwheel rigidity of her upper extremities. What is a reasonable intervention for this patient's condition?

   m. Increase the dose of risperidone
   n. Begin an anticholingeric medication like benztropine
   o. Add a second atypical antipsychotic medication
   p. Begin a beta-blocking medication like propranolol

Appendix A: Tables with Possible Answers to Vignettes

Vignette 20.1.2

Facts	Hypotheses	Information needed	Learning issues
Unkempt appearance	A mood disorder seems less likely since she denies mood problems	What are the results of her toxicology screen?	What are delusions and hallucinations?
Denies mood problems	A substance-induced problem seems less likely since she denies use of alcohol and illicit substances (although must keep in mind that people do not necessarily admit to their substance use)	Could she be abusing a substance that would be missed by a routine toxicology screen?	How does a positive family history of schizophrenia affect the likelihood of a person having schizophrenia?
Denies drug and alcohol abuse		Does she have a family history of psychiatric illness?	
Seems distracted but denies unusual perceptions	This could be the new onset of schizophrenia		

Vignette 20.2.1: Kenneth Crabb

Facts	Hypotheses	Information needed	Learning issues
44-year-old man with decreased need for sleep	This presentation could be related to a general medical condition or to the abuse of an illicit substance	How are his vital signs? Anything abnormal on physical exam? Any abnormalities on laboratory studies? Is his toxicology screen consistent with his stated history?	What are other types of delusions?
Grandiosity	Since he was previous taking risperidone and divalproex, this may be a recurrence of some preexisting psychiatric illness		What are thought process disorders?
Jumbled thoughts			
Rapid speech that is difficult to interrupt	His level of irritability and agitation increases his risk for violence	How does this episode compare with prior episodes?	
Medication nonadherence		Has he ever been violent or attempted suicide?	
Marijuana and alcohol use		What was his mental state and functioning like when on medications and not using drugs and alcohol?	
Irritable mood			

Vignette 20.2.3

Facts	Hypotheses	Information needed	Learning issues
Patient was admitted and started back on his previous medications	He meets criteria for schizoaffective disorder.	What other medications has he been tried on? What were his responses?	What are negative symptoms?
He improved but then began isolating and looked emotionless	His prior medication regimen allowed him to live independently, but he continues to be bothered by psychotic symptoms	Has he ever been tried on clozapine? If not, would he be willing to begin a trial?	What is the neurobiology of psychosis?
Family reported that he has multiple manic episodes before		Has he ever been on a long-acting injectible antipsychotic medication?	What is the role of genetics and the environment in the etiology of psychotic disorders?
Between manic episodes, he remains psychotic with delusions and hallucinations in spite of treatment		Has he been involved in any substance abuse treatment programs? Is he open to the idea?	What are the symptoms of schizophrenia and schizoaffective disorder?
He lived independently			

Vignette 20.3.1: Sam Aloo

Facts	Hypotheses	Information needed	Learning issues
Patient presents with chief complaint of "skin worms"	It is unlikely that he contracted a parasite during his trip to Africa	Does he meet criteria for an anxiety disorder such as generalized anxiety disorder?	What are the symptoms of delusional disorder? What are the differential diagnoses?
Several months of having itchy sores on bilateral forearms and ventral thighs	Based on his prior history of excessive somatic concerns and the nature, location and symmetry of his skin lesions, this may be psychiatric in origin	Does he have other somatic concerns currently?	
Cannot resist picking and scratching sores	A prior history of excessive somatic concerns does not rule out a subsequent general medical problem but raises suspicion that an atypical presentation could be psychiatric in origin	How does he function in his daily life?	
History of recurrent somatic concerns		Why does he think his skin lesions are caused by worms?	

Facts	Hypotheses	Information needed	Learning issues
History of travel to Africa		Has he had any unusual sensory perceptions?	
He appears anxious		Has he had any delusions?	

Vignette 20.3.2

Facts	Hypotheses	Information needed	Learning issues
Produces fibrous material that he says are dead worms	This is more than a simple anxiety or somatic disorder	How does he respond to the information that there are no parasites present?	When is it necessary to confront a person's hallucinations and delusions, and how can it be done to preserve the therapeutic alliance?
He can feel them crawling under his skin and can see movement in his lesions	He is having frank hallucinations of a tactile and even visual nature	Is he flexible in his thinking? To what degree can he accept that there may be a psychiatric basis for his symptoms?	Does flexibility around delusional beliefs occur on a continuum?
Microscopic examination of "worms" reveals only fibrous tissue and no parasitic organism	He holds a fixed belief that he is infected by a worm-like parasite	How likely is it that he can comply with instructions to dress the lesions and leave them alone?	

Vignette 20.3.3

Facts	Hypotheses	Information needed	Learning issues
His skin lesions continue to be problematic	He is frankly delusional and requires antipsychotic therapy	Will he adhere to antipsychotic medication therapy?	What factors should be considered in the treatment of Mr. Aloo?
		What kind of psychological issues will arise in the course of psychotherapy?	
He produces another baggie of fibrous material	He meets criteria for delusional disorder	Can he stop picking at the lesions?	How can helping him work through his psychological conflicts through psychotherapy, even if seemingly unrelated to his somatic delusions, be helpful to his overall recovery?
He indicates a willingness to comply with antipsychotic therapy and psychotherapy	With his hallucinations, he could have schizophrenia	Are his hallucinations flowing from and intimately tied to his somatic delusions?	

Vignette 20.3.4

Facts	Hypotheses	Information needed	Learning issues
He improves on risperidone therapy	His anxiety and dysphoric mood were directly related to his somatic delusion	Does he have side effects to the risperidone?	What is the role of pharmacotherapy and other treatment modalities in the treatment of psychotic disorders?
His skin lesions are healing	His obsessive skin picking was also directly related to his somatic delusion	Does he see the improvement?	
His mood is improved as well			

Appendix B: Answers to Review Questions

1. B, 2. A, 3. D, 4. C, 5. A, 6. B

References

American Psychiatric Association. (2013). *Diagnostic and statistical manual of mental disorders* (5th Ed.). Arlington: American Psychiatric Press.

Bramness, J. G., Gundersen, Ø. H., Guterstam, J., Rognli, E. B., Konstenius, M., Løberg, E. M., Medhus, S., Tanum, L., & Franck, J. (2012). Amphetamine-induced psychosis—a separate diagnostic entity or primary psychosis triggered in the vulnerable? *BMC Psychiatry, 5*(12), 221.

Coid, J. W., Yang, M., Ullrich, S., Hickey, N., Kahtan, N., & Freestone, M. (2015). Psychiatric diagnosis and differential risks of offending following discharge. *International Journal of Law and Psychiatry,* Feb 5 pii: S0160-2527(15)00010-2. doi:10.1016/j.ijlp.2015.01.009.

Editor. (1988). Where next with psychiatric illness? *Nature, 336,* 95–96.

Fernandez-Egea, E., Bernardo, M., Donner, T., Conget, I., Parellada, E., Justicia, A., Esmatjes, E., Garcia-Rizo, C., & Kirkpatrick, B. (2009). Metabolic profile of antipsychotic-naive individuals with non-affective psychosis. *British Journal of Psychiatry, 194*(5), 434–438.

Fernandez-Egea, E., Garcia-Rizo, C., Zimbron, J., & Kirkpatrick, B. (2013). Diabetes or prediabetes in newly diagnosed patients with nonaffective psychosis? A historical and contemporary view. *Schizophrenia Bulletin, 39*(2), 266–267.

Hales, R. E., Yudofsky, S. C., & Roberts, L. W. (Eds.). (2014). *The American psychiatric publishing textbook of psychiatry* (6th Ed.). Washington, DC: American Psychiatric Publishing.

Hamlyn, J., Duhig, M., McGrath, J., & Scott, J. (2013). Modifiable risk factors for schizophrenia and autism—shared risk factors impacting on brain development. *Neurobiology of Disease, 53,* 3–9.

Javitt, D. C., Zukin, S. R., Heresco-Levy, U., & Umbricht, D. (2012). Has an angel shown the way? Etiological and therapeutic implications of the PCP/NMDA model of schizophrenia. *Schizophrenia Bulletin, 38*(5), 958–966.

Lehrer, D. S., & Lorenz, J. (2014). Anosognosia in schizophrenia: Hidden in plain sight. *Innovations in Clinical Neuroscience, 11*(5–6), 10–17.

Noetzel, M. J., Jones, C. K., & Conn, P. J. (2012). Emerging approaches for treatment of schizophrenia: Modulation of glutamatergic signaling. *Discovery Medicine, 14*(78), 335–343.
Palmer, B. A., Pankratz, V. S., & Bostwick, J. M. (2005). The lifetime risk of suicide in schizophrenia: A reexamination. *Archives of General Psychiatry, 62*(3), 247–253.
Radhakrishnan, R., Wilkinson, S. T., D'Souza, D. C. (2014). Gone to pot—a review of the association between cannabis and psychosis. *Frontiers in Psychiatry, 22*(5), 54.
Remington, G. (2008). Alterations of dopamine and serotonin transmission in schizophrenia. *Progress in Brain Research, 172,* 117–140.
Wykes, T. (2014). Cognitive-behaviour therapy and schizophrenia. *Evidence Based Mental Health, 17*(3), 67–68.

Chapter 21
Mood Disorders and Suicide

Frederick Duennebier, Daniel A. Alicata* and Anthony P. S. Guerrero

Mood disorders are ubiquitous. They are passed on via genetic risk, directly linked to other medical conditions, triggered by social events beyond our control, and resist treatment through our own subconscious defenses. With a continued shortage of psychiatrists, it is essential that providers are able to screen, identify, and potentially treat these mood conditions. The following chapter illustrates some of most important aspects of mood disorders, and at the end, the reader will be able to:

1. Discuss the epidemiology, clinical presentation, evaluation, differential diagnosis, and treatment of major mood disorders
2. Have an appreciation of the biological, psychological, and social impacts of major mood disorders
3. Have a familiarity with the issues surrounding suicide

Case Vignette 21.1.1 Richard Scott
Mr. Scott, a 38-year-old restaurant owner, comes to your primary care clinic for a routine, annual follow-up. Mr. Scott initially denies any new health concerns. He is up to date with his yearly flu shot and his vital signs are all within normal limits. While going over his review of systems, he admits to having had some unintentional weight loss over the past few months and felt more tired than usual.

* Co-first editor of the book.

F. Duennebier (✉)
Department of Psychiatry, John A. Burns School of Medicine, University of Hawai‘i,
47-251 Ahaolelo Road, Kaneohe, HI 96744, USA
e-mail: fduenn@gmail.com

D. A. Alicata · A. P. S. Guerrero
Department of Psychiatry, John A. Burns School of Medicine, University of Hawai‘i,
1356 Lusitana Street, University Tower 4th Floor, Honolulu, HI 96813, USA
e-mail: alicatad@dop.hawaii.edu

A. P. S. Guerrero
e-mail: GuerreroA@dop.hawaii.edu

D. Alicata et al. (eds.), *Problem-based Behavioral Science and Psychiatry*,
DOI 10.1007/978-3-319-23669-8_21

Please proceed with the problem-based approach using the worksheet located in the appendix of Chap. 1!

Please fill in the facts, your hypotheses, further information needed, and learning issues for Learning Issue Table 21.1.1.

Learning Issue Table 21.1.1

FACTS	HYPOTHESES	INFORMATION NEEDED	LEARNING ISSUES

Fatigue is unfortunately a common consequence of everyday life, and weight loss, when intentional, is frequently celebrated by physicians. Together, however, prolonged and unexplained fatigue and weight loss raise concern for a number of serious conditions to evaluate further in your differential. Compared to diabetes, HIV, or cancer, a mood disorder might be overlooked in a busy primary care setting. Because of this, it is important to remember that depression is common, can lead to profound consequences of social impairment, productivity loss, increases the risk of comorbid medical conditions, and greatly increases health-care costs (Sadock and Sadock 2009).

Consider the following differential diagnostic categories for chronic fatigue and weight loss:

- Infections including HIV, tuberculosis, hepatitis, and tick-borne diseases
- Psychiatric concerns including mood disorders, stress-related disorders, alcohol, and substance use disorders
- Endocrine disorders including diabetes and thyroid disease
- Medication related including side effects and intoxications
- Gastrointestinal disorders including impaired absorption or nutrient loss
- Cardiopulmonary disorders including Congestive heart failure (CHF) and chronic obstructive pulmonary disease (COPD)
- Malignancies including lung and prostate cancer

Of the psychiatric disorders, you would want to distinguish between major depressive disorder (MDD), dysthymia, bipolar disorder, mood conditions related to other medical conditions, substance use effects, and adjustment disorders or other trauma-related disorders. Also, keep in mind that multiple medical conditions can directly precipitate a mood disorder. Similarly, many medications have an association with triggering a mood disorder. Examples of both are listed in Table 21.1.

Table 21.1 Medications and medical conditions associated with depression. (Adapted from Anawati 2008)

Medications	*Analgesics* (e.g., ibuprofen, indomethacin, opioids, phenacetin)
	Antibiotics (e.g., ampicillin, sulfamethoxazole, clotrimazole, tetracycline, griseofulvin, metronidazole, nitrofurantoin, streptomycin)
	Antihypertensive agents (e.g., hydralazine, methyldopa, prazosin, propanolol, reserpine, clonidine)
	Antineoplastic agents (e.g., bleomycin, vincristine, vinblastine)
	Steroids and hormones (e.g., corticosteroids, oral contraceptives, prednisone, triamcinolone)
	Stimulants and appetite suppressants (amphetamine and fenfluramine)
Medical conditions	*Neurologic*: chronic subdural hematoma, dementia, epilepsy, Huntington's disease, migraine headaches, normal pressure hydrocephalus, narcolepsy, Parkinson's disease, stroke, temporal lobe epilepsy, and Wilson's disease
	Infectious: encephalitis, HIV, infectious hepatitis, influenza, mononucleosis, subacute bacterial endocarditis, syphilis, trauma, and tuberculosis
	Neoplasms: bronchogenic carcinoma, CNS tumors, pancreatic cancer, and lymphoma
	Metabolic/endocrine: Addison's disease, anemia, Cushing's disease, diabetes, hepatic disease, electrolyte abnormalities (e.g., hypokalemia or hyponatremia), hypoparathyroidism, hypopituitarism, hypothyroidism, menses-related, pellagra, porphyria, thiamine/B12/folate deficiencies, and uremia
	Collagen vascular disease: rheumatoid arthritis, Sjögren's arthritis, and systemic lupus erythematosus
	Cardiovascular: chronic heart failure
	Respiratory: obstructive sleep apnea

Case Vignette 22.1.2 Continuation

You recall that Mr. Scott has no known medical conditions, that he takes no medications, and that his family history is significant only in that his father died of lung cancer. He also had basic labs completed a year ago, all within normal limits. He has not traveled outside of the country or gone camping in the recent past. He denies smoking or illicit drug use including IV drugs, and admits to only an occasional beer or two on the weekend. You ask about unprotected sex, which he denies. He mentions, however, that 2 months ago his wife of 7 years left him. "So basically I've been sleeping alone ever since," he says.

You explore his symptoms further, and Mr. Scott describes feeling down most days since they separated, tired all the time from waking up earlier than usual, having little interest in anything outside of work, and decreased appetite with a 5-pound weight loss. He shares that he cannot stop feeling responsible about his failing marriage, and that work is the only thing that makes him feel better but recently his performance at the restaurant has been declining, as he cannot seem to concentrate. He denies any recent thoughts of suicide but recalls when his father died 2 years ago that he felt depressed for months and thought about ending his life. He denies any history of prolonged periods of grandiosity, decreased need for sleep, pressured speech or flight of ideas, or increased risk-taking behaviors.

You do a thorough physical exam and find nothing concerning including no abnormal lung sounds, heart murmurs, lymphadenopathy, thyromegaly, edema, and no abnormal findings on digital rectal exam including being hemoccult negative.

You have him complete the Patient Health Questionnaire (PHQ-9) in the waiting room, which you score at 16, in the moderately severe depression range. You ask if he would be interested in talking to a psychiatrist to which he replies, "No way, those guys are just drug pushers," and adds that he also has no interest in therapy. You order additional labs and schedule a follow-up appointment in a month.

STOP

Please proceed with the problem-based approach using the worksheet located in the appendix of Chap. 1!

Please fill in the facts, your hypotheses, further information needed, and learning issues for Learning Issue Table 21.1.2.

Learning Issue Table 21.1.2

FACTS	HYPOTHESES	INFORMATION NEEDED	LEARNING ISSUES

For Mr. Scott, do you feel that all the major concerns within the differential have been addressed? What labs would you order? Would you consider further imaging or an EKG? What else might you ask, and how would you phrase your questions in an open-ended way to best elicit useful information? How soon would you schedule follow-up?

An MDD seems plausible from the history gathered at this point. When considering a diagnosis of MDD, it is important to keep particular epidemiologic factors in mind. Of note, MDD has the highest lifetime prevalence (nearly 17 %) of the psychiatric disorders with a twofold higher prevalence in women than men (Sadock and Sadock 2009).

Risk factors include a personal or family history of previous depressive episodes and suicide attempts, female gender, comorbid medical illness, occurrence of major life changes or traumatic and stressful life events, active alcohol or substance abuse, and absence of social support and isolation (Sadock and Sadock 2009; U.S. DHHS 2013).

Table 21.2 Mood disorders. (Adapted from Anawati 2008; Sadock et al. 2015)

Depressive disorders
Disruptive mood dysregulation disorder
Major depressive disorder
Persistent depressive disorder (dysthymia)
Premenstrual dysphoric disorder
Substance/medication-induced depressive disorder
Depressive disorder due to another medical condition
Other specified depressive disorder
Unspecified depressive disorder
Bipolar and related disorders
Bipolar I disorder
Bipolar II disorder
Cyclothymic disorder
Substance/medication-induced bipolar and related disorder
Bipolar and related disorder due to another medical condition
Other specified bipolar and related disorder
Unspecified bipolar and related disorder

In 2013, the revision of the Diagnostic and Statistical Manual of Mental Disorders (DSM) from version DSM-IV-TR to DSM-5 has led to significant changes for mood disorders. To begin with, depressive disorders and bipolar-related disorders have been separated into their own distinct categories (see Table 21.2). Within each of these categories, there are a number of new diagnostic terms as well as removal of outdated classifications. For depressive disorders, persistent depressive disorder is an example of such a new diagnosis. It replaces the previous condition of dysthymic disorder by also incorporating aspects of MDD to describe a chronic process of dysthymic mood and major depression. Disruptive mood dysregulation disorder (DMDD) is a new diagnosis that is identified for children up to age 18 and is meant to address concerns of previously over-diagnosis of childhood bipolar disorder (please see Chap. 18: Disorders of Childhood). Premenstrual dysphoric disorder was also added, relating to cycles of affective, anxious, and somatic symptoms. While the category of MDD did not undergo significant changes, there are now allowances for possible mixed features of mania without meeting criteria for an actual manic or hypomanic episode, and the previous exclusion criteria of "bereavement" has also been removed. As with many conditions, the distinction of "Not otherwise specified" or NOS, has been replaced with "Unspecified Depressive Disorder" (American Psychiatric Association 2013).

An MDD can be distinguished from persistent depressive disorder (dysthymia) by duration of symptoms and reduced severity and impact on functioning. A bipolar diagnosis would require the history of at least one manic or hypomanic episode. An endorsement of substance use in the recent past may lead to a substance-induced disorder, but keep in mind that the mood disorder may come first and the substance use second as self-medication or detrimental coping strategy. Adjustment disorders are classified under the DSM-5 as a trauma and stress-related disorder (American Psychiatric Association 2013). While the symptoms may overlap, mood symptoms related to a period of adjustment after an acute stressor are limited in duration and severity.

Regardless of the tool used, a diagnosis of MDD requires meeting the DSM-5 criteria for the disorder. The commonly used mnemonic, SIGECAPS, is useful to remember for your clinical interview by asking, if, over the past 2 weeks, the person has had a depressed mood nearly every day, most of the day, a loss in function, plus concerns in at least four of the following areas (ICSI 2013):

Sleep difficulties (increased or decreased)
Interest deficit (anhedonia; necessary, if no depressed mood)
Guilt (including hopelessness, worthlessness, and regret)
Energy deficits
Concentration deficits
Appetite difficulties (increased or decreased)
Psychomotor agitation or retardation
Suicidal thoughts, intentions, or plans

Quantitative scales can also be useful as a diagnostic tool in a busy clinic. In a primary care setting, easy access to rating scales can become essential for the initial screening as well as continued tracking of symptoms for depression throughout treatment. Such scales include the PHQ-2 and PHQ-9, the Beck Depression Inventory (BDI), Hamilton Rating Scale for Depression (HAM-D), Montgomery Asberg Depression Rating Scale, and Center for Epidemiological Studies Depression Scale.

As with this vignette it is often the case that a psychiatric referral will not happen in a timely manner, not only due to the lack of availability and high demand, but also due to ignorance regarding treatment of mental health concerns, stigma against mental illness, cultural differences, and due to personal discomfort (Thornicroft 2008). If a referral does not seem possible, what would you, as the Primary care physician (PCP), be comfortable managing? What might be the best way to proceed for treatment for moderate depression?

Case Vignette 21.1.3 Continuation

Mr. Scott misses the next follow-up visit but returns 2 months later. You review the recent lab results; his thyroid studies, chemistry panel, inflammatory markers, and blood count are all within normal limits, Rapid plasma reagin (RPR) is negative, as well as his urine drug screen (he declined an HIV test).

He apologizes for the missed appointment, and while avoiding eye contact shares: “Actually, I almost didn’t make it at all. A month ago, she handed me the divorce papers. I started drinking really bad that night … I just couldn’t get it out of my head that I screwed everything up, that it was all over … so I impulsively took a handful of vicodin, too. I didn’t expect to wake up but I did. So I guess that’s another failure.” He laughs, dismissively adding, “I’ve already tossed out all the alcohol and the rest of the pills. I tried taking a few days off from work, but now work is all I’ve got.”

Mr. Scott clarifies that he is glad the attempt was not completed. He admits to passive thoughts of suicide as recently as a week ago but without intent or plan, and no thoughts to harm others. He denies having access to guns, pills, or alcohol in his apartment.

Please proceed with the problem-based approach using the worksheet located in the appendix of Chap. 1!

Please fill in the facts, your hypotheses, further information needed, and learning issues for Learning Issue Table 21.1.3.

Learning Issue Table 21.1.3

FACTS	HYPOTHESES	INFORMATION NEEDED	LEARNING ISSUES

In 2010, suicide was ranked as the third leading cause of death for persons 15–24 years of age, second for persons 25–34 years of age, fourth for persons 35–54 years of age, and eighth for persons 55–64 years of age, with an average of 105 deaths a day for that year at an estimated combined cost of $34.6 billion (CDC 2015). Of depressed patients, approximately 60 % will have thoughts of suicide and up to 15 % will have a completed suicide attempt. While women have a higher risk of depression and have more suicide attempts than men, men more frequently die by suicide. An endorsement of a recent suicide attempt, therefore, should be taken very seriously (Sadock et al. 2015).

Depending on the resources available, a primary care physician might be at the front line for assessing safety and taking the steps necessary for urgent management. This may include making the difficult decision of initiating voluntary versus involuntary care. In general, this decision is based on providing the least restrictive setting possible for further treatment while maintaining safety (Riba and Ravindranath 2010). As each US state has different guidelines related to patient rights, safety, and acuity, it is important to be familiar with the mental health laws of your state.

To make a determination of imminent dangerousness and safety, it is important to acknowledge any history of previous suicide attempts, as well as any current suicidal thoughts, intent, and the lethality of any potential plan. For instance, is there a difference between planning the attempt for weeks versus deciding to take the pills impulsively? Would it be more concerning if he took a handful of pills and stopped only because the bottle was empty, or if he believed that the same number of pills was enough, and stopped despite having twice as many pills in the bottle? What if he had access to a gun instead? Similarly, timing the event when no one else is home versus contacting someone for help during or just after the act could lead to entirely different assessments of safety. A patient may also not be willing, or able, to be forthcoming about important information, and collateral may be sparse in an acute setting. Ultimately, therefore, your decision may be based on erring towards safety with a lack of reliable history.

An example of concerns that may lead to inpatient admission include (Riba and Ravindranath 2010):

- Comorbid psychosis
- The attempt was violent, near-lethal, or premeditated
- There was/is refusal of help, or avoidance of rescue or discovery
- The patient regrets surviving or is increasingly distressed
- Male gender, older than 45 years of age
- Limited family or social supports or housing
- Impulsive behavior, severe agitation, and poor judgment
- Medically unstable or needing further workup including acute change in mental status with metabolic, toxic, infectious, or other etiology
- Continued suicidal ideation and intent, with a specific plan with high lethality
- Need for a secure setting for specific treatment (e.g., ECT)

Given the known history for Mr. Scott, what would lead you towards involuntary commitment to a psychiatric facility? What evidence suggests that he may be safe with outpatient intervention? How would you assess his risk of using alcohol as a coping skill? Would you ask him to sign a safety contract?

Case Vignette 21.1.4 Continuation

You review with Mr. Scott the possible warning signs that he is again entering a crisis, environmental triggers, and choices he can make to improve his ability to make safe decisions, such as abstaining from alcohol. Notably, he only endorses guilt about his recent drinking when you ask the CAGE questionnaire (Ewing 1984; need to cut down, annoyance with criticism, guilt about drinking, use of alcohol as an "eye opener"; refer to Appendix C, Chapter 19—Substance-Related and Addictive Disorders). You also have him list personal coping strategies he would agree to implement if necessary; you ask Mr. Scott to list people, places, and activities that could keep his thoughts away from distressing emotions, and close family friends that he could talk to help resolve a crisis if suicidal thoughts return. You also give him the phone numbers to his area's crisis hotline, the national suicide prevention lifeline, and review directions to the nearest urgent care clinic and emergency department; he agrees to put this information on his refrigerator. He admits that going for walks helps him calm down, and shares that he called his sister for the first time in years shortly after his attempt and would agree to do so again when he is feeling distressed. He also states that he would likely use the crisis hotline in the future now that he knows about it.

Before he leaves, you again have him fill out the PHQ-9, which you score at 21, or severe depression. You again recommend seeing a psychiatrist, which he again declines. You discuss the seriousness of what he is going through and ask if he would consider being assessed for inpatient psychiatric admission, which he also declines. He agrees, however, to consider starting an antidepressant. You discuss the pros, cons, and alternative treatment options, and Mr. Scott agrees to start a selective serotonin reuptake inhibitor (SSRI) and see you for follow-up in 1 week.

Please proceed with the problem-based approach using the worksheet located in the appendix of Chap. 1!

Please fill in the facts, your hypotheses, further information needed, and learning issues for Learning Issue Table 21.1.4.

Learning Issue Table 21.1.4

FACTS	HYPOTHESES	INFORMATION NEEDED	LEARNING ISSUES

If you have determined that Mr. Scott is safe to treat on an outpatient basis, how do you help him remain safe? Reducing the risk of future crises begins by limiting exposure to environmental triggers and risk factors such as avoiding isolation, alcohol, and access to pills. Should prevention fail, a crisis plan may be necessary. One example is a step-wise plan of action that he agrees to implement when suicidal thoughts arise. Often a safety plan would start with recognizing warning signs of a crisis, individual actions and coping strategies he might take to reduce distress, followed by social supports and distractions, close family and friends who can to help resolve the crisis, and ultimately involvement of professional support systems should other strategies fail (SAMHSA 2015). It is worth noting that there continues to be controversy surrounding the use of safety contracts signed by the patient. Evidence that this leads to any improved outcome for the patient is very limited, and such a contract does not reduce any legal liability for the clinician (Garvey et al. 2009).

Following an assessment for acute dangerousness, treatment guidelines for moderate-to-severe depression currently begin with pharmacologic intervention using an antidepressant in combination with an evidence-based psychotherapy (Fig. 21.1). Psychoeducation, increased psychosocial support, and behavioral strategies such as increased exercise are also key components of management in this acute phase in treatment (ICSI 2013). Based on acuity, specific symptom clusters, and complications, other modalities may also be necessary, such as use of an antipsychotic, anticonvulsants, or electroconvulsive therapy (ECT) (Tazman and Mohr 2011).

Deciding on a specific medication is a similar process as with other medical conditions, such as factoring in patient preference, response to prior medication, potential drug interactions, half-life, cost, disease severity, comorbid conditions, and a discussion of risks and side effects versus anticipated benefits. Most often first-line treatment begins with an SSRI, serotonin norepinephrine reuptake inhibitor (SNRI), mirtazapine, or bupropion. Tricyclic antidepressants (TCAs) and monoamine oxidase inhibitors (MAOIs) are also used; however, increased side ef-

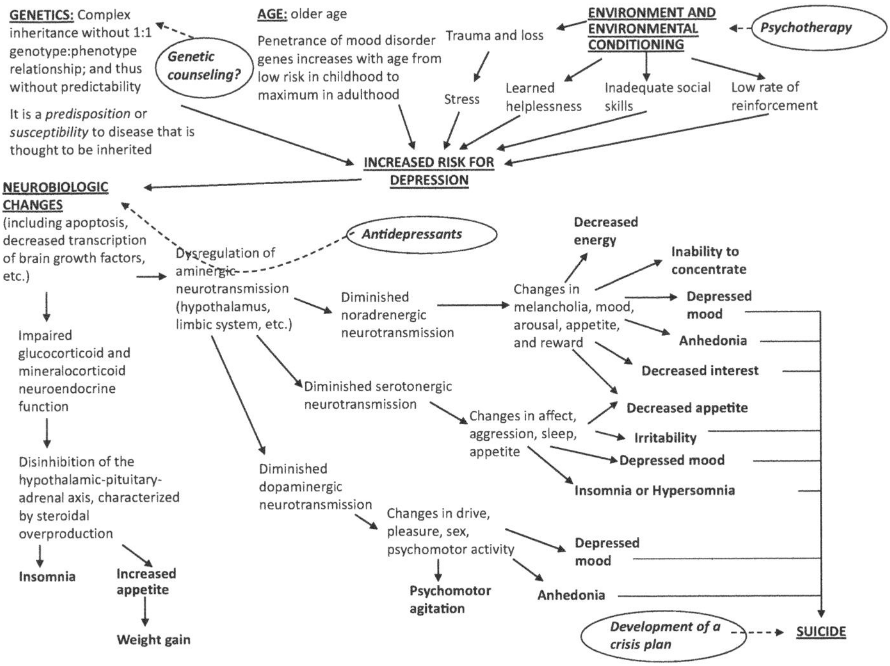

Fig. 21.1 Mechanistic diagram showing the pathophysiology of depression. Treatment options are *circled* and connected via *dashed lines*. (Adapted from Anawati 2008)

fect and risk profiles have led to a focus on specific populations for these classes of medications (American Psychiatric Association 2010; U.S. DHHS 2012). Table 21.3 lists the classes, mechanism of action, and adverse effects of commonly used antidepressants.

Case Vignette 21.1.5 Conclusion
Mr. Scott again misses his next appointment. You feel relieved, therefore, when he comes on time today, 5 months since his separation with his wife and 1 month since starting the SSRI. You have him fill out the PHQ-9 in the waiting room, which you score at 16, again within the moderate depression range. He admits to a few occasions of passive suicidal thoughts but none in the past 2 weeks. He feels that reconnecting with his sister and a few friends have helped a great deal, as well as starting a routine of walking to work every day for exercise. Mr. Scott shares that, "when I'm with others I'm okay, but the hardest part is when I'm alone. I just can't stop feeling like a failure."

He is not sure if the medication has been helping, but his sister has told him he seems to have more energy. You again discuss the risks and benefits of medications, importance of adherence, and time course of action once on a therapeutic dose. He agrees to schedule an appointment with a psychiatrist to potentially continue medications and to discuss cognitive behavioral therapy (CBT).

Table 21.3 Pharmacology of antidepressant medications. (Adapted from Anawati 2008; Ferrando et al. 2014; Sadock et al. 2015; Stahl 2013, 2014)

Pharmacologic class, examples, and indications	MOA	Adverse effects
All antidepressants		Patients should be counseled about the potential for rare, serious side effects, including allergic or other life-threatening reactions; increase in suicidal ideations; and unmasking of mania
Selective serotonin reuptake inhibitors	Inhibit reuptake of serotonin from the synaptic cleft by blocking reuptake transporters; more serotonin selectivity at lower doses	Significantly fewer adverse effects than other antidepressants, SSRIs may cause insomnia, agitation, sedation, GI distress, and sexual dysfunction
Citalopram, escitalopram, fluoxetine, fluvoxamine, paroxetine, sertaline	Many SSRIs inhibit various cytochrome P450 isoenzymes (the reader is encouraged to consult available resources including Flockhart 2007)	
First-line agents for depression; also used in various anxiety disorders such as panic disorder and OCD	They are better tolerated than tricyclics and have high safety in overdose. Shorter half-life SSRIs may be associated with discontinuation symptoms when abruptly stopped	
TCAs	All TCAs block reuptake of NE and are antagonists at histamine-1, alpha-1, and muscarinic cholinergic receptors; they also block voltage-sensitive sodium channels	Drowsiness, insomnia, OSH, agitation, CA, weight increase, GI distress, anticholinergic[a] Overdose may be fatal, dose titration is needed
Norepinephrine reuptake inhibitors	More selective for norepinephrine reuptake inhibition	
Desipramine, protriptyline, nortriptyline, and maprotiline		
Norepinephrine and serotonin reuptake inhibitors	Serotonin and norepinephrine reuptake inhibition	
Amitriptyline, doxepin, imipramine, and trimipramine		
Mixed action agents		
Amoxapine	Amoxapine—norepinephrine reuptake inhibitor, serotonin-2A and dopamine-2 antagonist	
Clomipramine	Clomipramine—parent drug is potent serotonin reuptake inhibitor, active metabolite is potent norepinephrine reuptake inhibitor	
Used in depression, anxiety disorders, and as adjuncts in bulimia and chronic pain disorders		

Table 21.3 (continued)

Pharmacologic class, examples, and indications	MOA	Adverse effects
MAOIs	Block deamination of monoamines by inhibiting monoamine oxidase, thus increasing cytoplasmic levels of serotonin and norepinephrine in the presynaptic neuron	MAOIs: tyramine toxicity: indirect sympathomimetic effects stimulate release of stored catecholamine when foods with tyramine are consumed (e.g., cheese, red wine, fava beans, cured meats)
(e.g., phenelzine, tranyl-cypromine)		MAOIs + SSRIs: serotonin syndrome[b]
Effective for refractory depression and refractory panic disorder, also good for depression with atypical features (e.g., psychosis), and other anxiety disorders including social phobia and OCD		MAOIs + TCAs: hypertensive crisis[c]
Norepinephrine-dopamine reuptake inhibitors	Like amphetamines, inhibits norepinephrine and dopamine reuptake	Insomnia or agitation, GI distress. Twice-a-day dosing with sustained release. No sexual dysfunction or weight gain
Bupropion		Slightly greater tendency (versus the other antidepressants) of lowering the seizure threshold, particularly in patients with eating disorders
Indications: depression, smoking cessation aid, seasonal affective disorder, and ADHD		
Serotonin-norepinephrine reuptake inhibitors	Selective inhibitor of serotonin and norepinephrine reuptake	Sleep changes, GI distress, and discontinuation syndrome
Venlafaxine, desvenlafaxine, and duloxetine		Higher dose may cause hypertension. Dose titration is needed. Abrupt discontinuation may result in discontinuation symptoms
Indications: depressive disorders, anxiety disorders, ADHD, and chronic pain management		

Table 21.3 (continued)

Pharmacologic class, examples, and indications	MOA	Adverse effects
Serotonin modulators	Nefazodone—Serotonin-2A and 2C antagonist, serotonin and norepinephrine reuptake inhibition	Sedation. Dose titration is needed. No sexual dysfunction
Pre- and postsynaptic active agents		
Nefazodone		
Mixed action agents	Trazodone—Serotonin-2A, 2C and histamine-1 antagonist, serotonin reuptake inhibition	Drowsiness, OSH, CA, GI distress, and weight gain. Priapism is possible
Trazodone		
Indications: refractory major depression, insomnia, PTSD, and chronic pain		
Norepinephrine-serotonin modulators	Alpha-2, serotonin-2A, 2C, 3 and histamine-1 antagonist	Sedation, weight gain. No sexual dysfunction
Pre- and postsynaptic active agents		
Mirtazapine		
Indications: depressive disorders, especially patients who need to gain weight		

CA cardiac arrhythmia, *OSH* orthostatic hypotension, *5-HT* serotonin, *NE* norepinephrine, *DA* dopamine, *GI* gastrointestinal, *SSRI* selective serotonin reuptake inhibitor, *OCD* obsessive-compulsive disorder, *TCA* tricyclic antidepressant, *MAOI* monoamine oxidase inhibitor, *ADHD* attention deficit hyperactivity disorder, *AE* adverse effects, *MOA* Mechanism of action

[a] Dry mouth, blurred vision, urinary hesitancy, and constipation

[b] Serotonin syndrome is typically seen with combined use of MAOIs and SSRIs, initially consisting of lethargy, restlessness, confusion, flushing, diaphoresis, tremor, and myoclonic jerks, and eventually can result in hyperthermia, hypertonicity, rhabdomyolysis, renal failure, convulsions, coma, and death

[c] Hypertensive crisis can result in headache, tachycardia, nausea, cardiac arrhythmias, and even stroke

Overcoming and subsequently preventing major depressive episodes can become a long and difficult struggle for a patient. For Mr. Scott, repeated no-shows to appointments and previous refusal of treatment may raise concern in the future for medication-adherence problems and resistance to therapy, ultimately placing him at high risk of a prolonged course of recovery. Frequent and consistent follow-up is thus a part of routine treatment for severe depression (American Psychiatric Association 2010). A successful trial on an antidepressant is contingent on adherence for at least 4–6 weeks and only after increasing the dose to a therapeutic level. If stabilization of symptoms is achieved, medication maintenance should then continue for at least 6 months—longer if there is a history of previous episodes or other concerning risk factors. Treatment response rates for a reduction in symptoms for moderate-to-severe depression range from 50 to 75 %, and studies suggest that remission rates range between 28 and 33 % (Tazman and Mohr 2011; Trivedi and Rush 2006).

Without the use of an antidepressant for stabilization, there may be up to a 50–80 % chance of a recurrence after the first depressive episode, and there is a 20 % chance of long-term chronicity. Once a patient has suffered three or more episodes, up to 90 % may expect to have more episodes in the future (Sadock and Sadock 2009; ICSI 2013). With maintenance pharmacologic treatment, the risk of relapse decreases to 29 % in the first year, and by 50 % for the following second and third years (Tazman and Mohr 2011).

Psychotherapy is an equally important arm of treatment for major depression. Combining the use of an antidepressant with an evidence-based therapy not only leads to higher response and remission rates compared to medication or therapy used alone but also keeps patients in active treatment longer than if medications are used in isolation (Pampallona et al. 2004; Cuijpers et al. 2009; Sadock and Sadock 2009).

Therapy modalities frequently used include CBT, interpersonal psychotherapy, marital and family therapy, psychodynamic therapy, problem-solving therapy, and mentalization-based therapy. Mr. Scott's frequent endorsement of hopelessness suggests that CBT would be a beneficial approach. As an evidence-based, time-limited psychotherapy, CBT focuses on identifying distorted cognitions such as "I am a failure," and reframing these thoughts to produce lasting emotional and behavioral change. For Mr. Scott, as for many people, a constant belief that you are a failure may lead to profound emotional distress and unhappiness, as well as create dysfunctional behaviors such as withdrawing from social supports and decreased success at work. The goal of CBT would be for Mr. Scott to challenge this core belief and see himself and his surroundings in a more realistic and positive way. This would then lead to less emotional distress in the future and a higher level of functioning (Beck 2011).

Case Vignette 21.2.1 Virginia Mayson
You are the Emergency department (ED) physician working nights this summer in a small hospital just outside of Seattle, Washington. You begin your shift, noting the strange look the nurse gives you as he hands you your first patient's chart. You look down to read about Mrs. Mayson, a 42-year-old physicist who walked in alone with complaints of a headache. Entering the room, you begin introducing yourself, but Mrs. Mayson immediately talks over you to say, "Are you the doctor? Good! I've been here for hours. Look, I am visiting Seattle to introduce my design for a free energy machine based off of vacuum generators and pressure turbines. I'm going to give the designs to the world to use for free, but the oil companies are on to me and I think they've finally found me, and they want to kill me," she says all of this in one breath, adding, "I might be putting everyone here in danger, so maybe I should just leave," as she gets up to go.

STOP

Please proceed with the problem-based approach using the worksheet located in the appendix of Chap. 1!

Please fill in the facts, your hypotheses, further information needed, and learning issues for Learning Issue Table 21.2.1.

Learning Issue Table 21.2.1

FACTS	HYPOTHESES	INFORMATION NEEDED	LEARNING ISSUES

Bipolar and Related Disorders
The ED physician in the vignette faces an interesting challenge: a patient with a seemingly simple chief complaint (headache) whose initial mental status findings (apparently increased rate and amount of speech, grandiose and paranoid thoughts, and behaviors—leading to abruptly trying to leave the ED) make it difficult to conduct a history and physical assessment in the usual manner. Because of the challenges that such a patient may present the physician with, whether in an emergency, outpatient, or other setting, it may be tempting to not try to further assess the patient and what exactly the psychiatric disturbance may be, leading to a lost opportunity to help a patient who may be at risk for other complications.

Differential Diagnosis

In the previous vignette, we encountered a patient with fatigue and depressed mood, whereas in this vignette, the patient has many of the opposite symptoms. It may be tempting to jump to the conclusion of a "manic episode" or "manic depression," leading to the apparent expansive mood via the brain-mediated mechanisms illustrated in Fig. 21.2. Indeed, bipolar disorder is not uncommon, with a 12-month prevalence of 2.6% according to the National Institute of Mental Health (NIMH 2015). The onset is usually in late adolescence or early adulthood.

It is important to ensure that several differential possibilities are considered, including substances and other medical conditions that may activate the same common brain mechanisms. Other psychiatric conditions that may be considered include attention-deficit hyperactivity disorder (with talkativeness and increased motor activity); anxiety disorders (with restlessness and poor concentration); personality disorders (with poor affect regulation); and schizophrenia and other psychotic disorders (particularly if there are delusions or other psychotic symptoms that are *not* concurrent with a mood disturbance) (Table 21.4).

Consequently, a thorough history, considering neurologic, endocrine, and infectious conditions and a general examination are necessary (Table 21.5).

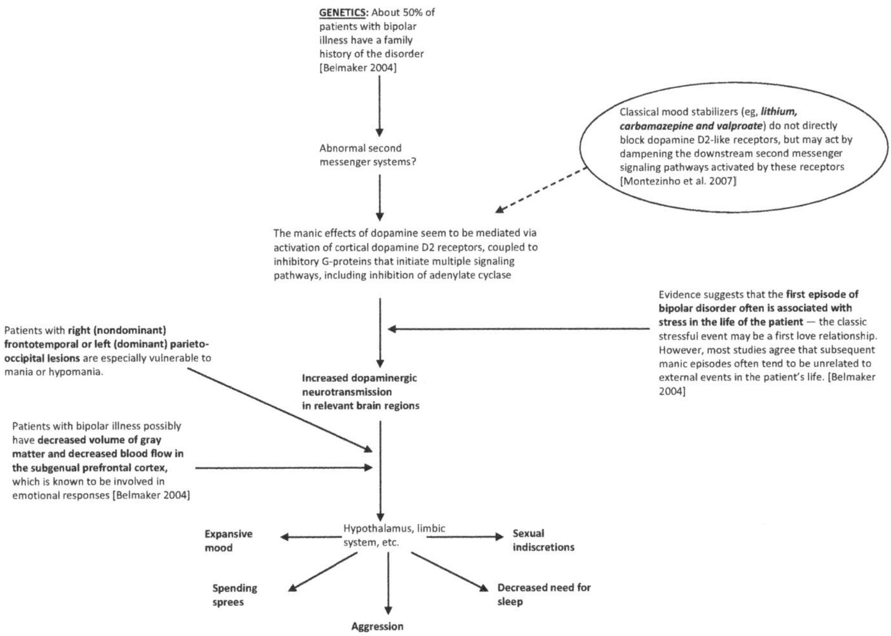

Fig. 21.2 Mechanistic diagram showing a proposed model for the pathophysiology of bipolar disorder. Treatment options are noted by *dashed lines*. (Adapted from Anawati 2008)

Table 21.4 Substance/medication-induced bipolar and related disorder, selected substances and treatments associated with secondary mood disorders. (Adapted from Anawati 2008; Ketter and Chang 2014)

Substances	Alcohol
	Illicit substances (e.g., amphetamines, cocaine, hallucinogens, inhalants, opioids, phencyclidine)
Psychiatric treatments	Anxiolytics, sedatives, and hypnotics (e.g., barbiturates, benzodiazepines)
	Antidepressants (e.g., serotonin-norepinephrine reuptake inhibitors, selective serotonin reuptake inhibitors, monoamine oxidase inhibitors, tricyclics)
	Stimulants (e.g., methylphenidate)
	Typical antipsychotics (e.g., haloperidol)
	Other somatic therapies (e.g., electroconvulsive therapy, light therapy)
General medications	Analgesics (e.g., indomethacin, opiates)
	Anti-infectives (e.g., interferon, isoniazid, zidovudine)
	Antineoplastics (e.g., vincristine, vinblastine)
	Cardiac drugs (e.g., hydralazine, propranolol, reserpine)
	Endocrine agents (e.g., corticosteroids, hormonal contraceptives)
	Neurological agents (e.g., anticholinergics, baclofen, levodopa)

Table 21.5 Bipolar and related disorder due to another medical condition, selected general medical conditions associated with secondary mood disorders. (Adapted from Anawati 2008; Ketter and Chang 2014)

Neurological conditions	Cerebral trauma
	Cerebral tumor
	Cerebrovascular infarction
	Dementia
	Epilepsy
	Multiple sclerosis
	Parkinson's disease
Endocrine conditions	Hypercortisolism (Cushing's disease/syndrome)
	Hypocortisolism (Addison's disease)
	Hyperthyroidism
	Hypothyroidism
Infectious conditions	AIDS
	HIV infection
	Infectious mononucleosis
	Influenza
	Tertiary syphilis (general paresis)
	Toxoplasmosis
	Viral hepatitis

Case Vignette 21.2.2 Continued

You take advantage of this brief moment to reintroduce yourself and calmly ask her to have a seat. You note that her hospital gown is on backwards, her hair is unkempt, and that she has dozens of diagrams sketched out on paper littered throughout the room. You ask her about her headache which she waves off dismissively, saying that Jesus showed her how to create the free energy machine and cured her of all illnesses as well.

You reassure her that she is safe here, and she calms enough for you to attempt a physical exam. As you work, she distractedly talks about how her church helped her hide from the oil companies who have been trying to kidnap her. You finish your exam and find no physical concerns. You try to find a pause to talk to her again as the nurse walks in to tell you that her husband has arrived. You excuse yourself, noting that she has returned to scribbling notes on a piece of paper while talking despite no one else being in the room.

STOP

Please proceed with the problem-based approach using the worksheet located in the appendix of Chap. 1!

Please fill in the facts, your hypotheses, further information needed, and learning issues for Learning Issue Table 21.2.2.

Learning Issue Table 21.2.2

FACTS	HYPOTHESES	INFORMATION NEEDED	LEARNING ISSUES

In diagnosing bipolar and related disorders, it is important to understand the DSM-5 definitions of a manic episode and hypomanic episode. A manic episode is defined according to the following criteria:

- A distinct period (≥1 week or any other duration if hospitalization needed) of elevated, expansive, or irritable mood, along with increased goal-directed activity or energy
- At least three (or four if the mood is only irritable) of increased self-esteem/grandiosity; decreased need for sleep; talkativeness; flight of ideas/racing thoughts; increased goal-directed activity or psychomotor agitation; and excessive activities with high potential for painful consequences
- Impairing or necessitating hospitalization to manage danger; or with psychotic features

- Other substances or medical conditions ruled out

While a hypomanic episode is similar, except:

- The mood change lasts at least 4 consecutive days.
- The episode, while leading to behaviors uncharacteristic of the patient when not ill and while observable by others, is not severe enough to cause "marked" impairment or to necessitate hospitalization or be associated with psychotic features.

According to the DSM-5, there are various subcategories under the general category of bipolar and related disorders: bipolar I disorder (at least one manic episode); bipolar II disorder (with at least one hypomanic episode *and* one major depressive episode *but* never a manic episode, and with distress or impairment related to the symptoms or unpredictability caused by mood alternation); cyclothymic disorder (at least 2 years in adults and 1 year in children and adolescents of numerous distressing/impairing hypomanic and depressive symptoms not meeting criteria for either a hypomanic episode or major depressive episode, and present at least half of the time, and never without a break of more than 2 months); substance/medication-induced bipolar and related disorder; bipolar and related disorder due to another medical condition; and other specified bipolar and related disorder.

However, as noted earlier (and not uncommonly with several psychiatric disorders, and as described in Chap. 17 on interviewing and mental status examination), the very illness itself often impairs the patient's insight and makes a detailed assessment difficult; therefore, it is important to obtain collateral information and do serial observations.

Case Vignette 21.2.3 Continued
Mrs. Mayson's husband has clearly been in a panic. "I'm so glad she's here!" he says. He states that he has been looking for her for hours, and that she had left early in the afternoon mumbling something about getting electrical equipment. "I tried everything to keep her inside, but she snuck out when I wasn't looking," he says. "Then I get a call from our credit card company that someone's purchased three thousand dollars of stuff at Home Depot! I drive over there and describe my wife, and they say she left with some guy who said he was going to take her to a hospital … You have no idea how scared I've been."

You find out that Mrs. Mayson and her husband have been married for 15 years, and that he has never known her to behave like this before. They arrived here on vacation 6 days ago from New Orleans, and she was scheduled to present a paper at a conference today. "She said she's a physicist? What? No … she's a history professor and her paper was on international affairs. When we first got here, she was irritated about how hard it was to sleep at night with jet lag, and with the sun up for so long at these latitudes over the summer. Then she said she didn't have time to sleep, and has since been staying up all night working on her talk. Today she decided to not present it, anyway …" her husband says. "It's probably a good thing. For the past 5 days she's making less and less sense and acting like she's on drugs or something."

You ponder what your next steps should be.

Please proceed with the problem-based approach using the worksheet located in the appendix of Chap. 1!

Please fill in the facts, your hypotheses, further information needed, and learning issues for Learning Issue Table 21.2.3.

Learning Issue Table 21.2.3

FACTS	HYPOTHESES	INFORMATION NEEDED	LEARNING ISSUES

As with the management of any other psychiatric condition, safety is a top priority, and attention must be paid to all aspects of the biopsychosocial formulation. Further labs should be targeted towards substance abuse screening as well as specific medical etiologies for mood disturbances (Tables 21.4 and 21.5). Several medications, as enumerated in Table 21.6, can address the specific portions of the pathophysiological mechanism as described in Fig. 21.2. Psychosocial interventions focus on providing adequate support and safety for the patient with limited insight, and psychotherapy has an important role in minimizing and preventing the stress that could further destabilize brain functioning and in facilitating compliance with what will need to be ongoing treatment.

Table 21.6 Treatment of bipolar and related disorders. (Adapted from Anawati 2008; Ketter and Chang 2014; Stahl 2013, 2014)

Pharmacologic agent	MOA and pharmacokinetics	Adverse effects	Clinical assessments and labs to monitor
Lithium Established treatment for acute mania and bipolar maintenance therapy that with chronic treatment appears to decrease suicidal behavior and suicide	Main MOA involves G proteins by blocking inositol-1-phosphatase in neurons, with subsequent interruption of the phosphatidylinositol second messenger system	Weight gain: Renal: nephrogenic diabetes insipidus, glomerular and interstitial fibrosis and nephron atrophy (patients need to maintain adequate fluid and sodium intake, and caution is indicated in the setting of protracted sweating, diarrhea, infection, and fever)	Baseline pregnancy test, electrocardiogram (in patients over 40 years of age), and renal (blood urea nitrogen, serum creatinine, and electrolytes) and thyroid (thyroid-stimulating hormone, TSH) indices, with reevaluation of renal and thyroid indices at 3 and 6 months and then every 6–12 months thereafter, and as clinically indicated; serum lithium concentrations are commonly assessed at steady state, which occurs at about 5 days after a dosage change, and then as indicated by inefficacy or adverse effects. More frequent laboratory monitoring is prudent in the medically ill and in patients with abnormal indices
	Excreted unchanged by the kidney; half-life: 20 h Monitor drug levels to keep in 0.8–1.2 mEq/L range	Dermatological: acneiform and maculopapular eruptions, psoriasis, and folliculitis	
		Thyroid: hypothyroidism	
		Cardiac: ranging from benign ECG T wave changes to clinically significant sinus node dysfunction or sinoatrial block, ventricular irritability	
		Teratogen: FDA Pregnancy Category D	

Table 21.6 (continued)

Pharmacologic agent	MOA and pharmacokinetics	Adverse effects	Clinical assessments and labs to monitor
Valproate Demonstrated efficacy for acute manic and mixed episodes in adults, but not in patients under 18 years of age	Suppresses high frequency, repetitive neuronal firing by blocking voltage-dependent sodium channels and also affects neuronal signal transduction through actions on protein kinase C Also increases brain GABA levels by inhibition of GABA catabolism by transaminases	Common dose-related adverse effects with valproate include gastrointestinal (nausea, vomiting, dyspepsia, and diarrhea), hepatic (transaminase elevations), CNS (tremor, sedation, and dizziness), and metabolic (weight gain and osteoporosis) problems and hair loss	Clinical assessments with valproate therapy include a baseline physical examination and routinely querying patients at baseline and during treatment regarding hepatic and hematological disorders and adverse effects. Laboratory monitoring during valproate therapy commonly includes baseline complete blood count, differential, platelets, and hepatic indices, and reevaluation every 6–12 months and as clinically indicated
	Metabolized by liver, but not affected much by P450; half-life is 6–16 h; highly protein bound, ideal serum level is 50–125 μg/mL	The US prescribing information for valproate includes boxed warnings regarding the risks of hepatotoxicity, teratogenicity, and pancreatitis	Serum valproate concentrations are typically assessed at steady state and then as clinically indicated by inefficacy or adverse effects
		Other warnings include the risks of hyperammonemic encephalopathy in patients with urea cycle disorders, somnolence in older adults, thrombocytopenia, hypothermia, multiorgan hypersensitivity reactions, polycystic ovarian syndrome, and suicidality (an anticonvulsant class warning)	
		Valproate, like the other mood stabilizers, is a teratogen (FDA Pregnancy Category D)	

Table 21.6 (continued)

Pharmacologic agent	MOA and pharmacokinetics	Adverse effects	Clinical assessments and labs to monitor
Carbamazepine Demonstrated efficacy for acute manic and mixed episodes in adults, but complexity of use (related to drug interactions and side effects) and lack of a maintenance indication make it less commonly used than other mood stabilizers	Alters neurotransmission by inhibiting presynaptic Na+ channels; also inhibits glutaminergic neurotransmission	Common dose-related adverse effects with carbamazepine involve CNS (diplopia, blurred vision, fatigue, sedation, dizziness, and ataxia) or gastrointestinal system (nausea and vomiting) problems	Clinical assessment include a baseline physical examination and routinely querying patients at baseline and during treatment regarding hepatic and hematological disorders and adverse effects

Table 21.6 (continued)

Pharmacologic agent	MOA and pharmacokinetics	Adverse effects	Clinical assessments and labs to monitor
	Metabolized by the liver (CYP3A4); excreted renally; P450 inducer; initially half-life is 25–65 h, then can decrease to 12–17 h	Risks of serious dermatological reactions in patients with the HLA-B*1502 allele (Asians should be genetically tested and, if HLA-B*1502 is positive, should not be treated with carbamazepine unless benefit clearly outweighs risk), aplastic anemia (16/million patient-years), and agranulocytosis (48/million patient-years)	Laboratory monitoring includes baseline complete blood count, differential, platelets, hepatic indices, and serum sodium In contemporary practice, clinically indicated (e.g., when a patient becomes ill with a fever) monitoring is emphasized. Patients who have abnormal or marginal indices at any point merit careful, scheduled, and clinically indicated monitoring
	Titrate-to-serum level of 8–12 μg/mL		Serum carbamazepine concentrations are typically assessed at steady state, and then as indicated by inefficacy or adverse effects
		Other warnings in the prescribing information include the risks of teratogenicity, increased intraocular pressure due to mild anticholinergic activity, and suicidality (an anticonvulsant class warning). Carbamazepine can cause hematological (benign leukopenia, benign thrombocytopenia), dermatological (benign rash), electrolyte (asymptomatic hyponatremia), and hepatic (benign transaminase elevations) problems	
		Carbamazepine, like the other mood stabilizers, is a teratogen (FDA Pregnancy Category D	

Table 21.6 (continued)

Pharmacologic agent	MOA and pharmacokinetics	Adverse effects	Clinical assessments and labs to monitor
Lamotrigine Approved for bipolar maintenance treatment in adults	Affects Na+ channels to modulate the release of glutamate and aspartate; also has a weak inhibitory effect on 5HT receptors	Common adverse events in patients with bipolar disorders in clinical trials were headache, benign rash, dizziness, diarrhea, dream abnormality, and pruritus	Patients need to be advised of lamotrigine adverse effects and drug interactions. Clinical assessments with lamotrigine therapy include a baseline physical examination and routinely querying patients regarding rash at baseline and during treatment
	Hepatically metabolized with subsequent renal excretion; half-life: 25 h	Lamotrigine can cause CNS (headache, somnolence, insomnia, dizziness, and tremor) and gastrointestinal (nausea and diarrhea) adverse effects	
		The US prescribing information for lamotrigine includes a boxed warning regarding the risk of serious rashes requiring hospitalization, which have included Stevens–Johnson syndrome. The risk of rash is higher in patients under age 16 years and may be higher when lamotrigine is coadministered with valproate, when exceeding the recommended initial lamotrigine dose, and when exceeding the recommended lamotrigine dose escalation. Benign rash may be seen in 10 % of patients, but because any rash is potentially serious, discontinuation of lamotrigine is required unless the rash is clearly not drug related	
		Patients should be advised that if they fail to take lamotrigine for five half-lives, gradual reintroduction is necessary. Rashes have been reported with rapid reintroduction	
		Other warnings in the prescribing information include the following risks: suicidality (an anticonvulsant class warning), hypersensitivity reactions (with fever and lymphadenopathy, but not necessarily rash), acute multiorgan failure, blood dyscrasia, aseptic meningitis, medication errors (confusion with other medications), lower and higher lamotrigine serum concentrations when given with hormonal contraceptives and valproate, respectively, binding in the eye and other melanin-containing tissues, withdrawal seizures in bipolar disorder patients; for this reason, lamotrigine should be tapered over 2 weeks unless safety concerns demand abrupt discontinuation	

Table 21.6 (continued)

Pharmacologic agent	MOA and pharmacokinetics	Adverse effects	Clinical assessments and labs to monitor
[a]Second-generation antipsychotics (SGAs)	Antagonist of serotonin-2A, 2C, dopamine-1, 2, 3, 4, alpha-1, histamine-1, and muscarinic-1 receptors	Common adverse reactions in adult acute mania trials with oral olanzapine monotherapy included somnolence (35 versus 13 % with placebo, number needed to harm (NNH) = 5), dry mouth (22 versus 7 % with placebo, NNH = 7), and dizziness (18 versus 6 % with placebo, NNH = 9)	Fasting blood sugar and lipids
Olanzapine Approved for treatment of schizophrenia, acute bipolar mania, and maintenance treatment of bipolar disorder	Hepatic metabolism via CYP1A2; half-life is 21–50 h; levels are decreased by tobacco use and carbamazepine	In 13 placebo-controlled adult olanzapine monotherapy studies with 8-week median exposure, at least 7 % weight gain was seen in 22.2 % of patients versus 3 % with placebo (NNH = 6). In long-term adult olanzapine monotherapy studies, at least 7 % weight gain was seen in 64 % of patients. Weight gain appears even more problematic in adolescents than in adults. In placebo-controlled adolescent olanzapine acute monotherapy studies, at least 7 % weight gain was seen in 40.6 % of patients versus 9.8 % (NNH = 4). In long-term adolescent olanzapine monotherapy studies, at least 7 % weight gain was seen in 89 % of patients. Thus, olanzapine can cause weight gain, diabetes, and hyperlipidemia, with the risk (as with clozapine) being greater than with other SGA	
		Olanzapine has not been associated with congenital malformations in humans (FDA Pregnancy Category C)	
[b]Quetiapine Adult acute mania and schizophrenia trials	Antagonist of serotonin-2A, dopamine-2, alpha-1 and 2, and histamine-1 receptors	Common adverse reactions in adult acute mania and schizophrenia trials with quetiapine monotherapy included somnolence (18 versus 8 % with placebo, NNH = 10) and at least 7 % weight gain (21.1 versus 6.6 % with placebo, NNH = 7).	Fasting blood sugar and lipids Eye examinations

Table 21.6 (continued)

Pharmacologic agent	MOA and pharmacokinetics	Adverse effects	Clinical assessments and labs to monitor
Pediatric acute mania trial	Hepatic metabolism via CYP3A4; half-life is 6 h	In a pediatric acute mania trial, quetiapine monotherapy was associated with at least 7 % weight gain in 11.5 % of patients versus 0.0 % with placebo (NNH = 9)	
		In a 26-week pediatric open follow-up study, quetiapine monotherapy was associated with at least 7 % weight gain in 45 % of patients. Thus, quetiapine can cause weight gain, diabetes, and hyperlipidemia, with the risk considered intermediate—less than with clozapine and olanzapine but more than with ziprasidone and aripiprazole Quetiapine has not been associated with congenital malformations in humans (FDA Pregnancy Category C)	
[c]Risperidone Adult acute mania/schizophrenia trials Pediatric acute mania, schizophrenia, and autism trials	Dopamine-2, 3, 4, serotonin-2A, 7, alpha-1, 2 receptor antagonist	Common adverse reactions in adult acute mania trials with risperidone monotherapy at dosages ≤ 6 mg/day included parkinsonism (25 versus 9 % with placebo, NNH = 7), akathisia (9 versus 3 % with placebo, NNH = 17), and sedation (6 versus 2 % with placebo, NNH = 25)	Fasting blood sugar and lipids
		In adult acute mania/schizophrenia trials, at least 7% weight gain was seen with risperidone dosages ≤8 mg/day in 8.7 % of patients versus 2.9 % with placebo (NNH = 18) and with risperidone dosages > 8 mg/day in 20.9 % of patients versus 2.9 % with placebo (NNH = 6)	
		In pediatric acute mania, schizophrenia, and autism trials, at least 7 % weight gain was seen with risperidone dosages ≤6 mg/day in 32.6 % of patients versus 6.9 % with placebo (NNH = 4)	
		Risperidone raises prolactin levels even at low doses	
		Risperidone has not been associated with congenital malformations in humans (FDA Pregnancy Category C)	

Table 21.6 (continued)

Pharmacologic agent	MOA and pharmacokinetics	Adverse effects	Clinical assessments and labs to monitor
[d]Ziprasidone Adult acute mania trials Adjunctive (added to lithium or valproate)	Serotonin-2A, 1B, 1D, 7, and dopamine-2, 3 receptor antagonist	Common adverse reactions with oral ziprasidone monotherapy included somnolence and extrapyramidal symptoms (both 31 versus 12 % with placebo, NNH=6)	In patients with acute mania, akathisia is commonly accompanied by and at times difficult to distinguish from agitation and anxiety. These overlapping symptoms may be attenuated with adjunctive benzodiazepine therapy
		Common adverse reaction in an adjunctive (added to lithium or valproate) maintenance trial was tremor	In clinical practice, lower (e.g., 80 mg/day) compared with higher (e.g., ≥ 80 mg/day) ziprasidone dosages may increase the risk of akathisia, so optimal titration of this agent may involve avoiding lower dosages to prevent akathisia or abruptly increasing to higher dosages if akathisia develops at lower dosages
		Risks of obesity, diabetes, and hyperlipidemia with ziprasidone were similar to those with aripiprazole and less than with other SGAs	
		Ziprasidone and aripiprazole, compared with risperidone, olanzapine, and quetiapine, cause less sedation and weight gain but more akathisia	
		Ziprasidone has not been associated with congenital malformations in humans (FDA Pregnancy Category C)	
Aripiprazole Adult acute mania trials	Dopamine-2 receptor partial agonist	Common adverse reactions in adult acute mania trials with oral aripiprazole monotherapy included akathisia (13 versus 4 % with placebo, NNH=12) and sedation (8 versus 3 % with placebo, NNH=20)	Aripiprazole-related akathisia (like ziprasidone-related akathisia) may respond to benzodiazepines
Pediatric acute mania and schizophrenia trials	Serotonin-2A, 7 receptor antagonist, 1A receptor partial agonist	Adult acute mania trials, oral aripiprazole monotherapy was associated with at least 7 % weight gain in 2.2 % of patients versus 2.7 % with placebo (NNH=−200)	

Table 21.6 (continued)

Pharmacologic agent	MOA and pharmacokinetics	Adverse effects	Clinical assessments and labs to monitor
Adult and pediatric monotherapy or adjunctive (added to lithium or valproate) therapy		Common adverse reactions in pediatric acute mania trials with oral aripiprazole monotherapy included somnolence (23 versus 3 % with placebo, NNH = 5) and extrapyramidal symptoms (20 versus 3 % with placebo, NNH = 6)	
		In pediatric acute mania and schizophrenia trials, oral aripiprazole monotherapy was associated with at least 7 % weight gain in 5.2 % of patients versus 1.6 % with placebo (NNH = 28)	
		In open-label extensions of adolescent schizophrenia and pediatric bipolar disorder, 32.8 % of patients gained ≥7 % of their weight	
		Aripiprazole has not been associated with congenital malformations in humans (FDA Pregnancy Category C)	
Asenapine Adult acute mania trials Monotherapy and adjunctive therapy	Dopamine-2, 3, 4; serotonin-2A, 2C, 6, 7; histamine-1 and alpha-2 receptor antagonist	Common adverse reactions with oral asenapine monotherapy included somnolence (24 versus 6 % with placebo, NNH = 6), dizziness (11 versus 3% with placebo, NNH = 13), and 7 % weight gain in 5.8 % of patients versus 0.5 % with placebo (NNH = 19)	The warnings and precautions in US prescribing information for asenapine, in addition to those mentioned earlier for multiple SGAs, include Electrocardiograph (EKG) abnormalities (in common with quetiapine and ziprasidone; see earlier "Quetiapine" section for risk-management recommendations) and hypersensitivity reactions (anaphylaxis, angioedema, hypotension, tachycardia, swollen tongue, dyspnea, wheezing, and rash)
		Asenapine has not been associated with congenital malformations in humans (FDA Pregnancy Category C)	Asenapine (in common with ziprasidone), unlike other SGAs, lacks a warning or precaution regarding hyperlipidemia/dyslipidemia

Table 21.6 (continued)

Pharmacologic agent	MOA and pharmacokinetics	Adverse effects	Clinical assessments and labs to monitor
Lurasidone Adult acute schizophrenia trials	Dopamine-2, 4; serotonin-1A, 2A, 7; alpha-2A receptor antagonist	Common adverse reactions with lurasidone monotherapy included somnolence (17 versus 7 % with placebo, NNH = 10) akathisia (13 versus 3 % with placebo, NNH = 10), and at least 7 % weight gain in 4.8 % of patients versus 3.3 % with placebo (NNH = 67)	Lurasidone is a cytochrome P450 3A4 (CYP3A4) substrate, so coadministration with strong CYP3A4 inhibitors and inducers is contraindicated
		Not associated with congenital malformations in humans or animals (FDA Pregnancy Category B)	

ECG electrocardiogram, *FDA* Food and Drug Administration, *NNH* number needed to harm, *SGA* second-generation antipsychotics

[a] SGAs—The warnings and precautions in US prescribing information for multiple SGAs can be accessed at http://www.pdr.net/

Additional FDA prescribing information for risperidone, quetiapine, and ziprasidone can be accessed at:

[b] Quetiepine—http://www.accessdata.fda.gov/drugsatfda_docs/label/2009/022047s011s016s017s019s022lbl.pdf. Accessed 11 May 2015

[c] Risperidone—http://www.accessdata.fda.gov/drugsatfda_docs/label/2014/020272s073,020588s062,021444s048lbl.pdf. Accessed 11 May 2015

[d] Ziprasidone—http://www.accessdata.fda.gov/drugsatfda_docs/label/2014/020825s053,020919s040,s021483s013lbl.pdf. Accessed 11 May 2015

Case Vignette 21.2.4 Continued

Her basic labs come in as you review Mrs. Mayson's health history with her husband, noting that all findings are within normal limits including a negative drug screen. He knows of no past medical conditions, psychiatric history, or drug use. He has never known her to have problems with depression or mania in the past. They both drink a few glasses of wine on weekends and do not smoke. He admits that she may be drinking a little more coffee than usual, "but nothing too out of the ordinary." He also recalls that her father saw a psychiatrist and took medications for some kind of mood problem years ago, and that her brother was in a psychiatric hospital as a kid, but he is waiting for a call back from her parents to find out why.

You return to Mrs. Mayson's room accompanied by her husband. She is delighted to see him and greets him rather inappropriately as he tries to guide her back to the hospital bed. You discuss the possible diagnosis of a manic episode, which she feels is impossible and reminds you that God has cured her of such things.

After talking to her parents and confirming that this sounds similar to what her brother experienced, Mr. Mayson tells you that they have a flight back to New Orleans early tomorrow morning, and that her parents will be coming to pick them up. They will also call first thing tomorrow morning to schedule an urgent appointment with the family's psychiatrist. Mrs. Mayson agrees to go back as she has decided that coming here was against God's plan. She also agrees to see the psychiatrist as she remembers that he has helped her family in the past. You also consider admission to a local inpatient psychiatric ward; however, Mrs. Mayson refuses, and Mr. Mayson would rather have her family's support back home. He agrees to not leave her side until they meet her parents at the airport. You discuss the risks and benefits of a PRN (abbreviation for *pro re nata,* a Latin phrase meaning, "as needed") neuroleptic with both Mr. and Mrs. Mayson. She agrees to consider it if it will also help her sleep, but she hopes it would not ruin her good mood.

On a positive note, with adequate treatment, many patients may be relatively symptom-free in between mood episodes, and there are several features of Mrs. Mayson's case that may portend a more positive prognosis, including previous good functioning, otherwise good health, and availability of psychosocial support.

Review Questions

1. Which of the following patients presents the *lowest* statistical risk for suicide?

   a. A 25-year-old single white male with a history of poorly controlled schizophrenia, and two previous suicide attempts
   b. A married 35-year-old white female who is the mother of two children and has a history of dysthymia successfully treated with sertraline (Zoloft)
   c. A 65-year-old recently widowed black male who has a history of alcohol abuse and dependence
   d. A 75-year-old white female with terminal breast cancer

2. Which of the following biological factors is most commonly associated with suicidal behavior?

   a. Low CSF levels of serotonin metabolite
   b. Low CSF levels of norepinephrine metabolite
   c. High CSF levels of epinephrine metabolite
   d. High CSF levels of dopamine metabolite
   e. High CSF levels of glutamic acid

3. Which of the following substances would represent a concern if administered concomitantly with an SSRI?

   a. Ginkgo biloba
   b. Piper methysticum
   c. Valeriana officinalis
   d. Omega-3 fatty acids
   e. Hypericum perforatum

4. A 50-year-old fireman became clinically depressed after sustaining a myocardial infarction. The most appropriate medication to prescribe would be:

   a. Nortriptyline
   b. Methylphenidate
   c. Venlafaxine
   d. Sertraline
   e. Phenelzine

The next three questions pertain to the following case vignette:

A 25-year-old woman, referred to her primary care physician at the insistence of concerned others, presents with pressured speech, irritability, insomnia, and a rapid train of creative ideas. She recently went on an impulsive buying spree and ran up $5000 on her credit card in 1 day. For a period of several weeks she impulsively had several sexual encounters with men she met in bars which was uncharacteristic for her usual conservative behavior. During the course of the interview she also exhibits a mild degree of paranoid ideation and is angry about having to see a physician.

5. At this point, based on the information provided, and assuming that she has no other significant psychiatric or medical history, which of the following is the most reasonable diagnosis?

   a. Major depressive disorder
   b. Bipolar disorder, type I
   c. Bipolar disorder, type II
   d. Cyclothymic disorder
   e. Schizoaffective disorder

6. The patient is referred to a psychiatrist, who initiates treatment with divalproex. Soon after starting this medication, the patient calls her primary care physician, complaining of a generalized rash. The most appropriate management would be to:

   a. Discontinue the medication and instruct the patient to continue with regular psychiatric follow-up
   b. Continue the medication and prescribe topical steroids
   c. Discontinue the medication and arrange for immediate medical examination
   d. Continue the medication and prescribe benzoyl peroxide
   e. Start carbamazepine and gradually taper the divalproex

7. In this condition, there is often a major psychosocial stressor that precedes the first episode. Later in the course of the illness, the significance of psychosocial stressors diminishes, and the interval between episodes of the illness:

   a. Lengthens
   b. Shortens
   c. Becomes progressively more irregular
   d. Becomes related to seasonal variation
   e. Does not alter in a predictable manner

8. A patient with newly diagnosed bipolar I disorder begins treatment with lithium. After 2 months of treatment, despite overall improvement, he complains of fatigue, tiredness, constipation, weight gain, and increased depression. The most likely reason is:

   a. Hypocalcemia
   b. Elevated prolactin
   c. Hypercortisolism
   d. Hypothyroidism
   e. Hypomagnesemia

Appendix A: Tables with Possible Answers to the Vignettes

Case Vignette 21.1: Richard Scott

Learning Issue Table 21.1

Facts	Hypotheses	Information needed	Learning issues
Mr. Scott, a 38-year-old restaurant owner, comes to your primary care clinic for a routine, annual follow-up	Concerns include diabetes, HIV, cancer, a mood disorder, are there others?	What labs would you order?	If a referral does not seem possible, what would you, as the PCP, be comfortable managing?
	Have major concerns in the differential been addressed?	Would you consider further imaging or an EKG?	What might be the best way to proceed for treatment for moderate depression?
	Primary care integration (PCI): what is the role of psychiatry?	What else might you ask, and how would you phrase your questions in an open-ended way to best elicit useful information?	
While going over his review of systems, he admits to having unintentional weight loss and fatigue	PCP might be at the front line for assessing safety and taking the steps necessary for urgent management		As each US state has different guidelines related to patient rights, safety, and acuity, it is important to be familiar with the mental health laws of your state
He mentions that 2 months ago his wife of 7 years left him			Given the known history for Mr. Scott, what would lead you towards involuntary commitment to a psychiatric facility?
He denies any recent thoughts of suicide, but recalls when his father died 2 years ago that he felt depressed for months and thought about ending his life		How soon would you schedule follow-up?	What evidence suggests that he may be safe with outpatient intervention?
			How would you assess his risk of using alcohol as a coping skill?
			Would you ask him to sign a safety contract?
Mr. Scott misses the next follow-up visit, but returns 2 months later			Is there a role for psychopharmacogenomics?

PCI primary care integration, *PCP* Primary care physician

Case Vignette 21.2 Virginia Mayson

Learning Issue Table 21.2

Facts	Hypotheses	Information needed	Learning issues
Mrs. Mayson, a 42-year-old physicist who walked in the Emergency department (ED) alone with complaints of a headache	Important to ensure that several differential possibilities are considered	Comprehensive evaluation and physical examination	How would you describe the patient's Mental status examination (MSE)?
She immediately talks over you to say, "Are you the doctor? Good! I've been here for hours. Look, I am visiting Seattle to introduce my design for a free energy machine based off of vacuum generators and pressure turbines. I'm going to give the designs to the world to use for free, but the oil companies are on to me and I think they've finally found me, and they want to kill me," she says all of this in one breath, adding, "I might be putting everyone here in danger, so maybe I should just leave," as she gets up to go		After considering Mrs. Mayson's differential diagnosis and indications for pharmacotherapy, what baseline labs and screens would you request?	Consider Mrs. Mayson's biopsychosocial formulation
You soon have the opportunity to speak with Mr. Mayson and find out that they have been married for 15 years, and that he has never known her to behave like this before			How would you assess Mrs. Mayson's safety concerns?
			What do neuroimaging studies demonstrate with bipolar illness?
			What is the mechanism of action of mood stabilizing agents; second-generation antipsychotic medications?
			What is the role of psychotherapy in bipolar disorder?
They arrived here on vacation 6 days ago from New Orleans, and she was scheduled to present a paper at a conference today			How would you provide informed consent to the family regarding pharmacotherapy efficacy, side effects, adverse events, acute and chronic management, and routine laboratory evaluations?
			Is there a role for pharmacogenomics?
When we first got here, she was irritated about how hard it was to sleep at night with jet lag, and with the sun up for so long at these latitudes over the summer. Then she said she didn't have time to sleep, and has since been staying up all night working on her talk			What psychosocial interventions would you consider for the family?

Appendix B: Answers to Review Questions

Answers

1. b
2. a
3. e
4. d
5. b
6. c
7. b
8. d

References

American Psychiatric Association. (2010). Practice guideline for the treatment of patients with major depressive disorder. http://psychiatryonline.org/pb/assets/raw/sitewide/practice_guidelines/guidelines/mdd.pdf. Accessed 3 April 2015.

American Psychiatric Association. (2013). *Diagnostic and statistical manual of mental disorders* (5th ed.). Arlington: American Psychiatric Association.

Anawati, M. (2008). Mood disorders and suicide. In A. Guerrero & M. Piasecki (Eds.), *Problem-based behavioral science and psychiatry*. New York: Springer (Science + Business Media, LLC, 233 Spring Street).

Beck, J. S. (2011). *Cognitive behavior therapy: Basics and beyond* (2nd ed.). New York: Guilford.

Belmaker, R. H. (2004). Medical progress: Bipolar disorder. *New England Journal of Medicine, 351*, 476–486.

Centers for Disease Control and Prevention (CDC). (2015). National center for injury prevention and control. Updated: February 11, 2015. Injury prevention & control: data & statistics (WISQARS). http://www.cdc.gov/injury/wisqars/index.html. Accessed 3 April 2015.

Cuijpers, P., Dekker, J., Hollon, S. D., & Andersson, G. (2009). Adding psychotherapy to pharmacotherapy in the treatment of depressive disorders in adults: A meta-analysis. *The Journal of Clinical Psychiatry, 70*(9):1219–1229.

Ewing, J. A. (1984). Detecting alcoholism: The CAGE questionnaire. *Journal of the American Medical Association, 252,* 1905–1907.

Ferrando, S. J., Owen, J. A., & Levenson, J. L. (2014). Psychopharmacology. In R. E. Hales, S. C. Yudofsky, & L. W. Roberts (Eds.) *The American psychiatric publishing textbook of psychiatry* (6th ed.) Arlington: American Psychiatric Association.

Flockhart, D. A. (2007). Drug interactions: Cytochrome P450 drug interaction table. Indiana University School of Medicine (2007). "/clinpharm/ddis/clinical-table/." Accessed 10 April 2015.

Garvey, K. A., Penn, J. V., Campbell, A. L., Esposito-Smythers, C., & Spirito, A. (2009). Contracting for safety with patients: Clinical practice and forensic implications. *Journal of the American Academy of Psychiatry and the Law, 37*(3):363–370.

Institute of Clinical Systems Improvement (ICSI). (2013). Healthcare guidelines. Adult depression in primary care. Updated September 2013. https://www.icsi.org/_asset/fnhdm3/Depr-Interactive0512b.pdf. Accessed 3 April 2015.

Ketter, T. A., & Chang, K. D. (2014). Bipolar and related disorders. In R. E. Hales, S. C. Yudofsky, & L. W. Roberts (Eds.) *The American psychiatric publishing textbook of psychiatry* (6th ed.). Arlington: American Psychiatric Association.

Montezinho, L. P., Mork, A., Duarte, C. B., Penschuck, S., Geraldes, C. F., & Castro, M. M. (2007). Effects of mood stabilizers on the inhibition of adenylate cyclase via dopamine D(2)-like receptors. *Bipolar Disorder, 9*(3):290–297.

National Institute of Mental Health (2015). http://www.nimh.nih.gov/health/statistics/prevalence/bipolar-disorder-among-adults.shtml, https://www.nimh.nih.gov/health/topics/bipolar-disorder/index.shtml. Accessed 5 June 2015.

Pampallona, S., Bollini, P., Tibaldi, G., Kupelnick, B., & Munizza, C. (2004). Combined pharmacotherapy and psychological treatment for depression: A systematic review. *Archives of General Psychiatry, 61*(7), 714–719.

Riba, M. B., & Ravindranath, D. (Eds.). (2010). *Clinical manual of emergency psychiatry.* Washington DC: American Psychiatric Publishing, Inc.

Sadock, B. J., & Sadock, V. A. (2009). *Kaplan and Sadock's comprehensive textbook of psychiatry* (10th ed., Vols. I & II). New York: Lippincott Williams & Wilkins.

Sadock, B. J., Sadock, V. A., & Ruiz, P. (2015). *Kaplan and Sadock's synopsis of psychiatry: Behavioral sciences/clinical psychiatry, 11th ed. Mood disorders* (pp. 347–386). Philadelphia: Wolters Kluwer.

Stahl, S. (2013). *Stahl's essential psychopharmacology, neuroscientific basis and practical applications* (4th ed.) New York: Cambridge University Press.

Stahl, S. (2014). *Prescriber's guide, Stahl's essential psychopharmacology* (5th ed.) New York: Cambridge University Press.

Substance Abuse and Mental Health Services Administration (SAMHSA). (2015). National suicide prevention lifeline. http://www.suicidepreventionlifeline.org/learn/safety.aspx. Accessed 3 April 2015.

Tasman, A., & Mohr, W. K. (Eds.). (2011). *Fundamentals of psychiatry.* Hoboken: Wiley.

Thornicroft, G. (2008). Stigma and discrimination limit access to mental health care. *Epidemiologia e psichiatria sociale, 17*(1):14–19.

Trivedi, M. H., & Rush, A. J. (2006). Evaluation of outcomes with citalopram for depression using measurement-based care in STAR*D: Implications for clinical practice. *The American Journal of Psychiatry, 163*(1):28–40.

U.S. Department of Health & Human Services. (2012). Agency for healthcare research and quality. National guideline clearinghouse. Diagnosis and treatment of depression in adults: 2012 clinical practice guideline. http://www.guideline.gov/content.aspx?id=39432#Section420. Accessed 3 April 2015.

U.S. Department of Health & Human Services. (2013). Agency for healthcare research and quality. National guideline clearinghouse. Adult depression in primary care. http://www.guideline.gov/content.aspx?id=47315. Accessed 3 April 2015.

Chapter 22
Anxiety Disorders, Obsessive-Compulsive and Related Disorders, Trauma- and Stressor-Related Disorders

Gretchen Gavero

Anxiety is one of the most common presenting symptoms in psychiatry and general medical practice. It can serve as a window into various causes of distress. Anxiety can manifest as an isolated episode (such as in panic attack) or as a debilitating and chronic illness (such as in obsessive-compulsive disorder, OCD, or posttraumatic stress disorder, PTSD). *Diagnostic and Statistical Manual of Mental Disorders, Fifth Edition (DSM-5)* defines fear as "the emotional response to real or perceived threat" and anxiety as "the anticipation of future threat" (APA 2013). Anxiety disorders exhibit excessive fear and anxiety associated with situations or objects. Note that both fear and anxiety are necessary components of our "fight and flight response" as humans. When the response is out of proportion, persistent, and falls beyond the cultural context, anxiety and fear may interfere with one's functioning, hence a disorder. To emphasize the diversity of the etiology of anxiety, the conditions that fall under "Anxiety Disorders" in *Diagnostic and Statistical Manual of Mental Disorders, Fourth Edition, Text Revision (DSM-IV TR*; APA 2000) were recategorized into three separate chapters in *DSM-5* (APA 2013) as follows (Table 22.1):

At the end of this chapter, the reader will be able to:

1. Discuss the epidemiology, mechanisms, clinical presentation, clinical evaluation, differential diagnosis, and treatment of common anxiety disorders, obsessive-compulsive and related disorders, and trauma- and stressor-related disorders.
2. Describe the mechanisms of action and potential adverse effects of anxiolytics.

G. Gavero (✉)
Department of Psychiatry, University of Hawai'i John A. Burns School of Medicine,
1356 Lusitana Street, University Tower 4th Floor, Honolulu, HI 96813, USA
e-mail: gaverog@dop.hawaii.edu

D. Alicata et al. (eds.), *Problem-based Behavioral Science and Psychiatry*,
DOI 10.1007/978-3-319-23669-8_22

Table 22.1 *Diagnostic and Statistical Manual of Mental Disorders, Fifth Edition (DSM-5)* revision of anxiety disorders (APA 2013)

Anxiety disorders
Separation anxiety disorder
Selective mutism
Specific phobia
Social anxiety disorder (social phobia)
Panic disorder
Agoraphobia
Generalized anxiety disorder
Substance/medication-induced anxiety disorder
Anxiety disorder due to another medical condition
Other specified anxiety disorder
Unspecified anxiety disorder
Obsessive-compulsive and related disorders
Obsessive-compulsive disorder
Body dysmorphic disorder
Hoarding disorder
Trichotillomania (hair-pulling disorder)
Excoriation (skin-picking) disorder
Substance/medication-induced obsessive-compulsive and related disorder
Obsessive-compulsive and related disorder due to another medical condition
Other specified obsessive-compulsive and related disorders
Unspecified obsessive-compulsive and related disorders
Trauma- and stressor-related disorders
Reactive attachment disorder
Disinhibited social engagement disorder
Posttraumatic stress disorder
Acute stress disorder
Adjustment disorders
Other specified trauma- and stressor-related disorder
Unspecified trauma- and stressor-related disorder

Case Vignette 22.1.1 Anjelique A

Your psychiatric consult-liaison team was requested to evaluate Anjelique, a 55-year-old female who is currently admitted to the medical floor for management of chest pain. She initially presented with symptoms of tachycardia, chest discomfort that is non-tender to palpation, shortness of breath, and tachypnea. She states that she is feeling "nervous."

Please proceed with the problem-based approach using the worksheet located in the appendix of Chap. 1!

Table 22.1.1

FACTS	HYPOTHESES	INFORMATION NEEDED	LEARNING ISSUES

A differential diagnosis should include:

- Cardiac event or arrhythmia
- Substance intoxication or overdose
- Anxiety due to a general medical condition
- Panic attack or disorder
- Generalized anxiety disorder
- Hyperthyroidism
- Hypoglycemia

Case Vignette 22.1.2 Continuation

You obtain further history: Anjelique reveals that she usually has feelings of nervousness and finally decided to go to the hospital since it has worsened over the past year. She describes herself as "always being on edge" with increasing irritability. She often feels anxious for days at a time. She feels easily fatigued despite having a "stress-free job." She is having difficulty concentrating at work because she is "worried about too many things." She describes constantly planning for the future. She was encouraged by her supportive husband to get a medical checkup. He reminds her not to worry too much about things that have not happened. She denies any major recent stressors or significant life events.

Anjelique has a past medical history of diabetes mellitus type II, which is currently managed with Metformin 500 mg po daily. Her most recent hemoglobin A1C is 2.0. She has no other medical conditions. She has a surgical history of an elective C-section at 25 years old after a normal, healthy pregnancy. She denies use of cigarettes, alcohol, and other drugs. She drinks one cup of decaffeinated coffee every morning. Family psychiatric history is positive for a sister with panic disorder. There is no family history of thyroid disorders. She is currently married to her husband of 30 years and has a 25-year-old daughter. She is working as an office manager for a successful realty company.

Physical exam on initial presentation reveals—vital signs: temperature 98.7, heart rate (HR) 105, blood pressure (BP) 130/72, respiratory rate (RR)

25, O_2 saturation 99 % on room air. General appearance: a 55-year-old female who is well groomed, appearing anxious, in moderate distress. Skin: mildly diaphoretic. Cardiovascular (CV) exam: Tachycardia, with regular rhythm. No murmurs. Respiration: No accessory muscle use, tachypnea. The remainder of the physical exam is negative. An accucheck reveals glucose level of 103 mg/dL. Urine toxicology and urinalysis are negative. Complete metabolic profile, thyroid-stimulating hormone (TSH), and thyroxine (T4) have no abnormalities. Electrocardiogram (ECG) shows sinus tachycardia with non-specific T-waves. Overnight observation ruled out cardiac etiology.

STOP

Please proceed with the problem-based approach using the worksheet located in the appendix of Chap. 1!

Table 22.1.2

FACTS	HYPOTHESES	INFORMATION NEEDED	LEARNING ISSUES

Anjelique's presentation is consistent with generalized anxiety disorder (GAD). While GAD has multiple medical comorbidities, her medical work-up currently rules out medical causes of her anxiety. GAD is characterized by excessive anxiety or worry occurring most days of the week for at least 6 months. Patients with GAD are often apprehensive about the future or various situations/events. The worry is difficult to control and is associated with at least three of the following six symptoms: (1) restlessness or feeling keyed up/on edge, (2) easily fatigued, (3) difficulty concentrating or mind going blank, (4) irritability, (5) muscle tension, and (6) sleep disturbance. It is important to perform a comprehensive medical history in patients with GAD, as there may be associated medical conditions that are often seen with anxiety.

In panic disorder, panic attacks are recurrent and may occur "out of the blue." There is a fear of having more attacks causing avoidance of situations that one believes would trigger an attack. The fear is intense, abrupt, peaks within minutes, and is associated with physical discomfort (i.e., shortness of breath, choking sensation, and palpitations), feelings of unreality ("derealization") or detachment from self ("depersonalization"), or fear of losing control or dying. Panic attacks are not limited to panic disorders and are commonly present in other psychiatric disorders. While agoraphobia (intense fear/anxiety of being exposed in at least two of the following situations: public transportation, open or enclosed spaces, being in crowds, or outside of the home alone) was considered a specifier in *Diagnostic and Statistical Manual of Mental Disorders, Fourth Edition (DSM-IV)*, note that in *DSM-5*, agoraphobia is now recognized as a diagnosis separate from panic disorder to acknowledge that there are people who experience agoraphobia without panic attacks.

In the USA, the 1-year prevalence of panic disorder in adults/adolescents is approximately 2–3 %. For GAD, the prevalence is 2.9 % in adults and 0.9 % in adolescents. For both conditions, females are twice more likely than males to have these disorders.

Case Vignette 22.1.3 Continuation

You obtain further history: Anjelique mentions, "that pill calmed me down a lot." She was given one dose of Lorazepam 1 mg in the emergency department (ED). She experienced a quick relief of her anxiety soon after taking the medication. She expresses desire to start a medication that can help with her anxiety; however, she is concerned about being addicted to any pills. She asked for your advice on alternative options.

Please proceed with the problem-based approach using the worksheet located in the appendix of Chap. 1!

Table 22.1.3

FACTS	HYPOTHESES	INFORMATION NEEDED	LEARNING ISSUES

Benzodiazepines are considered "anxiolytics" which bind to the benzodiazepine receptor sites at the gamma-aminobutyric acid (GABA)-A ligand-gated chloride receptor. Benzodiazepines increase the frequency of GABA channel opening, thereby increasing the inhibitory effects of GABA. This action occurs in the amygdala-centered fear circuits, hence alleviating symptoms in anxiety disorders. Although benzodiazepines may help in acute anxiety episodes or panic attack due to the rapid onset of action, they are reserved for short-term use due to their addictive potential. If needed for long-term maintenance, some recommend that benzodiazepines need to be continued 6 months after the resolution of symptoms before tapering off slowly. The pharmacology of benzodiazepines is summarized in Table 22.2.

The first-line treatment for GAD and long-term management of panic disorder is serotonin-selective receptor inhibitors (SSRIs). SSRIs are antidepressants that act on the 5-hydroxytryptamine (5-HT) system, which are not properly regulated in GAD and panic disorder.

Table 22.2 Pharmacology of benzodiazepines

Benzodiazepine	Pharmacokinetics	Adverse effects
Alprazolam (Xanax®) *short-acting*	Hepatic metabolism via CYP3A4; half-life about 6 h but XR formulation can go up to 27 h; fast to intermediate onset	Common: Sedation, dizziness, ataxia, forgetfulness, confusion; may also cause paradoxical hyperexcitability, nervousness
Lorazepam (Ativan®) *short/mid-acting*	Renal metabolism, liver is only affected when hepatic dysfunction is severe; half-life 10–20 h; intermediate onset	Life threatening side effects: respiratory depression especially in combination with CNS depressants
Diazepam (Valium®) *long-acting*	Hepatic metabolism via CYP450; half-life 20–50 h; accumulates with multiple dosing; fast onset	Alprazolam: Associated with less sedation but has a high incidence of inter-dosing anxiety
Clonazepam (Klonopin®) *long-acting*	Hepatic metabolism via CYP3A4; half-life is up to 18–50 h; slow onset	

CYP3A4 cytochrome P450 3A4, *CNS* central nervous system

Psychotherapy is another mode of treatment that has been studied to improve anxiety. Cognitive distortions, selective attention to negative details, classical conditioning that reinforces negative views, and coping make cognitive behavioral therapy (CBT) an effective mode of treatment in patients with GAD and panic disorder. If the anxiety is related to unresolved unconscious conflicts related to parents or early caregivers (i.e., overprotective parent or early loss of parent), psychodynamic psychotherapy may have a role. Newer forms of therapy such as mindfulness-based stress reduction are also gaining popularity in addressing anxiety disorders. Studies have shown that a combination of medications and psychotherapy can be an effective treatment for anxiety disorders. The mechanism below summarizes the pathophysiology of panic/anxiety disorder, which also shows the area of action of various treatment modalities (Fig. 22.1):

Case Vignette 22.2.1 Damian D.

Damian is a 62-year-old widowed male with no past psychiatric history who presents to your outpatient psychiatric clinic and complains of "anxiety." He first noticed this 9 months ago. He reports increasing anxiety when leaving the house for groceries or doctor's appointments. He is also often worried about his family, especially when they are travelling, fearful that they may experience an accident or fall ill. Prior to this, he has been socially active and was involved in regular recreational activities with his friends. Medical history is positive for arthritis. He takes multivitamins daily and no other medications. Surgical history is positive for appendectomy in his 20s. He has his own consulting business, which is currently thriving; he works from home. He lives alone, previously lived with his daughter who moved to another state about a

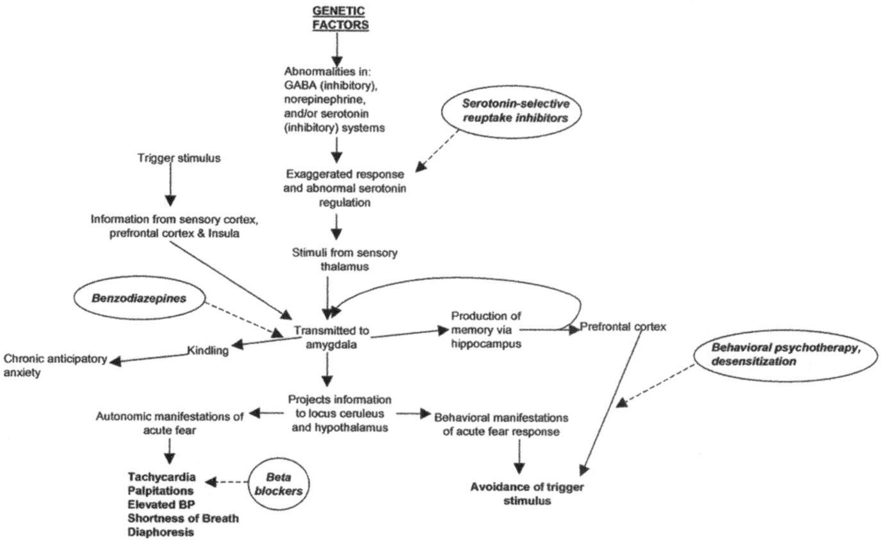

Fig. 22.1 Pathophysiology of anxiety/panic disorder. (Source: Anwati M. 2008. *Problem-Based Behavioral Science and Psychiatry, 1st Ed*)

year ago. He denies any substance use or smoking history. He does not drink coffee but drinks tea every morning. He had a recent physical exam and medical work-up from his family doctor and he was told that he is "healthy as a 20-year-old," and all his tests are negative.

Please proceed with the problem-based approach using the worksheet located in the appendix of Chap. 1!

Table 22.2.1

FACTS	HYPOTHESES	INFORMATION NEEDED	LEARNING ISSUES

Damian's current presentation lacks significant medical contributors to his anxiety. You may remember from earlier discussion that anxiety can represent various psychiatric disorders. At this point, a differential diagnosis should include:

- Generalized anxiety disorder
- Phobia or agoraphobia
- Social anxiety disorder

- Bereavement
- Depression
- Separation anxiety disorder

Case Vignette 22.2.2 Continuation

You obtain further information: Damian reveals that spending time with his daughter and his friends helped him cope when he lost his wife 10 years ago. His daughter recently married and moved out of the house into another state about a year ago. She visits him about once a month, which he appreciates very much especially that she lives 2-h flight away. He notices excessive worry that she may get into an accident when she is travelling. When she visits, he prefers to stay home with her rather than go out of the house. When she is away, Damian is hesitant to leave the house worrying that he may miss her phone call and has given up most of his outdoor activities because of this. He continues to enjoy his hobbies at home. He is happy about his daughter's marriage and new life. He denies feeling depressed, just "severely anxious" and hopes to overcome his anxiety and return to his normal activities.

Please proceed with the problem-based approach using the worksheet located in the appendix of Chap. 1!

Table 22.2.2

FACTS	HYPOTHESES	INFORMATION NEEDED	LEARNING ISSUES

Social anxiety disorder or social phobia is when one experiences excessive anxiety and fear of situations that call for social interactions. One may avoid situations where he/she may be judged by others. A prominent belief is that others may reject or humiliate him/her. As a result, there is a tendency to avoid situations that may cause fear of being negatively evaluated by others. This description is not consistent with Jon's presentation.

Damian's symptoms are suggestive of the diagnosis of separation anxiety disorder. In *DSM-5,* this diagnosis was moved from the section "Disorders Usually First Diagnosed in Infancy, Childhood, or Adolescence" in order to recognize it as an anxiety disorder that may also have an adult onset. In the USA, the 12-month prevalence of separation anxiety disorder is 0.9–1.9 % in adults, 1.6 % in adolescents, and about 4 % in children. About half of adult cases of separation anxiety have onset in childhood; separation anxiety in children or spouses is common. In children, studies have shown genetic heritability of separation anxiety disorder.

The diagnostic feature of separation anxiety disorder is a "developmentally inappropriate and excessive fear/anxiety concerning separation from attachment figures." This distinguishes this diagnosis from other anxiety disorders. The duration of fear/anxiety/avoidant behaviors must be at least 4 weeks in children/adolescents and at least 6 months in adults. Symptoms must include at least three of the following: recurrent/excessive distress when anticipating/experiencing separation from attachment figures, persistent/excessive worry about losing or harm to attachment figure or events that may cause separation from attachment figure, reluctance to go out due to separation or being alone (in children, school refusal is common), repeated nightmares about the separation, or repeated complaints of physical symptoms when separation is anticipated.

Like GAD and panic disorder, separation anxiety along with other anxiety disorders is treated with psychotherapy with or without the use of medications (antidepressants, anxiolytics such as benzodiazepines, sometimes atypical antipsychotics).

Case Vignette 22.3.1 Jon

Jon is a 31-year-old male who was referred to your outpatient psychiatric clinic by his primary care physician (PCP) for anxiety. He recently quit his work due to severe anxiety. He worked as a pizza deliveryman and describes having habits that interfere with his job tasks. He has had multiple minor car accidents (bumper scratches, rear-ending other cars) and driving tickets, explains that during his deliveries, his mind has been preoccupied with counting items on the road such as cars, signs, and light posts. He fears that if he does not count, he will encounter a problem on his delivery. He notes that he has had fascination with counting since he was young; however, it has now begun to affect his work.

Please proceed with the problem-based approach using the worksheet located in the appendix of Chap. 1!

Table 22.3.1

FACTS	HYPOTHESES	INFORMATION NEEDED	LEARNING ISSUES

Jon's symptoms suggest a diagnosis of obsessive-compulsive disorder (OCD). *Obsessions* are repetitive/persistent, intrusive thoughts, images, or urges that one attempts to ignore or neutralize with another thought or by performing an action. Such actions are called *compulsions,* which are repetitive behaviors (e.g., checking) or mental acts (e.g., counting) that one feels are necessary to reduce the distress from the obsessions. Common themes of obsession/compulsions include: contamination/cleaning, symmetry, taboo thoughts, and harm. Avoidant behaviors to minimize triggers for obsessions and compulsions are common. At times, individuals with OCD feel that a compulsion is necessary in order to prevent harm related to the obsession. There is a severe anxiety, discomfort, or nagging feeling of incompleteness if rituals are not performed. The Yale-Brown Obsessive Compulsive Scale (Y-BOCS) is a common tool used in identifying symptoms. In OCD, one is usually aware that the obsessions and compulsions are excessive and unreasonable; they are time-consuming and may cause significant impairment in functioning. In *DSM-5,* the diagnosis of OCD is further specified as having good or fair insight, poor insight, absent insight/delusional beliefs, or tic related. Most patients with OCD are encountered in primary care setting (APA 2013).

The 12-month prevalence of OCD in the USA is 1.2%, with a slightly higher rate in female adults than males; in childhood, prevalence is higher in males than females. The course of OCD can be episodic and if untreated, may be chronic. It is highly comorbid with anxiety and mood disorders. Individuals with OCD are also more likely to exhibit other OCD-related disorders (body-dysmorphic disorder, trichotillomania, and excoriation disorder). OCD may also be associated with schizophrenia spectrum of illness, Tourette's disorder, and eating disorders.

Neuroimaging studies reveal that there is hyperactivity in the ventral cognitive loop in the brain, which includes the orbitofrontal cortex, the caudate nucleus, and the dorsomedial thalamus. A mechanistic diagram of OCD pathophysiology is presented below (Fig. 22.2a, b):

In children, OCD may present as a manifestation of pediatric autoimmune neuropsychiatric disorders associated with streptococcal infections (PANDAS). This condition may be similar in mechanism to other nonsuppurative post-group A beta hemolytic streptococcal (GABHS) complications such as rheumatic fever. In addition to the presence of OCD and/or tic disorder, other diagnostic features of PANDAS include pediatric onset, abrupt onset with episodic course of symptom severity, related GABHS infections, and associated neurological abnormalities. With prompt treatment of the infection, the psychiatric symptoms (e.g., OCD, anxiety, and tic) may resolve as quickly as in 2 weeks.

Case Vignette 22.3.2 Continuation

You obtain further information: Jon relays that he had multiple repetitive behaviors that began in his teenage years, including washing his hands multiple times a day for at least 5 min at a time; he estimates doing this about 15–20 times a day. He fears that he will contract a disease or cause others to fall ill if he does not wash his hands for a long time. Because of this and other ritualistic behaviors, he saw a psychotherapist for about 3 months while he was in college. He was able to decrease some of his behaviors since then; however, he notices that since his recent stress, they have begun to occur

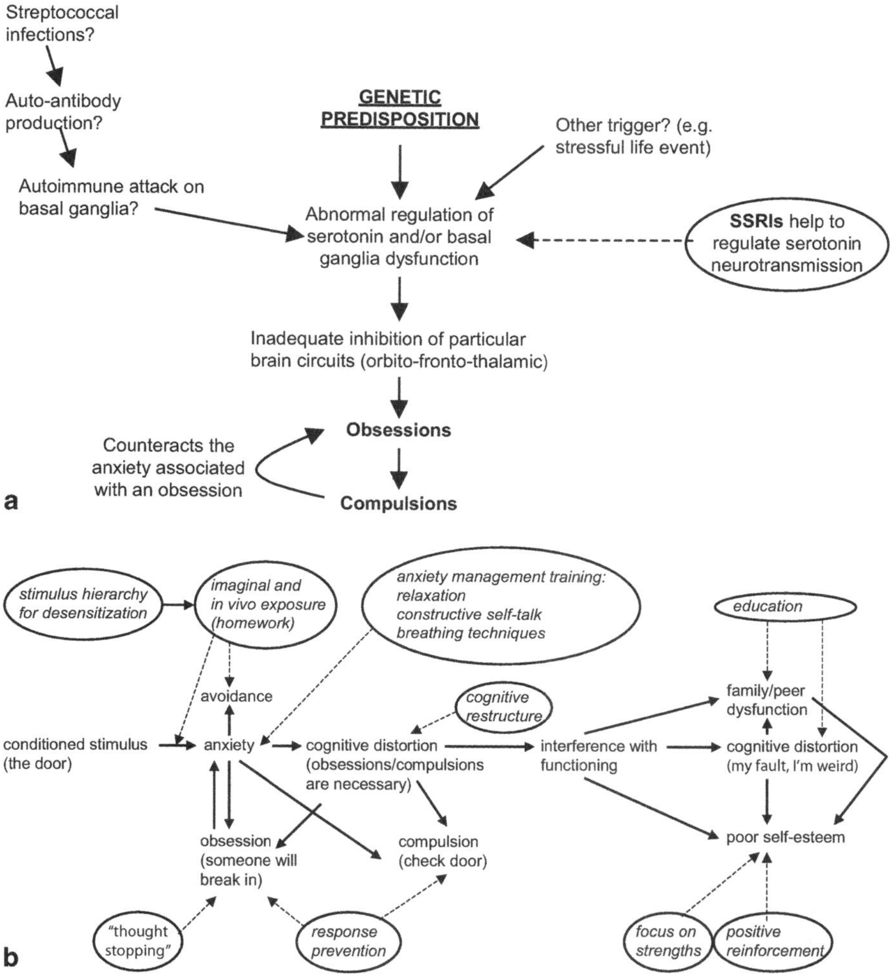

Fig. 22.2 Pathophysiology of obsessive-compulsive disorder *(OCD)*, from both a neurobiologic (**a**) and psychosocial (**b**) perspective. (Source: Anwati M. 2008. *Problem-Based Behavioral Science and Psychiatry, 1st Ed*)

more often. Jon denies any other psychiatric or medical history. No one in his family has ever been diagnosed with a psychiatric illness; however, he mentions that his mother has an unusual "hoarding behavior." They also share the habit of checking the house doors multiple times to ensure they are locked. Jon denies any use of alcohol or other drugs. His physical exam, including recent basic labs, is unremarkable.

Please proceed with the problem-based approach using the worksheet located in the appendix of Chap. 1!

Table 22.3.2

FACTS	HYPOTHESES	INFORMATION NEEDED	LEARNING ISSUES

A combination of pharmacotherapy and psychotherapy is recommended for the treatment of OCD. If the symptoms are mild, psychotherapy alone may be sufficient. First-line pharmacologic treatment of OCD includes serotonin-reuptake inhibitors (SSRIs), including clomipramine, paroxetine, sertraline, fluoxetine, and citalopram; for OCD, high doses of SSRIs are often required. When a patient achieves a good treatment response with medication, it is recommended for pharmacotherapy to continue for 12–18 months before attempting to discontinue medication.

Case Vignette 22.3.3 Continuation

Jon admits feeling severely stressed since he has been unemployed. Since then, he noticed an increased urge to check the news online every time he comes home, to see if there were any hit-and-run accidents in his area because of the fear that he caused a motor vehicle accident (i.e., hit a pedestrian) on the way home. At times, he could spend up to 2 h searching for evidence that he did not cause harm to anyone. This has obviously caused him severe distress. Jon feels very frustrated; he knows that his thoughts are irrational but cannot resist compulsively checking the news. He worries that medications may not be enough to address his concerns and asks for a referral to resume psychotherapy.

Please proceed with the problem-based approach using the worksheet located in the appendix of Chap. 1!

Table 22.3.3

FACTS	HYPOTHESES	INFORMATION NEEDED	LEARNING ISSUES

Cognitive and behavioral therapies are common treatment modalities for OCD. Exposure and response prevention (ERP) therapy is a specific type of behavior therapy that is the first-line of treatment for OCD, with good response as monotherapy or in combination with medications. ERP involves a hierarchal inventory of the obsessions and compulsions, and individuals are gradually exposed from the least anxiety-provoking to the most anxiety-provoking stimuli that trigger their OCD symptoms. Avoiding exposure to the stimuli (such as when one gives in to the compulsion or neutralizing act), although initially reducing acute distress, causes one to be hypersensitive to the triggers of anxiety and essentially further feeds the obsession-compulsion cycle. In ERP, individuals learn ways to cope with the anxiety brought upon by the obsessions while resisting the compulsions.

Case Vignette 22.4.1 Zinnia Z.

Zinnia is a 22-year-old graduate student who presents to your outpatient clinic complaining of difficulty with sleep. She has difficulty with sleep onset and has broken sleep, often wakes up from bad dreams most nights of the week with trouble getting back to sleep. She has done well in school but recently finds it difficult to concentrate on finishing her schoolwork. She was doing well up until the beginning of the last semester 3 months ago when she failed to submit her projects on time and had to ask for due date extensions. Her PCP has prescribed her Ambien, but she discontinued this due to one episode of sleepwalking.

STOP

Please proceed with the problem-based approach using the worksheet located in the appendix of Chap. 1!

Table 22.4.1

FACTS	HYPOTHESES	INFORMATION NEEDED	LEARNING ISSUES

At this point, the differential information should include:

- Primary insomnia
- Caffeine or substance-induced disorder
- Adjustment disorder (i.e., graduate school)
- PTSD
- Acute stress disorder

- Anxiety due to a general medical condition (i.e., hyperthyroidism)
- Other anxiety disorder
- Depression

Case Vignette 22.4.2 Continuation

You obtain further information: Zinnia has no past psychiatric history or family history of anxiety, depression, or suicide. She describes a good childhood; she enjoys learning and has always done well in school. She currently lives alone in her own apartment and denies any substance use. She has no known medical condition and takes no medications. Past medical history is positive for a broken wrist after a car accident about 9 months ago. She was a passenger involved in a motor vehicle accident, where the car flipped after the driver lost control causing her injury. She mentions she eventually returned to an active social life, however, notices that she often gets anxious when riding in a car with others. Since the accident, she tries to avoid going to events that require driving. If she has to go somewhere far, she prefers to drive herself than let others drive while she is a passenger. She also notes that she is often "hyper-alert" when driving.

STOP

Please proceed with the problem-based approach using the worksheet located in the appendix of Chap. 1!

Table 22.4.2

FACTS	HYPOTHESES	INFORMATION NEEDED	LEARNING ISSUES

Zinnia's symptoms are related to the traumatic experience of the motor vehicle accident and her symptoms are consistent with the diagnosis of PTSD. In PTSD, there is exposure to death (actual or threatened), serious injury, or sexual violence in one of the following ways: direct experience, as a witness, learning that the event occurred to a close family member or friend, or repeated/extreme exposure to details of event such as those experienced by first responders (e.g., police officers). There are four major symptom clusters in PTSD: reexperiencing the event (e.g., flashbacks), heightened arousal (e.g., sleep disturbance or hypervigilance), avoidance (e.g., avoiding memories or triggers), and negative thoughts and mood/feelings (e.g., estrangement or decreased interest in activities). Some individuals also experience feelings of detachment ("depersonalization") or unreality of surroundings ("derealization"). In Zinnia's case, the diagnosis of PTSD is specified to have "delayed expression" since at least 6 months have passed before the onset of symptoms. A diagnosis of acute stress disorder is appropriate if the symptoms occur and resolve within 1 month of the traumatic event. The diagnostic criteria for PTSD in children have unique features such as the presence of "PTSD preschool subtype" to specify diagnosis in children under 6 years old. There are various screening tools such as the "Trauma History Questionnaire (THQ)" and "PTSD Checklist" that may help in diagnosing PTSD.

The 12-month prevalence of PTSD in adults is 3.5 %; rates in children are varied due to the different developmental stages. PTSD rates are higher in veterans and individuals whose occupations involve risk of exposure to traumatic events (e.g., firefighters). The prevalence and duration of PTSD is higher in female adults than males. Cultural considerations are important in understanding PTSD, as studies have shown variable rates across ethnicities (e.g., higher rates in Latinos and lower rates in Asian Americans compared to non-Latino whites). The risk and prognosis of PTSD is contributed by pretraumatic factors (e.g., childhood temperamental problems, exposure to prior trauma), peritraumatic factors (e.g., perceived life threat or severity of trauma), and posttraumatic factors (e.g., coping skills, social support). Careful assessment of suicide risk and safety is imperative in PTSD just as in other psychiatric disorders.

The areas of the brain implicated in PTSD include the amygdala, hippocampus, and prefrontal cortex; traumatic stress is associated with functional and possible structural changes in these areas. There are no conclusive data regarding heritability of PTSD. What is clear is that there is an abnormal noradrenergic activity in individuals with this disorder (e.g., studies showing high levels of urine norepinephrine in Vietnam War veterans). PTSD causes an increased sympathetic nervous system and cortisol response. Figure 22.3 illustrates the suggested pathophysiology of PTSD.

Case Vignette 22.4.3 Continuation

Zinnia proceeded to describe further details of the accident. She also realized that her nightmares are usually related to the accident and her injury. You explain that her symptoms are consistent with PTSD and discussed the treatment options. She was open to starting medications and also requested a referral for psychotherapy. In addition, you discussed immediate interventions to address her sleep by educating her about good sleep hygiene. You also explained the prognosis of her condition. She was grateful after learning that there is hope for her condition and looks forward to performing well in academics once again.

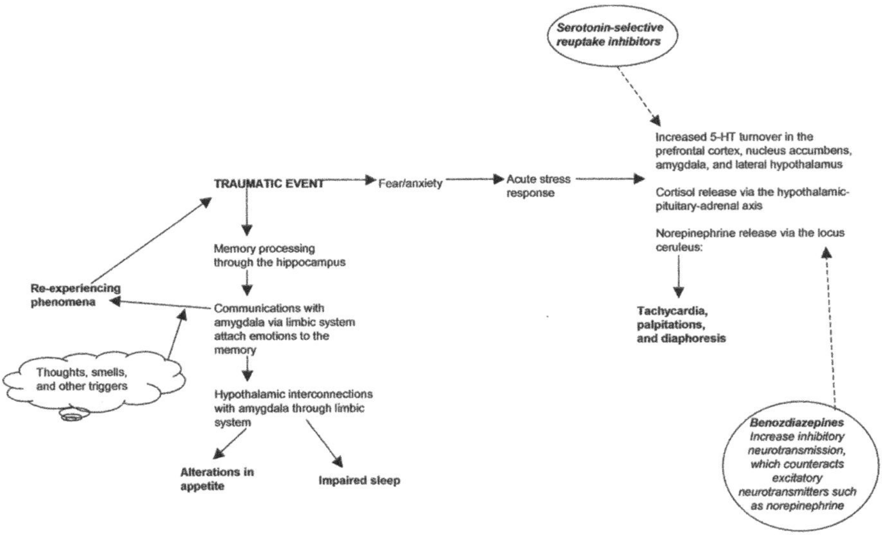

Fig. 22.3 Pathophysiology of posttraumatic stress disorder *(PTSD)*. (Source: Anwati M. 2008. *Problem-Based Behavioral Science and Psychiatry, 1st Ed*)

	Please proceed with the problem-based approach using the worksheet located in the appendix of Chap. 1!

Table 22.4.3

FACTS	HYPOTHESES	INFORMATION NEEDED	LEARNING ISSUES

Antidepressants such as SSRIs and Venlafaxine (a serotonin-norepinephrine reuptake inhibitor) are most commonly used as first-line pharmacotherapy of PTSD. Benzodiazepines may also be used to treat acute symptoms, such as in anxiety disorders; however, it should be used in caution as some studies suggest that it may interfere with learning strategies to cope with trauma. Other medications used include mirtazapine, tricyclic antidepressants, monoamine oxidase inhibitors, antipsychotics, and anticonvulsants, prazosin.

Psychotherapy plays an important role in the treatment of PTSD in both adults and children. In adults, CBT is considered the first-line mode of therapy. Just like in the previous case of OCD, this form of therapy focuses on reframing cognitive distortions related to negative self-perception and safety by processing emotions related to the trauma and decreasing avoidant behaviors. The behavioral part of the therapy may also include exposure and response prevention in addition to activities planning. Specific forms of CBT used in PTSD include prolonged exposure therapy and cognitive processing therapy. Other forms of therapy used are eye movement desensitization and reprocessing (EMDR). Strong social support is very important for individuals with PTSD, especially soon after the trauma.

22.1 Review Questions

1. The most common type of psychotherapy used for treatment of anxiety disorders, OCD, and PTSD is:
   a. Psychodynamic psychotherapy
   b. Psychoanalysis
   c. Cognitive-behavioral therapy
   d. Motivational interview
   e. Hypnosis
2. Which of the following statements is true about acute stress disorder?
   a. The trauma occurred within 1 month of the onset of symptoms
   b. The symptoms resolve within 1 month from the traumatic event
   c. Both a and b
3. Which of the following disorders is not included in the obsessive-compulsive and related disorders category?
   a. Body dysmorphic disorder
   b. Separation anxiety disorder
   c. Hoarding disorder
   d. Trichotillomania
   e. Excoriation disorder
4. Which of the following benzodiazepine-onset of action pair is correct:
   a. Lorazepam-slow onset
   b. Diazepam-slow onset
   c. Clonazepam-slow onset
   d. Alprazolam-intermediate onset
   e. Alprazolam-fast onset
5. The differential diagnosis of a panic attack may include:
   a. Myocardial infarction
   b. Substance-induced reaction
   c. Generalized anxiety disorder
   d. Adjustment disorder
   e. All of the above

Appendix A: Tables with Possible Answers to the Vignettes

Case Vignette 22.1: Anjelique A.

Table 22.1.1

Facts	Hypotheses	Information needed	Learning issues
55-year-old female	Cause may be medical or psychiatric	What pertinent medical history may be contributing to current symptoms?	What is the differential diagnosis for chest pain?
Physical symptoms: chest pain nontender to palpation, tachycardia, tachypnea, dyspnea		What was the precipitating event?	What are the signs and symptoms of a panic attack?
Feeling nervous			

Table 22.1.2

Facts	Hypotheses	Information needed	Learning issues
Symptom duration at least 1 year	Anjelique may have had a panic attack; intensity of worries may be related to an anxiety disorder	How does she cope with her panic/anxiety?	What psychiatric disorders are associated with panic attack?
Prominent anxiety and worry despite lack of stressful situations	She may be genetically predisposed to mental illness given positive family history, specifically; she may be suffering from an anxiety disorder like her sister	Is she compliant with her medications?	
Medical conditions are well managed			What are the features of an anxiety disorder?
Hospitalized for cardiac observation, which was essentially negative?			What medical comorbidities are associated with anxiety disorders?

Table 22.1.3

Facts	Hypotheses	Information needed	Learning issues
Lorazepam caused quick relief	Benzodiazepine relieves anxiety but may be addictive	Is there any history that may suggest risk for addiction	What are the pertinent properties of benzodiazepines? (i.e., mechanism, onset of action)
			Which benzodiazepines have low/high addictive properties?

Case Vignette 22.2: Damian D.

Table 22.2.1

Facts	Hypotheses	Information needed	Learning issues
62-year-old male, widowed, no past psychiatric history	Damian may be suffering from an anxiety disorder.Since he has been well up until several months ago, there may have been a precipitating event that caused his current symptoms	What significant life changes has Damian experienced lately?	What is agoraphobia?
Has arthritis but generally healthy		When did his wife pass away?	What are possible causes of Damian's anxiety?
Used to live with daughter, now lives alone		Does he continue to enjoy his hobbies?	
Anxiety is worsening, interfering with responsibilities involving leaving the house		What is preventing him from leaving the house?	
Worries about family			

Table 22.2.2

Facts	Hypotheses	Information needed	Learning issues
Onset of symptoms was shortly after his daughter left the house	Damian has a strong social support and expresses good motivation to transcend his symptoms; he may be able to overcome his symptoms with psychotherapy alone	What helped him in the past when he experienced a "loss?"	What treatment is available to address separation anxiety in adults?
No depression			

Case Vignette 22.3: Jon

Table 22.3.1

Facts	Hypotheses	Information needed	Learning issues
31-year-old male with anxiety	Jon may be suffering from OCD and likely has other related thoughts or behaviors that may be causing distress	What other obsessions does Jon have?	What are the features of OCD?
Preoccupation with counting		Are there other compulsive behaviors associated with his thoughts?	How do "obsessions" and "compulsions" differ from each other?
Serious consequences due to current symptoms: lost job, driving tickets, car accidents		Did he have recurrent infections as a child?	What medical conditions may be associated with OCD?
		Is there family history of mental illness?	

OCD obsessive-compulsive disorder

Table 22.3.2

Facts	Hypotheses	Information needed	Learning issues
Jon had multiple ritualistic/repetitive behaviors that began in his teenage years	Psychotherapy was effective in Jon's OCD-related behaviors in the past and may be helpful again	Any allergies to medications?	What medications are indicated in treatment of OCD?
Ritualistic/repetitive behaviors occupied over 1 h per day	He may have been genetically predisposed to psychiatric condition as evidenced by a positive family history of similar symptoms	Is Jon willing to take medications or resume therapy?	Is there a genetic predisposition to OCD?
Psychotherapy was effective in decreasing symptoms		What other obsessions or compulsions has Jon experienced since he noticed worsening of his symptoms?	
Behaviors recurred since stress level increased			
Jon's mother exhibited "hoarding behavior"			
No substances or acute medical issues			

OCD obsessive-compulsive disorder

Table 22.3.3

Facts	Hypotheses	Information needed	Learning issues
Obsessions include fear that he may have caused harm to others	Heightened stress level from recent life changes (unemployment) may have contributed to exacerbation of OCD symptoms	How is Jon coping with his condition now?	What is the prognosis of OCD?
Compulsions include checking the news in search for evidence		Is he willing to commit time and effort in engaging in psychotherapy to help alleviate his symptoms?	Are there specific modes of therapy that are helpful in OCD?
Significant distress in obsessions and significant amount of time spent in compulsions			

OCD obsessive-compulsive disorder

Case Vignette 22.4: Zinnia Z.

Table 22.4.1

Facts	Hypotheses	Information needed	Learning issues
22-year-old female	Symptoms may be related to a primary sleep disorder or stress related	Was there any stress or particular situation related to onset of symptoms?	What are possible causes of sleep problems?
Sleep problems: onset, frequent awakening, nightmares		How is her sleep hygiene?	What conditions may be associated with nightmares?
Problems with concentration		Does she use any caffeine or stimulants?	What conditions may be associated with concentration problems?
			What are other side effects of sleep aids aside from sleepwalking?

Table 22.4.2

Facts	Hypotheses	Information needed	Learning issues
No personal or family psychiatric history	Recent car accident may be causing trauma-related stress	Has she sought any treatment right after the accident?	What are the features of PTSD?
Car accident in the recent past caused physical injury		Does she have intrusive memories of her trauma?	How does PTSD differ from acute stress disorder?
Anxiety associated with driving			

PSTD posttraumatic stress disorder

Table 22.4.3

Facts	Hypotheses	Information needed	Learning issues
Trauma experienced was the car accident, which currently continues to manifest in acute symptoms	Medications and psychotherapy may help relieve PTSD symptoms	Does she have any allergies to medications?	What mode of psychotherapy is commonly used in PTSD?

PSTD posttraumatic stress disorder

Appendix B: Answers to Review Questions

1. c, 2. c, 3. b, 4. c and e, 5. e

References

American Psychiatric Association. (2013). *Diagnostic and statistical manual of mental disorders* (5th ed.). Arlington: American Psychiatric Association.

Hales, R. E., Yudofsky, S. C., Roberts, L. W. (2014). *The American psychiatric publishing textbook of psychiatry* (6th ed.). Arlington: American Psychiatric Association.

Massachusetts General Hospital and McLean Hospitals Residents and Faculties. (2010). *The Massachusetts General Hospital/McLean Hospital residency handbook of psychiatry*. Philadelphia: Lippincott Williams & Wilkins.

Sadock, B. J., Sadock, V. A., Ruiz, P. (2009). Anxiety disorders. In *Kaplan and Sadock's comprehensive textbook of psychiatry*. (9th ed., pp. 1839–1926). Philadelphia: Lippincott Williams & Wilkins.

Stahl, S. (2014). *Prescriber's guide, Stahl's essential psychopharmacology* (5th ed.). New York: Cambridge University Press.

Chapter 23
Somatic Symptom and Related Disorders

Catherine McCarthy and Jason Reinhardt

> *Trying to suppress or eradicate symptoms on the physical level can be extremely important, but there's more to healing than that; dealing with psychological, emotional and spiritual issues involved in treating sickness is equally important.*
>
> Marianne Williamson

The prominence of somatic symptoms associated with significant clinical distress and functional impairment is the hallmark of illness within the class of disorders called somatic symptom and related disorders (American Psychiatric Association 2013). Patients suffering from these conditions more commonly present in primary care or acute care settings (American Psychiatric Association 2013). It is only after initially presenting in this setting that they are able to receive necessary psychiatric mental health support (American Psychiatric Association 2013). Somatic symptom disorder, illness anxiety disorder, conversion disorder(functional neurological symptom disorder), psychological factors affecting other medical conditions, factitious disorder, other specified somatic symptom and related disorders, and unspecified somatic symptom and related disorders belong to this diagnostic class. Due to the diagnostic and treatment challenge that these disorders present, physician awareness becomes crucial for early diagnosis.

C. McCarthy (✉)
Department of Family and Community Medicine, University of Nevada School of Medicine, 123 17th Street, Reno, NV 89557, USA
e-mail: Mccarthy@medicine.nevada.edu

J. Reinhardt
Department of Psychiatry, University of Nevada School of Medicine, Mailstop 0354, Reno, NV 89557, USA
e-mail: jreinhardt@medicine.nevada.edu

D. Alicata et al. (eds.), *Problem-based Behavioral Science and Psychiatry*,
DOI 10.1007/978-3-319-23669-8_23

23.1 Objectives

At the end of the chapter the reader will be able to:

1. Apply the Diagnostic and Statistical Manual of Mental Disorders, 5th Edition (DSM-5) criteria for somatic symptom and related disorders to clinical vignettes

Vignette 23.1.1 Presenting Situation: Janelle Miller
At 11 a.m. on Thanksgiving Day, Janelle Miller, a 28-year-old married white woman, presents to the emergency department where you are on duty. Her chief complaint is bilateral leg paralysis. Mrs. Miller states she had no previous health problems. She lives with her husband and two children (3 and 5 years old). Mrs. Miller was preparing Thanksgiving Day dinner when she decided to sit down. When she tried to get up, she could not use her legs. The patient then called her husband, and he came to her aid. He brought her to the emergency department for further evaluation. The patient was concerned that dinner would not be ready for the family and friends that are visiting later that evening.

2. Identify the elements of a complex medical history that are suggestive of somatic symptom and related disorders
3. Describe treatment strategies for patients with somatic symptom and related disorders

Please proceed with the problem-based approach using the worksheet located in the appendix of Chap. 1!

Table 23.1.1

FACTS	HYPOTHESES	INFORMATION NEEDED	LEARNING ISSUES

Case 23.1.2 Continuation

Mrs. Miller denies any significant past medical history. She had two healthy pregnancies and normal vaginal deliveries. She sees her primary care physician yearly for physical exams which have always been normal.

She denies any past psychiatric history and appears a bit upset with this area of questioning. She had never been hospitalized in a psychiatric hospital. She had never attempted suicide. She had never been diagnosed with a psychiatric illness.

Mrs. Miller states that she drinks a glass of wine a couple times a year on special occasions. She denied any drinking recently as well as the use of any illicit drugs. She does not use any tobacco products.

Social History: Mrs. Miller has two older brothers who are both healthy. She was raised by both parents, and she described her childhood as good. As early as 6 years of age she was expected to help with household chores because both her parents had demanding careers. Starting at the age of 14 she was responsible for making dinner for her older brothers, including meal planning, preparing, and cleanup. Mrs. Miller graduated high school and had a variety of jobs including a waitress and housekeeper in the local hotel industry. She is currently unemployed and is happy to stay at home with her young children. She describes herself as happily married; she feels safe in her marriage and denies any abuse. She has been married for 6 years. Her husband is a long-distance truck driver, and Mrs. Miller is often alone with her children for up to a week at a time.

STOP

Please proceed with the problem-based approach using the worksheet located in the appendix of Chap. 1!

Table 23.1.2

FACTS	HYPOTHESES	INFORMATION NEEDED	LEARNING ISSUES

23.2 Learning Issues

Mrs. Miller's case highlights several common aspects of conversion disorder (functional neurological symptom disorder; American Psychiatric Association 2013). This is a disorder in which a patient may present with one or more symptoms of various types. These include motor symptoms such as weakness or paralysis; gait abnormalities; tremor or dystonic movements; and abnormal limb posturing. Sensory symptoms may include altered, diminished or absent skin sensation, vision, or hearing. The precise prevalence of conversion disorder (functional neurological symptom disorder) is unknown. The incidence of individual persistent conversion symptoms is reported in the DMS-5 as an estimated two to five cases per 100,000 per year and is two to three times more common in females (American Psychiatric Association 2013).

Case 23.1.3 Continuation

Mrs. Miller's physical exam reveals:

Vitals: Heart Rate (HR) 74, Blood Pressure (BP) 110/72, RR: 14, temp 98.4

General: Mrs. Miller is resting comfortably in her hospital bed. She has good hygiene and appears to be comfortable and in no distress.

Neurological: Mrs. Miller has bilateral leg paralysis. She cannot voluntarily move her legs when asked by the examiner or bear any weight when asked to stand. Mrs. Miller also lacks pin prick sensation up to her waist but has full sensation above her waist. Mrs. Miller's patellar and Achilles reflexes were 2+ bilaterally. Passive movement of her legs by the examiner reveals a ratchet-like weakness. The rest of Mrs. Miller's physical exam is unremarkable.

Mental Status Exam: Mrs. Miller is quite calm with regard to her paralysis and appears more concerned about her husband being able to finish dinner. She sits up during the interview. She describes her mood as "worried." Her affect is bright and seemed incongruent with her current physical symptoms. Mrs. Miller denies any thoughts of harming herself or others. She denies any auditory hallucinations or paranoid thoughts. She exhibits no signs of delusional systems. Mrs. Miller is alert and oriented and has no significant gaps in short, immediate, or long-term memory. She seems to have average intelligence, and she has no deficits in concentration or attention. Judgment and insight both appear good.

Complete Blood Count (CBC) and chemistry panel were all within normal limits.

MRI of brain was unremarkable, without evidence of acute pathology.

Please proceed with the problem-based approach using the worksheet located in the appendix of Chap. 1!

Table 23.1.3

FACTS	HYPOTHESES	INFORMATION NEEDED	LEARNING ISSUES

23.3 Learning Issues

Though it can be diagnosed at any age, conversion disorder is more common in adolescents and young adults (American Psychiatric Association 2013). Mrs. Miller also represented a typical presentation because she had specific stressors in her life due to holiday preparations and a lack of support in her social environment. This stress ultimately manifested itself as lower extremity paralysis. The diagnosis also requires that the symptoms cannot be better explained by neurological disease and should not be made simply because testing is unremarkable or because the symptoms seem "bizarre." There must be clinical findings that show clear evidence of incompatibility between symptoms and recognized neurological or medical conditions, as well as clinically significant distress in social, occupational, or other important areas of functioning. In addition to a complete medical work-up, it is important to obtain a thorough social history of a patient you suspect of having conversion disorder (functional neurological symptom disorder).

As with Mrs. Miller, the diagnosis does not require the judgment that the symptoms are not intentionally produced, as this is often not reliably determined.

In this vignette, medical testing ruled out stroke, malignancy, or other apparent pathology that might account for the paralysis in Mrs. Miller's presentation. The differential diagnosis for conversion disorder (functional neurological symptom disorder) includes potentially treatable medical conditions such as multiple sclerosis or intracranial mass, as well as other mental disorders comprising factitious disorder and malingering, dissociative disorders, body dysmorphic disorders, depressive disorders, and anxiety disorders.

Case 23.1.4 Conclusion
Mrs. Miller is admitted to the hospital for observation. In the hospital, Mrs. Miller receives Lorazepam (2 mg by mouth) to treat hypothesized underlying anxiety. She is praised when she tries to move her legs and strongly encouraged when any sign of progress is made. No physical cause for the paralysis is identified. Mrs. Miller has some toe movements before leaving the hospital but is discharged in a wheel chair.

Over the next few weeks, her husband took time off of work and was able to help her with all the household chores. Mrs. Miller slowly regained function of both her legs. Several months later with follow-up at her family doctor, she had a normal neurological exam.

23.4 Learning Issues

Consequently, as her husband took time off of work and helped her, her psychological needs were met. Slowly, the symptoms of the disorder resolved on their own with conservative management.

In clinical practice, conversion disorder (functional neurological symptom disorder) may be more difficult to recognize. Because this disorder manifests itself with one or more symptoms of various types, requiring altered voluntary motor and sensory function for diagnosis, any deficit may suggest a neurological or other general medical condition.

Unfortunately, not much is known about the mechanism of action of conversion disorder (functional neurological symptom disorder) or how to treat it (Allin et al. 2005). Physicians should avoid communicating a judgmental attitude. Collaboration with education is key at every point in management, and patients should be actively involved in setting treatment goals (Croicu et al. 2014). It is best to provide evidence-based treatment for underlying anxiety or depression as well as address the believed psychological stress that precipitated this episode (Croicu et al. 2014, Table 23.1).

Vignette 23.2.1 Lorraine Chun: Presenting Situation
You are a psychiatrist on the consult-liaison service of a teaching hospital. You were asked to evaluate Lorraine Chun, a 44-year-old woman with seven previous hospital admissions over the past 3 years. Ms. Chun was admitted to the hospital last night for intractable back pain that could not be managed as an outpatient. Ms. Chun has gone to the emergency department ten times over the past 3 months, and the ER staff decided to admit her for further evaluation. Ms. Chun was friendly but slightly annoyed when she realized a psychiatrist was sent to see her. "What—you people think this is all in my head?"

Table 23.1 Conversion disorder

Conversion disorder (functional neurological symptom disorder)		
Diagnostic criteria	Differential diagnosis	Treatment and management
One or more symptoms of altered voluntary motor or sensory function	Medical evaluation aimed at ruling out potential etiologies of presenting symptoms	Optimizing patient rapport is important during management and treatment
Clinical findings provide evidence of incompatibility between the symptom and recognized neurological or medical conditions	Be cognizant of co-occurring neurological and mental disorders	Recognize and treat underlying anxiety and depression with evidence-based interventions
The symptom or deficit is not better explained by another medical or mental disorder		Follow-up evaluation of presenting symptoms is important with support and intervention as indicated
The symptom or deficit causes clinically significant distress or impairment in social, occupational, or other important areas of functioning		

Please proceed with the problem-based approach using the worksheet located in the appendix of Chap. 1!

Table 23.2.1

FACTS	HYPOTHESES	INFORMATION NEEDED	LEARNING ISSUES

Case 23.2.2 Continuation

After building rapport, Ms. Chun is willing to discuss her history: "So you can understand I'm not crazy." Ms. Chun is single and lives with her mother and father. Both of her parents are elderly but in fairly good health. For as long as she can remember, Ms. Chun has been in poor health. As a teenager, she remembered having to go to the school nurse and her family doctor for severe abdominal pain on a regular basis. Though they could never find a cause of her pain, she missed many days of school and barely graduated high school.

She has worked at various locations as a cashier and administrative assistant. However, she feels that her multiple illnesses have held her back and made working difficult. During her twenties, patient experienced excessive menstrual bleeding. At the age of 31, she had a total hysterectomy. Since then, Ms. Chun has had four more surgeries in an effort to reduce adhesions and decrease chronic abdominal pain. She states none of the surgeries have really helped her and "new symptoms come up all the time."

Ms. Chun states that things really got bad in her thirties after she was rear ended by a car at a stop light. The car was only going around 5 mph but must have hit her "just right." She states that she had some "scans" that showed some disc degeneration. Ms. Chun also complains of numbness and tingling in her hands. Since then she has had two back surgeries. She was 37 when she received her last back surgery. Ms. Chun states the pain over the past year has been really bad and resists medications. She expects to "go under the knife again."

When asked about her living situation, Ms. Chun states she is the only daughter and has always lived with her parents because of her health problems. She feels her parents are very understanding and supportive. Ms. Chun has never been in a relationship. She states she just never has had any desire to have sex and so she figured there was not much point in having a boyfriend.

Currently, Ms. Chun complains of severe back pain that is not being relieved by narcotics. She states she also has abdominal pain that is diffuse. She also has been having severe headaches that could "kill a horse." She reports general aches and pains in all her joints, which are a little better with ibuprofen. More recently, she has noticed a difficulty with her balance. She said, "I just don't feel right when I'm walking, like my balance is off."

STOP

Please proceed with the problem-based approach using the worksheet located in the appendix of Chap. 1!

Table 23.2.2

FACTS	HYPOTHESES	INFORMATION NEEDED	LEARNING ISSUES

Case 23.2.3 Continuation

Ms. Chun's physical exam reveals:

- Vitals: BP 115/68, HR 72, RR 24, temp 98.6, pulse oximetry 98 % on room air.
- General: Ms. Chun is lying in hospital bed and appeared to be in discomfort.
- HEENT: tenderness to palpation of maxillary and frontal sinuses.
- Cardiovascular: regular without murmurs.
- Respiratory: slightly tachypneic; however, lungs were clear to auscultation bilaterally.
- Abdominal exam: She is obese. Several scars from abdominal surgeries are visible. Ms. Chun complains of diffuse abdominal tenderness on palpation. Abdominal exam is otherwise unremarkable.
- Back: Scars from past surgeries. She reports diffuse tenderness when spinus processes were palpated and more severe tenderness when her lower back was palpated.
- Neurological: normal reflexes. Normal strength bilaterally. Gait was normal.

Mental Status Examination

- General Appearance: Ms. Chun is a 44-year-old woman who looks her stated age. She is lying in a hospital bed wearing hospital gown. Her hygiene is fair. Her hair was unkempt; however, she was not malodorous and her nails were well groomed. She appears to be in discomfort.
- Attitude: Initially, Ms. Chun is guarded and angry that a psychiatric consult was requested. However, she becomes conversational during the course of the interview. She answers most questions but is short or evasive when psychological themes are asked.
- Speech: normal tone, volume, rate, and rhythm.
- Thought process: logical and goal directed.
- Thought content: Ms. Chun denies suicidal or homicidal ideation. She cannot believe "you would even ask me that." She denies auditory or visual hallucinations and has no paranoid ideation. There is no evidence of delusional systems.
- Cognition: She is alert and oriented with a 30/30 on her Mini Mental Status Exam. She has normal attention and concentration.
- Insight: poor.
- Judgment: fair.

STOP

Please proceed with the problem-based approach using the worksheet located in the appendix of Chap. 1!

Table 23.2.3

FACTS	HYPOTHESES	INFORMATION NEEDED	LEARNING ISSUES

Case 23.2.4 Conclusion

After you complete the psychiatry assessment, you meet with Ms. Chun's hospital team to discuss your findings. Everyone is in agreement that Mrs. Chun had somatic symptom disorder. For patients with this condition, it is important to have a single physician as a primary caretaker, and you recommend that Ms. Chun see her primary care doctor once a month. The monthly visit should be brief but should include a physical exam to address Ms. Chun's complaints. The goal of the primary care physician is to keep Ms. Chun from having unnecessary surgery, as it would only complicate her condition. At the request of the inpatient team, you contact the primary care doctor and inform her of your findings and recommendations.

Over the following year, Ms. Chun follows up with her primary care physician. Slowly, her doctor counsels her on the links between the mind and physical complaints. After several discussions with her doctor, Ms. Chun agrees to see a psychiatrist. She states she had "nothing else to lose," and she knows her primary doctor does not think she was crazy. Though she continues to have chronic pain and other somatic complaints, Ms. Chun does not have any back or abdominal surgeries over the next few years. Once Ms. Chun developed rapport with an outpatient psychiatrist, she required less frequent visits with her primary care provider.

23.5 Learning Issues

Ms. Chun provides an example of somatic symptom disorder (American Psychiatric Association 2013). She meets the criteria by having one or more distressing somatic symptoms that are distressing and significantly impact her day-to-day

Table 23.2 DSM-5 criteria for somatic symptom disorder

Diagnostic criteria somatic symptom disorder		
A. One or more somatic symptoms that are distressing or disrupt daily life	*B*. Persistent symptoms for more than 6 months	*C*. Excessive thoughts, feelings, or behaviors associated with symptom(s)

life. By definition the somatic symptom(s) must be present for at least 6 months. Therefore, a suspicion of this disorder requires a thorough medical and surgical history. Some of the complaints that the patient may have exhibited in the past may have resolved by the time of presentation. For patients with somatic symptom disorder, it is important to prevent the patient from undergoing surgery or other procedures without significant physical or objective evidence of correctable pathology (Smith 1991). Patients with this condition tend to be annoyed at the suggestions of seeing a psychiatrist since this appears to invalidate their experience of illness (Koelen et al. 2014). It is important to be respectful of the strong belief these patients have in their symptoms. The majority of these patients are first encountered by the primary care physician before being identified and referred for psychiatric evaluation (Rosendal et al. 2009). The primary care physician is usually in a critical role and needs to maintain rapport with the patient. If a patient with somatic symptom disorder decides to seek another provider, he or she could undergo further unnecessary and potentially risky tests and procedures. Frequent contact with primary care providers, initially as often as twice a week and later increased to monthly, appears to be the best means to prevent unnecessary trips to the emergency department and unwarranted procedures (Rosendal et al. 2009). A related goal of the primary care physician is to increase rapport with the somatic symptom disorder patient in order for the patient to agree to a psychiatric evaluation and treatment. If this transition is done well, it will aid in initiating good rapport with her outpatient psychiatrist.

Somatic symptom disorder is more common in women than in men: women outnumber men 5- to 20-fold (Creed 2004). It is unknown why this difference exists, but some have proposed that there is a tendency among physicians to more readily diagnose women with this condition (Creed 2004). Prevalence is estimated to be 5–7% in the general population, although it is likely higher in females (DSM-5).

Like other related somatic symptom disorders, the etiology of somatic symptom disorder in unknown. Also, based on its criteria, it is not a condition that can really be diagnosed until after patients have exhibited significant complaints and morbidity (Kellner 1987). In this case, Ms. Chun had several surgeries before a diagnosis of somatic symptom disorder was considered (Table 23.2).

Vignette 23.3.1 Presenting Situation: Denise Carson

It is a cold, snowy morning in January the first time Ms. Carson presents at the Family Medical Care office where you are finishing your last 6 months of residency. There were many patient cancellations that morning due to the weather. Ms. Carson has a list of nonspecific complaints to review with the doctor. She begins going over the list with the nurse, who listened patiently while she collected vital signs. The nurse had just joined the team at the office, and she liked it when the patients had a single chief complaint, such as a sore throat or cough. Feeling somewhat overwhelmed and tentative, the nurse politely informs Ms. Carson that she would send the doctor right in to see her because it seemed that she had a lot of important things to discuss with you.

After greeting Ms. Carson, you begin by asking what you can do for her today. She produces her crumpled up list and calmly states that she has a lot of important things to discuss. She begins with a complaint about headaches, which she says she has regularly had for many years. She mentions that she faints frequently, when the headaches get bad. She has even had a stroke. That was when she was 38, which was only 4 years ago. For more information about the history of a stroke you ask, "Was it from a clot or from a bleed?" She does not know, and her details are vague. She begins to talk about knee pain and bloody noses. You persist with more detailed information about the headaches "How often do you faint? Do you have any warning signs?" Ms. Carson states that she "faints all the time," and seems determined to move down her list. You attempt to structure the interview, but Ms. Carson resists this and ensues to the next item on her list. There is no emphasis given to major incidents such as syncope or stroke in comparison to the more minor complaints, such as her nosebleed or knee pain. To Ms. Carson they seem equivalent yet not necessarily bothersome, more like a routine laundry list of nuisances.

STOP

Please proceed with the problem-based approach using the worksheet located in the appendix of Chap. 1!

Table 23.3.1

FACTS	HYPOTHESES	INFORMATION NEEDED	LEARNING ISSUES

23.6 Learning Issues

It is important to differentiate between symptoms that are produced intentionally and those that are not intentionally produced. In somatic symptom disorder the medical symptoms are not voluntarily or deliberately produced (American Psychiatric Association 2013). In factitious disorders the symptoms are deceptively and voluntarily produced (American Psychiatric Association 2013).

Case 23.3.2 Continuation

You glance at your watch as you reach up to scratch your head and note with disbelief that you had already gone 5 min over the allotted 15-min office visit. "There are some tests I would like to order," you explain. After sharing and discussing information regarding the tests with Ms. Carson, you write an order for blood tests, an Electrocardiogram (EKG), and an echocardiogram. Ms. Carson feels cut short, finding herself in the hallway with her referrals and her check-out slip. She does not mind having the tests done and willingly agrees to sign consents to release information from other doctors she has visited. Her schedule was not particularly busy that day anyway, and it was still lightly snowing when she got outside to her car.

STOP

Please proceed with the problem-based approach using the worksheet located in the appendix of Chap. 1!

Table 23.3.2

FACTS	HYPOTHESES	INFORMATION NEEDED	LEARNING ISSUES

Case 23.3.3 Continuation

A follow-up visit with Ms. Carson was scheduled for the following Tuesday. Upon visiting with her, she seems satisfied with all of her test results, although somewhat confused. It was reassuring that the lab values were all within normal limits and that the EKG and echocardiogram were unremarkable, but she wonders "What should we do about the fainting?" You arrange for a tilt table test, to see if that would replicate her symptoms. You are still waiting for previous hospital records and were assured that they would arrive by the next appointment.

The next week Ms. Carson's cardiologist calls you to discuss the results of the tilt-table test. He sounds perplexed. Normally, if a patient has a drop in blood pressure on the tilt table, they may faint or experience syncope. She had an episode of syncope but her measured vital signs remained normal. The cardiologist noted that this was not consistent. The cardiologist went on to share that he performed a bit of "detective work" while Ms. Carson was "passed out." He lifted her limp arm above her head and then let go of her hand, positioned exactly overhead. Her hand fell, but somehow managed to miss her face. The cardiologist was suspicious of this clinical picture and recommended that Ms. Carson be evaluated by a psychiatrist.

Please proceed with the problem-based approach using the worksheet located in the appendix of Chap. 1!

Table 23.3.3

FACTS	HYPOTHESES	INFORMATION NEEDED	LEARNING ISSUES

23.7 Learning Issue

Factitious disorders involve the falsification of physical or psychological signs or symptoms, or the induction of injury or disease, associated with identified deception (American Psychiatric Association 2013). The deceptive behavior is evident even in the absence of obvious external rewards (American Psychiatric Association 2013). It is important for the clinician to make the distinction between a malingering patient and a factitious patient (Bass and Halligan 2014). Malingering can be differentiated from factitious disorder by the presence of intentional reporting of symptoms for personal gain (American Psychiatric Association 2013). The incentives may include obtaining disability or sick leave. In contrast, factitious disorder requires the absence of obvious rewards (American Psychiatric Association 2013).

Factitious disorder is divided into factitious disorder imposed on self and factitious disorder imposed on another (American Psychiatric Association 2013). The essential feature of these disorders is the falsification of medical or psychological signs and symptoms in oneself or others that are connected with the identified deception (American Psychiatric Association 2013). Making this diagnosis requires validating that the individual is taking surreptitious actions to distort, feign, or cause signs and symptoms of illness or injury in the absence of clear external rewards (American Psychiatric Association 2013). It is worth noting that preexisting medical conditions may be present; the deceptive behavior or fabrication of injury associated with deception creates a discernment of such individuals (or another) as more ill or disabled that can lead to disproportionate clinical intervention (American Psychiatric Association 2013).

Assessment of patients suffering with factitious disorder involves careful review of medical notes from all health-care facilities, noting any inconsistencies for investigation. Management of factitious disorders can be difficult with the key to success requiring negotiation and agreement of the diagnosis with the patient and commitment of that patient with treatment (Bass and Halligan 2014).

Case 23.3.4 Continuation

Almost 2 years passed before Ms. Carson has another appointment at your office. Her medical records never arrived from the office of the psychiatrist. A new, junior physician, Dr. Tanner, sees her and did not see the old chart. Ms. Carson does not complain of fainting or headaches nor did she mention her history of a stroke. At this visit her complaints center mostly on problems of bleeding. Apparently, her period past month had not stopped, and she has been bleeding for the past 5 weeks. The young, bright-eyed doctor suggests an endometrial biopsy to rule out uterine cancer. He explains the process to her with great patience, and she agrees without posing any questions. The procedure is uncomplicated, and she schedules to return the following week for her results.

At her next visit the following week, Dr. Tanner is delighted to share the good news of a normal pathology result. Ms. Carson shakes her head understandingly and then begins to describe new complaints: her gums have been bleeding when she brushes her teeth, and she has been having bloody noses.

There were bruises on her left arm, back, and stomach. She even had a bruise on her cheek. She had no idea how she acquired any of these bruises. Her doctor shows his concern. Had someone been abusing her? Ms. Carson adamantly denies abuse of any sort, ever. Dr. Tanner pondered over the bleeding, the bruising, and concerned about leukemia, he sends her to the lab for a blood count that day. The following week, again, Dr. Tanner is relieved to have good news to share with his patient. The blood count was within normal limits with no evidence of leukemia. After a moment, he begins to worry that she may have a bleeding disorder despite her normal blood counts. Ms. Carson assures him that there are no bleeding problems in her family. She did not drink alcohol or have a history of liver problems.

Please proceed with the problem-based approach using the worksheet located in the appendix of Chap. 1!

Table 23.3.4

FACTS	HYPOTHESES	INFORMATION NEEDED	LEARNING ISSUES

Case 23.3.5 Conclusion

During Ms. Carson's next visit, she reports blood in her urine and in her stool. Dr. Tanner tells her that one of her blood tests was abnormal. He asked her if she takes blood thinners, such as Coumadin® (warfarin) and she reports she does not. Dr. Tanner grows more and more confounded. He repeats the abnormal blood clotting test to confirm the accuracy and the result is unchanged. He considers the possibility that someone might be poisoning her and proceeds with a very detailed family and social history. She is a single mother, divorced, raising a teenaged son. Her relationship with her ex-husband is amicable. Her son has been in some trouble recently, but nothing out of the ordinary for a 15-year-old boy. The rest of her details seemed routine and unremarkable.

The next time Dr. Tanner sees Ms. Carson, she is in the emergency room. The previous evening, Ms. Carson began bleeding profusely after a bowel movement. The laboratory data showed that her blood clotting time was dangerously elevated. Blood transfusions stabilize her, and she is admitted to the hospital for observation. On her second day in the hospital, her blood test for the chemical brodifacoum is elevated. Brodifacoum tests for levels of rat poison which is similar to warfarin, a common blood thinner. Now Dr. Tanner understands why his patient was bleeding and bruising. Rather than feeling pleased about solving the mystery, he now has a bigger puzzle to solve. He decides to ask the police for protection while she was in the hospital because he fears for her life. The teenage son was the number one suspect in his mind. He gently reviews with her what the blood test meant and that she had a high level of rat poison in her system. She is oddly indifferent and does not seem concerned. Dr. Tanner is astonished. Ms. Carson remains agreeable. The next thought that he had seemed too improbable to even consider. Could she be taking the rat poison herself? She would have had to ingest at least 40 6-ounce boxes to achieve her current blood level. He asks her directly, and she denies it. He suggests that the psychiatric team visit with her in the hospital. She remained pleasant and was almost overly compliant. He made the call. The next morning Ms. Carson cannot be found. She had left the hospital.

Please proceed with the problem-based approach using the worksheet located in the appendix of Chap. 1!

23.8 Learning Issues

Ms. Carson intentionally produced her symptoms by ingesting rat poison. This is a distinction from the first two cases. In the first case of conversion disorder, the paralysis was involuntarily produced. Similarly, in the second case of somatic symptom disorder, the patient had an array of symptoms that were not intentionally produced (Table 23.3).

The prevalence of factitious disorders is not known but is estimated to range between 0.5 and 2% (Bass and Halligan 2014). The course of this disorder is usually one of intermittent episodes, with onset in early adulthood. Individuals with

Table 23.3 Differentiating somatic symptom disorder, factitious disorder, and malingering

Disorder	Symptoms	Benefit from symptoms
Somatic symptom disorder	Involuntary	Subconscious
Factitious disorder	Voluntary	No obvious external reward
Malingering	Voluntary	External personal gain (financial, time off work, litigation, etc.)

Table 23.4 Summary of factitious disorder

Factitious disorder		
Diagnostic criteria	Differential diagnosis	Treatment and management
Falsification of physical or psychological signs or symptoms, or induction of injury or disease, associated with identified deception	Specific distinction from malingering	Optimizing patient rapport is important during management and treatment
The individual presents himself or herself to others as ill, impaired, or injured	Careful review of medical notes from individual health-care history	Key to success requiring negotiation and agreement of the diagnosis with the patient and commitment of that patient with treatment
The deceptive behavior is evident even in the absence of obvious external rewards		
The behavior is not better explained by another mental disorder, such as delusional disorder or another psychotic disorder		

recurrent episodes and successive deceptive relationships with medical personnel may develop a lifelong pattern (American Psychiatric Association 2013). Many individuals presenting with factitious disorder are likely to be socially conforming young women in their 30s with stable social networks (Bass and Halligan 2014) (Table 23.4).

23.8.1 Conclusion

Somatic symptom and related disorders include the diagnosis of somatic symptom disorder, illness anxiety disorder, conversion disorder (functional neurologic function disorder), psychological factors affecting other medical conditions, factitious disorder, other specified somatic symptom and related disorder, and unspecified somatic symptom-related disorder. All of these diagnoses share the common feature of the prominence of somatic symptoms associated with significant impairment and distress. Disorders with somatic complaints are commonly seen in the offices of primary care providers.

23.9 Learning Questions

1. In diagnosing somatic symptom disorder which of the following is incorrect?
   a. The symptom(s) must be present for 6 months.
   b. The somatic symptom may be associated with a concurrent diagnosis.
   c. There cannot be a medical explanation for the symptom.
   d. There is significant distress and preoccupation with the symptom.
2. A patient is suspected of self-inflicting an injury after losing a football game and then uses it as an excuse to miss practice the next week. The likely diagnosis is.
   a. Anxiety disorder
   b. Conversion disorder
   c. Factitious disorder
   d. Somatic symptom disorder
3. You evaluate a young woman in the Emergency Room (ER) who has suddenly and inexplicably lost her vision. She has a chemistry final exam tomorrow but does not seem that worried that she will not be able to complete the exam. You are suspicious that she has.
   a. Somatic symptom disorder
   b. Conversion disorder
   c. Factitious disorder
   d. Posttraumatic stress disorder
4. You are rotating in family medicine and encounter a young man in clinic who has a long list of health concerns. He has no documented health history and appears healthy. You note that he has been seen twice this year for similar complaints and seems overly preoccupied that there might be a problem with his health. He likely has____________disorder.

Appendix A: Possible Answers to PBL Tables

Vignette 23.1: Janelle Miller

Table 23.1.1

Facts	Hypotheses	Information needed	Learning issues
Mrs. Miller is a 28-year-old female	Was there any physical injury?	What is her social history?	A complete history is important in patient evaluation
She has bilateral leg paralysis	Is there a metabolic etiology?	What is her psychiatric history?	
She has no previous health problems	Is there a psychological etiology?	What is her family history?	

Table 23.1.2

Facts	Hypotheses	Information needed	Learning issues
Mrs. Miller is adherent to primary care	Is there a psychological etiology that is stress related?	A physical exam must be conducted	What is the presentation of symptoms in conversion disorders?
She has no psychiatric history	Is there a metabolic etiology?	A mental status exam must be conducted	What are the common aspects of conversion disorder (functional neurological symptom disorder)?
She has no family history of similar presentation		Pertinent lab tests are needed	
She had an increased level of responsibility as a child			
She is happily married			
Her husband is gone often			
She acts as a single parent when her husband is gone			

Table 23.1.3

Facts	Hypotheses	Information needed	Learning issues
Mrs. Miller's vitals are within normal limits	There seems to be a psychological etiology	What is the persistence of symptoms?	Conversion disorder can be difficult to recognize
There is no acute distress, and she is alert and oriented	Her anxiety and fear seem to be playing a role	Does she experience resolution of symptoms after hospital admission?	Altered voluntary motor and sensory function are needed for diagnosis
She has bilateral leg paralysis			Must rule out possible medical etiology
She has decreased sensation			Importance of treating and managing possible co-occurring disorders
Ratchet-like weakness			
Her physical exam is otherwise unremarkable			
She has worried mood			
She denies suicidal ideation			
She denies psychotic symptoms			
Her lab and imaging results unremarkable for acute pathology			

Vignette 23.2: Lorraine Chun

Table 23.2.1

Facts	Hypotheses	Information needed	Learning issues
Ms. Chun has "intractable" back pain (>6 months)	Is the etiology musculoskeletal?	What are the results of prior diagnostic studies?	It is important to be respectful of patient's beliefs about her symptoms
She frequently seeks medical care at the ER	Is there a neurological etiology?	What do reports from previous specialty consultations indicate?	It is necessary to rule out potential medical etiologies
	Is there a psychiatric etiology?		

Table 23.2.2

Facts	Hypotheses	Information needed	Learning issues
Ms. Chun has an extensive history of medical conditions, including chronic pain and severe headaches	Does she have factitious disorder?	A complete history and physical examination are needed	It is important to assess unexplained symptoms
She has had multiple surgeries	Does she have somatic symptom disorder?	A mental status examination is needed	Pay attention to lack of positive findings on physical examination

Table 23.2.3

Facts	Hypotheses	Information needed	Learning issues
Ms. Chun has a history of many physical complaints	Ms. Chun may be depressed	Is there any past history of false information or deceptive behavior?	Criteria of four pain symptoms in somatic symptom disorder
She has multiple pain complaints: abdominal pain, back pain, headaches, and arthralgias	She may have factitious disorder	Is there any medical basis of symptoms?	Centrality of medically unexplained symptoms
	She may be malingering		
	She may have somatic symptom disorder		

Vignette 23.3: Denise Carson

Table 23.3.1

Facts	Hypotheses	Information needed	Learning issues
Ms. Carson has headaches	Is there any neurological etiology?	Clarification on and confirmation of medical history	It is important to differentiate between symptoms that are produced intentionally and those that are not intentionally produced
She faints frequently	Is there a metabolic etiology?	Lab tests	Somatic symptom disorder versus factitious disorder
She reports a history of stroke		EKG	
She has many equally important medical concerns	Is there any psychological etiology?	Echocardiogram	

Table 23.3.2

Facts	Hypotheses	Information needed	Learning issues
Ms. Carson agreed to sign a release of information	Is there a neurological etiology?	Is her reported medical history confirmed by her medical record?	Somatic symptom disorder versus factitious disorder
Tests are ordered	Is there a metabolic etiology?	What do lab tests, EKG, and echocardiogram indicate?	
	Is there a psychological etiology?		

Table 23.3.3

Facts	Hypotheses	Information needed	Learning issues
Her lab tests were within normal limits	A psychological etiology is likely	Why would Ms. Carson alter her symptoms?	How can a diagnostician differentiate between somatic symptom disorder and factitious disorder?
Her EKG was unremarkable for pathology	Does she meet criteria for somatic symptom disorder?	Are her symptoms intentional or unintentional?	How can a diagnostician differentiate between malingering and factitious disorder?
Her echocardiogram was unremarkable for pathology	Does she meet criteria for factitious disorder?	Are the medical records consistent with the patient's report?	What are the types of factitious disorder?
Her cardiologist is concerned			Careful review of medical records
The tilt-table test was ordered, with inconsistent results			

Table 23.3.4

Facts	Hypotheses	Information needed	Learning issues
It has been 2 years since her last visit	Is the etiology psychological?	A repeat blood count is needed	Recognizing overall presentation and pattern of patient symptoms
Your office was unable to obtain medical records	Has she been physical abused?	Additional social history is needed	Intentional versus unintentional symptoms
Her reported history was inconsistent with her prior visit	Does she have a clotting disorder?	Additional medical history is in order	Factitious disorder diagnosis, treatment, and management
She presents a new concern of vaginal bleeding	Does she have leukemia?	Why would the patient alter her symptoms?	
She has a normal biopsy result	Did she ingest a poison?	Are the symptoms intentional or unintentional?	
She has an additional, new concern at follow-up			
She has new bruising			
Her blood count is within normal limits			
She has no history of alcohol use or liver problems			

Appendix B: Answers to Learning Questions

1. C
   Rationale: A somatic symptom disorder diagnosis does not require that the somatic symptoms are medically unexplained; symptoms may or may not be associated with another medical condition.
2. C
   Rationale: Factitious disorder imposed on self is the falsification of a physical or psychological symptom, or induction of injury associated with an identified deception.
3. B
   Rationale: Conversion disorder (functional neurologic symptom disorder) includes one or more symptoms of altered voluntary motor or sensory function that is not compatible with medical explanation.
4. Illness anxiety
   Rationale: Illness anxiety disorder includes a preoccupation with having or acquiring a serious illness, and there is a high level of anxiety about health.

References

Allin, M., Streeruwitz, A., & Curtis, V. (2005). Progress in understanding conversion disorder. *Neuropsychiatric Disease and Treatment, 1*(3), 205.

American Psychiatric Association. (2013). *Diagnostic and statistical manual of mental disorders: DSM-5* (5th ed.). Washington, DC: American Psychiatric Association.

Bass, C., & Halligan, P. (2014). Factitious disorders and malingering: Challenges for clinical assessment and management. *The Lancet, 383*(9926), 1422–1432.

Creed, F., & Barsky, A. (2004). A systematic review of the epidemiology of somatization disorder and hypochondriasis. *Journal Psychosomatic Research, 56,* 391.

Croicu, C., Chwastiak, L., & Katon, W. (2014). Approach to the patient with multiple somatic symptoms. *Medical Clinics of North America, 98*(5), 1079–1095.

Kellner, R. (1987). Hypochondriasis and somatization. *JAMA, 258,* 2718.

Koelen, J. A., Houvteen, J. H., Abbass, A., et al. (2014). Effectiveness of psychotherapy for severe somatoform disorder: Meta-analysis. *British Journal of Psychiatry, 204,* 12–19

Rosendal, M., Burton, C., Blankenstein, A. H., et al. (2009). Enhanced care by generalists for functional somatic symptoms and disorders in primary care. *The Cochrane Database of Systematic Reviews,* 2013, Issue 10. Art No.:CD008142. doi:10.1002/14651858.CD008142.pub2.

Smith, G. R. (1991). Somatization disorder in the medical setting. Washington, DC: American Psychiatric Press Inc.

Chapter 24
Personality Disorders

M. Nathan Mason, Negar Nicole Jacobs* and Latha Pai

Personality disorders (PDs) are a challenging yet intriguing set of psychiatric diagnoses. Some have suggested that 14% of adults in the USA have at least one PD (Grant et al. 2004). Given the high prevalence of PDs in patient populations, it is incumbent on clinicians to familiarize themselves with the identification and evidence-based management of such disorders. This familiarity may decrease unnecessary medical expenditures as well as other undesirable outcomes, such as litigation. This chapter will review the PDs officially recognized by the current *Diagnostic and Statistical Manual* (5th ed.; DSM-5; American Psychiatric Association 2013; Fig. 24.1).

Objectives:

By the end of this chapter, the reader will be able to:

1. Describe the morbidity and mortality resulting from PDs
2. Diagnose a PD according to DSM-5 criteria
3. Summarize treatment approaches for PDs

PDs are persistent, maladaptive patterns of inner experience and behavior. These patterns lead to distress or impairment in a patient's life, such as strife within

---

Whenever I climb, I am followed by a dog called "Ego." Friedrich Nietzsche

*Co-first editor of the book.

M. N. Mason (✉)
Department of Psychiatry, University of Arizona College of Medicine, 1202 Albany Way, Rocklin, CA 95765, USA
e-mail: mnathanmason@gmail.com

N. N. Jacobs
Psychiatry and Behavioral Sciences, School of Medicine, University of Nevada, 401 W. Second Street, Suite 201, Reno, NV 89503, USA
e-mail: nnjacobs@medicine.nevada.edu

L. Pai
Psychiatry, Mental health services (116), Veterans affairs Sierra Nevada health care system, 975 Kirman Avenue, Reno, NV 89502, USA
e-mail: Latha.pai@va.gov

D. Alicata et al. (eds.), *Problem-based Behavioral Science and Psychiatry*,
DOI 10.1007/978-3-319-23669-8_24

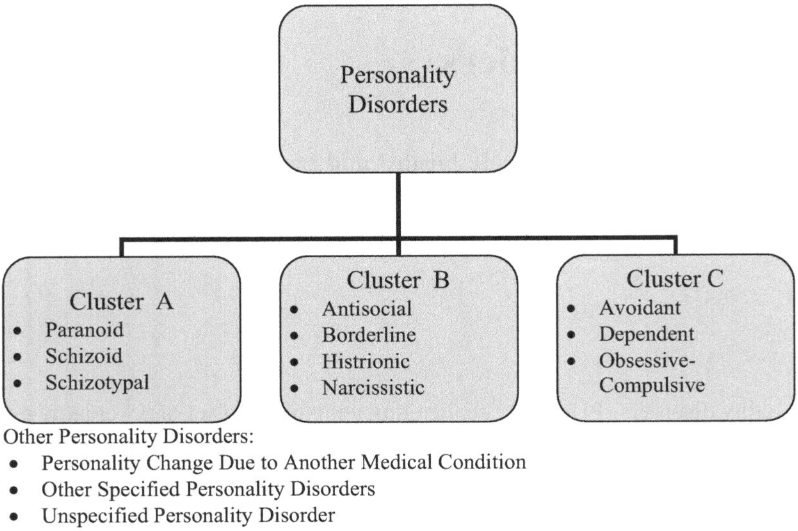

Fig. 24.1 Overview of personality disorders

romantic relationships, difficulty with coworkers and others in one's community, and other interpersonal problems. Depending on the type of PD, such patients may suffer a disconcerting sense of self, lack of self-direction and self-reflection, a lack of empathy, or a failure to establish and maintain satisfying, emotionally intimate relationships. Many people who meet criteria for a PD do not view themselves as the source of their suffering. They are more likely to externalize their problems, blaming other people. In general, psychotherapy is the treatment of choice for PDs (Verheul and Herbrink 2007). Psychotherapy tends to outperform pharmacotherapy for the PDs (Paris 2011).

The National Epidemiologic Survey on Alcohol and Related Conditions (NESARC) was a recent population-based study of over 40,000 Americans. It concluded that over 14 % of Americans suffer from at least one PD (Grant et al. 2004). However, until 2007, studies on the prevalence of PDs looked at study populations which were not representative of the general American public. As well, a myriad of various assessment tools were employed in earlier studies. Because of this, the National Institute of Mental Health (NIMH) funded a nationally representative study of the general public, utilizing the well-regarded International Personality Disorder Examination (IPDE), a semi-structured clinical tool. The results demonstrated that 9.1 % of Americans have a PD as defined by DSM-IV (Lenzenweger et al. 2007). Due to their high prevalence in the general population, it is not surprising PDs are especially prevalent in those engaged with mental health services. One study employed the Structured Interview for DSM-IV Personality to interview 859 psychiatric outpatients upon initial presentation for treatment (Zimmerman et al. 2005). When only considering patients diagnosed with one of the ten official PDs, 31.4 % of psychiatric outpatients ruled in. However, when patients with PD not otherwise specified were included, the prevalence jumped to 45.5 %. About 15 % of psychiatric hospitalizations are motivated primarily by problems related to a PD rather than another mental disorder (Loranger 1990). Approximately half the remaining inpatients suffer from a comorbid PD in addition to their principal mental disorder.

The behavioral patterns associated with PDs affect the person in multiple aspects of life and are inflexible. Like all psychiatric diagnoses, the diagnosis of a PD is made when the symptoms rise to the level of clinical impairment or distress. The nature of this type of disorder is chronic, and aspects that contribute to this disorder start developing during childhood or adolescence.

Most people with PDs exhibited the traits of the disorder in adolescence or earlier. Clinicians generally are reluctant to diagnose a PD in someone under the age of 18. Such a diagnosis in someone under eighteen requires the diagnostic criteria to be manifest for at least 1 year. One notable exception is that DSM-5 specifically prohibits the diagnosis of antisocial personality disorder (ASPD) in those under the age of 18. Rather, they are diagnosed with conduct disorder.

PDs are grouped into three "Clusters": Cluster A, odd or eccentric; Cluster B, dramatic, emotional, or erratic; and Cluster C, anxious or fearful. Comorbidity among the PDs is common.

Cluster A Odd or eccentric

Paranoid personality disorder
Schizoid personality disorder
Schizotypal personality disorder

Case 24.1.1 Presenting Situation: Leslie Danforth

Leslie Danforth is a 24-year-old individual brought to your outpatient psychiatry clinic by her mother, who states she is frustrated by her daughter's behavior. Specifically, Leslie's mother is "fed up" by her daughter's inability to "get along" with people and hold a job long enough to live independently. Coming to see a psychiatrist is the "last resort."

Leslie's chief complaint is, "I am fed up with my mother trying to rule my life!" During the introductions, the patient appears uncomfortable and looks around the interview room. She intermittently glances behind her. She finally requests that her chair be moved to a position where she can watch the door. Her mother is in tears.

STOP

Please proceed with the problem-based approach using the worksheet located in the appendix of Chap. 1!

Table 24.1.1

FACTS	HYPOTHESES	INFORMATION NEEDED	LEARNING ISSUES

Case 24.1.2 Continuation

Leslie's mother tells you that her daughter lives with her because she has difficulty keeping a job. Leslie quickly interrupts her mother and asserts that her mother has always been against her, right from childhood and has favored all the other siblings over her. She adds (defensively) that it is never her fault when she leaves a job. Her bosses are "always" at fault. She has held a number of jobs as executive assistant and has been fired several times for going through confidential files and mail of colleagues. She reports that her peers would never be honest with her about the projects she would work on. She is confident that she was fired because she discovered too many "secrets" that would make her employer look bad.

Her mother states that her daughter has two broken engagements in the last 3 years. Again, Leslie quickly interrupts to state that both her fiancés were cheating on her, and she could never marry someone she cannot trust. When questioned about how she knew of the infidelities, Leslie snaps, "I do not need proof! I just know they were cheating on me!" She converses with logical, spontaneous speech. She denies the use of any illicit drugs. She denies any auditory or visual hallucinations. She denies any history of a head injury.

Please proceed with the problem-based approach using the worksheet located in the appendix of Chap. 1!

Table 24.1.2

FACTS	HYPOTHESES	INFORMATION NEEDED	LEARNING ISSUES

Learning Issues

Leslie Danforth's presentation is suggestive of paranoid PD. The case information did not present sufficient information about her motives and thinking to meet full criteria, so the diagnosis would reflect the limits of the database: paranoid personality traits or rule out paranoid PD. Estimates of the prevalence of this PD in the general population range from 2.3 to 4.4% (Kessler et al. 2004).

DSM-5 specifies that a diagnosis of this PD requires four or more of the following findings: (nondelusional) suspiciousness of harm, exploitation, or deception; preoccupation with unjustified doubts; reluctance to confide in others; tendency to read negative meanings into benign remarks and events; tendency to bear grudges; tendency to perceive attacks on one's character; and recurrent suspiciousness regarding fidelity of partner (APA 2013). Psychologically, the defense mechanisms most commonly employed by persons with this PD include fantasy, projection, and acting out.

Case 24.1.3 Conclusion

Leslie's laboratory results from a general physical examination she had 3 months ago (complete blood count (CBC), chemistry panel, and thyroid panel) were all within normal limits. Her urine drug screen is negative. You suggest that some of her experiences with relationships sound as if she might have gone through some difficult times. She agrees. You venture to offer a follow-up meeting to see if you can understand those times better and to see if there are any supports or services the you or the clinic might offer to her. She agrees to a follow-up appointment in 2 weeks. She does not show up for this appointment, and you never hear from her again.

Please proceed with the problem-based approach using the worksheet located in the appendix of Chap. 1!

Table 24.1.3

FACTS	HYPOTHESES	INFORMATION NEEDED	LEARNING ISSUES

Learning Issues: Other Cluster A Personality Disorders and Treatment of Cluster A Personality Disorders

The PDs in Cluster A generally represent eccentric or odd behavioral patterns, which may be especially prominent in schizoid PD and schizotypal PD. People with these disorders tend to often be isolated and rarely present for treatment of their own volition. The prevalence of schizoid PD has trended to showing an increase at 4.9% (Grant et al. 2004). The occupational choices of people with schizoid PD (if they work outside the home) tend be solitary, such as employment as night security guard. In order to diagnose an individual with schizoid PD, four or more of the following criteria must be met: lacks desire for and enjoyment of close relationships; almost always opts for solitary activities; has little, if any, interest in sexual encounters with another person; takes pleasure in few, if any, activities; lacks close friends/confidants outside of first degree relatives; seems indifferent to the praise or criticism of others; and shows emotional coldness, detachment, or flattened affectivity (APA 2013). Fantasy is the psychological defense mechanism most commonly employed by persons with this PD.

The third PD in Cluster A is schizotypal PD. People with this disorder tend be have odd thoughts as well as eccentric and unusual behaviors and speech. They may be noticeable because of their unusual appearance reflected in what they choose to wear. Although schizotypal PD may superficially resemble a psychotic disorder, the odd beliefs are not full-blown delusions. Approximately 3.9% of the population has this PD (per NESARC; Grant et al. 2004). Epidemiologic studies suggest a link between schizotypal PD and schizophrenia. Schizotypal PD is more prevalent in families of schizophrenia probands than in the general population. As well, schizophrenia is more prevalent among the blood relatives of schizotypal PD probands. There is an increased concordance for schizotypal PD in identical twins compared to nonidentical twins. Not dissimilar to schizoid PD, individuals with schizotypal PD most commonly rely upon the defense mechanism of fantasy.

Several lines of evidence suggest a shared neurobiological basis with schizophrenia, including similarities in anatomy, neuropathology, neurophysiology, neurocognition, and upon gross physical examination (Nelson et al. 2013). Magnetic resonance imaging (MRI) studies show both conditions have associated increased cerebrospinal fluid, decreased temporal cortical volume and grey matter, and decreased caudate volumes. Both schizotypal PD and schizophrenia are associated with decreased metabolic activity of the temporal lobes although the finding is more pronounced in schizophrenia. Both have elevated cerebrospinal fluid levels of homovanillic acid, a major metabolite of dopamine. Both have similar patterns of cognitive deficits, involving sustained attention, verbal learning, visual processing, and working memory.

A diagnosis of schizotypal PD requires five or more of the following DSM-5 criteria: ideas of reference (nondelusional); odd beliefs or magical thinking; unusual perceptual experiences; odd thinking and speech; suspiciousness/paranoia; inappropriate affect; odd behavior, lack of close friends/confidants outside of first degree relatives; and excessive social anxiety that does not decrease with familiarity and tends to be associated with paranoia (APA 2013).

Proper diagnosis of Cluster A PDs is important since each has a unique pattern of response to treatment. The current literature suggests psychotherapy or sociotherapy (support groups) offers no benefit to paranoid PD. It is uncertain if psychotropic medications improve the longitudinal course of this disorder, but they can certainly aid with decreasing symptoms. In general—with all the PDs—any somatic treatment is focused on mitigating symptom clusters such as cognitive-perceptual disturbances, affective dysregulation, or impulse-behavior dyscontrol. Nonetheless, if a patient with paranoid PD suffers an overtly psychotic decompensation, antipsychotic medications may have a role in controlling the symptom profile and improving quality of life and functionality in day-to-day activities for the patient. With schizotypal PD, the literature again provides no support that psychotherapy is helpful. It is unclear if sociotherapy is beneficial. Some suggest that psychotropics may be modestly helpful in the longitudinal course of this disorder, although scientifically rigorous data are absent. For example, an open-label study suggested that olanzapine could decrease symptoms and improve overall functioning in schizotypal PD (Keshavan et al. 2004). Finally, there is growing interest in non-neuroleptic psychotropics for the treatment of this disorder. McClure et al. (2007) reported the results of a parallel-design, double-blind, placebo-controlled trial, concluding that the α_{2A} agonist guanfacine improved context processing in schizotypal patients. Schizoid PD has a treatment response profile which is unique among the PDs. Recent meta-analysis suggests that both psychotherapies and sociotherapies can decrease symptomatology in this disorder (Verheul and Herbrink 2007). However, pharmacotherapy offers no added benefit but can act as an adjunct to psychotherapy-based approaches.

Case 24.2.1 Presenting Situation: Brendan Ryles

Brendan Ryles is a 36-year-old man who is brought to the county hospital emergency department where you are on call. He is wearing handcuffs with a police escort from the county jail. His chief complaint is, "There was a little misunderstanding when I was handling my business."

Mr. Ryles demonstrates several contusions and cuts. He has several bleeding lacerations on his face and body. You also notice several healed scars. He appears agitated and angry and bellows: "Fix me!" At this point, the police escorts pull him back and request that he be patient.

You carefully clean and suture Mr. Ryles after appropriate local anesthesia. While you are suturing, he tells you in a conversational tone that he has been in prison for arson, armed robberies, and attempted murder.

Mr. Ryles says he grew up in a dysfunctional family where his father regularly "beat up" his mother. He says he was suspended from junior high school for fighting and never went back to school. He was put into foster care early on, and he says he has always gotten into trouble. He laughs as he recounts how he enjoyed making life miserable for his foster parents and was continuously moved from one care facility to another. Mr. Ryles finally ran away at age 14 after stealing money and some expensive electronic items. He was arrested for this crime and put in a juvenile facility. He says he enjoys cheating people who are "too dumb not to cheat." Mr. Ryles reports that he drives even though he has a suspended driver's license for reckless driving and endangering others. His most recent accident involved a fatality that eventually led to his current incarceration, where he is awaiting adjudication. "I've gotta go to court on that—they could strike me out."

Mr. Ryles has never been married and has six children with one on the way. He reports he got into a fight this time with two other inmates because they did not allow him to cut into the food line. He says he got angry and punched someone, and this altercation evolved into to a fistfight with several inmates. When living "on the streets," Mr. Ryles drinks a 12-pack of beer daily and smokes approximately 30 cigarettes daily. He says he has used multiple drugs including methamphetamines, phencyclidine, marijuana, and pain medications. "I love my OCs," he says, smugly referring to the long-acting preparation of oxycodone.

Please proceed with the problem-based approach using the worksheet located in the appendix of Chap. 1!

Table 24.2.1

FACTS	HYPOTHESES	INFORMATION NEEDED	LEARNING ISSUES

Learning Issues: Cluster B Personality Disorders

Patients with Cluster B personality diagnoses tend to have more contact with medical professionals than those from other clusters because of the associated high-risk behaviors which lead to medical or legal consequences. Genetic factors contribute to the finding that both borderline personality disorder (BPD) and ASPD sometimes run in family pedigrees.

Cluster B Dramatic, emotional, or erratic

Antisocial personality disorder (ASPD)
Borderline personality disorder (BPD)
Histrionic personality disorder
Narcissistic personality disorder

ASPD is strongly associated with criminal behavior. However, an absence of criminal convictions does not rule out the diagnosis. Also strongly associated with this disorder are the psychoactive substance use disorders. Mr. Ryles presents with a history that is highly suggestive of the diagnosis. The diagnosis of ASPD requires three or more of the following DSM-5 criteria: failure to conform to social norms and laws; deceitfulness; impulsivity; irritability and aggressiveness; disregard for safety; irresponsibility; and lack of remorse (APA 2013). DSM-5 mentions this disorder may have a prevalence of 0.2–3.3% (APA 2013). Psychologically, persons with ASPD rely heavily upon the defense mechanisms of denial and acting out.

Scientists are beginning to unravel the biology of ASPD and (Minzenberg et al. 2007) related social phenomena (Spitzer et al. 2007). Recently, a group reported the results of functional magnetic resonance imaging (fMRI) studies of the brains of people who matched behavioral responses with hypothetical vignettes under study conditions (Yang et al. 2009). Available responses entailed either abiding by consensus social norms or violating them. Some vignettes entailed circumstances where serious rule violations may have been punished, whereas other stories suggested there was no possibility of punishment. That is, study participants were asked to ponder what they would do if only they could "get away with it." These types of thoughts were consistently mapped to a few brain regions. This supports a recent model that suggests that dysfunction of brain structures such as the amygdala, within the temporal lobe, would impair one's ability to associate cause and effect, especially regarding punishment for specific behaviors (Yang et al. 2009).

As opposed to all other PDs, the individual diagnosed with ASPD must be at least 18 years of age. This disorder is unique among the PDs because it has a requirement of a preceding childhood disorder: conduct disorder before age 15 years (see Chap. 18).

24.2.2 Case Conclusion
Mr. Ryles returned to jail. He received lock-up orders to house in "administrative segregation" as a consequence for unprovoked violence.

STOP

Please proceed with the problem-based approach using the worksheet located in the appendix of Chap. 1!

Table 24.2.2

FACTS	HYPOTHESES	INFORMATION NEEDED	LEARNING ISSUES

ASPD has a unique treatment response profile. Current meta-analysis suggests psychotherapies or pharmacotherapies have nothing to offer persons with this disorder (Hofmann et al. 2012). However, select sociotherapies may be modestly helpful. Since prevalence appears to be higher in samples affected by adverse socioeconomic or sociocultural factors, improving this might aid in treatment.

Case 24.3.1 Presenting Situation: Sharon Young
While working as a resident on a university's consult-liaison team, you are called to consult on a 22-year-old white woman admitted two days ago after overdosing on diphenhydramine and acetaminophen. Ms. Young is on the

medical floor and is very reluctant to talk to "the shrinks." She appears irritable and states she doesn't think she is "crazy" or needs to see "a head doc." With questioning, Ms. Young responds that she took a handful of each medication so she could kill herself. At this point in the interview, she becomes quite upset, starts crying, and yells at you to leave her room and to leave her alone.

You leave the room and read through the patient's chart which was previously unavailable. You read that Ms. Young has had multiple visits to the emergency room (ER) for past suicidal thoughts and four attempts. The attempts were all medication overdoses at sublethal dosages. Ms. Young also has a history of self-inflicted superficial cuts to her forearms. The cutting and overdosing behaviors appear to coincide with a failed relationship or problems in school.

STOP

Please proceed with the problem-based approach using the worksheet located in the appendix of Chap. 1!

Table 24.3.1

FACTS	HYPOTHESES	INFORMATION NEEDED	LEARNING ISSUES

Learning Issues: Borderline Personality Disorder

Sharon Young's case illustrates some of the difficulties facing patients with BPD: chaotic relationships, episodes of depressive feelings, self-harming behaviors, and poor skills in solving problems. DSM-5 estimates a prevalence rate between 1.6 to as high as 5.9 % (APA 2013). Its prevalence in primary care settings is about 6 %, 10 % in an outpatient mental health clinic, and about 20 % among psychiatric inpatients. About 10 % of patients with this disorder eventually die at their own hands of suicide. BPD patients may have brief periods of psychosis, usually paranoid beliefs, during extreme stress. Nonlethal self-harm can be prominent in this disorder and is called "parasuicidal" behavior to distinguish it from a suicide attempt with full lethal intent that may have been aborted or interrupted.

Biological research in BPD has found abnormalities in rapid eye movement (REM) sleep cycles and endocrine abnormalities involving the adrenal and thyroid glands. Recent neuroimaging studies suggest that patients with this disorder process neutral visual information (such as photos of neutral facial expressions) as though they were threats (Daros et al. 2013).

In order to diagnose an individual with BPD, he or she must report at least five of the following DSM-5 criteria: frantic effort (to the point of self-injurious behavior) to avoid abandonment; a pattern of intense and unstable relationships alternating between extremes of idealization and devaluation; identity disturbance; impulsivity; recurrent self-injurious behavior; affective instability; chronic feelings of emptiness; inappropriate intense anger; transient paranoid ideation; or severe dissociative symptoms (APA 2013). Persons with BPD employ suboptimal defense mechanisms, most commonly splitting, projection, and projective identification.

24.3.2 Continuation

Ms. Young's past medication trials over the past 10 years include various antipsychotic medications and a large number of antidepressants. Her list of medications also included valproic acid for "mood stability" and a benzodiazepine for anxiety.

The next morning, Ms. Young is lying down in her bed flipping through the channels on the television. She had been crying and appears sullen with poor eye contact. When you question her about her mood, she looks at the floor and tells you she is not feeling good and is very depressed. You ask about her suicide attempt, and Ms. Young begins crying, explaining that her boyfriend had left her for someone else. She said she had tried so hard and wonders, "How could he ever leave me? How can he do this to me? After everything we have been through together!" She said he told her that he could not tolerate her behavior or her mood swings. She confronted him about an affair and cut her wrist telling him that he needs to stop talking to his other girlfriend. That is when he stormed out of the apartment. She then took the pills and hoped her boyfriend would feel bad about the way he treated her and come back. She reports that talking about that night makes her think about hurting herself.

Please proceed with the problem-based approach using the worksheet located in the appendix of Chap. 1!

Table 24.3.2

FACTS	HYPOTHESES	INFORMATION NEEDED	LEARNING ISSUES

An important diagnosis to consider in patients with dramatic and destructive behaviors is bipolar disorder. The mood instability for BPD represents a lifelong "trait." On the other hand, patients with bipolar disorder invariably suffer relatively discrete "states" which differ from their baseline euthymia. On average, even an untreated person with bipolar affective disorder enjoys euthymia approximately half their life. Such persons with bipolar affective disorder invariably demonstrate elevations of mood and usually have major depressive mood episodes as well (see Chap. 22). In truth, most symptomatic time for bipolar patients is in the depressive phase.

24.3.3 Conclusion

You arrange an "intake" appointment for Ms. Young at the community mental health center. You describe the dialectical behavior therapy (DBT) program as "made to order" for her. Ms. Young attends the intake appointment and reluctantly agrees to enroll in the DBT program. She attends almost all of the individual and group sessions and becomes increasingly interested in learning new behaviors and ways of coping with her emotions.

Table 24.3.3

FACTS	HYPOTHESES	INFORMATION NEEDED	LEARNING ISSUES

Linehan et al. (2006) suggest that patients with this disorder are best treated in outpatient programs that offer DBT. This therapy treats patients individually and in groups and focuses on building skills and finding ways to manage intensely uncomfortable emotions without self-harm (Koerner and Linehan 2000). There is some evidence that medications such as antidepressants, mood stabilizers, and the newer antipsychotics may confer some benefits, especially in the short term.

Learning Issues: Other Cluster B Personality Disorders
Patients with histrionic PD are often dramatic in their appearance and behavior. In the general medical setting, a histrionic patient may engage medical professionals with a charming (or even seductive) manner and entertaining or implausible descriptions of symptoms. Patients with this disorder may display suggestibility and present with the symptoms of illnesses featured in the media. There is a considerable overlap between this PD and somatization disorder as well as conversion disorder (see Chap. 23). Roughly 2 % of the general population meets criteria for histrionic PD. The diagnosis of histrionic PD requires five or more of the following per DSM-5: discomfort in situations where one is not the center of attention; inappropriate seductive or provocative interactions with others; rapidly shifting and shallow emotions; use of physical appearance to draw attention to self; impressionistic speech; self-dramatization; suggestibility; and the tendency to consider relationships to be more intimate than what they are in reality (APA 2013). Histrionic patients mostly use defense mechanisms such as denial, repression, and dissociation.

Meta-analyses (Leichsenring and Leibing 2003; Perry et al. 1999) suggest that psychotherapy can be significantly helpful for this disorder, but sociotherapy or psychopharmacology have no proven efficacy.

Individuals with narcissistic PD are likely to be demanding and dissatisfied patients. This disorder includes distorted beliefs about self-importance that can lead to inappropriate anger when confronted with the mundane realities of medical care such as waiting for appointments and completing redundant paperwork. Rejection, whether real or perceived, is another potential source of inappropriate anger. In order to diagnose an individual with this disorder per DSM-5, at least five or more of the following must be present: grandiose self-importance; preoccupations with fantasies of success, power, brilliance, beauty, or love; belief that one is unique and only understandable by other special people; need for excessive admiration; sense of entitlement; personal exploitativeness; lack of empathy; envy or belief that others are envious of self; and arrogance (APA 2013). Narcissistic individuals mostly use defense mechanisms such as devaluation, idealization, and omnipotence. In terms of response to treatment, this PD shares the same profile as histrionic PD: Psychotherapy can be quite helpful, but sociotherapy or medication has no proven role.

Case 24.4.1 Presenting Situation: Carol Jennings
Mrs. Jennings is a 34-year-old woman who is referred to you by her obstetrician/gynecologist (Ob/Gyn) for marital and work problems. Her chief complaint is, "I made an appointment because my doctor told me to." She is the

general manager of a local manufacturing company. Before she sits down in your office chair, she pulls a sanitizing wipe from her purse and wipes the chair. When she is seated comfortably on the chair, she looks at her watch and starts talking.

Mrs. Jennings describes her job as a source of both great pride and frustration. She describes her career path as a "pursuit of perfection" and views herself as "very disciplined." She is annoyed if the employees under her supervision do not keep their desks or calendars well organized. She tries to help out with suggestions and offers of help to stay late with them to arrange their desks. She is planning on installing a mandatory time management system on the company server. She says she instead gets curt remarks from ungrateful people who tell her she is driving them "nuts" with her micromanagement. She shakes her head in disbelief that anyone would make a choice to be inefficient.

Please proceed with the problem-based approach using the worksheet located in the appendix of Chap. 1!

Table 24.4.1

FACTS	HYPOTHESES	INFORMATION NEEDED	LEARNING ISSUES

Learning Issues: Cluster C Anxious or fearful

Obsessive-compulsive personality disorder (OCPD)
Avoidant personality disorder
Dependent personality disorder

Carol Jennings displays many behaviors and attitudes consistent with OCPD. According to NESARC, this is the most common PD, occurring in 2.1–7.9% of all Americans (Grant et al. 2004). She attempts to impose her values of organization and time management on others and has little insight into how this creates conflicts. Her family and employees likely find her rigid and controlling.

The criteria for OCPD include four or more of the following: excessive preoccupation with details, rules, lists, or organization to such an extreme that the functional point of the activity is lost; perfectionism that interferes with task completion; excessive devotion to productivity to the exclusion of leisure and not out of economic necessity; overconscientiousness and inflexibility; inability to discard objects, including those without sentimental value; reluctance to delegate; miserliness; and rigidity/stubbornness (APA 2013). Individuals with OCPD mostly use defense mechanisms such as isolation of affect and reaction formation.

24.4.2 Continuation and Conclusion

Mrs. Jennings describes her personal life as "married with one son." She says that her husband is a great guy—if only he would listen to her. A recent fight was over his repeated requests for an extended (10-day) family vacation as part of a family reunion. She told him why this is impossible for her. Mrs. Jennings keeps her 12-year-old son on a "strict leash." She feels her home would be a mess if both her husband and son were given too much responsibility. She has made it easy for them by placing a recyclable and a trash can in strategic places in each room and describes how her laundry room has special baskets for formal clothes, casual clothes, sportswear, etc. Mrs. Jennings has conflict with her son over his wardrobe. She fails to understand why he refuses to wear "perfectly good clothes that still fit" and insists on spending money for new school clothes.

Mrs. Jennings repeatedly questions why she was in your office paying a large co-pay instead of being with her colleagues or her husband. She demonstrated no insight into her role in the problems at work and home and declined to "waste time and money" on therapy appointments.

Please proceed with the problem-based approach using the worksheet located in the appendix of Chap. 1!

Table 24.4.2

FACTS	HYPOTHESES	INFORMATION NEEDED	LEARNING ISSUES

The diagnosis of OCPD is distinct from the similarly named obsessive-compulsive disorder (OCD). Although both disorders may include preoccupation with order as well as anxiety, patients with OCD recognize their preoccupations as problematic and dysfunctional (see Chap. 23).

Learning Issues: Other Cluster C Personality Disorders
Patients with avoidant PD are shy and sensitive. This PD occurs in about 2.4% of Americans (Grant et al. 2004). A fear of criticism and rejection may dissuade them from seeking personal and professional goals. This disorder is distinct from schizoid PD (Cluster A), in which there is no desire for relationships (as opposed to shyness and sensitivity in spite of the desire for relationships). Avoidant PD demonstrates a unique pattern of response to treatment. Such patients can enjoy a robust response to psychotherapy and a modest response to sociotherapy, but it is unclear if they benefit from medications.

The diagnosis of avoidant PD requires four or more of the following DSM-5 criteria: avoidance of job-related activities that involve interpersonal contact because of fears of disapproval; unwillingness to become involved with people unless certain of being liked; restraint with intimate relationships because of fear of being ridiculed; preoccupation with criticism or rejection in social situations; inhibition in interpersonal situations because of self-perceived inadequacy; self-perception of being unappealing or inferior; and reluctance to take risks that may lead to embarrassment (APA 2013). Fantasy and projection are the defense mechanisms mostly utilized by avoidant persons.

Dependent PD occurs in 0.49–0.6% of individuals within the USA (Grant et al. 2004; Lenzenweger et al. 2007). The hallmark of this disorder is an inability to assert an independent choice. Passive and developmentally immature behaviors can lead to parents to care for an adult child well after same-age peers have left home and started their own families. The treatments for dependent PD include insight-oriented therapy, behavioral therapy, assertiveness training, family therapy, and group therapy. High levels of separation anxiety or panic attacks may benefit from serotonergic antidepressants.

The diagnosis of dependent PD requires five or more of the following DSM-5 criteria: difficulty making everyday decisions without excessive guidance; need for others to assume responsibility for major areas of one's life; difficulty expressing disagreement out of unrealistic fear of loss of support; difficulty doing things on one's own because of lack of confidence; tendency to take excessive measures to secure nurturance and support from others; discomfort or helplessness when alone; tendency to seek another relationship as a source of care and support when one relationship ends; and unrealistic preoccupation with fears of being left alone to take care of oneself (APA 2013). Not dissimilar to avoidant PD, those with dependent PD mostly employ projection and fantasy as defense mechanisms.

24.1 Review Questions

For questions 1–5, please match the following illness with its associated clinical presentation.

a. Histrionic personality disorder
b. Schizotypal personality disorder
c. Avoidant personality disorder
d. Dependent personality disorder
e. None of the above

1. Family history often includes relatives with schizophrenia
2. Inappropriate provocative interactions with others
3. Inability to assert an independent choice
4. Delusional beliefs
5. Significant anxiety in social situations, notwithstanding desire for social relationships

Appendix A: Answers to Case Questions

Table 24.1.1: Leslie Danforth

What are the facts?	What are your hypotheses?	What do you want to know next?	What specific information would you like to learn about?
If true, Leslie's mother's assertion that she has difficulty "getting along" could speak to a lack of empathy on Leslie's part, as well as impairment in emotional intimacy	Leslie's problems with intimacy and self-direction, along with suspiciousness, could be suggestive of a Cluster A PD	How long have Leslie's problems lasted? Were they present prior to age 18?	What are the diagnostic criteria for the Cluster A PDs, and how do they differ from one another?
An inability to "hold a job" could speak to lack of self-direction		Pertinent questions to be addressed include the patient's identity, what sort of goals she makes, how she understands others' motivations and behaviors, and if she has any positive, emotionally intimate relationships	

What are the facts?	What are your hypotheses?	What do you want to know next?	What specific information would you like to learn about?
Looking around the room, glancing behind herself, and watching the door suggests suspiciousness, which is a facet of detachment		Does Leslie have any auditory or visual hallucinations? Are her thoughts and speech disorganized? Are there any other pertinent positives in her mental status exam?	
		A thorough psychological history is in order	

PD personality disorder

Table 24.1.2

What are the facts?	What are your hypotheses?	What do you want to know next?	What specific information would you like to learn about?
Her thoughts and speech are not disorganized	Without disorganization, hallucinations, fixed delusions, or abulia, this case is looking more like a Cluster A PD	One needs to inquire about possible psychoticism, other aspects of detachment, and substance use	What are the diagnostic criteria for the Cluster A PDs, and how do they differ from one another?
Leslie denies hallucinations, drug use, and head injuries		Collateral information about her beliefs and behaviors is in order	
The fact she was engaged speaks against abulia or the sort of pronounced lack of will which is observed in patients with schizophrenia			
Leslie has a history of feeling that others are against her, doubts others' honesty, accused her fiancés of infidelity, and has trouble trusting others			

PD personality disorder

Table 24.1.3

What are the facts?	What are your hypotheses?	What do you want to know next?	What specific information would you like to learn about?
Leslie's symptoms are not due to substance use, and her lab reports are normal	Leslie likely has paranoid PD	Would Leslie be willing to engage in treatment?	How do you differentiate between schizophrenia and some of the Cluster A PDs?
Leslie agrees to a follow-up appointment but does not show up for this appointment			What are the treatments for Cluster A PDs such as paranoid PD, and how effective are they?

PD personality disorder

Table 24.2.1: Brendan Ryles

Facts	Hypotheses	Information needed	Learning issues
Brendan is brought in by the police and has a criminal history, extending back into adolescence	Brendan's criminal behavior, family history, and impulsivity are suggestive of ASPD	Does Brendan meet the other diagnostic criteria for ASPD?	What are the diagnostic criteria for ASPD?
Brendan has a history of family dysfunction and lack of regard for authority			What does the literature suggest regarding the biology of ASPD?
Brendan is agitated and impatient			
Brendan drinks excessively and uses illicit drugs			

ASPD antisocial personality disorder

Table 24.2.2

Facts	Hypotheses	Information needed	Learning issues
Brendan is returned to jail, then to prison	Brendan meets criteria for ASPD	Will Brendan participate in treatment?	How do patients with ASPD respond to treatment?
He is held in segregation due to unprovoked violence		Is treatment beneficial for patients with ASPD?	Are there effective treatments for ASPD?

ASPD antisocial personality disorder

Table 24.3.1: Sharon Young

Facts	Hypotheses	Information needed	Learning issues
Ms. Young is admitted secondary to a suicide attempt and has a history of multiple suicide attempts	Ms. Young's self-injurious behavior, affective lability, and chronic history of difficulties in coping suggest a diagnosis of BPD	Does Ms. Young meet the other diagnostic criteria for BPD?	What are the diagnostic criteria for BPD?
Ms. Young's affect is labile			What is known about the biologic aspects of patients with BPD?
Ms. Young has a history of cutting and overdosing in response to interpersonal or academic problems			

BPD borderline personality disorder

Table 24.3.2

Facts	Hypotheses	Information needed	Learning issues
Ms. Young does meet other diagnostic criteria for BPD, including frantic efforts to avoid abandonment, unstable relationships, mood swings, and anger	Ms. Young has BPD	More information is needed about her "mood swings"	How can a diagnostician differentiate between BPD and bipolar disorder?
Ms. Young's medication history includes antipsychotics and antidepressants, as well as a mood stabilizers and an anxiolytic	Her affective lability may be part of her BPD or it may be bipolar disorder		

BPD borderline personality disorder

Table 24.3.3

Facts	Hypotheses	Information needed	Learning issues
Ms. Young engages in DBT	She will learn new skills to cope with her symptoms in DBT	What is DBT and how effective is it?	Treatments for BPD, including DBT and psychotropic medications
		What are the other personality disorders in Cluster B?	Other Cluster B personality disorders, such as histrionic personality disorder and narcissistic personality disorder

DBT dialectical behavior therapy, *BPD* borderline personality disorder

Table 24.4.1: Carol Jennings

Facts	Hypotheses	Information needed	Learning issues
Mrs. Jennings is referred due to marital and work problems	Mrs. Jennings has some compulsive behaviors consistent with OCPD	What are her other symptoms?	What are the diagnostic criteria for OCPD?
She is overly concerned with details, cleanliness, time, and perfection		Does she meet full criteria for OCPD?	What is the prevalence of OCPD?
She is disciplined, rigid, and inflexible			
Her imposition of perfectionistic standards on others causes interpersonal problems			

OCPD obsessive-compulsive personality disorder

Table 24.4.2

Facts	Hypotheses	Information needed	Learning issues
Mrs. Jennings's rigidity and inflexibility with her family are causing interpersonal conflict and impairments in family functioning	Mrs. Jennings likely has OCPD, but OCD must be ruled out	Does she meet criteria for OCD, or are her symptoms better accounted for with a diagnosis of OCPD?	How can a diagnostician differentiate between OCD and OCPD?
She is excessively concerned with organization			What are the other Cluster C personality disorders?
She is miserly and has an inability to discard her son's old clothes			
She lacks insight into how her behaviors are negatively affecting her colleagues and family			
She refuses treatment			

OCPD obsessive-compulsive personality disorder, *OCD* obsessive-compulsive disorder

Appendix B: Answers to Review Questions

1. b
2. a
3. d
4. e
5. c

References

American Psychiatric Association. (2013). *Diagnostic and statistical manual of mental disorders* (5th ed.). Washington, DC: American Psychiatric Association.

Daros, A. R., Zakzanis, K. K., & Ruocco, A. C. (2013). Facial emotion recognition in borderline personality disorder. *Psychological Medicine, 43*(9), 1953–1963.

Grant, B. F., Hasin, D. S., Stinson, F. S., Dawson, D. A., Chou, S. P., Ruan, W. J., & Pickering, R. P. (2004). Prevalence, correlates, and disability of personality disorders in the United States: Results from the national epidemiologic survey on alcohol and related conditions. *Journal of Clinical Psychiatry, 65*(7), 948–958.

Hofmann, S. G., Asnaani, A., Vonk, I. J. J., Sawyer, M. A., & Fang, A. (2012). The efficacy of cognitive behavioral therapy: A review of metaanalyses. *Cognitive Therapy and Research, 36*(5), 427–440.

Keshavan, M., Shad, M., Soloff, P., & Schooler, N. (2004). Efficacy and tolerability of olanzapine in the treatment of schizotypal personality disorder. *Schizophrenia Research, 71*(1), 97–101.

Kessler, R. C., Berglund, P., Chiu, W. T., Demler, O., Heeringa, S., Hiripi, E., Jin, R., Pennell, B. E., Walters, E. E., Zaslavsky, A. L., & Zheng, H. (2004). The U.S. National Comorbidity Survey replication (NCS-R): Design and field procedures. *International Journal of Methods in Psychiatric Research, 13*(2), 69–92.

Koerner, K., & Linehan, M. M. (2000). Research on dialectical behavior therapy for patients with borderline personality disorder. *The Psychiatric Clinics of North America, 23*(1), 151–167.

Leichsenring, F., & Leibing, E. (2003). The effectiveness of psychodynamic therapy and cognitive behavior therapy in the treatment of personality disorders: A meta-analysis. *The American Journal of Psychiatry, 160*(7), 1223–1232.

Lenzenweger, M. F., Lane, M. C., Loranger, A. W., & Kessler, R. C. (2007). DSM-IV personality disorders in the National Comorbidity Survey replication. *Biological Psychiatry, 62*(6), 553–564.

Linehan, M. M., Comtois, K. A., Murray, A. M., Brown, M. Z., Gallop, R. J., Heard, H. L., Korslund, K. E., Tutek, D. A., Reynolds, S. K., & Lindenboim, N. (2006). Two-year randomized controlled trial and follow-up of dialectical behavior therapy vs therapy by experts for suicidal behaviors and borderline personality disorder. *Archives of General Psychiatry, 3*(7), 757–766.

Loranger, A. W. (1990). The impact of DSM-III on diagnostic practice in a university hospital. A comparison of DSM-II and DSM-III in 10,914 patients. *Archives of General Psychiatry, 47*(7), 672–675.

McClure, M. M., Barch, D. M., Romero, M. J., Minzenberg, M. J., Triebwasser, J., Harvey, P. D., & Siever, L. J. (2007). The effects of guanfacine on context processing abnormalities in schizotypal personality disorder. *Biological Psychiatry, 61*(10), 1157–1160.

Minzenberg, M., Fan, J., New, A. S., Tang, C., & Siever, L. J. (2007). Fronto-limbic dysfunction in response to facial emotion in borderline personality disorder: an event-related fMRI study. *Psychiatry Research, 155*(3), 231–243.

Nelson, M. T., Seal, M. L., Pantelis, C., & Phillips, L. J. (2013). Evidence of a dimensional relationship between schizotypy and schizophrenia: A systematic review. *Neuroscience & Biobehavioral Reviews, 37*(3), 317–327.

Paris, J. (2011). Pharmacological treatments for personality disorders. *International Review of Psychiatry, 23,* 303–309.

Perry, J. C., Banon, E., & Ianni, F. (1999). Effectiveness of psychotherapy for personality disorders. *American Journal of Psychiatry, 156*(9), 1312–1321.

Spitzer, M., Fischbacher, U., Hermberger, B., Gron, G., & Fehr, E. (2007). The neural signature of social norm compliance. *Neuron, 56*(1), 185–196.

Verheul, R., & Herbrink, M. (2007). The efficacy of various modalities of psychotherapy for personality disorders: A systematic review of the evidence and clinical recommendations. *International Review of Psychiatry, 19*(1), 25–38.

Yang, Y., Raine, A., Narr, K. L., Colletti, P., & Toga, A. W. (2009). Localization of deformations within the amygdala in individuals with psychopathy. *Archives of General Psychiatry, 66*(9), 986–994.

Zimmerman, M., Rothschild, L., & Chelminski, I. (2005). The prevalence of DSM-IV personality disorders in psychiatric outpatients. *The American Journal of Psychiatry, 162,* 1911–1918.

Chapter 25
Neurocognitive Disorders

June C. Lee, Russ S. Muramatsu and Junji Takeshita

We hope you are continuing to enjoy learning about the different categories of psychiatric diagnoses! This chapter covers neurocognitive disorders (NCDs) that affect medically vulnerable and elderly patients and that highlight the close connection between body, brain, and behavior. At the end of this chapter, the reader will be able to:

1. Understand the concepts of cognition and memory and recognize when there is a change from baseline status
2. Compare and contrast normal age-associated forgetfulness, mild neurocognitive disorder (mNCD), major neurocognitive disorder (MNCD), delirium, and depression
3. Present a differential diagnosis for MNCD and delirium
4. Explain a comprehensive approach to evaluating a suspected NCD using a combination of history of illness, screening scales, and laboratory and imaging tests
5. Discuss the treatment of NCDs with a focus on MNCD due to Alzheimer's disease and delirium

J. C. Lee (✉) · J. Takeshita
Department of Psychiatry, University of Hawai'i John A. Burns School of Medicine, 1356 Lusitana Street, University Tower 4th Floor, Honolulu, HI 96813, USA
e-mail: jlee@dop.hawaii.edu

J. Takeshita
e-mail: takeshitaj@dop.hawaii.edu

R. S. Muramatsu
VA Pacific Islands Healthcare System, 459 Patterson Road, Honolulu, HI 96819, USA
e-mail: russ.muramatsu@va.gov

D. Alicata et al. (eds.), *Problem-based Behavioral Science and Psychiatry*,
DOI 10.1007/978-3-319-23669-8_25

Case Vignette 25.1.1 Presenting Situation Eli Thompson

Mr. Thompson is a 76-year-old man with a history of hypertension and diabetes. He "retired" 2 years ago from his full-time work of 35 years as a commercial house painter and has lived alone for the past year since his wife passed away from a hemorrhagic stroke. With hard work and dedication, he advanced through the ranks of his job and eventually succeeded in starting his own company with ten full-time employees. Over the years, he spent more time getting new "jobs" rather than painting himself. He has always been quite proud of his accomplishments.

Over the past year, his adult son and daughter have become increasingly concerned with some of his behavior and in the past 2 months have begun to seriously question whether he can continue to live alone. His children noticed that he occasionally forgets the names of his grandchildren. Additionally, he is frustrated that he "can't do things like the old days," and he would say, "My memory is not like it was before." Most concerning is that he seems to be having problems with his medications. They noticed sometimes he forgets to take them and sometimes he takes the wrong ones or the wrong amount. As Mr. Thompson's primary care provider, you see him in your office with his daughter.

STOP

Please proceed with the problem-based approach using the worksheet located in the appendix of Chap. 1!

Please fill in the facts, your hypotheses, further information needed, and learning issues for Learning Issue Table 25.1.1.

Learning Issue Table 25.1.1

FACTS	HYPOTHESES	INFORMATION NEEDED	LEARNING ISSUES

At this point, the primary concern voiced both by Mr. Thompson and his family is a change in cognition. Before going any further, it is important to understand what is meant by cognition. The term cognition (Latin: *cognoscere,* "to know") is used in several ways to describe mental processes such as memory, attention, perception, action, problem solving, and mental imagery. The Diagnostic and Statistical Manual of Mental Disorders, Fifth Edition (DSM-5), defines specific cognitive domains, which form the basis of the various NCDs. These cognitive domains are complex attention, executive function, learning and memory, language, perceptual-motor, and social cognition (American Psychiatric Association 2013).

There is a large array of biopsychosocial factors that could potentially affect someone's cognition. For example, almost every disorder in DSM-5 could likely affect cognition. Patients with schizophrenia typically have cognitive problems as well as a thought disorder. In this chapter, we will limit our discussion primarily to the disorders classified under NCDs, emphasizing MNCD and delirium. The DSM-5 (American Psychiatric Association 2013) classifies delirium, the syndromes of mNCD and MNCD, and their etiological subtypes as a group of disorders in which "the primary clinical deficit is in cognitive function that is acquired rather than developmental" (see Table 25.1).

Once a cognitive problem is suspected, the first step is obtaining an accurate history from the patient, family, and caregivers. The focus of the history is on the chronology of the cognitive changes including onset, course, progression, and

Table 25.1 Neurocognitive disorders

Delirium
Substance intoxication delirium
Substance withdrawal delirium
Medication-induced delirium
Delirium due to another medical condition
Delirium due to multiple etiologies
Other specified delirium
Unspecified delirium
Major and mild neurocognitive disorders
Major or mild neurocognitive disorder due to Alzheimer's disease
Major or mild frontotemporal neurocognitive disorder
Major or mild neurocognitive disorder with Lewy bodies
Major or mild vascular neurocognitive disorder
Major or mild neurocognitive disorder due to traumatic brain injury
Substance/medication-induced major or mild neurocognitive disorder
Major or mild neurocognitive disorder due to HIV infection
Major or mild neurocognitive disorder due to prion disease
Major or mild neurocognitive disorder due to Parkinson's disease
Major or mild neurocognitive disorder due to Huntington's disease
Major or mild neurocognitive disorder due to another medical condition
Major or mild neurocognitive disorder due to multiple etiologies
Unspecified neurocognitive disorder

Table 25.2 Neurocognitive disorder continuum

	Normal memory	Normal age-related decline	Mild neurocognitive disorder	Major neurocognitive disorder
Memory deficits	None	Trace, may be transient	Mild, may be reversible	Moderate to severe, typically nonreversible
Other cognitive deficits	None	None	Possible	Definite
Psychometric performance	Normal		1.5 standard deviation below mean for age	
Level of function	Independent	Independent	Independent	Dependent

associated symptoms. A complete "data set" is the most efficient way to narrow down the differential diagnosis from which eventually you will hopefully attain the best diagnosis. Mr. Thompson, for example, had a noticeable change in his behavior and cognition about 1 year ago, which coincided with the death of his wife. You might consider a diagnosis of a depressive disorder that is presenting with memory and concentration problems. On the other hand, a history of onset of cognitive problems as a young adult might suggest acute lead toxicity from exposure to lead-based paint.

Identifying Mr. Thompson's baseline level of cognition and functioning is helpful to figure out the progression and severity of the problems. It also has some role in predicting performance on testing and prognosis. While Mr. Thompson's formal educational level was only a high school diploma, he demonstrated an above average intellect and resourcefulness as a successful business owner. Educational attainment is not the best indicator of intelligence for older individuals as many elderly have limited formal education.

Upon closer inspection, you might suspect that his problems with cognition started even earlier. Often, family members only recognize a problem when the symptoms have become obvious. Looking back, there are sometimes subtle clues that indicate the process started much earlier. In Mr. Thompson's case, you might wonder why he retired 2 years ago. Could he have had early MNCD or mNCD? Was he having difficulty keeping track of his business? Could this be just part of "normal" aging in a 74-year-old (Feldman and Jacova 2005)? Table 25.2 lists other possibilities.

Case Vignette 25.1.2 Continuation

Further history reveals that Mr. Thompson has no personal history of depression or other psychiatric conditions. He has never used tobacco or any illicit drugs. He has been treated with an antihypertensive and oral hypoglycemic medication for the past 10 years. He has no family history of NCDs or other neuropsychiatric disorders. He denies any other symptoms or problems including problems with movement, falls, or hallucinations.

While he admits that he still misses his wife, he feels he is over his acute grief and has not become tearful or overwhelmingly sad for 6 months or more. In fact, other than sleep problems he does not endorse any other symptoms of depression including suicidality. He spends his time reading and working in his yard. His favorite past time, however, since his early twenties, was to "kick back" with his friends after a hard day's work and enjoy a "few" beers.

Please proceed with the problem-based approach using the worksheet located in the appendix of Chap. 1!

Please fill in the facts, your hypotheses, further information needed, and learning issues for Learning Issue Table 25.1.2.

Learning Issue Table 25.1.2

FACTS	HYPOTHESES	INFORMATION NEEDED	LEARNING ISSUES

Here we get additional information that could be used to help with continued evaluation of what type or types of NCDs we are dealing with.

At this point, a diagnosis of depression, although important to consider and differentiate from NCDs, is low on the list of potential diagnoses. Alcohol intoxication or withdrawal delirium is a possibility given Mr. Thompson's alcohol use history. However, there is no evidence of a delirium at this time as his level of attention and awareness has been stable without fluctuation. His cognitive deficits seem more significant than just "normal" aging. The most likely diagnosis is an early-stage MNCD. Table 25.3 reviews differentiating factors between depression, MNCD, and delirium (Arnold 2004; Potter and Steffens 2007) (see Table 25.3).

In the DSM-5, the term "dementia" was retained from the DSM-IV-TR for continuity and is included under the newly named term "major neurocognitive disorder." Although there are many different MNCDs as defined in the DSM-5, all share common characteristics, including evidence of significant objective cognitive decline in one or more cognitive domains (complex attention, executive function, learning and memory, language, perceptual-motor or social cognition) that cause functional impairment, that represent a decline from previous functioning, that are not better explained by another mental disorder, and that do not exclusively occur during a delirium (American Psychiatric Association 2013).

Table 25.3 Differentiating the "3 D's"

	Dementia	Depression	Delirium
Precipitating event	Uncommon (depends on type)	Sometimes may have a psychosocial stressor	Present usually a change in medical condition or medications
Age of onset	Uncommon below age 60	Any age	Any age
Rate of onset	Insidious months to years	Moderately acute weeks to months	Acute hours to days
Fluctuations	Stable throughout the day may be worse at night ("sundowning")	Hourly to daily worse in morning	Minutes to hourly worse at night
Course	Progressive decline	Resolves with treatment, may reoccur or be chronic	Resolves with treatment
Duration	Lifetime (for nonreversible causes)	Moderate weeks to months	Short hours to weeks
Consciousness	Intact	Intact	Altered
Memory complaints	May be denied by patient	Common	None
Memory performance	Worse than self-assessment does not improve with cues normal effort	Better than self-assessment improves with retrieval cues decreased effort "don't know"	Usually no self-assessment does not improve with cues variable effort
Family history	Often noncontributory	Common to have a family history of mood disorders	Generally noncontributory
Personal history	Possible risk factors may be present	Common to have a history of stressors	Generally noncontributory

Table 25.4 Etiologies of major neurocognitive disorder. (Adapted from Gray and Cummings 1996)

Category	Example
Degenerative	Major neurocognitive disorder due to Alzheimer's disease, Parkinson's disease
Vascular	Multiple infarcts
Myelinoclastic	Multiple sclerosis
Inflammatory	Systemic lupus erythematosus
Infectious	Syphilis, HIV infection
Toxic	Alcohol related
Metabolic	Hepatic encephalopathy
Traumatic	Subdural hematoma, traumatic brain injury
Neoplastic	Meningioma
Hydrocephalic	Normal pressure hydrocephalus
Psychiatric	Schizophrenia

Case Vignette 25.1.3 Continuation

Mr. Thompson's Mini Mental State Examination (MMSE) testing reveals a score of 26 out of 30. He missed three points on orientation and one point on recall. His clock-drawing test was without errors, although he was somewhat slow in completing it. Throughout the testing, Mr. Thompson seemed motivated to perform well. Laboratory results were as follows: nonreactive rapid plasma reagin RPR, low normal vitamin B12 level, normal folate level, normal thyroid-stimulating hormone TSH level, and normal chemistries and complete blood count CBC. Heavy metal screening including lead is normal. You had debated testing for HIV but decide against it. A non-contrast computed tomography (CT) scan of the brain is significant only for some mild cortical atrophy and "periventricular white matter changes."

The DSM-5 added a new diagnosis in the NCD chapter named "mild neurocognitive disorder" (mNCD) which is recognized as a less severe form of cognitive impairment. In mNCD, there is evidence of mild cognitive decline in one or more cognitive domains, but the cognitive deficits do not cause functional impairment. Much of our understanding of mNCD has been attained from research on mild cognitive impairment (MCI). MCI is a broad term, which is defined as a syndrome with a slight impairment in cognitive function (often memory) with otherwise normal functioning. Patients with MCI, especially amnestic MCI, have a greater risk of developing MNCD. However, not all patients with MCI progress to dementia and some patients remain stable or even improve (Levey et al. 2006).

It is important to realize that MNCD can include features beyond just a memory problem. Now that we are pretty sure that we are dealing with an MNCD, we must now review all of the potential etiologies. Giving a diagnosis of "major neurocognitive disorder" is akin to giving a diagnosis of "fever," which is present in a variety of illnesses. In Mr. Thompson's case, certain potential etiologies include alcohol, lead exposure, and vascular events (see Table 25.4). There are also a few that need to be ruled out with laboratory tests and brain imaging.

Please proceed with the problem-based approach using the worksheet located in the appendix of Chap. 1!

Please fill in the facts, your hypotheses, further information needed, and learning issues for Learning Issue Table 25.1.3.

Learning Issue Table 25.1.3

FACTS	HYPOTHESES	INFORMATION NEEDED	LEARNING ISSUES

The MMSE, not to be confused with a Mental Status Examination (MSE), is a 30-point screening test for MNCD that can be used in the clinical setting. It has been perhaps the most utilized and recognized cognitive screening test, although other tests such as the Montreal Cognitive Assessment (MoCA) and the Saint Louis University Mental Status Examination (SLUMS) are also being used (Folstein et al. 1975). In the MMSE, each question tests a specific area of cognition, for example, memory, language, and visual–spatial orientation, which can be correlated with functioning of a specific area in the brain. The lower the score, the more severe the cognitive problem.

There are several important points to remember. The MMSE is purely a screening test; it does not diagnose MNCD. Further cognitive testing is necessary in combination with history and labs to confirm a diagnosis of MNCD. There are several reported limitations with the MMSE. For example, the questions overemphasize memory and do not even test for executive functioning. Performance on the MMSE is affected by culture and educational level. Someone who has more "educational reserves" may continue to score high on the MMSE while having significant change in cognitive ability from baseline. Even problems with vision or hearing must be taken into account as they could affect performance.

The MMSE score can be used to categorize the severity of the cognitive deficit. The true value of the test, however, is to track performance over time and thereby be able to evaluate the progression of disease or success of treatment. In general, a score greater than 26 is considered normal; 20–26 suggests mild MNCD; 10–19 suggests moderate MNCD; and 10 suggests severe MNCD. On average, without treatment, people with MNCD will lose 2–4 points each year.

The Clock-Drawing Test is another screening test for MNCD. Patients are presented with a circle drawn on a piece of paper. They are told, "This circle represents a clock face." They are then asked to, "Fill in the numbers to look like a clock and then set the time to 10 past 11." Shulman (2000) indicates that the cognitive skill necessary for completion of this task include (a) comprehension, (b) planning, (c) visual memory and reconstruction, (d) visual–spatial abilities, (e) motor programming and execution, (f) numerical knowledge, (g) abstract thinking, (h) inhibition of the tendency to be pulled by perceptual features of the stimulus, and (i) concentration and frustration tolerance. It can be used similarly as the MMSE to track changes over time.

Other cognitive screening tests include the SLUMS and the MoCA. The MoCA and SLUMS were developed to screen patients with mild cognitive problems and who usually perform normally on the MMSE. Both tests have comparable sensitivities and specificities with the MMSE in detecting dementia, and they are better than the MMSE at detecting mNCD (Nasreddine et al. 2005; Tariq et al. 2006). The SLUMS is a 30-point clinician-administered test similar to the MMSE with additional tasks such as a clock-drawing task, animal naming, digit span, and immediate recall of facts from a paragraph. The MoCA is a 30-point clinician-administered test with tasks screening for executive functioning such as a clock-drawing task, alternation task adapted from the trail-making B task, phonemic fluency, and two-item verbal abstraction task. The SLUMS has cutoff scores for mNCD and dementia, whereas the MoCA has a cutoff score of 26 for cognitive impairment. Therefore, it may be practical to administer the MoCA or SLUMS rather than the MMSE to patients with mild cognitive problems with no functional impairment to screen for mNCD.

Standard laboratory and imaging tests for major neurocognitive impairment are shown in Table 25.5. Heavy-metal screening is typically not done but ordered in this case as the patient was a painter and may have had exposure to lead-based paint. The most likely diagnosis for Mr. Thompson at this point is MNCD due to Alzheimer's disease. A definitive diagnosis can only be made at autopsy.

Please proceed with the problem-based approach using the worksheet located in the appendix of Chap. 1!

Table 25.5 Laboratory and imaging evaluation for major neurocognitive disorder. (Adapted from Kawas 2003; Knopman et al. 2001)

Routine	*Nonroutine*
CBC	Syphilis screening
Glucose	Lumbar puncture
Serum electrolytes	EEG
BUN/creatinine	Genetic testing for DLB or CJD
Serum B12 levels	APOE genotyping for DAT
Thyroid function tests	SPECT
Liver function tests	Linear or volumetric MRI or CT
CT imaging	
MRI	
Not enough evidence	
Other genetic markers for AD	
CSF or other biomarkers for AD	
Tau mutations for FTD	
AD gene mutations in FTD	

CT computed tomography, *MRI* magnetic resonance imaging, *EEG* electroencephalography, *AD* alzheimer's disease, *FTD* frontotemporal dementia, *CSF* cerebrospinal fluid, *DLB* dementia with Lewy bodies, *CJD* creutzfeldt-Jakob disease, *APOE* apolipoprotein E, *DAT* dementia of the Alzheimer's type, *SPECT* single-photon emission computerized tomography

Case Vignette 25.1.4 Continuation

Two weeks later, you receive a call from Mr. Thompson's daughter who is distraught. She tells you that she is at her father's house and just now found him lying on the floor moaning in pain. You tell her to call 911. In the emergency room, an X-ray reveals that Mr. Thompson has fractured his hip. His daughter tells her brother on the phone, "See I told him to get rid of that ugly living room area rug…I knew he would trip on that one day…" Mr. Thompson was admitted to the orthopedic service, and you see him the next day to manage his general medical problems.

Upon greeting him in his hospital room, you realize that he is not himself. He thinks he is at home and shares with you how people were outside his window last night trying to break into his house to steal his money. He is unable to give the correct date, month, or year for that matter. Looking at the nursing notes, you learn that he had been severely agitated and combative with staff requiring him to be physically restrained during the night. An electrocardiogram reveals some tachycardia but normal corrected QT interval (QTc). You believe that his tachycardia is due to agitation rather than alcohol withdrawal and decide to give an antipsychotic rather than a benzodiazepine. You are concerned about QTc as antipsychotics can prolong QTc. After the addition a very low dose of antipsychotic medication, his confusion improves, and eventually it is tapered off. One-week post-surgery, Mr. Thompson is ready for discharge.

Please fill in the facts, your hypotheses, further information needed, and learning issues for Learning Issue Table 25.1.4.

Learning Issue Table 25.1.4

FACTS	HYPOTHESES	INFORMATION NEEDED	LEARNING ISSUES

Mr. Thompson had another, more dramatic change in his cognition. His confusion is much worse, and there are new symptoms of delusions and hallucinations. The time course of worsening symptoms and onset of new symptoms are too sudden to be consistent with progression of the MNCD. Also, it is too much of a coincidence that this presentation coincides with the hip fracture, hospitalization, and surgery. Notice again the importance of understanding the chronology of symptoms in narrowing the differential diagnosis.

An acute delirium best explains Mr. Thompson's presentation. Possible etiologies include alcohol withdrawal, pain medications, or the surgery itself. Like with MNCD, there are many different causes of delirium (see Table 25.6). Irrespective of etiology, delirium as defined in the DSM-5 includes the following characteristics: disturbance of attention and awareness, a disturbance in cognition (e.g., memory deficit, disorientation, language, visuospatial ability, or perception), acute onset with fluctuating course, the disturbances are not better explained by an MNCD, and there is evidence that the disturbance is a direct consequence of another medical condition, substance intoxication or withdrawal, exposure to a toxin, or due to multiple etiologies (American Psychiatric Association 2013).

Table 25.6 Etiologies of delirium: "I WATCH DEATH". (Adapted from Wise and Trzepacz 1996)

Category	Example
Infectious	Encephalitis
Withdrawal from drugs	Alcohol
Acute metabolic disorder	Electrolyte disturbance
Trauma	Closed-head injury
CNS pathology	Seizure
Hypoxia	Hypotension
Deficiencies in vitamins	Thiamine
Endocrinopathies	Hyper-/hypoglycemia
Acute vascular insults	Stroke
Toxins or drugs	Medications
Heavy metals	Lead

CNS central nervous system

Delirium can be categorized into hyperactive, hypoactive, and mixed delirium. Physicians are far more likely to be called by nursing staff for the hyperactive form (as was the case with Mr. Thompson). While the exact pathophysiology underlying delirium is not known, one hypothesis is that there is a decreased level of acetylcholine and an increased level of dopamine present. In addition to treating the underlying etiology, the most common pharmacologic treatment of delirium, especially when agitation is present, is low doses of antipsychotic medications, particularly haloperidol (Friedman et al. 2014). Atypical antipsychotics may also be used (Wang et al. 2013). The exception to this is the presence of alcohol or sedative hypnotic withdrawal or seizures, which should be primarily treated with benzodiazepines. In Mr. Thompson's case, haloperidol was used with good success.

Case Vignette 25.1.5 Continuation

Mr. Thompson is admitted to a nursing home for rehabilitation. His children have the long-term plan to sell his house and move him into an assisted living facility. On repeat MMSE testing, he scores 23 out of 30. Mr. Thompson has great difficulty settling in to his new environment. He is unhappy about sharing a room with another person. He is irritable towards both the staff and his family and asks everyone "Why can't I go home?" The physical therapist expressed concerns that he was not progressing as fast as she thought he should in therapy. When asked about his progress, he replies, "Don't ask me…how should I know…I don't even know why I'm here really…."

Mr. Thompson's score on the Geriatric Depression Scale (GDS) is 9 out of 15, highly suspicious for the presence of a depression. Mr. Thompson denies feeling depressed but is willing to take an antidepressant medication, "Go ahead…whatever you think…you're the doctor." You prescribe low dose of a selective serotonin reuptake inhibitor (SSRI) and spend time listening to his concerns. Two weeks later, Mr. Thompson seems to be in a little better mood; his family also noticed a small change. By 4 weeks, his mood had changed considerably. He is no longer so irritable and is even beginning to like his living environment. At the end of 8 weeks, he has made so much progress in therapy that the treatment team began planning for discharge back to the community.

STOP

Please proceed with the problem-based approach using the worksheet located in the appendix of Chap. 1!

Please fill in the facts, your hypotheses, further information needed, and learning issues for Learning Issue Table 25.1.5.

Learning Issue Table 25.1.5

FACTS	HYPOTHESES	INFORMATION NEEDED	LEARNING ISSUES

Again, Mr. Thompson has had a change in his cognitive functioning as seen by his MMSE score and clinical presentation. MNCD, delirium, and depression are, as usual, the primary differential considerations. As before, the progression is abrupt. Delirium is not likely, although residual cognitive deficits post-delirium is a possible problem. The most likely problem at this point, however, is a dementia syndrome of depression. Terms such as "pseudodementia" were previously used to describe this syndrome. Historically, clinicians believed that treating the depression would result in resolution of cognitive deficits although data that are more recent suggest a close relationship between depression and dementia (Lyketsos 2010). In elderly patients, depression after nursing home placement is not uncommon and may present with atypical symptoms. Depression is also common in the early phases of a MNCD. Citalopram may be particularly beneficial in managing the behavioral symptoms of Alzheimer dementia as well as depression (Pollack et al. 2007).

Elderly patients commonly have many physical illnesses and symptoms, which overlap with neurovegetative symptoms such as changes in weight, sleep, or fatigue. Focusing on the other symptoms of depression such as suicidal thoughts, feelings of guilt, or feelings of hopelessness can be more helpful. It is also important to realize that depression is not an inevitable and untreatable outcome of either aging or nursing home placement.

The GDS is a screening test for depression in the elderly patient. There are two versions of the scale: a 30-point version and a shorter 15-point version (Brink et al. 1982; Sheikh and Yesavage 1986). The questions differentiate depression from depression-like symptoms from other physical illnesses. The higher the score, the more likely the patient is depressed.

Please refer to Chap. 21 for more specific information on major depressive disorder. Depression and MNCD can occur very independently of each other. They can both occur at the same time in a person but be independent of each other. MNCD can be associated with or be a cause of depression. Depression is a risk factor for

MNCD, may be a prodrome to MNCD, cause cognitive deficits itself, and worsen the physical and functional symptoms of MNCD (Potter and Steffens 2007). Screening for depression is a recommended part of routine workup for MNCD (Knopman et al. 2001).

Case Vignette 25.1.6 Conclusion

A year and a half later, Mr. Thompson shows up in your outpatient clinic with his daughter. “I’m living by myself now,” he says smiling, although you know from his daughter that he is in an assisted living facility and requires hired caregivers to assist with daily activities such as medication management. His MMSE today indicates a score of 20/30, and there is no indication of depression or acute confusion. You spend the rest of the time talking to Mr. Thompson and his daughter educating them on the course of illness and what to expect in the future.

STOP

Please proceed with the problem-based approach using the worksheet located in the appendix of Chap. 1!

Please fill in the facts, your hypotheses, further information needed, and learning issues for Learning Issue Table 25.1.6.

Learning Issue Table 25.1.6

FACTS	HYPOTHESES	INFORMATION NEEDED	LEARNING ISSUES

With the delirium and depression resolved, Mr. Thompson’s underlying MNCD continues to slowly progress, as indicated by his declining MMSE score. As part of the treatment plan, you discuss the use of medications such as acetylcholinesterase

Table 25.7 General stages of major neurocognitive disorder

Mild (early stage)	Memory loss and/or other cognitive deficits are noticeable
	Can compensate and may continue to function independently
Moderate (mid-stage)	Memory and other cognitive deficits worsen
	Accompanied by personality and physical changes
	More dependent on others
Severe (late stage)	Deterioration of the personality
	Loss of control of bodily functions
	Total dependence on others

inhibitors and N-methyl-D-aspartate (NMDA) antagonists with Mr. Thompson and his daughter.

The primary pathophysiologic process underlying MNCD due to Alzheimer's disease is the production of abnormal proteins in the brain and the subsequent development of beta-amyloid plaques and neurofibrillary tangles. These abnormalities correlate with neuronal dysfunction and ultimately degeneration of a cluster of neurons that produce acetylcholine (nucleus basalis of Meynert). This decreases the production of the neurotransmitter acetylcholine, which is thought to play a role in cognition. Acetylcholinesterase inhibitors, like donepezil, while not affecting the underlying pathophysiology or reversing dementing diseases, help limit the degradation of the existing acetylcholine and therefore slow down the effects of the disease. Acetylcholinesterase inhibitors are typically more effective in the early phase of Alzheimer's disease but can be used in later stages. NMDA antagonists such as memantine, reserved for moderate-to-severe stages, work on a different neurotransmitter, glutamate. Glutamate is involved in the release of calcium from neurons. Too much calcium causes death of the cell, and memantine interferes with this process. Behavioral symptoms such as agitation, delusions, and hallucinations are common during the course of Alzheimer's disease and respond to some degree with medications such as citalopram, prazosin, and antipsychotics (Pollack et al. 2007; Sink et al. 2005; Wang et al. 2009). Antipsychotics should be used with caution given the increased risk of diabetes, stroke, extrapyramidal symptoms, and death (Schneider et al. 2005, 2006).

Table 25.7 describes the stages of MNCD due to Alzheimer's disease and the common progression of the illness. Dividing the disease into stages can help families plan for the future. Realize, however, that no two patients are alike; the type of symptoms and rate of progression may differ. People with MNCD due to Alzheimer's disease live for an average of 10 years after the diagnosis, and most die from complications such as pneumonia and decubitus ulcers.

We close with a summary diagram (Fig. 25.1) and biopsychosocial–cultural–spiritual formulation (Table 25.8) of Mr. Thompson's case.

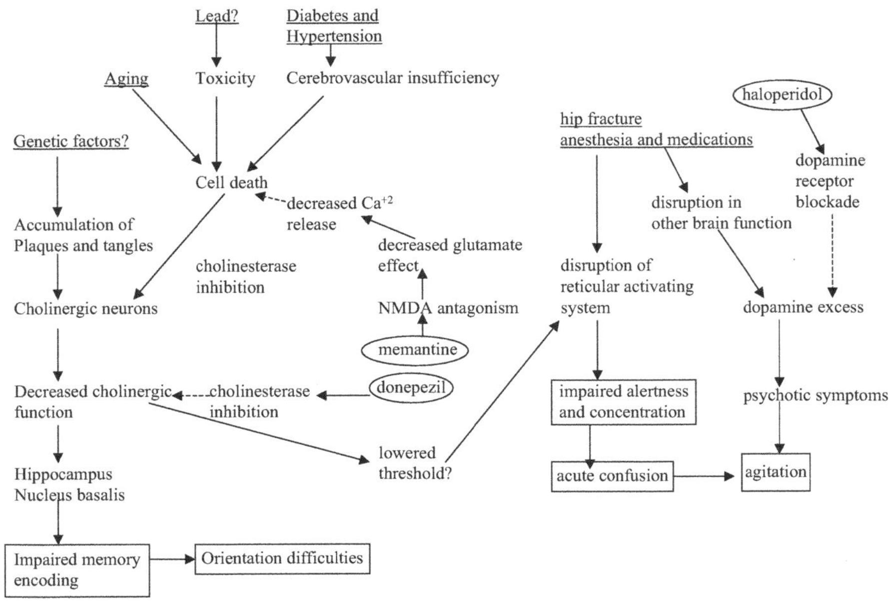

Fig. 25.1 Mechanistic case diagram of the case "Mr. Thompson"

Table 25.8 Biopsychosocial formulation of the case "Mr. Thompson"

	Biological		Psychological		Social	
	Factor	*Intervention*	Factor	*Intervention*	Factor	*Intervention*
Predisposing factors	History of heavy alcohol use and exposure of lead paint	*Stopped drinking and no longer paints*	Death of his wife 1 year ago	*None*	Less immediate social support after wife's death	
	Diabetes and hypertension	*Oral hypoglycemic and antihypertensive medications*	Loss of his job due to retirement	*None*		
Precipitating factors	Cognitive decline and memory problems	*Comprehensive evaluation*	Role transition from independent to dependent	*Individual counseling*	Inappropriate level of care	*Hospital and then nursing home admission*
					Inadequate environment	*Education of family*

Table 25.8 continued

	Biological		Psychological		Social	
Perpetuating factors	Delirium and depression	*Haloperidol to treat delirium*		*Medication and supportive therapy*	Need for increased care and supervision	*Change in living environment*
	Worsening MNCD	*SSRI to treat depression*	Dealing with loss and change			*Education of family*
		Acetylcholinesterase inhibitors and NMDA antagonists				

SSRI selective serotonin reuptake inhibitor, *NMDA* N-methyl-D-aspartate, *MNCD* major neurocognitive disorder

25.1 Review Questions

1. In evaluating a patient with cognitive deficits which of the following is most useful:

(a) Obtaining serum anticholinergic level
(b) Administering the GDS
(c) Getting an adequate history
(d) Checking MMSE
(e) Ordering a CT of head

2. The MMSE is most useful for which of the following:

(a) Diagnosing MNCD
(b) Evaluating frontal lobe functioning
(c) Determining progression of cognitive deficits
(d) Screening tool for mania
(e) Evaluating which patients should be given an acetylcholinesterase inhibitor

3. Delirium is differentiated from MNCD by which of the following feature:

(a) Fluctuating attention and awareness
(b) Severity of cognitive deficits
(c) Relationship with psychosocial stressors
(d) Improved cognitive examination with cues
(e) Family history

4. Memantine helps with cognition through the following neurotransmitter:

(a) Acetylcholine
(b) Dopamine

(c) Norepinephrine
(d) Serotonin
(e) glutamate

Appendix A: Tables with Possible Answers to the Vignettes

Case Vignette 25.1: Presenting Situation Eli Thompson

Learning Issue Table 25.1.1

Facts	Hypotheses	Information needed	Learning issues
76–year-old man with hypertension and diabetes	Depressive disorders	Obtain history from patient, family, and caregivers	What are the different presentations of normal memory, normal age-related decline, mild neurocognitive disorder, and MNCD? (See Table 25.2)
Behavior and memory changes (forgets name of grandchildren and medications)	MNCDs	Identify baseline level of cognition and functioning	
Death of his wife a year ago	Mild neurocognitive disorders		
Retirement 2 years ago	Normal aging		
	Delirium		

MNCD major neurocognitive disorder

Learning Issue Table 25.1.2

Facts	Hypotheses	Information needed	Learning issues
Alcohol use history	Major neurocognitive disorders	Cognitive testing	What are the differentiating factors between depression, MNCD, and delirium? (see Table 25.3)
No history of depression	Depression	Laboratory testing (CBC, BMP, RPR, vitamin B12, folate, TSH)	What are the potential etiologies of MNCD? (See Table 25.4)
No illicit drug use	Delirium	Imaging of the brain (non-contrast CT of the brain)	

BMP basic metabolic panel

Taking antihypertensive and oral hypoglycemic medication	Alcohol intoxication or withdrawal delirium		
No family history of neurocognitive disorders			
No movement problems, falls, or hallucinations			
Sleep problems			
No depressive symptoms			

CT computed tomography, *MNCD* major neurocognitive disorder

Learning Issue Table 25.1.3

Facts	Hypotheses	Information needed	Learning issues
MMSE score 26/30	MNCD due to Alzheimer's disease	Neuropsychological testing	What are the standard laboratory and imaging tests for MNCD? (See Table 25.5)
Clock-Drawing Test was normal	Major frontotemporal neurocognitive disorder		What is the MMSE and Clock-Drawing Test?
Lab results normal	Major vascular neurocognitive disorder		
Heavy-metal screening normal			
Non-contrast CT scan of the brain significant for mild cortical atrophy and periventricular white matter changes			

CT computed tomography, *MMSE* Mini Mental State Examination, *MNCD* major neurocognitive disorder

Learning Issue Table 25.1.4

Facts	Hypotheses	Information needed	Learning issues
Hip fracture after fall	Acute delirium due to alcohol withdrawal, pain medications, or surgery	Medication list	What are the common causes of delirium? (See Table 25.6)
Disorientation, delusions, and hallucinations		Laboratory testing (CBC, BMP, urinalysis, urine toxicology screen)	What is the treatment of delirium?

Severe agitation and combativeness with staff			
Antipsychotic medication used for agitation			

Learning Issue Table 25.1.5

Facts	Hypotheses	Information needed	Learning issues
MMSE score was 23/30	Depression	Response to SSRI medication (repeat GDS)	What is the GDS?
Irritability with staff and family	Major neurocognitive disorder		What is the treatment for geriatric depression?
GDS scored 9 out of 15 points	Delirium		
SSRI prescribed for depression			

SSRI selective serotonin reuptake inhibitor, *GDS* Geriatric Depression Scale, *MMSE* Mini Mental State Examination

Learning Issue Table 25.1.6

Facts	Hypotheses	Information needed	Learning issues
Mr. Thompson living in an assisted living facility	Major neurocognitive disorder due to Alzheimer's disease	Obtain more information on functional status	What is the pathophysiology of Alzheimer's disease?
MMSE score was 20/30			What are the stages of Alzheimer's disease? (See Table 25.7)

MMSE Mini Mental State Examination

Appendix B: Answers to Review Questions

Answers:

1. C
2. C
3. A
4. E

References

American Psychiatric Association. (2013). Diagnostic and statistical manual of mental disorders DSM-5 Fifth Edition.

Arnold, E. (2004). Sorting out the 3 D's: Delirium, dementia, depression. *Nursing, 34,* 36–42.

Brink, T. L., Yesavage, J. A., Lum, O., Heersema, P., Adey, M. B., & Rose, T. L. (1982). Screening tests for geriatric depression. *Clinical Gerontologist, 1,* 37–44.

Feldman, H. H., & Jacova, C. (2005). Mild cognitive impairment. *The American Journal of Geriatric Psychiatry, 13,* 645–655.

Folstein, M. F., Folstein, S. E., & McHugh, P. R. (1975). Mini Mental State: A practical method for grading the cognitive state of patients for the clinician. *Journal of Psychiatric Research, 12,* 189–198.

Friedman, J. I., Soleimani, L., McGonigle, D. P., Egol, C., & Silverstein, J. H. (2014). Pharmacological treatments of non-substance-withdrawal delirium: A systematic review of prospective trials. *The American Journal of Geriatric Psychiatry, 171,* 151–159.

Gray, K. F., & Cummings, J. L. (1996). *Dementia. Textbook of consultation-liaison psychiatry* (pp. 68). Washington, DC: Rundell/Wise.

Kawas, C. H. (2003). Early Alzheimer's disease. *The New England Journal of Medicine, 349,* 1056–1063.

Knopman, D. S., DeKosky, S. T., Cummings, J. L., Chui, H., Corey-Bloom, J., Relkin, N., Small, G. W., Miller, B., Stevens, J. C. (2001). Diagnosis of dementia (an evidenced based review): Report of the quality standards subcommittee of the American Academy of Neurology. *Neurology, 56,* 1143–1153.

Levey, A., Lah, J., Goldstein, F., Steenalnd, K., & Bliwise, D. (2006). Mild cognitive impairment: An opportunity to identify patients at high risk for progression to Alzheimer's disease. *Clinical Therapeutics, 28,* 991–1001.

Lyketsos, C. G. (2010). The Interface between depression and dementia: Where are we with this important frontier? *The American Journal of Geriatric Psychiatry, 18,* 95.

Nasreddine, Z. S., Phillips, N. A., Bédirian, V., Charbonneau, S., Whitehead, V., Collin, I., et al. (2005). The Montreal cognitive assessment (MoCA): A brief screening tool for mild cognitive impairment. *Journal of the American Geriatrics Society, 53,* 695–699.

Pollock, B. G., Mulsant, B. H., Rosen, J., Mazumdar, S., Blakesley, R. E., Houck, P. R., et al. (2007). A Double-blind comparison of citalopram and risperidone for the treatment of behavioral and psychotic symptoms associated with dementia. *The American Journal of Geriatric Psychiatry, 15,* 942–952.

Potter, G. G., & Steffens, D. C. (2007). Contribution of depression to cognitive impairment and dementia in older adults. *The Neurologist, 13,* 105–117.

Schneider, L. S., Dagerman, K. S., & Insel, P. (2005). Risk of death with atypical antipsychotic drug treatment for dementia: Meta-analysis of randomized placebo-controlled trials. *Journal of the American Medical Association, 294,* 1934–1943.

Schneider, L. S., Dagerman, K., & Insel, P. S. (2006). Efficacy and adverse effects of atypical antipsychotics for dementia: Meta-analysis of randomized, placebo-controlled trials. *The American Journal of Geriatric Psychiatry, 14,* 191–210.

Sheikh, J. I., & Yesavage, J. A. (1986). *Geriatric depression scale (GDS): Recent evidence and development of a shorter version. Clinical gerontology: A guide to assessment and intervention* (pp. 165–173). New York: The Haworth Press.

Shulman, K. I. (2000). Clock-drawing: Is it the ideal cognitive screening test? *International Journal of Geriatric Psychiatry, 15,* 548–561.

Sink, K. M., Holden, K. F., & Yaffe, K. (2005). Pharmacological treatment of neuropsychiatric symptoms of dementia a review of the evidence. *Journal of the American Medical Association, 293,* 596–608.

Tariq, S. H., Tumosa, N., Chibnall, J. T., Perry, M. H. 3rd, & Morley J. E. (2006). Comparison of the Saint Louis University mental status examination and the mini-mental state examination for detecting dementia and mild neurocognitive disorder-a pilot study. *The American Journal of Geriatric Psychiatry, 14,* 900–910.

Wang, L. Y., Shofer, J. B., Rohde, K., Hart, K. L., Hoff, D. J., McFall, Y. H., et al. (2009). Prazosin for the treatment of behavioral symptoms in patients with Alzheimer's disease with agitation and aggression. *The American Journal of Geriatric Psychiatry, 17,* 744–751.

Wang, H. R., Woo, Y. S., & Bahk, W. M. (2013). Atypical antipsychotics in the treatment of delirium. *Psychiatry and Clinical Neurosciences, 67,* 323–331.

Wise, M. G., & Trzepacz, P. T. (1996). *Delirium (confusional states). Textbook of consultation-liaison psychiatry* (pp. 268). Washington, DC: Rundell/Wise.

Chapter 26
Sleep–Wake Disorders

Ole J. Thienhaus and Justin B. Otis

Insomnia and poor sleep are among the most common reasons patients consult their primary care physician. However, the diagnosis of insomnia is nonspecific and is easily confused with parasomnias and hypersomnias. Thus, the clinician must fully assess the sleep problem and rule out a primary or underlying condition (Taylor et al. 2007) before treating sleeplessness symptomatically with a sedative hypnotic (medication to induce sleep). The three cases in this chapter illustrate insomnia as well as less common sleep disorders.

At the end of this chapter the reader will be able to:

1. Describe a differential diagnosis for symptoms of insomnia.
2. Identify the behaviors associated with parasomnias.
3. Develop a plan for assessment of daytime hypersomnia

Vignette 26.1.1 Presenting Situation: Maria Thompson
Maria Thompson is a 36-year-old married woman who is the mother of two preteen boys. She comes to your primary care office with the complaint of "not sleeping." Until a few years ago, she never noticed any sleeping problems, although she describes herself as a light sleeper. Currently, she says that her insomnia causes her to toss and turn for at least 2 h most nights. She grows increasingly worried about not getting enough sleep before she is finally able to fall asleep. During the night, she wakes up for no apparent reason, or because of a trivial noise or minimal urge to use the bathroom. Then she cannot go back to sleep as she thinks about the difficult problems in her home.

"But I, being poor, have only my dreams; I have spread my dreams under your feet; Tread softly because you tread on my dreams."William Butler Yeats—*He Wishes for the Cloths of Heaven*

J. B. Otis (✉) · O. J. Thienhaus
University of Arizona College of Medicine at South Campus Psychiatry, 2800 E Ajo Way, Tucson, AZ 85711, USA
e-mail: Justin.Otis@uahealth.com

D. Alicata et al. (eds.), *Problem-based Behavioral Science and Psychiatry*,
DOI 10.1007/978-3-319-23669-8_26

Please proceed with the problem-based approach using the worksheet located in the appendix of Chap. 1!

Table 26.1.1

FACTS	HYPOTHESES	INFORMATION NEEDED	LEARNING ISSUES

26.1 Learning Issues: Insomnia

Epidemiology Insomnia is defined as any combination of symptoms including difficulty falling asleep, frequent nighttime awakenings, and early morning awakening. It is one of the most common complaints among primary care patients and is estimated to affect over 60 million Americans each year. Up to 20 % of individuals in the primary care setting report significant insomnia symptoms, and it is more common in woman than men with an estimated ratio of 1.44:1 (APA 2013).

Differential Diagnosis A thorough clinical history and examination are the most critical elements that direct a clinician toward a differential diagnosis. Difficulty in sleeping (insomnia/dyssomnia) should be distinguished from excessive sleepiness (hypersomnia). The type of insomnia (e.g., difficulty falling asleep as opposed to early morning awakening) can be determined by specific, clarifying questions. Table 26.1 briefly details several of the more common dyssomnias that should be considered on differential diagnosis. Medical, psychiatric, and other secondary causes should be also considered and ruled out. Alcohol or sedative use, caffeine use, smoking, and mood disorders may cause insomnia, and are part of a thorough history. Possible underlying medical problems, such as endocrine disorders may be identified on physical examination and targeted laboratory tests. A sleep study is the ideal way to objectively measure the quality of a patient's sleep and monitor for physiologic events disturbing sleep.

Table 26.1 Dysomnias

Dysomnias	Diagnostic features	Special features
Primary insomnia	1 month or more of poor sleep	Rule out substances, mood disorders, pain, environmental causes
Primary hypersomnia	1 month or more of excessive sleep	Rule out substances, endocrine, mood, and causes
Narcolepsy	Cataplexy, hallucinations, sleep paralysis, and sleep attacks	Polysomnogram and multiple sleep latency test
Obstructive sleep apnea	Interruptions of breathing during the night, periods of low blood oxygenation	Excessive soft tissue in oropharynx. Desaturation of blood triggers brief awakenings for breathing
Central sleep apnea	Interruptions of breathing during the night, periods of low blood oxygenation	Dysfunction of thalamus due to neurological disorder
Circadian rhythm sleep disorder	Mismatch of sleep–wake cycle and environment	Includes shift work, jet lag
Nocturnal myoclonus	Jerking movements of legs while sleeping	May have symptoms during the day as well
Restless leg syndrome	Uncomfortable leg sensations that interfere with sleep	
Kleine–Levin syndrome	Periodic hypersomnia with episodic increases in appetite and sexual activity	Affects mainly adolescent males

Vignette 26.1.2: Continuation

Mrs. Thompson has already tried to adjust her sleep time, at the suggestion of a magazine article, and goes to bed at least an hour after her husband. When she wakes up, she has a hard time going back to sleep and often finishes out the night on the living room couch so as not to disturb her husband. She awakens early in the morning, but feels exhausted and worn out. “Often it’s hard to get up and started on the day.” Coffee helps, but by noon, she is ready to “crawl back into bed,” if only she felt she actually could get back to sleep. The patient believes that her two boys have begun to worry about her. Her husband is at times solicitous about her health and at other times irritated with her perceived “laziness.” He wonders “if we’ll ever have sex again.”

A few months ago another physician checked Mrs. Thompson’s thyroid status (which was normal), and prescribed sleeping pills. First, she tried hydroxyzine, then zolpidem. Later, she tried a low dose of trazodone. Mrs. Thompson says that all these medications “made me even more tired,” but none helped her sleep through the night.

Mrs. Thompson says that she has always been in good health. The two childbirths were the only times she was in the hospital. After the second baby, she had “the blues” for a while, but it resolved in a few weeks. She denies any family history of psychiatric illness. Her mother, who died of cervical cancer at the age of 41, also had sleeping problems, but Mrs. Thompson thinks this was related to the cancer.

Mrs. Thompson does not drink alcohol and has never used illicit drugs. She takes no prescription or over-the-counter medications. She appears somewhat tense at the beginning of the interview, but when asked about her feeling "at a dead end," she suddenly burst into tears. She is worried about her failures as a wife and mother. She has been withdrawing from activities she could and would be doing with her family. Mrs. Thompson used to enjoy running a book club with neighborhood friends; however, after her second son was born she stopped. At first, it was because she was busy taking care of the baby, but later because she just did not feel like doing it anymore.

Mental Status Examination: Mrs. Thompson is alert and fully oriented. Her affect is dejected, tearful, and weary, but she responds to supportive comments and maintains stable eye contact. She describes her mood as "worried." There is no evidence of any cognitive impairment, thought disorder, or perceptual disorder. She denies feeling suicidal.

STOP

Please proceed with the problem-based approach using the worksheet located in the appendix of Chap. 1!

Table 26.1.2

FACTS	HYPOTHESES	INFORMATION NEEDED	LEARNING ISSUES

Mrs. Thompson's tearful effect, sense of failure, and anhedonia (lack of pleasure), suggest that the original complaint of insomnia is likely a symptom of a major depressive episode (please refer to Chap. 21 for further discussion of mood disorders). As with other common generalized symptoms such as fatigue and weight loss, insomnia should not be reduced to a purely symptom-based diagnostic label. The original treatments geared toward sleep were ineffective because they did not address the primary cause of Mrs. Thompson's insomnia.

Case Vignette 27.1.3: Conclusion
After further questioning, you discover that Mrs. Thompson meets criteria for major depressive disorder with five out of nine criteria in the DSM-5 lasting longer than 2 weeks. After discussion of several treatment options, she agrees to a trial with an antidepressant and a limited supply of a benzodiazepine. In addition, she appreciates that the latter medicine may only have a limited role in her improvement and that psychological interventions, family therapy, and supportive counseling regarding stress management and coping could be the most important with her recovery. She agrees to schedule an appointment with a local therapist covered by her insurance plan. You see Mrs. Thompson weekly for a month, and then schedule a 3 month follow-up appointment. She reports improvements in mood, sleep, and energy, and has started to see her therapist.

26.2 Learning Issues

Treatment Treatment of insomnia targets underlying primary pathology whenever present. For example, successful treatment of a depressive disorder will improve related sleep problems. In primary insomnia or when coexisting diagnoses have only an aggravating effect, the clinical target is insomnia. First-line interventions include improving sleep hygiene and the practice of relaxation techniques (Morgenthaler et al. 2006). Proper sleep hygiene includes going to bed and rising at the same time each day, avoiding caffeine, alcohol, television (or other blue light), and exercise in the evening, and sleeping in the same quiet, dark environment that is used only for sleeping (Morgenthaler et al. 2006) . Sleep medications can assist these interventions and build a positive reward experience. Hypnotic medications exert their effects in one of three neurotransmitter systems: the histamine receptors such as diphenhydramine and hydroxyzine (most over-the-counter sleep aids), the gamma-aminobutyric acid (GABA) receptors (benzodiazepines and GABA allosteric agonist *Z* drugs), or the melatonin receptors (ramelteon; Taylor et al. 2006) . In short-term situations where insomnia results from a time-limited stress exposure (e.g., during a hospital stay), pharmacologic intervention can be justified as the first choice of treatment. Long-term use of sleep medications remains controversial because of the potential for abuse and dependence with most hypnotics. Ramelteon and eszopiclone (allosteric GABA agonist) have been shown to maintain long-term effectiveness for insomnia with minimal risk of dependence (Taylor et al. 2006) .

Vignette 26.2.1 Presenting Situation: Vickie Sippets
Vickie is a 17-year-old high school student seen in clinic with her parents. Vickie's mother explains she and her husband are worried about their daughter, who started sleepwalking about 6 weeks earlier. At first they thought Vickie was waking up to use the bathroom, and was so groggy she would

not respond. When it started happening nearly every night, they decided to get up, lead her back to her room, and wake her up. Several minutes into the interview, Vickie speaks for the first time, and tells you she is quite puzzled and cannot explain how she ended up out of bed.

Please proceed with the problem-based approach using the worksheet located in the appendix of Chap. 1!

Table 26.2.1

FACTS	HYPOTHESES	INFORMATION NEEDED	LEARNING ISSUES

26.3 Learning Issues

26.3.1 Parasomnias

Epidemiology Parasomnias are less common than insomnias and mostly affect children and young adults. Somnambulism (sleepwalking disorder) is by far the most common parasomnia with an estimated prevalence of 5–15 % among children in the USA (Szelenberger et al. 2005). It is classified as a non-REM sleep arousal disorder in the DSM-5 (APA 2013). Table 26.2 describes the stages of sleep. Sleepwalking is most likely to occur during stage III or IV sleep. Table 26.3and 26.4 describe some typical features of common parasomnias and other abnormal sleep behaviors.

Table 26.2 Stages of sleep

Sleep stage	EEG findings	Clinical findings
Stage I	Low voltage, fast waves	Light sleep, easily aroused
Stage II	Sleep spindles and K complexes	Easily awakened; metabolism slows
Stage III and IV	Slow delta waves	Deep sleep, no muscle movement, difficult to awaken. Sleep stage for sleepwalking, enuresis, and night terrors
REM (rapid eye movement)	Highly active, with small and irregular waves similar to waking state	4–5 distinct periods in 90 min cycles during night of sleep, increased in the last one third of the night; Dreams occur

Table 26.3 Parasomnias

Parasomnias	Diagnostic features	Special features
Sleepwalking	Repeated episodes of walking during sleep, difficult to wake	Amnesia for episode
Sleep terror	Awakenings related to intense fear state	Patient not alert, no recall of a dream, awakens with a scream, usually early in sleep cycle
Nightmare disorder	Awakenings related to vivid nightmares	Patient is alert upon awakening

Table 26.4 Related sleep diagnoses

Nocturnal bruxism	Teeth clenching and grinding during the night	May require mouth guard to protect teeth
Nocturnal enuresis	Bed wetting after the age of 6	Primary: no history of nocturnal bladder control Secondary: previous bladder control
Sleep hyperhidrosis	Night sweats	May be related to menopause, some serious illnesses

Differential Vickie's presentation suggests somnambulism, which is a primary sleep disorder (Lee-Chiong 2005). Other possibilities need to be considered, and the differential diagnosis includes a seizure disorder with psychomotor phenomena (partial complex seizures), and a factitious disorder (Eisensehr and Schmidt 2005). In a factitious disorder, the patient assumes a sick role in order to obtain gratification of certain psychological needs of which he or she is not consciously aware (see Chap. 23 on Somatic Symptom Disorders for more information on factitious disorder).

Vignette 26.2.2: Continuation

History: Vickie and her mother report that there is no past history of any psychiatric problems. Her performance in school is above average and she enjoys sports. She broke up with her boyfriend a couple of months earlier and has not been dating since. She denies any use of drugs or alcohol. She denies any current or past sexual activity. Vickie hopes to go to college to study psychology.

You ask Vickie's parents to step out for a moment, and then gently ask Vickie further questions about her personal life. She continues to endorse her same convictions and history. She reiterates that she is confused about what is going on, and states that she has not taken any alcohol or drugs.

Mental Status Examination: Vickie is a young woman in no acute distress. She appears age-appropriate in her development and intellectual function. There is no evidence of psychosis or cognitive impairment.

STOP

Please proceed with the problem-based approach using the worksheet located in the appendix of Chap. 1!

Table 26.2.2

FACTS	HYPOTHESES	INFORMATION NEEDED	LEARNING ISSUES

26.4 Learning Issues

Diagnosis The key to diagnosis in sleep disorders is an electrophysiological evaluation known as a polysomnogram or sleep study. During the assessment, an electroencephalogram (EEG) records wave patterns during both non-REM sleep (stages I–IV) and rapid eye movement (REM) sleep, while an electromyogram (EMG) measures muscle activity. Additionally, respiratory rate, heart rate, and blood oxygenation are recorded during periods of sleep and wakefulness. A sleep study with polysomnographic EEG data would show, in a case of somnambulism, an onset of motor phenomena coinciding with deep non-REM sleep (stages III and IV, also called delta sleep) early in the night, with REM sleep closer to the morning (Guilleminault et al. 2006). In order to diagnose a partial complex seizure disorder, also called temporal lobe epilepsy or psychomotor seizure disorder, a sleep-deprived EEG is performed with nasopharyngeal leads to detect abnormal electrical activity in deep brain structures. When a patient has an abnormal EEG, neurologists will further evaluate for the cause of the abnormal activity and will treat the patient with antiseizure medications. If the polysomnogram does not offer a clear diagnosis, psychological testing may be useful to determine if personality factors would make the patient more likely to communicate her distress by developing physical symptoms.

Treatment With somnambulism, the first intervention is education. Acknowledgement and avoidance of priming factors including sleep deprivation, poor sleep hygiene, and ingestion of certain medications, such as propranolol, antiarrhythmics, sedative hypnotics, and antihistamines, may reduce the frequency of episodes (Pressman 2007). Other factors that may trigger episodes include stress, anxiety, migraines, caffeine intake, or a full bladder. If a patient does not respond to these interventions, low-dose antidepressants or clonazepam may be effective at reducing occurrences (Reite and Weissberg 2014).

Vignette 26.2.3: Conclusion
Vickie's sleep study supports a working diagnosis of somnambulism. When Vickie and her parents return, you explain that sleepwalking is a fairly common occurrence in children and young adults, and usually resolves spontaneously. You further warn that because she is not awake during her motor activities at night there is a possibility that Vickie could harm herself. It is therefore important to make her environment safer, for example, by blocking staircases and locking away knives. You go on to explain that the incidence of somnambulism may increase with anxiety, stress, and unresolved conflicts such as the breakup with her boyfriend. Her parents accept this with some hesitancy, but agree after further reassurance that they can return if the problem worsens or does not go away.

Vignette 26.3.1 Presenting Situation: Randolph Jegniff
Mr. Randolph Jegniff, an obese 30-year-old recently married man, comes to your primary care clinic at his wife's suggestion. He reports that during their recent honeymoon his wife noticed that "the little naps I take" occur frequently and without any warning: "She was driving the car, and talking to me, when suddenly, I was gone." His wife told him that he "looked funny" when I fell asleep "like I had collapsed." Sometimes, he would briefly just "slump down like he'd been hit on the head" and she wondered if he'd gone asleep again, except he seemed to be alert, and straightened up his posture again after a few seconds.

Please proceed with the problem-based approach using the worksheet located in the appendix of Chap. 1!

Table 26.3.1

FACTS	HYPOTHESES	INFORMATION NEEDED	LEARNING ISSUES

26.5 Learning Issues: Hypersomnias

Differential and Epidemiology The details in the case above suggest narcolepsy with cataplexy, abrupt loss of muscle tone, a type of hypersomnia (Dauvilliers et al. 2007). Other possibilities include sleep apnea, a petit mal seizure disorder, as well as problems adjusting to alternating sleep–wake times, sometimes called *shift worker syndrome* (Ohayon et al. 2002).

Narcolepsy is more rare than parasomnias or insomnias with a prevalence of less than 10 % (Longstreth et al. 2007). If left untreated, it has the potential to cause serious functional impairment; however, it has an excellent prognosis with treatment.

Sleep apnea is another relatively common hypersomnia. Its prevalence has been reported between 9–24 % in men aged 30–60, and 4–9 % for women of the same age (Rowley 2014). Sleep apnea may lead to a host of related symptoms including impaired cognition, mood problems, hypertension, and increased risk for cardiovascular events (Lee et al. 2008). It is also strongly correlated with diabetes mellitus (Nieto et al. 2000; Caples et al. 2005). A rare cause of hypersomnia is Kleine–Levin syndrome. This is a primary hypersomnia affecting adolescents with sleep attacks that can last for 2 days with periods of irritability, hypersexuality, and confusion.

Vignette 26.3.2: Continuation

History: Mr. Jegniff is a postdoctoral student at the nearby college. He denies any medical problems. He admits to an occasional glass of wine, but no recreational drugs since his late teenage years when he occasionally smoked marijuana. He characterizes himself as a light sleeper who needs "lots of naps during the day." Mr. Jegniff remembers a few embarrassing occasions when he briefly fell asleep while teaching classes. At those times, he considered such episodes "a wake-up call" to try and get more sleep during the night. Mr. Jegniff and his wife concur that he does not snore at night. He does not wake-up to catch his breath, or have periods of not breathing for several seconds.

Physical Examination: 30-year-old obese male with a 15-in. neck circumference, oral pharyngeal cavity appears clear and unobstructed. Jaw line is of normal prominence. No other abnormal findings.

STOP

Please proceed with the problem-based approach using the worksheet located in the appendix of Chap. 1!

Table 26.3.2

FACTS	HYPOTHESES	INFORMATION NEEDED	LEARNING ISSUES

26.6 Learning Issues

Diagnosis The key to differential diagnostic understanding with narcolepsy is a sleep study with polysomnographic EEG data. This examination will provide data regarding latency of sleep onset which is reduced in narcolepsy from an average of 20 min to 5 min or less. Sleep EEGs may also show brief intrusions of REM sleep during *twilight* periods. This abnormal REM activity is responsible for the sleep paralysis and hypnogogic (falling asleep) and hypnopompic (waking up) hallucinations associated with narcolepsy. The decreased latency of sleep onset in narcolepsy is accompanied by electromyographic findings suggestive of cataplexy. The EEG would also be helpful in the diagnosis of sleep apnea as well as a petit mal seizure disorder. With Mr. Jegniff, a larger neck circumference, crowded pharynx, small non-prominent jaw (retrognathia), and a history of snoring would support a diagnosis of obstructive sleep apnea. A history of periodic respiratory cessation followed by waking or other catching of breath would support investigation of a much less common condition called central sleep apnea.

Treatment Once diagnosed, patients must start taking precautions to avoid complications. For instance, a person with untreated narcolepsy should not drive. The condition itself is otherwise benign and with treatment there are usually no limitations to patient functioning. However, this vulnerability must be kept in mind, so when a patient with a history of narcolepsy undertakes intercontinental travel or starts variable shift work, the patient, family, and physician ought to prepare for a possible relapse.

Narcolepsy appears to be the result of deficient hypocretin production in the brain. In the research laboratory, CSF levels of the neurotransmitter hypocretin are low or nonexistent in narcolepsy (Siegel and Boehmer 2006). Modafinil is a compound that seems to indirectly stimulate hypocretin secretion. It also has histamine and dopamine agonist properties resulting in improved wakefulness (Siegel and Boehmer 2006). The R-enantiomer of modafinil and armodafinil has also been approved for the treatment of narcolepsy. Traditionally, stimulants such as methylphenidate have been used as well. Tricyclic antidepressants can reduce the incidence of cataplexy, as does sodium oxybate (the same compound as the club drug gamma-hydroxybutyric acid, GHB).

Sleep apnea often improves with weight loss, although many patients require positive pressure oxygen during the night to maintain normal blood oxygenation levels. Alternative treatments include using a mandibular advancing device or undergoing a uvulopalatopharyngoplasty (UPPP), a surgical intervention that involves removal of the soft palate tissue in order to improve nighttime airflow (Rowley 2014) .

Case Vignette 26.3.3 Conclusion

Mr. Jegniff is scheduled for a sleep study. The results of the study come back strongly suggestive of narcolepsy. His treatment begins conservatively with a well-designed sleep hygiene schedule. Mr. Jegniff needs to go to bed approximately the same time every night, avoid sleep-delaying activities or stimulants, sleep in the same room, and get up at around the same time every morning. You explain that this will reduce the frequency of sleep attacks and minimize functional impairment due to narcolepsy. Change in his sleeping habits during his vacation likely caused his symptoms to worsen. In addition, you discuss prescription of modafinil (Provigil) or armodafinil (Nuvigil) to increase his daytime alertness, especially after he demonstrates desire to regain the confidence to drive.

26.7 Self-Assessment Questions

1. The most common form of insomnia is:
    a. Insomnia due to major depressive disorder
    b. Insomnia due to hyperthyroidism
    c. Restless leg syndrome
    d. Primary insomnia
    e. Shift worker syndrome
2. In the differential diagnosis of somnambulism, factitious disorder can be detected
    a. By psychological evaluation
    b. By a specific EEG pattern
    c. By polygraph test
    d. By waking up the patient
    e. By examination of the CSF
3. In the treatment of narcolepsy, the most important element in improving symptom control is
    a. Modafinil in the morning
    b. Cognitive behavioral therapy
    c. Sleep hygiene
    d. Aversive conditioning
    e. Methylphenidate
4. In the diagnostic assessment of persons with insomnia, which factor is not usually of importance?
    a. Total sleeping time
    b. Daytime sleepiness
    c. Sleep onset latency
    d. Coexisting psychiatric problems
    e. Socioeconomic class
5. Which of the following factors does not increase risk for obstructive sleep apnea?
    a. Neck circumference greater than 17 cm
    b. Mallampatti classification scores of 3 or 4
    c. Presence of retrognathia
    d. Chronic obstructive pulmonary disease
    e. Obesity
6. Which is the most sensitive symptom in diagnosing major depressive disorder?
    a. Suicidal ideation
    b. Depressed mood
    c. Sleep disturbances

   d. Poor energy
   e. Guilt

7. To prepare for clinical interview of patients presenting with chief complaints relating to sleep or energy, prepare a complete list of factors for proper sleep hygiene.

Appendix A—Possible Answers to Clinical Vignettes

Table 26.1.1: Maria Thompson

Facts	Hypotheses	Information needed	Learning issues
36-year-old woman, married, mother of two preteens	She is overwhelmed with perceived family obligations, and stress leads to abnormalities in cortisol regulation/PHA feedback?	What does *overwhelmed* mean?	What are the different types and causes of insomnia?
Trouble falling asleep (2 h)	Trouble falling asleep and awakenings with concerns about problems and adequacy could point toward a mood or anxiety disorder?	Were there any periods when she did NOT have sleep problems?	What is the epidemiology of insomnia?
Trouble staying asleep	Use of substances to cope with stress having negative effects on sleep?	Assessment of sleep hygiene?	What should be considered as differential diagnoses?
Cannot go back to sleep once awakened	Medical etiology?	Are there any other signs and symptoms of a mood disorder?	What would a sleep study tell us about her sleep patterns?
Worried about household problems		Any PMH suggestive of endocrine abnormalities, manic or hypomanic episodes, substance abuse?	
		Lab: Thyroid panel	

Table 26.1.2

Facts	Hypotheses	Information needed	Learning issues
Intervention of adjusting sleep time has failed	Symptoms suggestive of a major depressive episode as a cause for sleep impairment	Are there any recent stressors?	What are the symptoms of a major depressive episode?

Early morning awakenings feeling exhausted and worn out	Excessive caffeine or other substance use in response to stress as an etiology for sleep dysfunction	History and family history of psychiatric illness?	What are the interventions for impaired sleep that do not require medications?
Difficulty getting motivated for her day		Evaluation for other symptoms of depression?	What are the components of proper sleep hygiene?
Daytime sleepiness		Other substance use history?	How do sleep medications exert their effects?
Caffeine use			
Perceived *laziness*			
Lack of sexual desire/ intimacy			
Normal TSH			
Failed trials of zolpidem, trazodone, hydroxyzine			

Table 26.2.1: Vickie Sippets

Facts	Hypotheses	Information needed	Learning issues
17-year-old female sleepwalking beginning 6 weeks ago	Experiencing sleep arousal disorder due to multiple possible factors including recent stress	Psychiatric history and family history	What are the different stages of sleep?
Not responsive during episodes	Substance use contributing to disruption in sleep	Substance abuse history	In what stages of sleep would somnambulism or sleepwalking occur?
No recollection of events	Psychiatric etiology for sleep disturbances including major depression, anxiety, PTSD	Recent life stressors or changes	What are parasomnias? What are the differential diagnoses for parasomnias?
		History of sleep disturbances as a child	What are the sleep architecture changes associated with psychiatric illness and substance use?

PTSD posttraumatic stress disorder

Table 26.2.2

Facts	Hypotheses	Information needed	Learning issues
No past psychiatric history	Non-REM sleep arousal disorder secondary to recent emotional stress of breakup with boyfriend	Polysomnographic data assessing movement and sleep abnormalities in a controlled setting	What is a sleep study, and how can it help diagnose a sleep disorder?

Normal intellectual functioning	Anxiety or depressive symptoms not addressed during clinical interview contributing to sleep loss	More extensive psychiatric interviewing regarding depressive and anxiety symptoms	What are the primary causes of non-REM sleep arousal disorders?
Recent stress of breakup with boyfriend			What patient population does somnambulism primarily affect?
Denies any drug use or alcohol			What are the treatments for somnambulism?
No current sexual activity			
Normal mental status examination			

Table 26.3.1: Randolph Jegniff

Facts	Hypotheses	Information needed	Learning issues
30-year-old obese male	Fatigue from recent honeymoon with expected increase in sleep drive	Full sleep history including hygiene and quality	What is the normal physiologic response to sleep deprivation?
Frequent *little naps*	Psychiatric illness causing impaired sleep	Substance use history	Which stage of sleep is associated with muscle paralysis?
Looking funny and collapsing asleep, slumping down	Abnormal intrusion of sleep in form of narcolepsy or other hypersomnia	Psychiatric history and family history	What is the most common chief complaint of patients diagnosed with narcolepsy?
Short period of somnolence followed by abrupt return of consciousness and muscle tone	Substance use or intoxication altering level of consciousness	Recent history of activities while on honeymoon	What is the association between narcolepsy and insomnia?
	Sleep apnea causing decreased quality of sleep	History of gasping, snoring, and other descriptors for sleep apnea	What are the types of sleep apnea?

Table 26.3.2

Facts	Hypotheses	Information needed	Learning issues
Postdoctoral student	Frequent naps and intrusion of sleep into daytime due to hypersomnia with cataplexy	Polysomnogram study and multiple sleep latency test to evaluate for apnea and decreased REM latency	How is narcolepsy diagnosed?

No medical problems	Central sleep apnea or obstructive sleep apnea contributing to poor quality of sleep		Which neck circumference increases risk for apnea?
Occasional glass of wine			What are relieving and exacerbating factors for narcolepsy and what are treatments options? What are the treatments for sleep apnea?
Frequent naps			
Falling asleep while teaching classes			
No snoring, catching his breath			
15 in. neck with clear oropharynx			

Appendix B—Answers to Self-assessment Questions

1. D—Primary insomnia
2. A—Psychological evaluation
3. C—Sleep hygiene
4. E—Socioeconomic class
5. D—Chronic obstructive pulmonary disease
6. C—Sleep disturbances
7. Proper sleep hygiene includes going to bed and rising at the same time each day, avoiding caffeine, alcohol, television (or other blue light), and exercise in the evening, and sleeping in the same quiet, dark environment that is used only for sleeping.

References

American Psychiatric Association. (2013). *Diagnostic and statistical manual of mental disorders* (5th edn.). Washington, DC: American Psychiatric Publishing.

Caples, S. M., Gami, A. S., & Somers, V. K. (2005). Obstructive sleep apnea. *Annals of Internal Medicine, 142,* 187–197.

Dauvilliers, Y., Arnulf, I., & Mignot, E. (2007). Narcolepsy with cataplexy. *Lancet, 369,* 499–511.

Eisensehr, I., & Schmidt, D. (2005). Epilepsie und Schlafstörungen. *MMW – Fortschritte der Medizin, 147*(2), 54–57.

Guilleminault, C., Kirisoglu, C., da Rosa, A. C., Lopes, C., & Chan, A. (2006). Sleepwalking, a disorder of NREM sleep instability. *Sleep Medicine, 7,* 163–170.

Lee, W., Nagubadi, S., Kryger, M. H., & Mokhlesi, B. (2008). Epidemiology of obstructive sleep apnea: A population-based perspective. *Expert Review of Respiratory Medicine, 2*(3), 349–364. doi:10.1586/17476348.2.3.349.

Lee-Chiong, T. L. Jr. (2005). Parasomnias and other sleep-related movement disorders. *Primary Care, 32,* 415–434.

Longstreth, W. T. Jr, Koepsell, T. D., Ton, T. G., Hendrickson, A. F., & van Belle, G. (2007). The epidemiology of narcolepsy. *Sleep, 30,* 13–26.

Morgenthaler, T., Kramer, M., Alessi, C., Friedman, L., Boehlecke, B., Brown, T., et al. (2006). American Academy of Sleep Medicine: Practice parameters for the psychological and behavioral treatment of insomnia: An update. An American Academy of Sleep Medicine Report. *Sleep, 29,* 1415–1419.

Nieto, F. J., Young, T. B., Lind, B. K., et al. (2000). Association of sleep-disordered breathing, sleep apnea, and hypertension in a large community based study - Sleep Heart Health Study. *JAMA: The Journal of the American Medical Association, 283,* 1829–1836.

Ohayon, M. M., Lemoine, P., Arnaud-Briant, V., & Dreyfus, M. (2002). Prevalence and consequences of sleep disorders in a shift worker population. *Journal of Psychosomatic Research, 53,* 577–583.

Pressman, M. R. (2007). Factors that predispose, prime, and precipitate NREM parasomnias in adults: Clinical and forensic implications. *Sleep Medicine Review, 11,* 5–33.

Reite, M., & Weissberg, M. (2014). Sleep-Wake Disorders. In R. E. Hales, S. C. Yudofsky, & L. W. Roberts (Eds.), *The American psychiatric publishing textbook of psychiatry* (pp. 607–644). Washington, DC: American Psychiatric Publishing.

Rowley, R. (2014). Obstructive sleep apnea-hypopnea syndrome. Medscape by WebMD LLC. http://www.emedicine.com/med/topic2697.htm. Accessed 3 March 2015.

Siegel, J. M., & Boehmer, L. N. (2006). Narcolepsy and the hypocretin system—where motion meets emotion. *National Clinical Practice of Neurology, 2,* 548–556.

Szelenberger, W., Niemcewicz, S., & Dabrowska, A. J. (2005). Sleepwalking and night terrors: Psychopathological and psychophysiological correlates. *International Review of Psychiatry, 17,* 263–270.

Taylor, J. R., Vazquez, C. M., & Campbell, K. M. (2006). Pharmacologic management of chronic insomnia. *Southern Medicine Journal, 99,* 1373–1377.

Taylor, D. J., Mallory, L. J., Lichstein, K. L., Durrence, H. H., Riedel, B. W., & Bush, A. J. (2007). Comorbidity of chronic insomnia with medical problems. *Sleep, 30,* 213–218.

Chapter 27
Feeding and Eating Disorders

Hy Gia Park

Eating disorders and obesity are problems that dramatically affect psychological and physical well-being. These disorders carry some of the highest mortality rates in psychiatry.

At the end of this chapter, the reader will be able to:

1. Describe the medical approach to a patient presenting with an eating disorder
2. Compare the epidemiology, pathophysiology, *Diagnostic and Statistical Manual of Mental Disorders, Fifth Edition* (DSM-5) diagnostic criteria, clinical course, treatment and prognosis for anorexia nervosa (AN), bulimia nervosa (BN), and binge eating disorder (BED)
3. Discuss how to evaluate and manage a patient with obesity

Case Vignette 27.1.1 Olga Mathias
Olga Mathias is a 15-year-old female in the 9th grade at a local private school. Her concerned parents brought her to the emergency room for "weakness and almost passing out while getting out of bed this afternoon". Olga concurs with her mother's story but thinks that her mother is completely blowing this situation out of proportion. "It's really not that big of a deal. My mom is such a control freak. She just has to get involved in every part of my life! Can I go home now?!" she shouts angrily.

History obtained from Olga reveals that she has not eaten for the past 2 days prior to this near-syncopal episode. "You'd be stressed too if you maintained a 4.25 GPA! I also have an upcoming gymnastics competition but since I'm here I can't really expect to win, can I?" she says in a strained tone. Her mother chimes in, "See, she really has just not been herself since starting high

H. G. Park (✉)
Arahant Health Services, LLC, 950 S. Cherry St., Suite 410, Denver, CO 80246, USA
e-mail: hparkmd.arahant@gmail.com

D. Alicata et al. (eds.), *Problem-based Behavioral Science and Psychiatry*,
DOI 10.1007/978-3-319-23669-8_27

school. She is always sad or irritable, sleeps in late, spends a lot of time by herself, and exercises constantly. If she shows up for meals, she'll often open a can of kidney beans, eat very little of it but drinks ten glasses of water and spends most of her time cutting up the food into tiny pieces and moving the pieces around her plate. She'll use an entire roll of paper towels in 2 days because she uses them to cover her plate and hide food." Her parents note that she has probably lost about 40 lb in the past 4 months.

STOP

Please proceed with the problem-based approach using the worksheet located in the appendix of Chap. 1!

Please fill in the facts, your hypotheses, further information needed, and learning issues for Learning Issue Table 27.1.1.

Learning Issue Table 27.1.1

FACTS	HYPOTHESES	INFORMATION NEEDED	LEARNING ISSUES

At this point, an eating disorder is an obvious diagnosis. Eating disorders are a complex set of illnesses that encompass a wide spectrum of abnormal eating patterns and can occur in all stages of life, from infancy to the elderly. The disturbances in eating behavior involve the manner, type, quantity, and rate of consumption of food. These disorders have a number of co-occurring psychiatric and medical conditions. The diagnoses of specific eating disorders are established in the DSM-5 (see Table 27.1).

The three main eating disorders are AN, BN, and BED. These conditions are characterized by a persistent disturbance of eating or eating-related behavior that significantly impacts physical health and impairs psychosocial functioning.

Eating disorders have previously been considered diseases of the Western, industrialized world, particularly the USA, Canada, Europe, Australia, New Zealand, and South Africa. However, globalization and cultural influences have resulted in an increase occurrence of eating disorders in non-Western countries. Prevalence ratios by gender are skewed toward females with male–female prevalence ratios ranging from 1:6 to 1:20. The lifetime prevalence of AN, BN, and BED is estimated to be

Table 27.1 Feeding and eating disorders recognized in the DSM-5

Name of disorder	Description of disorder
Pica	Persistent eating of nonnutritive substances, such as clay, lead, feces, and hair
Rumination disorder	Repeated regurgitation and rechewing of food after feeding
Avoidant/restrictive food intake disorder	Persistent failure to eat adequately to meet appropriate nutritional and/or energy needs as evidenced by significant failure to gain weight or weight loss, significant nutritional deficiency, dependence on enteral feeding or nutritional supplements
Anorexia nervosa (subtypes: restricting vs. binge eating/purging)	Restriction of food intake leading to persistent low body weight accompanied by intense fear of weight gain and becoming fat and disturbed body image
Bulimia nervosa	Recurrent episodes (at least once per week for 3 months) of binge eating and inappropriate compensatory methods (including self-induced vomiting, laxative use, fasting, and excessive exercise) to avoid weight gain and absence of anorexia nervosa
Binge eating disorder	Recurrent episodes (at least once per week for 3 months) of binge eating that causes marked distress and involves eating alone, rapidly, when not hungry, and until uncomfortably full resulting in negative affect afterward, and absence of compensatory behavior as in bulimia nervosa and anorexia nervosa
Other specified feeding or eating disorder	Disorders of eating that do not meet the criteria for any specific eating disorder and the specific reason why criteria were not met is communicated
Unspecified feeding or eating disorder	Disorders of eating that do not meet the criteria for any specific eating disorder and the specific reason why criteria were not met is not communicated

DSM-5 Diagnostic and Statistical Manual of Mental Disorders, Fifth Edition

0.9, 0.9–1.5, and 1.9%, respectively, in women and 0–0.3, 0.1–0.5, and 0.3%, respectively, in men (Smink et al. 2012). AN, BN, and BED generally develop during adolescence or young adulthood (APA 2013).

Although Olga probably has an eating disorder, there are other diagnoses to consider:

- Other medical conditions (usually not associated with excessive worry about weight or body image)
- Major depressive disorder (usually not associated with desire to lose weight or fear of gaining weight).
- Psychotic disorders (there may be fear that food has been poisoned as part of paranoid ideation; however, there is usually no impairment in body image, desire to lose weight, or fear of gaining weight. Also, these patients tend to have bizarre thinking and behavior about things other than food).
- Social anxiety disorder (usually not restricted to reluctance to eat in public).
- Obsessive-compulsive disorder (obsessions occur in other areas besides food, weight, and body image; food rituals are not intended for weight loss).

So, further evaluation is needed.

Case Vignette 27.1.2 Continued

You meet with Olga and her family to gather more information. Her parents report that she began changing her eating habits about 2 years ago. She would diet often, only eat salads for dinner, spend a lot of time in front of the mirror, complain that she was too fat, and wear baggy clothes. When asked, Olga reports that her ideal body weight is 80 lb, and she thinks that her thighs and abdomen are too big. She states that she wakes up at 6 a.m. every morning to run 4 miles. She admits to occasional binge eating (donuts, cookies) and purging by vomiting. Olga continues to insist that she feels fine and that she wants to go home.

Olga is reluctant at first to be examined, but she eventually obliges with much coaxing. She appears thin and pale, with dark sunken eyes. She was dressed in a loose-fitting T-shirt and baggy jeans. Her vital signs are as follows: temperature 97.1 °F, pulse 52/min, blood pressure 84/64, respiratory rate 16/min, weight 88.6 lb, height 63 in., and body mass index (BMI) 15.7. The remainder of the physical examination is remarkable for lanugo (soft, downy hair on her chest and arms), thinning hair, slight peripheral edema, and loss of subcutaneous fat. The mental status examination reveals poor cooperation and eye contact, rapid and loud speech, angry and tearful affect, poor concentration, and poor insight and judgment. Her laboratory findings are hemoglobin (Hb) 8.2, mean corpuscular volume (MCV) 90, leukocyte count 3500, serum Na^+ 130, and serum glucose 55.

Olga's parents admit their unwilling child to the inpatient psychiatric unit where she remains for the next 3 months. During the course of her hospitalization, she participates in the treatment, which includes a cardiac evaluation, weight restoration through gradual refeeding, psychoeducation, as well as individual and family psychotherapies. Olga grows increasingly irritable and repeatedly asks to be discharged. "I don't need doctors, nurses, psychiatrists, and dietitians. I'm totally fine so let me go home!" After her weight has been restored to near her ideal weight, Olga starts taking the medication fluoxetine. Two weeks later, she is discharged home on the condition that she has weekly follow-up visits with her pediatrician, a nutritionist, and a therapist.

STOP

Please proceed with the problem-based approach using the worksheet located in the appendix of Chap. 1!

Please fill in the facts, your hypotheses, further information needed, and learning issues for Learning Issue Table 27.1.2.

Learning Issue Table 27.1.2

FACTS	HYPOTHESES	INFORMATION NEEDED	LEARNING ISSUES

Based on Olga's presentation, the criteria for AN are met, and the most appropriate diagnosis would be AN and binge eating/purging type. Of note, AN has a worse prognosis than BN and BED.

One of the trademarks in AN is impaired insight into the nature of their illness. Patients are often brought in for medical attention by loved ones. Although accurate histories are not easily obtained from the patient, their accounts, along with collateral sources of information (e.g. family members, friends, and teachers), paint pictures of a preoccupation with food, weight, calories, and physical appearance. Patients with AN develop rituals around the consumption of food such as eating slowly, cutting foods into small pieces, rearranging the food on the plate, and even hiding food in clothing. Other elements that reflect a preoccupation with weight are strict exercise routines, constant weighing on scales, repeated checking in mirrors, purging behavior including excessive use of laxatives, and social withdrawal. Adolescents with AN will have delayed psychosocial development and adults will report decreased libido (Halmi 2007).

Histories of patients with BN, on the other hand, will reveal an abnormal eating pattern of binge eating and fasting that typically develops during or after an episode of dieting to lose weight. During binges, there is a sense of loss of control as patients with BN may consume large volumes of high caloric foods in a short time and often in secrecy. Binges are terminated by interruption, fatigue, abdominal discomfort, or feelings of depression, guilt, and disgust. Because of their fear of weight gain and excessive preoccupation on body shape and weight, patients will fast for long periods of time in between the binges and use inappropriate compensatory behaviors, such as vomiting, misuse of laxatives, diuretics, and enemas, and overexercise. Additionally, these patients tend to have an impaired ability to sense satiety after meals (APA 2013; Halmi 2007). Of the BN patients, 10–15% eventually cross over to AN and some will have multiple incidences of crossovers between BN and AN (APA 2013).

Table 27.2 Common signs and symptoms of eating disorders

Anorexia nervosa	Bulimia nervosa	Binge eating disorder
Loss of subcutaneous fat tissue	Normal weight or overweight	Normal weight, overweight, or obese
Orthostatic hypotension	Dental enamel erosions[a]	Hypertension
Bradycardia	Erosions on the dorsum of the hands (Russell's sign)[a]	
Amenorrhea	Enlargement of the salivary glands[a]	
Alopecia	Gastroesophageal reflux[a]	
Lanugo-like body hair	Dyspepsia[a]	
Hypothermia	Metabolic hypokalemic alkalosis[a]	

[a] Can be seen in both binge/purge subtype of anorexia nervosa and purging subtype of bulimia nervosa

In contrast to patients with BN, the onset of binge eating in BED patients is preceded by dysfunctional dieting and is not associated with the recurrent use of inappropriate compensatory behavior. Episodes of out of control binge eating are similar to the ones seen in BN and are typically characterized by rapid eating, eating until uncomfortably full, eating when not physically hungry, and eating alone. Furthermore, they are also accompanied by marked distress as feelings are shame, embarrassment, disgust, depression, and guilt often arise. Crossover from BED to other eating disorders is uncommon (APA 2013).

Patients suffering from eating disorders will present clinically with a wide range of symptoms. Those with less severe illness may have nonspecific complaints, such as fatigue, dizziness, and lack of energy. Patients with AN will often wear loose-fitting clothes in an attempt to hide their emaciated bodies. In order to conceal their true weight, patients with AN patients may fluid load, put weights in their pockets, or wear multiple layers of clothing before stepping on a scale. Additional signs and symptoms of patients with AN and BN are presented in Table 27.2. Eating disorders are associated with a variety of abnormal laboratory findings, presented in Table 27.3 (APA 2013, 2006; Halmi 2007; Yager and Andersen 2005).

Medical complications from eating disorders are primarily a consequence of starvation and weight loss in AN, the form and frequency of purging behavior in BN, and being overweight and obese in BED. As shown in Table 27.4, the resulting complications from these disorders affect multiple organ systems of the body (APA 2006; Halmi 2007; Mitchell and Crow 2006).

There are few randomized clinical trials that evaluate treatments for eating disorders. This is in part due to the intrinsic difficulties associated with studying this population, which is resistant to treatment and has high dropout rates and incomplete hospitalization courses. As a result, we lack a standard of care for treating patients with eating disorders.

Table 27.3 Common laboratory findings in eating disorders

Anorexia nervosa	Bulimia nervosa	Binge eating disorder
Chemistry	*Chemistry*	*Chemistry*
Decreased K^+, Na^+, Cl^-, Mg^{+2}, P^{+3} and Zn^{+2}	Decreased K^+, Na^+, Cl^-, Mg^{+2}, P^{+3}	Elevated serum cholesterol, glucose, triglyceride
Metabolic alkalosis	Metabolic alkalosis (with vomiting)/acidosis (with laxative abuse)	*EKG*
Elevated serum amylase, BUN, cholesterol	Elevated serum amylase	Left shifts of the P wave QRS and T wave axes
Abnormal liver function test	*Urinalysis*	Changes in P wave morphology
Hematologic	Increased urine specific gravity and osmolality	Low QRS voltage
Anemia	*EKG*	Various markers of left ventricular hypertrophy
Leucopenia	Prolonged QT and PR intervals	T wave flattening in the inferior and lateral leads
Decreased serum ferritin, B12, folate, and niacin (in severe cases)	Depressed ST segment	Prolonged QT interval
Endocrine	Widened QRS complex	
Low estrogen	*Brain imaging*	
Low testosterone (in males)	Cortical atrophy	
Low-normal T4; Low T3	Enlarged ventricles	
Prepubertal patterns of LH, FSH secretion	Decreased gray and white matter	
Increased serum cortisol	*DEXA*	
EKG	Osteopenia	
Bradycardia or arrhythmia	Osteoporosis	
QTc prolongation		
Increased PR interval		
First-degree heart block		
ST-T wave abnormalities		
Brain imaging		
Enlarged ventricles		
Decreased gray and white matter		
DEXA		
Osteopenia		
Osteoporosis		

BUN blood urea nitrogen, *EKG* electrocardiogram, *DEXA* dual-energy X-ray absorptiometry, *LH* luteinizing hormone, *FSH* follicle stimulating hormone

Table 27.4 Complications from eating disorders

Central nervous system	Cognitive impairment; anxious, depressed, irritable mood; seizures; peripheral neuropathy
Skin	Xerosis, lanugo-like body hair, hair loss, acne; carotenoderma (yellowish skin), acrocyanosis (bluish hands or feet), purpura, stomatitis, nail abnormalities
Cardiovascular	Cardiomyopathy and cardiac failure secondary to ipecac abuse, hypertension, arrhythmias, congestive heart failure, cardiac arrest
Pulmonary	Pneumomediastinum
Gastrointestinal	Benign parotid hyperplasia, gastric dilatation, esophageal or gastric rupture, delayed gastric emptying, impaired sense of hunger and satiety, delayed small bowel transit time, pancreatitis, necrotizing colitis; constipation, gallbladder disease
Musculoskeletal	Muscle wasting, peripheral myopathy, arrested skeletal growth, osteopenia, and osteoporosis leading to pathologic fractures
Hematologic	Thrombocytopenia, clotting factor abnormalities
Endocrine and metabolic	Severe electrolyte abnormalities, vitamin deficiency, thyroid dysfunction, high cholesterol level, type 2 diabetes mellitus
Renal	Renal failure
Reproductive	Infertility, miscarriages, pregnancy complications

27.1 Anorexia Nervosa

Treatment of AN requires a multidimensional treatment approach with medical management, psychoeducation, psychotherapy, and medication. The treatment team includes a primary care physician, a dietitian, nurses and a psychiatrist, a psychologist, or a therapist trained in treating patients with eating disorders (APA 2006; Yager and Andersen 2005). The treatment setting is typically determined by the severity of the illness. Options include outpatient care, day programs, residential programs, general psychiatric units, specialized eating disorder inpatient units, and medical intensive care units. Treatment on an outpatient basis is best reserved for patients who have had the illness for less than 6 months, with no binging or purging and active family involvement (APA 2006).

Medical management of patients with AN is complex due to the effects of starvation and the medical interventions themselves. Physicians must closely monitor vital signs, intakes and outputs, electrolyte status, cardiopulmonary and gastrointestinal function, and physical activity. Weight restoration through refeeding with adequate calories is the first intervention taken since it facilitates the success of other interventions in the treatment plan. Refeeding reduces apathy, lethargy, and obsessions related to food and body image. Weight gain of 1–3 lb weekly in the inpatient setting and a 0.5–2 lb weekly in the outpatient setting is typical. Refeeding syndrome occurs in approximately 6% of patients and includes abdominal pain, bloating, and peripheral edema or more serious complications such as cardiopulmonary, neurological, and neuromuscular dysfunction (Yager and Andersen 2005).

Behavioral treatments are an essential component for treating AN. These interventions include individual and family psychotherapy, nutritional counseling, and group therapies. They are often employed despite minimal evidence-based support for their use.

Although it is not a primary treatment modality, fluoxetine appears to decrease relapse episodes and depressive symptoms and helps maintain weight gain in weight-restored patients. Atypical antipsychotics, such as olanzapine and risperidone, may help with weight gain, decrease obsessional and distorted thoughts, decrease anxiety, and even improve insight.

27.2 Bulimia Nervosa

The primary objectives in the treatment of BN are to treat the associated medical complications and to break the binge–purge cycles with medications and psychotherapy. Medical management of complications addresses oral and dental care, associated gastrointestinal illnesses, bone health, and electrolyte and acid–base imbalances (e.g., hypokalemic metabolic alkalosis; Mehler 2003). Psychiatric management of BN typically involves cognitive behavioral therapy (CBT) as first-line treatment since it is one of the few treatments that has consistently been shown to be effective in randomized controlled trials, especially if administered by a trained professional (Halmi 2007). CBT can be used in group or individual settings and aims to challenge the core beliefs that drive the illness and break the circle of destructive thoughts, feelings, and binge–purge behaviors.

Antidepressants can be effective adjuvant interventions in reducing the severity of bulimic symptoms, including binge eating and purging behaviors, obsessive thoughts related to food, weight and body shape, relapse rates, and symptoms of depression and anxiety. Fluoxetine is the only Food and Drug Administration (FDA)-approved pharmacologic agent for the treatment of BN. Bupropion is specifically contraindicated for patients with eating disorders. The combination of antidepressants and CBT appears to be most effective in reducing the frequency of binging and purging (Mehler 2003). Eating disorder support groups and twelve-step programs such as Overeaters Anonymous may also be helpful during treatment and relapse prevention (APA 2006).

27.3 Binge Eating Disorder

CBT and interpersonal therapy (IPT) remain the treatments of choice for BED patients. Compared to behavioral weight loss (BWL) treatment, CBT and IPT produce the greatest degree of remission from binge eating, depression, overvaluation of body shape and weight, and improvement in psychosocial functioning. There are no current evidence-based pharmacologic treatments recommended for treatment of BED (Wilson 2011).

Knowing the chronic nature of AN, we wonder how well Olga will follow up with outpatient therapy.

Case Vignette 27.1.3 Continued
Olga stops going to her appointments after only 2 weeks after discharge. In the course of 1 year, Olga is reluctantly brought in to the emergency room on two occasions for syncopal episodes. Each time, she unwillingly is admitted for medical stabilization, weight restoration, and psychosocial support, but she does not adhere to treatment after discharge. Olga is angry with her parents for forcing her into treatment. Her parents are beside themselves, blaming themselves for her condition and feeling helpless as they watch her spiral into a skeletal version of her former self. They decide to send her to an intensive residential program for eating disorders despite Olga's resistance. One year later, a very emaciated and angry Olga is brought in again to the emergency room by her parents for "heart problems" from binge–purge behaviors.

Please proceed with the problem-based approach using the worksheet located in the appendix of Chap. 1!

Please fill in the facts, your hypotheses, further information needed, and learning issues for Learning Issue Table 27.1.3.

Learning Issue Table 27.1.3

FACTS	HYPOTHESES	INFORMATION NEEDED	LEARNING ISSUES

In general, follow-up studies conducted 6 years after disease onset show that eating disorders develop into chronic illnesses with high rates of medical morbidity and mortality. Among patients with AN, approximately 25 % of patients recover, 25 % show no change in their condition, and the remainder of patients show some slight improvement. The prognosis for patients with BN similarly shows that half of these patients have residual features even after treatment. Compared to AN and BN, BED appears to have higher rates of remission in both natural course and treatment outcome studies (APA 2013; Wonderlich et al. 2009). The high rates of morbidity from these diseases correlate to high mortality rates; compared to all other psychiatric disorders, eating disorders have the highest death rates. The crude mortality rate for AN is 5.1 deaths per 1000 people, BN is 1.7 deaths, and BED is 2.9 deaths (Suokas et al. 2013). Death most often results from suicide or the effects of starvation in AN and BN (Yager et al. 2006). Of patients with BN, 25–35 % attempt suicide, as opposed to 3–20 % of patients with AN (Franko and Keel 2006), but the rate of death from suicide is higher among patients with AN.

Several factors are prognostic predictors in eating disorders. For example, a shorter duration of illness and age of onset between the ages of 12 and 18 are associated with better outcomes (Halmi 2007). On the other hand, lower body weights at diagnosis, vomiting, binge eating, alcohol and substance abuse, depression, and chronic illness carry a poor prognosis.

How did this bright, athletic teenager develop an eating disorder, and how will you effectively manage her treatment?

There is a strong genetic link in eating disorders. The risk of AN, BN, and BED is increased among first-degree biological relatives of individuals with these disorders as well as in families with depression, substance abuse, and obesity (APA 2006, 2013). Investigators have identified genes that may be linked to eating disorders. Two genes on chromosome 1 called the opioid delta receptor (OPRD1) and serotonin 1D (human 5-hydroxytryptamine (serotonin) receptor 1D; HTR1D) genes appear to be linked to AN. BN may be linked to genes on chromosomes 10 and 14 (Halmi 2007). There are not yet any genetic polymorphisms or neurotransmitter/peptide findings that are clearly and consistently related to BED (Wonderlich et al. 2009).

Changes in neuroendocrine functions also play an important role in the development of eating disorders. Corticotrophin-releasing hormone (CRH), a strong anorectic hormone, is increased in underweight and dieting individuals. Dysregulation of serotonergic, norepinephrine, and dopaminergic pathways, as well as the dysfunction in a wide range of peptides (e.g. leptin, ghrelin), is thought to be linked to AN, BN, and BED, although the exact role of these substances is unknown (Halmi 2007; Wonderlich et al. 2009).

In childhood and adolescence, depression, bipolar disorder, dysthymia, and anxiety disorders (particularly overanxious disorder, obsessive compulsive disorder, and social anxiety disorder) are common mental disorders that are comorbid with eating disorders. Alcohol or substance abuse and impulsivity are also common, particularly in BN where 30 % of patients have comorbid alcohol or stimulant use (APA 2013; Halmi 2007; Yager and Andersen 2005).

Psychological factors that contribute to the development of eating disorders include dysfunctional family dynamics, personality traits, and life stressors. Over- or underinvolvement of parents in their child's life appears to be a risk factor (Yager and Andersen 2005). There is an association between eating disorders and personality disorders such as borderline, avoidant, and obsessive–compulsive. Traits such as perfectionism, competitiveness, negative self-evaluation, and rigidity are commonly found in these patients (APA 2006). Stressful life events, whether normative or traumatic, can precipitate eating disorders. Normative events in an individual's development may include the onset of puberty, the start of college, and the beginning of a new relationship. Traumatic events include sexual abuse, loss of a loved one, the breaking up of a relationship, and illness (Halmi 2007).

27.4 Social Factors

Cultural and social ideals of beauty strongly impact the development of eating disorders. Certain types of professionals, such as female models, ballet dancers, figure skaters, gymnasts, and male body builders and wrestlers, are at increased risk for eating disorders (APA 2006).

With the information provided above, please take this opportunity to complete a bio-psycho-social-cultural-spiritual formulation that will guide Olga's treatment planning (refer to Fig. 27.1).

The bio-psycho-social-cultural-spiritual formulation allows you to target interventions at the predisposing, precipitating, or perpetuating factors for eating disorders.

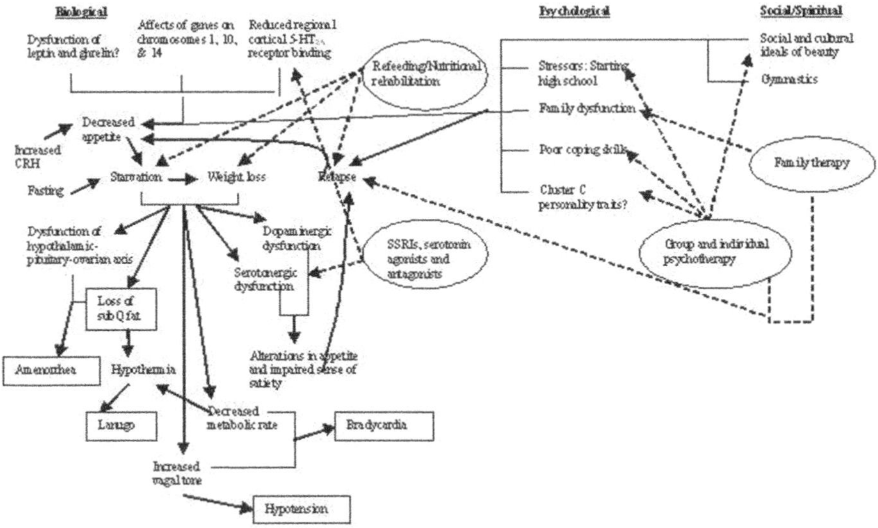

Fig. 27.1 Bio-psycho-social-cultural-spiritual formulation of case vignette, "Olga"

Next, we present a brief case on obesity, which (like AN, BN, and BED) involves abnormal eating behaviors, significant medical complications, and a complex interplay of biological, psychological, and social factors.

Case Vignette 27.2.1 Mac
"Mac" is the 13-year-old son of one of your primary care patients. Your patient asks you to evaluate Mac because "I think he must have some emotional problem, because of his weight." He is 5 ft. tall and weighs 180 lb (BMI = 35). His diet includes fast food, candy, soda (from the refrigerator), and typical school lunches.

STOP

Please proceed with the problem-based approach using the worksheet located in the appendix of Chap. 1!

Please fill in the facts, your hypotheses, further information needed, and learning issues for Learning Issue Table 27.2.1.

Learning Issue Table 27.2.1

FACTS	HYPOTHESES	INFORMATION NEEDED	LEARNING ISSUES

In adults, overweight is defined as BMI of 25–29.9, obesity is defined as BMI of 30.0–39.9, and severe obesity is defined as BMI greater than 40. In children and adolescents, obesity is defined as BMI greater than or equal to the 95th percentile for children of the same age and sex and severe obesity is defined as BMI greater than 120 % of 95th percentile. In the USA, the prevalence of obese children is currently 8.4 % among 2–5-year-olds, 18 % among 6–11-year-olds, and 21 % among 12–19-year-olds. The prevalence of severe obesity is 2% among 2–5-year-olds, 5 % among 6–11-year-olds, and 6.5 % among 12–19-year-olds. The prevalence of obesity in adults is now 34.9 % and 6 % are classified as severely obese (TFAH and RWJF 2014). The prevalence is higher in certain ethnic groups (including Pacific Islanders and other indigenous peoples exposed to Western diets). The risk of an obese child developing obesity (and associated cardiovascular and metabolic complications) increases with age. Early detection (through frequent monitoring of BMI during pediatric office visits) and intervention for obesity is part of routine pediatric practice.

Case Vignette 27.2.2 Continued

Mac denies symptoms suggestive of a mood, anxiety, or binge eating disorder.

Past medical and developmental history: Mother had a history of gestational diabetes mellitus. Birth weight was 9 lb. He was exclusively bottle-fed. He has been greater than 95th percentile in weight since infancy.

Family history: Everyone on the father's side of the family is overweight, including the father. Mother has a history of depression. Grandmother has a history of dementia.

Social history: He is the only child at home. The other adults are the parents and grandmother. He has minimal access to outdoor activities. He watches 4 h of TV per day. Father works two jobs. The mother cares for the grandmother.

Examination is significant for nasal speech, nasal congestion, and fidgeting.

Labs include a normal thyroid test.

The assessment of obesity requires screening for the general medical etiologies for (e.g., genetic and endocrine disorders) and complications of (e.g., diabetes, hypertension, hyperlipidemia, and obstructive sleep apnea syndrome) obesity. It is also important to screen for potential psychiatric comorbidities summarized in Table 27.5.

Table 27.5 Psychiatric comorbidities that should be screened for when evaluating a patient with obesity

Psychiatric condition	Relationship with obesity
Binge eating disorder	Increased caloric intake (without compensatory weight loss mechanisms) may lead to obesity
Major depressive disorder	Increased appetite may lead to increased caloric intake, which may, in turn, lead to obesity
Adjustment disorder	Obesity may lead to low self-esteem and social ostracism
Attention deficit hyperactivity disorder	Inattention, impulsivity, and suboptimal organizational skills may interfere with intended diets and activity schedules
Psychotic disorders, mood disorders, and other psychiatric conditions that require chronic medications	Medications may increase appetite and/or cause obesity through other mechanisms
Many psychiatric disorders	May interfere with judgment around food choices and/or ability to comply with weight loss regimens
	Associated poverty and untoward psychosocial circumstances may limit food choices and availability of healthy and safe activities

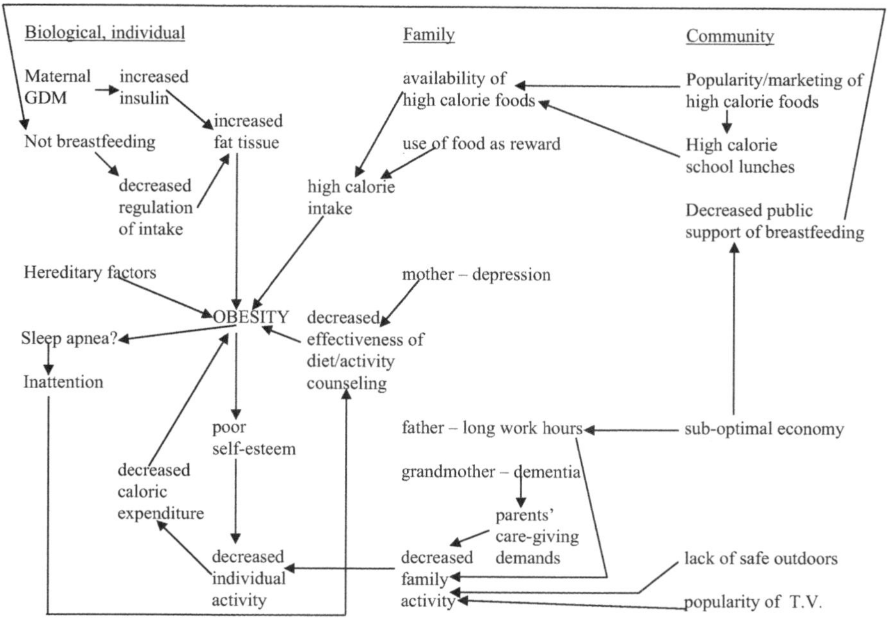

Fig. 27.2 Causative factors for obesity in the case of Mac

You need additional history in order to consider the biological, family, and societal factors that predispose to and perpetuate obesity. A diagram of the case of Mac is shown in Fig. 27.2 (Birch and Fisher 1998; Kohl and Hobbs 1998).

As Mac illustrates, treatment and prevention of obesity needs a comprehensive approach. In this specific case, treatment interventions may include addressing any comorbid sleep apnea and attentional difficulties, improving the family's capacity to adhere to diet and activity recommendations, and addressing potentially controllable community risk factors (such as unhealthy school lunches).

Options for treating obesity are summarized in Table 27.6.

Table 27.6 Individual-level interventions for treating obesity. (Adopted from Singhal et al. 2007)

First-line interventions
Goal setting (e.g., cessation of weight gain and/or modest weight loss) and monitoring of weight
Dietary counseling (e.g., regular meals and healthy meal choices)
Self-monitoring and anticipation of triggers for eating
Establishing healthful activity routines
Regular physician follow-up to monitor progress
Second-line interventions
Specialist referral
Consideration of medications:
Orlistat

Table 27.6 (continued)

First-line interventions
Blocks intestinal absorption of fat
Multivitamin supplementation is recommended
FDA-approved for patients older than 12 years
Sibutramine
Blocks reuptake of norepinephrine and serotonin)
FDA-approved for patients older than 12 years
Third-line interventions
Bariatric surgery: for severe obesity (BMI > 40) in adults and possibility in adolescents with complications

FDA Food and Drug Administration, *BMI* body mass index

27.5 Review Questions

1. Which of the following statements is *true* about the epidemiology of eating disorders:
   a. Anorexia nervosa is more common than bulimia nervosa.
   b. The prevalence of anorexia nervosa is approximately 3 %.
   c. The prevalence of anorexia nervosa is higher in developed countries.
   d. Anorexia nervosa and bulimia nervosa typically have their onset during adulthood.
   e. (b) and (c).
2. The first priority in the management of anorexia nervosa is:
   a. Initiation of a medication that reduces eating disordered behaviors, such as fluoxetine
   b. Medically supervised refeeding
   c. Initiation of a medication that promotes weight gain, such as olanzapine
   d. Exploration of childhood conflicts that have led to poor self-esteem and refusal of food
   e. None of the above
3. A 15-year-old female is brought to the pediatrician because she was caught "making herself vomit." She endorses recurrent episodes of binging and purging. She is also significantly underweight and fearful of becoming fat. She has not had any menstrual periods for the past 6 months. The most likely diagnosis is:
   a. Bulimia nervosa
   b. Anorexia nervosa, binge eating/purging type
   c. Anorexia nervosa, restricting type
   d. Eating disorder not otherwise specified
   e. Rumination disorder

4. A mother asks the pediatrician what can be done to ensure that her 1-year-old baby will not develop the problems of obesity that the two older teenage sons have. All of the following would be helpful to advise her *except*:

   a. Establishing regular family routines around meals
   b. Establishing regular family routines around physical activity
   c. Reducing exposure to television
   d. Bottle-feeding using commercially prepared formula
   e. Involving other family members in discussion about healthy diet and activity

5. Who are responsible for addressing the growing epidemic of obesity in the USA?

   a. Physicians
   b. Parents
   c. Lawmakers
   d. Food manufacturers
   e. All of the above, plus more

Appendix A: Tables with Possible Answers to the Vignettes

Case Vignette 27.1: Olga Mathias
Learning Issue Table 27.1

Facts	Hypotheses	Information needed	Learning issues
Olga Mathias is a 15-year-old female in the 9th grade at a local private school	One of the trademarks in AN is impaired insight into the nature of their illness	Thorough psychiatric, medical and pubertal evaluation (how do you optimize collateral information?)	Are there other diagnoses to consider?
Behaviors include food restriction and excessive exercise (deliberate drive for thinness)	Delayed psychosocial development	Physical/neurological exam	What are the criteria for inpatient hospitalization?
Rituals around the consumption of food	Treatment resistance, high dropout rates, and incomplete hospitalization courses	Vital signs (BMI)	What are the goals for inpatient treatment (medical management, cardiac evaluation, weight restoration, psychoeducation, psychotherapy, and psychopharmacology)?
Sad, irritable, isolation	Strong genetic link in eating disorders	Labs including CBC and electrolytes	What is the role of the multidimensional treatment approach, how does the team engage and maintain the patient and family in treatment?

Facts	Hypotheses	Information needed	Learning issues
40 lb weight loss in past 4 months	Neuroendocrine changes associated with eating disorders		How do you manage refeeding syndrome?
Concern about body image			What are the prognostic predictors in eating disorders?

AN anorexia nervosa, *BMI* body mass index, *CBC* complete blood count

Appendix B: Answers to Review Questions

1. c. 2. b. 3. b. 4. d. 5. e

References

American Psychiatric Association. (2006). *Practice guidelines for the treatment of patients with eating disorders* (3rd ed.). Washington, DC: American Psychiatric Publishing.

American Psychiatric Association. (2013). *Diagnostic and statistical manual of mental disorders* (5th ed.). Washington, DC: American Psychiatric Publishing.

Birch, L. L., & Fisher, J. O. (1998). Development of eating behaviors among children and adolescents. *Pediatrics, 101,* 539–549.

Franko, D. L., & Keel, P. K. (2006). Suicidality in eating disorders: Occurrence, correlates and clinical implications. *Clinical Psychology Review, 26,* 769–782.

Halmi, K. A. (2007). Anorexia nervosa and bulimia nervosa. In A. Martin & F. R. Volkmar (Eds.), *Lewis's child and adolescent psychiatry* (pp. 592–602). Philadelphia: Lippincott Williams & Wilkins.

Kohl, III H. W., & Hobbs, K. E. (1998). Development of physical activity behaviors among children and adolescents. *Pediatrics, 101,* 549–554.

Mehler, P. S. (2003). Bulimia nervosa. *The New England Journal of Medicine, 349,* 875–881.

Mitchell, J. E., & Crow, S. (2006). Medical complications of anorexia nervosa and bulimia nervosa. *Current Opinion in Psychiatry, 19,* 438–443.

Singhal, V., Schwenk, W. F., Kumar, S. (2007). Evaluation and management of childhood and adolescent obesity. *Mayo Clinic Proceedings, 82,* 1258–1264.

Smink, F. R. E., van Hoeken, D., & Hoek, H. W. (2012). Epidemiology of eating disorders: Incidence, prevalence and mortality rates. *Current Psychiatry Reports, 14,* 406–414.

Suokas, J. T., Suvisaari, J. M., Gissler, M., Lofman, R., Linna, M. S., Raevouri, A., & Haukka, J. (2013). Mortality in eating disorders: A follow-up study of adult eating disorder patients treated in tertiary care, 1995–2010. *Psychiatry Research, 210,* 1101–1106.

Trust for America's Health and Robert Wood Johnson Foundation. (2014). The state of obesity: 2014. Better policies for a healthier America.

Wilson, G. T. (2011). Treatment of binge eating disorder. *Psychiatric Clinics of North America, 34,* 773–783.

Wonderlich, S. A., Gordon, L. H., Mitchell, J. E., Crosby, R. D., & Engel, S. G. (2009). The validity and clinical utility of binge eating disorder. *International Journal of Eating Disorder, 42,* 687–705.

Yager, J., & Andersen, A. E. (2005). Anorexia nervosa. *The New England Journal of Medicine, 353,* 1481–1488.

Yager, J., Devlin, M. J., Halmi, K. A., et al. (2006). For the work group on eating disorders. *Practice guideline for the treatment of patients with eating disorders* (3rd ed.). Washington, DC: American Psychiatric Association.

Chapter 28
Sexual Disorders

Brandon Harsch

Ultimately, it is the desire, not the desired, that we love.
—Friedrich Nietzsche

This chapter will highlight three groups of disorders found in the *Diagnostic and Statistical Manual of Mental Disorders,* fifth edition (DSM-5) (APA 2013) including sexual disorders, gender dysphoria (formerly "gender identity disorder" in the *Diagnostic and Statistical Manual of Mental Disorders,* fourth edition; DSM-IV), and paraphilias. Many individuals do not seek care from their provider primarily for these disorders, and they may only be identified when they present for an associated medical or psychiatric condition.

At the end of this chapter, the reader will be able to:

1. Differentiate between medical and nonmedical causes for disorders related to sexual dysfunction
2. Discuss the epidemiology, clinical presentation, a differential diagnosis, and treatment options for gender dysphoria
3. Identify paraphilic behaviors and develop an appropriate differential diagnosis

Vignette 28.1.1: Presenting Information: Lynne Sparks
Lynne Sparks is a 51-year-old woman who was referred to your family medicine clinic for help regarding her "sexual problem." She is currently married to her husband of 23 years and describes their relationship as "strong" until recently. She states that she is still sexually attracted to her husband, but admits

B. Harsch (✉)
Department of Psychiatry, University of Nevada School of Medicine,
1664 N Virginia St, Reno, NV 89557, USA
e-mail: Brandon.Harsch@unchealth.unc.edu

D. Alicata et al. (eds.), *Problem-based Behavioral Science and Psychiatry,*
DOI 10.1007/978-3-319-23669-8_28

that her sexual desire has been progressively declining over the past year. Mrs. Sparks has not had sexual intercourse for approximately 3 months and is worried about the effect this will have on her marriage. She has noticed that lately she and her husband have been fighting more frequently, which is adding to her distress. Although she has been faithful to her husband, she expresses concern that he may leave her if things do not get better. She denies any recent life stressors such as loss of a job or loved one, trauma, or recent move.

STOP

Please proceed with the problem-based approach using the worksheet located in the appendix of Chap. 1!

Table 28.1.1

FACTS	HYPOTHESES	INFORMATION NEEDED	LEARNING ISSUES

28.1 Learning Issues

The patient's sexual concern is causing her a great deal of distress—enough to bring her to a physician to discuss this sensitive matter. Only 20 % of women with some form of sexual dysfunction seek medical care (Moreira et al. 2005). Additionally, sex can be a difficult subject for a physician to discuss with their patient, and many physicians feel uncomfortable obtaining a full sexual history. Discussing sex should begin with open-ended questions, and then focus on menstrual, obstetric, reproductive, and sexual history, including current relationships and a history of abuse or trauma (Frank et al. 2008). It is also important to get a thorough surgical and medical history including medication and substance use. The PLISSIT model can be applied to initiate the discussion and treatment of sexual dysfunction (Annon 1976):

1. Obtain **P**ermission to discuss sex with the patient
2. Provide **L**imited **I**nformation to dispel myths and discuss normal sexual functioning
3. Provide **S**pecific **S**uggestions for the patient's complaint
4. Consider **I**ntensive **T**reatment with therapy for complex issues

Table 28.1 Common medical and nonmedical causes of reduced sexual desire in women

Medical causes	Nonmedical causes
Lichen sclerosis	Female orgasmic disorder
Pelvic nerve damage (from hysterectomy)	SSRIs
PID	MDD
Diabetes mellitus	Female sexual interest/arousal disorder
MS	Genito-pelvic pain/penetration disorder (vaginismus, dyspareunia)
Vulvovaginal atrophy	
Endometriosis	
Thyroid dysfunction	

PID pelvic inflammatory disorder, *MS* multiple sclerosis, *SSRI* selective serotonin reuptake inhibitors, *MDD* major depressive disorder

Mrs. Sparks initially described a gradual decrease in her sexual desire, which could be caused by a number of different things, giving a broad differential diagnosis. There are both medical and nonmedical causes for sexual dysfunction that must be considered. Given her age, perimenopause and the related changes associated with decreased estrogen levels should be evaluated. A decrease in estrogen production can lead to vaginal atrophy characterized by symptoms of vaginal dryness, itching, and pain. These physical manifestations may result in reduced sexual desire in perimenopausal women. Table 28.1 lists common causes of reduced sexual desire in women.

Vignette 28.1.2: Continuation

After further questioning, Mrs. Sparks reveals that she has been experiencing pain associated with intercourse that began over a year ago. She had never experienced pain with intercourse prior to this. She did not think much about this at first, but admits that this pain has recurred many times since then, and may be gradually worsening. The pain was initially associated with deep penetration during sexual intercourse but is now triggered even by shallow penetration. She has become so "sensitive" that she has begun experiencing pain even when inserting a tampon. Mrs. Sparks admits that at first, the pain limited her ability to achieve orgasm, but now her fear of the pain has advanced to the point that she does not enjoy engaging in any sexual activity. She has tried to use a variety of lubricants but states that this was ineffective in alleviating the pain. A gynecological exam 1 month ago revealed no concerning pathological findings, but she reports that insertion of the speculum was excruciatingly painful—something she states had never been an issue before. She says that her doctor requested that she return to her primary care for evaluation of vaginal "muscle spasms."

She denies any trauma to her genital region, but reveals that she had a chlamydia infection that led to pelvic inflammatory disorder (PID) at the age of 19. She also mentions that her periods have become irregular and heavier over the past 2 years, with her last period occurring 3 months ago. During this time, she has also been experiencing hot flashes, feeling emotionally more labile, and crying more often. Mrs. Sparks admits that she has been attributing the pain and decrease in sexual desire to aging and nearing menopause, and states that she was "hoping it would just get better."

Please proceed with the problem-based approach using the worksheet located in the appendix of Chap. 1!

Table 28.1.2

FACTS	HYPOTHESES	INFORMATION NEEDED	LEARNING ISSUES

Mrs. Sparks, like many women, is having pain during intercourse. Approximately 15 % of North American women have experienced recurrent pain during intercourse at some point in their life (Lauman et al. 1999). Diagnosis of genito-pelvic pain/penetration disorder based on DSM-5 criteria requires one of the following four symptoms to be present for a period of at least 6 months (APA 2013):

1. Difficulty with vaginal penetration during sexual intercourse
2. Genito-pelvic pain during vaginal penetration attempts
3. Fear or anxiety of pain in anticipation of vaginal penetration
4. Tension of the pelvic floor muscles during vaginal penetration or sexual intercourse

Genito-pelvic pain/penetration disorder is often associated with other sexual dysfunctions. For example, a fear of pain associated with intercourse may decrease sexual desire for the painful activity and lead to orgasmic impairment. Some women with genito-pelvic pain disorder may even find all aspects of the sexual experience unsatisfying or distressing. A history of sexual and/or physical abuse has been implicated as a risk factor for developing genito-pelvic pain/penetration disorder, but new research has brought this association into question (Reed 2009).

Vignette 28.1.3: Conclusion

Based on the history Mrs. Sparks has given, you tell her that her decreased sexual desire is likely secondary to vaginismus, a form of genito-pelvic pain/penetration disorder. Because of the chronic course of her pain and her recent normal gynecological exam, you do not suspect a medical cause for her pain. You refer Mrs. Sparks to a sex therapist for cognitive behavioral therapy (CBT). You explain that CBT will help modify her thought patterns, emotions, and behaviors to decrease muscle tension and help alleviate the pain. You also recommend kegel exercises and the use of dilators to help with desensitization. You inform her that self-insertion of dilators of increasing diameter will also help her to better control her introital muscles which will allow her to gradually experience less pain with penetration.

In your discussion, you also inform Mrs. Sparks that she may be approaching menopause given her change in menstrual pattern and hot flashes. As she does not appear to have any contraindications to estrogen therapy, you recommend that she begin using an estrogen cream to reduce vaginal dryness and any associated pain. You inform her that you expect her sexual desire to improve once her discomfort with vaginal penetration resolves.

STOP

Please proceed with the problem-based approach using the worksheet located in the appendix of Chap. 1!

Table 28.1.3

FACTS	HYPOTHESES	INFORMATION NEEDED	LEARNING ISSUES

Vignette 28.1.4: Follow-Up

Mrs. Sparks returns to your clinic 2 months later for follow-up. She began CBT shortly after her last visit and reports that she is experiencing less pain between the therapy and the use of vaginal dilators. Her sexual desire and overall relationship with her husband have improved. It has now been 5 months since her last period and her hot flashes have become more frequent, however the estrogen cream has effectively reduced her vaginal dryness.

Table 28.2 DSM-5 classification of sexual disorders. (APA 2013)

Delayed ejaculation	Delay in or infrequency/absence of ejaculation
Erectile disorder	Difficulty in:
	Obtaining an erection during sexual activity *or*
	Maintaining an erection throughout sexual activity *or*
	Decreased erectile rigidity
Female orgasmic disorder	Delay in or infrequency/absence of orgasm, or reduced orgasmic intensity
Female sexual interest/arousal disorder	Lack of or significantly reduced sexual interest or arousal
Genito-pelvic pain/penetration disorder	Persistent or recurrent difficulty with vaginal penetration during intercourse *or*
	Vulvovaginal or pelvic pain with penetration *or*
	Fear or anxiety regarding pelvic pain in anticipation of, during, or as a result of vaginal penetration *or*
	Pelvic floor muscle contraction during attempted vaginal penetration
Male hypoactive sexual desire disorder	Persistent or recurrent deficiency or absence of sexual/erotic thoughts and sexual desire
Premature ejaculation	Persistent or recurrent ejaculation within 1 min following vaginal penetration *and* before the individual desires
Substance/medication-induced sexual dysfunction	Sexual function disturbance that develops:
	During or shortly after initiating a medication *or*
	Intoxication/withdrawal from a substance

Sexual disorders affect both men and women. See Table 28.2 for a list of DSM-5 sexual disorder classifications. Vaginismus and dyspareunia are two forms of genito-pelvic pain/penetration disorder that may present similarly. Dyspareunia is uncommon in premenopausal women and involves genital pain that occurs during sexual intercourse and is not due to vaginismus or inadequate lubrication. Vaginismus is an involuntary, spastic contraction of the vaginal muscles that causes pain upon vaginal penetration (Frank et al. 2008). The cause is often idiopathic, but may be associated with pelvic trauma from sexual assault, painful intercourse, or iatrogenic causes such as episiotomy, pelvic surgery, or a painful gynecological examination (Biggs 2011). Addressing the underlying cause is the first step in treating the disorder, as effective treatment may involve a multidimensional and multidisciplinary approach to address the physiological, emotional, and relational factors (Crowley et al. 2006). Physiological treatment of vaginismus involves self-treatment using vaginal dilators of increasing size to slowly train the vaginal muscles to remain relaxed during nonpainful penetration. Psychotherapy addresses the patient's fear associated with penetration to better understand the relationship between anxiety, muscle contraction, and pain, in order to regain conscious control over the pelvic muscles (Frank et al. 2008). Psychotherapy is tailored to the individual and including the woman's sexual partner is highly encouraged (Crowley et al. 2006).

Genito-pelvic pain complaints peak during early childhood and in the peri- and postmenopausal age ranges. During menopause, less estrogen is produced by the ovaries which leads to vaginal atrophy and decreased lubrication and sensation

(Frank et al. 2008). Therefore, it is especially important to rule out vulvovaginal atrophy in women whose estrogen is suspected of declining significantly. Additionally, women with vulvovaginal atrophy are more likely to report difficulties with achieving orgasm than women with other sexual disorders. Estrogen-based lubricants help improve vaginal dryness, but do not improve sexual desire. Before initiating estrogen therapy, it is important to ensure that the patient does not have a contraindication to treatment, such as an estrogen-responsive tumor.

Vignette 28.2.1: Presenting Information: Angel Bridges

Angel Bridges is a 38-year-old woman who is referred to your psychiatric lesbian, gay, bisexual, and transgender clinic. She appears distressed, stating that she has been feeling very depressed for quite some time. She proceeds to tell you the events that have brought her to your office today.

Ten years ago, Angel, born a male, had a wife of 8 years and two young children. As a struggle was waging within her over a feeling that she was trapped in the wrong body, she was falling further into depression and began having suicidal thoughts. Although she was born and raised as a boy and had normal secondary male sex characteristics, she was experiencing progressive anxiety and distress associated with being male. She reflects that at the age of 5, she preferred to dress like a girl and borrow her sister's clothing, but abruptly stopped these behaviors after her parents scolded her. She had not thought much about the significance of that experience until about 10 years ago when she began trying on her wife's clothes. She states that she enjoyed wearing her clothes and started to wish that she had breasts to better fill her bra. She began shaving her legs and armpits, waxing her chest, and scheduled laser hair removal appointments to rid herself of facial hair.

STOP

Please proceed with the problem-based approach using the worksheet located in the appendix of Chap. 1!

Table 28.2.1

FACTS	HYPOTHESES	INFORMATION NEEDED	LEARNING ISSUES

28.2 Learning Issues

Angel Bridges has discussed her developing incongruence between her natal sex and experienced gender, with a desire to attain the secondary sex characteristics of a female, rather than the male ones she possessed. While the diagnosis appears to be gender dysphoria, it is important to consider other potential explanations for her thoughts and behaviors. An initial differential diagnosis for symptoms of gender dysphoria includes:

1. Nonconformity to gender roles—It differs from gender dysphoria in that it does not involve a strong desire to be of another gender.
2. Transvestic disorder—A disorder in which cross-dressing behavior creates excitement sexually but does not involve a desire to be of another gender. However, it can be associated with gender dysphoria and is often a precursor to late-onset gender dysphoria in adults.
3. Body dysmorphic disorder—Focus on alteration or removal of a particular body part (i.e. penis, vagina, breasts, nose, etc.) due to the perception that it is abnormally formed.
4. Schizophrenia and other psychotic disorders—Delusions that the individual belongs to another gender in the presence of psychotic symptoms.

Gender dysphoria, formerly termed "gender identity disorder" in DSM-IV-TR, is described as the distressing incongruence between one's natal sex and his/her experienced gender (APA 2000). To understand this concept, it is essential to distinguish gender from sex: Sex refers to the biological basis of being male or female, whereas gender refers to the lived role of being a man/woman or boy/girl. See Table 28.3 for definitions of terms related to sex and gender. Because gender dysphoria varies with age, there are distinct diagnostic criteria for children and adolescents/adults. See Table 28.4 for these criteria. We will be primarily focusing on adolescent and adult dysphoria.

Cross-gender behaviors in children first present between the ages of 2 and 4 years, which is the time period children often begin developing gender-specific behaviors and interests. The ratio of individuals with persistent thoughts and behaviors into adolescence and adulthood is 2.2–30% in natal males and 12–50% in natal females (APA 2013). The onset of dysphoria often first occurs as early as puberty, but is not always present in childhood and may occur much later in life. Adolescent and adult gender dysphoria is divided into early and late onset. Early-onset gender dysphoria may persist into adolescence and adulthood, or there may be a period of time in which the dysphoria breaks and then recurs later in life. Those with late-onset dysphoria may or may not experience a desire to be of the opposite gender during childhood, and parents are often surprised due to the lack of "signs." Childhood gender dysphoria is higher in natal boys compared to natal girls, with a ratio of 2–4.5:1, and ranges from 1 to 6.1:1 in adult gender dysphoria (APA 2013).

Table 28.3 Definition of terms related to gender and sex

Sex	Being biologically male or female based on reproductive organs and function, including sex chromosomes, gonads, and nonambiguous internal and external genitalia
Gender	Male and female roles based on constructs defined by society and culture
Gender assignment	Also referred to as "natal gender," it is the initial designation as either male or female which usually occurs at birth
Gender identity	Social identification as male, female, or rarely another category
Transgender	A spectrum of individuals with either persistent or transient identification with a gender different than their assigned gender
Gender dysphoria	Affective and cognitive discontent with one's natal gender
Gender nonconformity	The difference between an individual's gender identity, role, or expression and societal or cultural norms
Transsexual	An individual who desires to or has undergone gender transition
Homosexual	An individual who is sexually attracted to people of one's own sex

Table 28.4 DSM-5 diagnostic criteria for gender dysphoria in children and adolescents/adults. (APA 2013)

Children	Adults and adolescents
At least six symptoms that occur for ≥6 months, and associated with distress or impairment in social and school domains	At least six symptoms that occur for ≥6 months, and associated with distress or impairment in social, school, and occupational domains
A strong desire to be of the other gender or an insistence that one is the other gender	A marked incongruence between one's experienced/expressed gender and his/her anticipated or acquired primary and/or secondary sex characteristics
A strong preference for cross-dressing or simulating female attire in boys. A strong preference for wearing only typical masculine clothing with a strong resistance to wearing typical feminine clothing in girls	A strong desire to be rid of, or prevent development of, one's primary and/or secondary sex characteristics because of a marked incongruence with one's experienced/expressed gender
Strong preference for cross-gender roles in make-believe play or fantasy play	A strong desire for the primary and/or secondary sex characteristics of the other gender
Strong preference for the toys, games, or activities stereotypically used or engaged in by the other gender	A strong desire to be of the other gender (or some alternative gender different from one's assigned gender)
Strong preference for playmates of the other gender	A strong desire to be treated as the other gender
Strong rejection of typically masculine toys, games, and activities and a strong avoidance of rough-and-tumble play in boys. Strong rejection of typically feminine toys, games, and activities in girls	A strong conviction that one has the typical feelings and reactions of the other gender
A strong dislike of one's sexual anatomy	
A strong desire for the primary and/or secondary sex characteristics that match one's experienced gender	

Vignette 28.2.2: Continuation

Ms. Bridges felt as though she identified more with being female and wished to shed the features that made her a male so that she could make the transition to a woman. Ten years ago, she also realized she was no longer sexually attracted to her wife and was actually much more attracted to men. She secretly began dating a man she met at the gym and began daydreaming of becoming his wife and running away to start her life anew. She admits that she feared her depression and suicidal thoughts would continue and potentially progress to suicide if she did not seek sex reassignment.

Although she was experiencing a significant amount of guilt regarding this decision and the threat it posed on her marriage and family, she decided to move forward. She proceeded to undergo psychiatric evaluation and hormonal therapy in order to initiate the transition toward becoming a woman. She also underwent endocrine and other laboratory evaluations for hormonal imbalances which revealed no abnormalities. She started a "trial" of living as a woman for 1 year so that she could eventually undergo surgical transformation. She began taking hormone supplements to start the process of ridding her of her "masculinity" and assuming a more feminine appearance.

Upset with Angel's decisions, her wife took the children and filed for divorce. She admits to an emotional struggle with the thought that "I let my family down," but found the twice weekly psychiatry and therapy appointments essential for helping her develop coping skills to manage all the changes taking place. After living as a woman and taking hormones for a year, she decided to proceed with reassignment surgery. She was referred to a urologist who performed the sex reassignment procedures which were completed successfully and without complications.

STOP

Please proceed with the problem-based approach using the worksheet located in the appendix of Chap. 1!

Table 28.2.2

FACTS	HYPOTHESES	INFORMATION NEEDED	LEARNING ISSUES

The World Professional Association for Transgender Health Standards of Care has established a set of criteria for initiating treatment to help an individual transition to the opposite sex. Before initiating either medical or surgical treatment for changing one's sex, a diagnosis of persistent gender dysphoria should be established. The individual must also have capacity for decision-making, be of legal age, and his/her mental and medical health must be well controlled. It is important to discuss the risks, benefits, and expectations associated with transitioning sexes as well as the financial expense associated with treatment. It is recommended that individuals live as the opposite gender either prior to or concurrently with hormone therapy for 1 year prior to being considered for surgical treatment. Exceptions to this include medical contraindications for hormonal therapy or if the patient is either unwilling or unable to take hormones. Of note, the only realized benefit from surgery is relief of symptoms associated with gender dysphoria, such as subjective well-being and sexual function, and has not been shown to improve any other facet of the individual's life (Coleman et al. 2012). Only 10–25 % of patients undergo sex reassignment surgery, largely due to the large financial expense associated with a lack of coverage by health insurance plans (Gooren and Tangpricha 2014). In addition, hormone treatment with gonadotropin-releasing hormone (GnRH) agonists used for male-to-female (MTF) transsexuals can be too expensive for many individuals.

Hormone therapy is used to suppress endogenous hormones of the individual's natal sex and induce secondary sex characteristics of the desired sex. Hormone therapy is continued even after surgical reassignment to maintain normal physiological levels in the desired sex. For MTF transsexuals, the goal of hormonal therapy is to eliminate sexual hair growth, induce breast development, and modify fat formation to appear more feminine. In addition, prostate and testicular atrophy will occur over many years. This is accomplished with medications that suppress androgen secretion or action, which include antiandrogens, progestins, estrogens, GnRH agonists, and 5-alpha reductase type II inhibitors. For female-to-male (FTM) transsexuals, the goals of hormone treatment with testosterone include obtaining masculine hair growth patterns including facial hair, as well as deepening the voice, decreasing breast glandular tissue and subcutaneous fat, increased libido, and up to 40 % will develop acne. Menses will typically stop a few months after initiating testosterone (Giltay and Gooren 2000).

Treatment can be administered to adolescents if it is thought that the gender dysphoria will persist into adulthood. Hormone therapy, considered a partially reversible treatment, can be used to delay development and spare the individual of going through puberty and developing secondary characteristics inconsistent with their identified gender. The Endocrine Society's Clinical Guidelines suggest that GnRH agonists should be used when boys or girls develop the first physical changes of puberty, but no earlier than Tanner stage 2 (Hembree et al. 2009). Individuals must then live as the opposite gender for at least a 2-year trial period. If the dysphoria persists, aggressive hormone therapy can be started at the age of 16 to initiate the gender transition process. Surgery is not considered until the individual is at least 18 years old (Nicholson and McGuiness 2014).

Vignette 28.2.3: Conclusion

Ms. Bridges tells you that she was very satisfied with the surgery and content with her decision. She states that the relationship with her boyfriend is still going strong and he has been very supportive and understanding of everything she has gone through. Despite her "dream" becoming reality and being in the "perfect" relationship, she reports that she has been struggling emotionally in her role as a female. She has been experiencing worsening anxiety and depression over the past few years and has been considering reverting back to a male. She hoped her initial unhappiness was intimately linked to the dysphoric feeling of living as a male when she so strongly desired to be a female, and is concerned that she will find herself in the same "deep depression" she was in prior to her transformation. She also has begun to self-medicate with marijuana and increasing amounts of alcohol. She is hopeful that you will be able to help improve her mood, reduce her self-harm behaviors, and control her substance use. She is amenable to medication and psychotherapy and consents to a trial of an antidepressant and referral to a therapist.

STOP

Please proceed with the problem-based approach using the worksheet located in the appendix of Chap. 1!

Table 28.2.3

FACTS	HYPOTHESES	INFORMATION NEEDED	LEARNING ISSUES

Of those who undergo gender reassignment with hormone therapy or surgery, 80 % experience improvement in their symptoms and distress from gender dysphoria, 78 % have improvement in psychological symptoms, 80 % have improvement in quality of life, and 72 % have improvement in sexual function (Murad et al. 2010). As these data describe, a proportion of individuals do not experience complete resolution of their emotional distress after undergoing transition. Suicide is a considerable risk even after reassignment, and long-term follow-up with a mental health professional is warranted. The overall mortality rate is 51 % higher in MTF compared to FTM transsexuals due to higher rates of drug abuse, HIV, cardiovascular disease, and suicide in the MTF transsexuals (Asscheman et al. 2013).

Vignette 28.3.1: Presenting Information: Kurt Dawson
Kurt Dawson is a 19-year-old patient you are asked to evaluate as a third-year medical student on the hospital psychiatric consultation-liaison service. Mr. Dawson has been in the hospital for 7 days and was just transferred out of the intensive care unit (ICU) yesterday after spending 5 days on life support. Prior to admission, he was found unconscious in his room by his mother with one end of a rope around his neck and the other around the ceiling fan. After combing through the patient's records with information provided by the mother, you discover that the patient has been feeling depressed and isolating himself more since starting college. There is a strong family history of depression, but Mr. Dawson has no history of depression or suicidal ideation in the past.

You walk into Mr. Dawson's room and find a young lethargic man lying in his hospital bed with obvious bruising around his neck. He is arousable and able to converse, so you sit down and start your interview.

Please proceed with the problem-based approach using the worksheet located in the appendix of Chap. 1!

Table 28.3.1

FACTS	HYPOTHESES	INFORMATION NEEDED	LEARNING ISSUES

28.3 Learning Issues

Based on the information that was obtained by the patient's mother on presentation, a suicide attempt appears to be a possibility. In addition, it is important to consider a differential diagnosis that includes a hypoxyphilic game known as the "choking game," especially in adolescents and young adults. Homicide/attempted murder and suicide/suicide attempt should also be considered as an asphyxiophilia-related incident can present similarly. As a result of the similar presentations, it is estimated that the true number of asphyxiophilia-related deaths is underestimated due to misclassifying the death as a suicide or homicide. In evaluating someone who has survived the incident, simply asking questions may lead you to a diagnosis. However, if the individual is deceased or unable to communicate, the diagnosis may be difficult to accurately obtain. Identifying clues related to the nature and cause of death can help narrow the differential and lead to appropriate classification of death. It is important to examine the scene for evidence of foul play, a presence/absence of a suicide letter, and what the patient was wearing at the time of death.

Case Vignette 28.3.2: Continuation

Mr. Dawson appears shy and guarded at first but begins to open up as you progress through the interview. With some prodding, he begins to recount the events that brought him to the hospital. He begins by telling you that he did not try to kill himself, despite how it may have appeared. He explains that since he was 16, he has been experimenting with hanging himself in order to experience a more intense orgasm while masturbating. You expect him to be hesitant to reveal such intimate details and are surprised by his willingness to discuss his sexual practices. He admits that he has tried this roughly a dozen times since he started, but it had never reached the point of unconsciousness before. Although he has a girlfriend who he is sexually active with, he explains that he enjoys and has continued to engage in autoerotic asphyxiation. He also mentions that he often fantasizes about being bound up and put into painful or demeaning situations. He further describes occasions when he and his girlfriend have role-played where he has her play a "bad" cop who interrogates and punishes him by verbally and physically beating him. He admits that she was hesitant to do this at first, but now appears to enjoy it as well. Although he has involved her in these fantasies, he has not told her or anyone else about his experiments with methods to restrict his breathing. He goes on to describe the event that nearly killed him.

He states that he usually uses a belt that he fastens around his neck and ties the loose end around his bedpost. He then leans forward until he feels close to passing out. Although he admits to understanding the risks if he were to pass out, he has been pushing himself closer and closer to the "edge." To get more leverage, he decided to secure a rope around the ceiling fan in his room. He is not able to recall exactly what happened this time, as he was unable to recognize his proximity to losing consciousness. He is however, thankful that his mother found him and cut him down in time.

Although he has always enjoyed the sensation he gets from this act, he found that certain things made his experience even more enjoyable. He began wearing women's clothing on occasion, and was wearing a dress and bra he borrowed from his girlfriend during this last autoerotic act. He also found that he enjoys watching himself as he masturbates, as it seems to make the experience more pleasurable and admits to positioning a mirror in his room to facilitate this.

Please proceed with the problem-based approach using the worksheet located in the appendix of Chap. 1!

Table 28.3.2

FACTS	HYPOTHESES	INFORMATION NEEDED	LEARNING ISSUES

Mr. Dawson has described the common features of the paraphilic disorder: sexual masochism with asphyxiophilia. A differential diagnosis for sexual masochism includes transvestic fetishism, sexual sadism disorder, hypersexuality, and alcohol/substance use disorders. Paraphilia is the term used to describe a persistent and intense sexual interest in something aside from genital stimulation or fondling with someone who is not physically mature, phenotypically normal, or a consenting human partner (APA 2013). This sexual interest is considered a disorder if it involves self-harm or potential harm to others, or causes the individual distress or impairment in a variety of functional settings. Paraphilias are comorbid with one another and individuals with one paraphilia will often manifest others. See Table 28.5 for a list of the most common paraphilias, as discussed in DSM-5 (APA 2013).

Sexual masochism is described as sexual arousal that results from being humiliated, beaten, bound, or otherwise made to suffer through fantasies, sexual urges or behaviors. The average age of onset for sexual masochism is 19, while its prevalence in the USA is unknown (Hucker 2012). An Australian study reports that 2.2 % of males and 1.3 % of females were involved in sexual masochistic activities over a 12-month period (Richters et al. 2008). Individuals with this disorder tend to do well socially and psychologically, are on average more educated, and have higher incomes than the general population (Hucker 2012). The importance of identifying sexual masochism, especially with asphyxiophilia, is the risk of accidental death associated with the practice of autoerotic actions.

Asphyxiophilia is a subgroup of behaviors within sexual masochism that involves sexual arousal from activities that result in restricted breathing. Nearly all reported cases of asphyxiophilia are males under the age of 40, although practicing these acts can begin with puberty. There are no specific signs or predisposing factors, and many individuals are involved in healthy sexual relationships. Behaviors that restrict breathing are often performed in solitary settings, such as a basement, and often when there is no one else in the home. The individual usually understands

Table 28.5 Paraphilic disorders

Paraphilia	Sexual arousal manifested as fantasies, urges, or behaviors from:
Voyeurism	Observing an unconsented individual who is naked, in the process of becoming naked, or involved in a sexual activity
Exhibitionism	Exposing one's genitals to an unconsented individual
Frotteurism	Rubbing or touching an unconsented individual
Sexual masochism	Acts of being beaten, bound, humiliated, or made to suffer
Sexual sadism	Causing physical or psychological suffering of an unconsented individual
Pedophilia	Sexual activity with a prepubescent child, generally less than age 13
Fetishism	The use of nonliving objects or a focus on nongenital body parts
Transvestism	Cross-dressing

the risks and often employs a safety mechanism to prevent death. However, this often only involves *subjective* judgment such that the individual will cease the activity when they feel close to losing consciousness (Hucker 2012).

Sexual arousal obtained from asphyxiation is gained from the process of restricting breathing rather than the subjective lack of oxygen (Hucker 2011). Methods for restricting breathing include compressing the chest, strangulation, choking, suffocation, and self-hanging. Suffocation may involve placing a plastic bag or mask over the head and face, or the use of volatile gases or vapors. Means of strangulation include hanging via noose, rope, or other ligature, often in an excessive and complex arrangement. Hanging is the most likely method to result in fatality (Hucker 2012).

Individuals may engage in hypoxia-inducing activities frequently; however, these activities are not typically performed on a daily basis. Many individuals describe sadistic or cross-gender fantasies. Asphyxiophilia is associated with other paraphilias including other masochistic forms, sadism, transvestic fetishism, and other fetishisms. While an association between asphyxiophilia and mood and anxiety disorders has not been established in fatal cases, it is reported to exist with living asphyxiophilia patients. About 60 % of living patients were noted to have made suicide attempts in the past (Hucker 2012).

Case Vignette 28.3.3: Continuation

Mr. Dawson begins feeling very fatigued, so you decide it would be best to return the following day to continue the interview. That night, you research sexual masochism to gain a better understanding of his disorder and ask more specific questions pertaining to it. You return the next morning to talk to Mr. Dawson and find that his mother is visiting him. You ask if he would like talk in private but surprisingly, he states that he feels comfortable talking about this in front of his mother. You start by filling the mother in on what Kurt discussed with you the day prior. You inform her that although he may have some underlying depression, it does not appear that this was a suicide attempt, but rather a sexual act that accidentally went too far. You explain that his behavior is not that uncommon and typically involves various methods of hanging. You tell her that sometimes these acts can lead to accidental death if the individual loses consciousness and cannot escape from their method of asphyxiation. She bursts into tears when you tell her that it was a fortunate circumstance that she found him before it was too late. When she regains her composure, she admits that she actually feels a great sense of guilt. She admits that although she called 911 when she first discovered her son, she promptly removed all evidence of his act including the pornography, and changed his clothes so that it would "look more like a suicide."

Please proceed with the problem-based approach using the worksheet located in the appendix of Chap. 1!

Table 28.3.3

FACTS	HYPOTHESES	INFORMATION NEEDED	LEARNING ISSUES

Identifying an accidental death from asphyxiophilia is not always straightforward, and the circumstances may be confused with suicide or homicide. Evaluation of the death scene can help elicit the cause of death. Specific findings consistent with death due to asphyxiation include evidence of sexual activity, such as pornographic materials, ligatures, clips, clamps, whips, dildos, and/or mirrors or cameras, so that the individual can observe him- or herself performing the act. When initially discovered, up to a quarter of men are found wearing women's clothing, while others may be nude or in bondage-style clothing (Hucker 2012). Family members or friends who find the deceased will often remove items, dress/redress them, and otherwise alter the scene to prevent potential embarrassment to the individual or family member. These alterations make it difficult to distinguish suicide from accidental death (Hucker 2012).

Case Vignette 28.3.4: Conclusion

Mr. Dawson admits that he is concerned about his sexual fantasies and behaviors and wants to know if there is anything that can be done to help him. He says, "This was too close of a call for me, and I'm afraid that next time I won't be so lucky." You tell him that his willingness to change is a good sign as many with this disorder are not willing. You refer him for CBT. Also, considering his depressive symptoms, you prescribe him a selective serotonin reuptake inhibitor (SSRI) which may have the dual benefit of also decreasing his sexual impulses.

STOP

Please proceed with the problem-based approach using the worksheet located in the appendix of Chap. 1!

Table 28.3.4

FACTS	HYPOTHESES	INFORMATION NEEDED	LEARNING ISSUES

Most paraphilias are chronic in nature and may last many years without treatment. The frequency of sexual acts may increase or decrease over time, but usually diminishes by the age of 60. Individuals with paraphilias are often unwilling to give up their methods of sexual satisfaction and may be identified only when being treated for a comorbid mood disorder. Initial treatment for sexual masochism and other paraphilias involves initiating CBT and pharmacologic therapy.

While there are no formal guidelines for the treatment of paraphilias, CBT and/or pharmacologic therapy should be initiated in all offenders. Animal studies have shown that serotonin and prolactin inhibit sexual arousal, while dopamine, norepinephrine, oxytocin, GnRH, testosterone, and estrogen/progesterone stimulate it. Thus, antidepressants such as SSRIs or tricyclic antidepressants (TCAs), antiandrogen hormones, and luteinizing hormone-releasing hormone (LHRH) are effective in the treatment of paraphilias. In sex offenders with a high risk of reoffending, such as those with multiple paraphilias, multiple victims, psychiatric illness, or deviant sexual interests, CBT and pharmacologic treatment should be initiated simultaneously. In those that partake in nonviolent paraphilias or are at low risk for reoffending, monotherapy with an SSRI or TCA is appropriate. SSRIs have a beneficial side effect profile that includes a reduced libido, and also treats mood symptoms or disorders, such as depression, which are highly comorbid with paraphilias. When considering dual combination therapy with a serotonergic and antiandrogenic in offenders such as pedophiles, progestogens such as cyproterone acetate or medroxyprogesterone acetate (MPA) should be used before trying LHRH agonists or estrogen (Guay 2009).

28.4 Conclusion

As has been illustrated in the preceding vignettes, sexual disorders, gender dysphoria, and paraphilias constitute an important group of disorders that may go unnoticed by medical professionals but can be associated with significant distress and risk. Identifying individuals with any of these conditions may not become apparent unless treatment is sought for an associated condition such as depression or physical or medical sequelae. These topics can be difficult to discuss with patients and are likely underreported for fear of embarrassment and other factors related to foregoing medical or psychiatric care. The PLISSIT approach and collateral interviews may help clinicians best serve their patients' needs.

28.5 Review Questions

1. A 32-year-old female patient of yours presents to your outpatient office with complaints of "vaginal pain." After talking with the patient, you learn that she has been having severe pain when she has sexual intercourse with her husband since the birth of her daughter 4 months ago. She suffered a third-degree laceration during an otherwise uncomplicated vaginal delivery. What is her likely diagnosis?
   a. Genito-pelvic pain/penetration disorder
   b. Vaginal pain secondary to trauma
   c. Dyspareunia
   d. Vulvovaginal atrophy
2. When you suspect that a patient has a sexual dysfunction, how should you initiate a discussion of their sexual history?
   a. Obtain permission to discuss sex with the patient
   b. Provide limited information to dispel myths and discuss normal sexual functioning
   c. Provide specific suggestions for the patient's complaint
   d. Consider intensive treatment with therapy for complex issues
   e. All of the above

3. A prepubescent child unhappy with his natal gender is evaluated by a psychiatrist. His symptoms meet criteria for gender dysphoria. What are his therapeutic options?
    a. Wait until the child is at least 18 before considering hormone or surgical therapy
    b. Initiate hormone therapy now to delay puberty
    c. Initiate hormone therapy at the first sign of physical changes associated with puberty, but not before Tanner stage 2
    d. Obtain a chromosome analysis prior to any treatment
4. Which of the following is a benefit of sex reassignment surgery?
    a. Reduced level of distress from gender dysphoria
    b. Improved sexual function
    c. Result in better psychological functioning
    d. All of the above
5. Match each paraphilia to the source of sexual arousal

Sexual masochism	Exposing one's genitals to an unconsented individual
Sexual sadism	Rubbing or touching an unconsented individual
Transvestism	Acts of being beaten, bund, humiliated, or made to suffer
Exhibitionism	Causing physical or psychological suffering of an unconsented individual
Fetishism	Use of nonliving objects or focus on nongenital body parts
Frotteurism	Cross-dressing

6. What are some clues that may help distinguish an accidental death related to asphyxiophilia from a suicide?

Appendix A: Tables with Possible Answers to Vignettes

Vignette 28.1: Lynne Sparks

Table 28.1.1

Facts	Hypotheses	What do you want to know next?	Learning issues
51-year-old female with a progressive decline in sexual desire for 1 year	Decreased libido due to:	Does she experience pain during intercourse?	What medical and nonmedical factors are associated with decreased libido?
Increase in marital conflict	MDD	Was there an inciting event, such as trauma or abuse?	How do you discuss sexual history with a patient?

Facts	Hypotheses	What do you want to know next?	Learning issues
No major life stressors	Medication side effect	Does she have a history of underlying medical conditions?	
Distress over this change	Thyroid dysfunction	Does she have depression? Is she being treated?	
Maintains sexual attraction to husband	Female sexual interest/arousal disorder	Is she still having periods? Are they consistent?	
	Marital discord	Does she smoke cigarettes? Does she drink alcohol?	
	Perimenopause		

MDD major depressive disorder

Table 28.1.2

Facts	Hypotheses	What do you want to know next?	Learning issues
Pain associated with vaginal penetration	Genito-pelvic penetration disorder (dyspareunia, vaginismus)	What types of lubricants has she used?	What are the criteria for diagnosing a genito-pelvic pain disorder?
Pelvic pain not improved with lubricant	Vulvovaginal atrophy	Has she engaged in therapy/counseling for this?	How does menopause status affect the prevalence of a sexual disorder?
Inability to achieve orgasm		Has therapy helped to reduce the pain?	
Periods becoming inconsistent and less frequent		Has the estrogen cream helped reduce vaginal dryness?	
History of PID Normal gynecological exam 6 months ago		How has her relationship with her husband improved? Less stress and anxiety?	

PID pelvic inflammatory disorder

Table 28.1.3

Facts	Hypotheses	What do you want to know next?	Learning issues
Experiencing less pain	Vaginismus	Will CBT and dilators be sufficient to eliminate the pain altogether, or will she need additional treatment?	What are the treatment options for genito-pelvic pain/penetration disorder?
Vaginal dryness improved with estrogen cream	Perimenopause		What are the different sexual disorders?

CBT cognitive behavioral therapy

Vignette 28.2: Angel Bridges

Table 28.2.1

Facts	Hypotheses	What do you want to know next?	Learning issues
38-year-old transgender born male, developed normal male secondary sex characteristics	Gender dysphoria Nonconformity to gender roles	Did she feel as though she was born in the wrong body and desire to be of the opposite gender?	Understand the difference between sex and gender
	Transvestic disorder	Did she feel that her body was abnormally formed?	What is the differential diagnosis for someone dissatisfied with their sex?
Preferred to wear dresses in childhood	Body dysmorphic disorder	Have there been features of psychosis?	When do signs of gender dysphoria first appear?
Was married to woman and had two children with her	Psychotic disorder	Did she experience sexual arousal when she would dress in women's clothes?	What are the criteria for diagnosing gender dysphoria?
Enjoyed wearing his wife's clothes		Has she sought hormonal or surgical treatment?	
History of anxiety and depression		Does she have a history of depression?	

Table 28.2.2

Facts	Hypotheses	What do you want to know next?	Learning issues
Left his wife and children	Depressive and suicidal thoughts due to gender dysphoria	What are the hormonal treatment options for transitioning from a male to female?	Understand the process for undergoing gender reassignment
Attracted to men		How has she adapted to her role as a female?	What are the desired effects of hormone therapy?
Underwent hormone therapy followed by surgical reassignment		How has her mood symptoms improved since reassignment?	At what age can hormone therapy first be given?

Table 28.2.3

Facts	Hypotheses	What do you want to know next?	Learning issues
In a supportive relationship	Unmet expectations from gender reassignment	What are her expectations moving forward?	What are the limitations of gender reassignment?
Depression and anxiety with multiple suicide attempts		Has she considered reverting back to being a male?	

Vignette 28.3: Kurt Dawson

Table 28.3.1

Facts	Hypotheses	What do you want to know next?	Learning issues
19-year-old male found unconscious by mother	Suicide attempt	Is he depressed, or ever had thoughts of suicide in the past?	Develop a differential diagnosis for someone with an apparent suicide attempt
History of depression	Attempted murder	Was this an attempt to end his life?	
No prior suicide attempts	Accidental sexual masochism with asphyxiophilia	Did someone do this to him?	
Required several days in ICU		Is there another explanation for hanging himself?	
		Has he done this before?	

ICU intensive care unit

Table 28.3.2

Facts	Hypotheses	What do you want to know next?	Learning issues
Sexual pleasure from hanging since age of 16	Asphyxiophilia-related accident with failure of subjective safety mechanism	Why did he not present to the hospital in his girlfriend's clothes?	What is a paraphilia?
Girlfriend with whom he is sexually active		What features are typically associated with sexual masochism?	What are the risks associated with sexual masochism?
Thankful he is alive			
Was wearing girlfriend's clothes			

Table 28.3.3

Facts	Hypotheses	What do you want to know next?	Learning issues
Mother lied to make it appear as though her son had tried to commit suicide	Sexual masochism with near-asphyxiophilia-related death, staged to look like a suicide by his mother	Why would his mom make it look like he tried to kill himself?	Paraphilias are not easily identified and may only present as part of another disorder
		What are some specific findings at the scene of an asphyxiophilia-related death?	

Table 28.3.4

Facts	Hypotheses	What do you want to know next?	Learning issues
Concerned about his behaviors	Sexual masochism with asphyxiophilia	How likely is he to give up his risky behaviors?	What is the treatment of sexual masochism and other paraphilias?

Appendix B: Key to Review Questions

1. B
2. E
3. C
4. D
5. 1-C; 2-D; 3-F; 4-A; 5-E; 6-B
6. Specific findings consistent with death due to asphyxiation include evidence of sexual activity such as pornographic materials, ligatures, clips, clamps, whips, dildos, and/or mirrors or cameras so that the individual can observe him or herself performing the act. Up to a quarter of men are found wearing women's clothing, while others may be nude or in bondage-style clothing.

References

American Psychiatric Association. (2000). Diagnostic and statistical manual of mental disorders (4th ed., text rev.). Washington, DC: American Psychiatric Association.

American Psychiatric Association. (2013). *Diagnostic and statistical manual of mental disorders* (5th edn.). Arlington: American Psychiatric Publishing.

Annon, J. (1976). The PLISSIT model: A proposed conceptual scheme for the behavioral treatment of sexual problems. *Journal of Sex Education and Therapy, 2*(2), 1–15.

Asscheman, H., Giltay, E. J., Megens, J. A., et al. (2011). A long-term follow-up study of mortality in transsexuals receiving treatment with cross-sex hormones. *European Journal of Endocrinology, 164,* 635.

Biggs, W. S. (2011). Medical human sexuality. In R. E. Rakel. (Ed.), *Textbook of family medicine* (pp. 1000–1011). Philadelphia: Saunders.

Coleman, E., et al. (2012). Standards of care for the health of transsexual, transgender, and gender-nonconforming people. *International Journal of Transgenderism, 13*(4), 165–232.

Crowley, T., Richardson, D., & Goldmeier, D. (2006). Recommendations for the management of vaginismus: BASHH special interest group for sexual dysfunction. *International Journal of STD and AIDS, 17*(1), 14–18.

Frank, J. E., Mistretta, P., & Will, J. (2008). Diagnosis and treatment of female sexual dysfunction. *American Family Physician, 77*(5), 635–642.

Giltay, E. J., & Gooren, L. J. (2000). Effects of sex steroid deprivation/administration on hair growth and skin sebum production in transsexual males and females. *The Journal of Clinical Endocrinology and Metabolism, 85,* 2913.

Gooren, L. G., & Tangpricha, V. (2014). Treatment of transsexualism. In: Snyder, P. J., Matsumoto, A. M. (Eds) UpToDate. Waltham, MA. http://www.uptodate.com. Accessed 24 Sep 2014.

Guay, D. R. P. (2009). Drug treatment of paraphilic and nonparaphilic sexual disorders. *Clinical Therapeutics, 31*(1), 1–31.

Hembree, W. C., Cohen-Kettenis, P., Delemarre-van de Waal, H. A., et al. (2009). Endocrine treatment of transsexual persons: An endocrine society clinical practice guideline. *The Journal of Clinical Endocrinology and Metabolism, 94,* 3132.

Hucker, S. J. (2011). Hypoxyphilia. *Archives of Sexual Behavior, 40,* 1323–1326.

Hucker, S. J. (2012). Paraphilia: Hypoxyphilia/auto-erotic Asphyxia. Forensic Psychiatry.ca. http://www.forensicpsychiatry.ca/paraphilia/aea.htm. Accessed 24 Aug 2014.

Laumann, E. O., Paik, A., & Rosen, R. C. (1999). Sexual dysfunction in the United States: Prevalence and predictors. *JAMA: The Journal of the American Medical Association, 281*(6), 537–544.

Moreira, Jr E. D., Brock, G., Glasser, D. B., et al. (2005). Help-seeking behavior for sexual problems: The global study of sexual attitudes and behaviors. *International Journal of Clinical Practice, 59,* 6–16.

Murad, M. H., Elamin, M. B., Garcia, M. Z., et al. (2010). Hormonal therapy and sex reassignment: A systematic review and meta-analysis of quality of life and psychosocial outcomes. *Clinical Endocrinology (Oxf), 72,* 214.

Nicholson, C., & McGuinness, T. M. (2014). Gender dysphoria and children. *Journal of Psychosocial Nursing, 52*(8), 27–30.

Reed, B. D. (2009). Dyspareunia and sexual/physical abuse. In A. T. Goldstein, C. F. Pukall, & I. Goldstein (Eds.), *Female sexual pain disorders* (pp. 213–217). Hoboken: Wiley-Blackwell.

Richters, J., De Visser, R. O., Rissel, C. E., Grulich, A. E., & Smith A. M. A. (2008). Demographic and psychosocial features of participants in bondage and discipline, "sadomasochism" or dominance and submission (BDSM): Data from a national survey. *Journal of Sexual Medicine, 5,* 1660–1668.

Chapter 29
Other Disorders

Anthony P. S. Guerrero

Welcome to the last chapter of this textbook! We sincerely hope that you have enjoyed this overview of the key topics in behavioral sciences and clinical psychiatry. To round out your learning, we will end with a glimpse of "other disorders" and hopefully review some of the other conditions and principles discussed elsewhere in this textbook.

At the end of this chapter, the reader will be able to:

1. Discuss the approach to "other" psychiatric symptom clusters that do not automatically lead to diagnosis of the disorders heretofore discussed.
2. Discuss the epidemiology, mechanisms, clinical presentation, clinical evaluation, differential diagnosis and treatment of dissociative disorders, impulse control disorders not previously discussed in other chapters, and other conditions that may be a focus of clinical attention.

Case Vignette 29.1.1 (Presenting Situation)
Hau'oli Smith is a 10-year-old female who is hospitalized for migraine headaches with significant pain and nausea requiring intravenous medications and fluid. Laboratory tests did not indicate any other medical problems besides the migraines. It was felt that her degree of pain is significantly more than what would be expected for this condition.

Nursing staff reported that Hau'oli seemed to most be in pain when her mother and stepfather were in the room together. She would otherwise seem "fine." Additionally, it had been noted that there were recent family stressors, including marital conflict between the mother and stepfather and the birth of a new sibling, who is now 3 months old. The mother had reported that, particularly

A. P. S. Guerrero (✉)
Department of Psychiatry, University of Hawai'i John A. Burns School of Medicine,
1356 Lusitana Street, University Tower 4th Floor, Honolulu, HI 96813, USA
e-mail: GuerreroA@dop.hawaii.edu

D. Alicata et al. (eds.), *Problem-based Behavioral Science and Psychiatry*,
DOI 10.1007/978-3-319-23669-8_29

in the last few months, Hau'oli has been crying more, arguing more, and complaining more of headaches. A psychiatric consultation was, therefore, requested to evaluate for "adjustment difficulties," to rule out "malingering" or other psychological component to the headaches, and to provide "counseling" if indicated.

Please proceed with the problem-based approach using the worksheet located in the appendix of Chap. 1!

At this point, diagnosis of an adjustment disorder, while only one of several diagnostic possibilities (to be discussed further), is a reasonable one to consider. An adjustment disorder involves clinically significant (e.g., socially, academically, or occupationally impairing or involving disproportionate distress) emotional/behavioral symptoms arising, within 3 months, from an identifiable stressor. As with many of the conditions you have learned thus far, these symptoms are not better explained by another condition, including bereavement. Finally, these symptoms should not persist beyond 6 months following the termination of the stressor or its sequelae. According to the Diagnostic and Statistical Manual of Mental Disorders, Fifth Edition (DSM-5), adjustment disorders should be further classified as being acute (lasting less than 6 months) or chronic (lasting 6 months or longer) and as being predominantly: with depressed mood, with anxiety, with mixed anxiety and depressed mood, with disturbance of conduct, with mixed disturbance of emotions and conduct, or unspecified.

Adjustment disorders, as discussed previously in "Anxiety Disorders, Obsessive-Compulsive and Related Disorders, Trauma- and Stressor-Related Disorders" (Chap. 22) are among the most common of the psychiatric disorders, with apparently increased prevalence in general medical and psychiatric settings. As previously noted, in considering the diagnosis of an adjustment disorder, it is significantly important to consider other (though perhaps less common) differential possibilities. For the case above, reasonable diagnoses to consider would have included:

- Major depression (e.g., with crying and irritability)
- Other trauma or stressor-related disorder (e.g., post-traumatic stress disorder)
- Child physical abuse, child sexual abuse, child neglect, or child psychological abuse (e.g., with unexplained somatic symptoms, family stressors that are not yet clarified)
- Anxiety disorder (e.g., separation anxiety disorder)
- Mood disorder secondary to other medical conditions (e.g., intracranial pathology)
- Somatic symptom disorder
- Malingering

Table 29.1 Organization of other conditions that may be a focus of clinical attention (please refer to The Diagnostic and Statistical Manual of Mental Disorders, Fifth Edition text for actual wording and codes)

Relational problems
Problems related to family upbringing (including parent–child or sibling relational problem, upbringing away from parents, child affected by parental relationship distress)
Other problems related to primary support group (including relationship distress with spouse or intimate partner, disruption of family by separation or divorce, high expressed emotion level within a family, and uncomplicated bereavement)
Abuse and neglect (initial encounter or subsequent encounter)
Child maltreatment and neglect problems (including child physical and sexual and psychological abuse, child neglect)
Adult maltreatment and neglect problems (including spouse or partner physical or sexual violence, spouse or partner neglect, spouse or partner psychological abuse, adult abuse by nonspouse or nonpartner)
Educational (academic or educational problem) and occupational problems (e.g., related to current military deployment or other problems)
Housing (homelessness; inadequate housing; discord with neighbor, lodger, or landlord; problem related to living in a residential institution) and economic (lack of adequate food or safe drinking water, extreme poverty, low income, insufficient social insurance or welfare support) problems
Other problems related to the social environment (phase of life problem, problem related to living alone, acculturation difficulty, social exclusion or rejection, target of adverse discrimination or persecution, unspecified problem related to social environment)
Problems related to crime or interaction with the legal system (e.g., crime victim, conviction, imprisonment/incarceration, problems related to prison release, other)
Other health service encounters for counseling and medical advice
Problems related to other psychosocial, personal, and environmental circumstances (e.g., religious/spiritual problem; problem related to unwanted pregnancy or multiparity; discord with social service provider; victim of terrorism or torture; exposure to disaster, war, or other hostilities; other
Other circumstances of personal history (e.g., personal history of psychological trauma, self-harm, or military deployment; lifestyle-related problem; adult or child/adolescent antisocial behavior)
Problems related to access to medical and other health care (unavailability/inaccessibility of health-care facilities or other helping agencies)
Nonadherence to medical treatment, overweight or obesity, malingering

The differential possibilities discussed above should stimulate us to recall the information we have learned in the previous chapters on "Mood Disorders and Suicide" (Chap. 21); "Violence and Abuse" (Chap. 7); "Anxiety Disorders, Obsessive-Compulsive and Related Disorders, Trauma- and Stressor-Related Disorders" (Chap. 22); and "Somatic Symptom and Related Disorders" (Chap. 23)! Do you recall which of these conditions are relatively more common than the others?

Two of the differential possibilities listed above are included in the important section of the DSM-5 called "Other Conditions That May Be a Focus of Clinical Attention." Table 29.1 summarizes the organization of these conditions. These conditions are listed because they may affect the diagnosis, course, prognosis, or treatment of a patient's mental disorder but are not mental disorders in and of themselves.

Malingering is a condition that we visited in Chap. 23. For review, according to the DSM-5, it involves "the *intentional* production of false or grossly exaggerated physical *or psychological* symptoms, motivated by *external incentives*." Usually, malingering is considered when physical symptoms or complaints are present; however, psychological symptoms (including psychosis) can also be malingered. Malingering is differentiated from a factitious disorder and many of the somatic symptom disorders (covered in Chap. 23) by the characteristics summarized in Table 29.2.

Because it is not clear that this patient is intentionally producing these symptoms, additional evaluation is necessary.

Case Vignette 29.1.2

You meet with Hau'oli and her family. While she is not worried that the headaches represent anything other than her migraines, her mother and stepfather report that they are somewhat concerned that these symptoms might indicate the presence of an "aneurysm," from which the patient's maternal great grandmother, who was close to the patient, died 5 months ago. You encourage them to discuss this concern with the medical team.

The family notes that, in the past few months, there have in fact been multiple stressors, including: the birth of the patient's half-sister (who is the only other child in the family), loss of the stepfather's job, increased marital conflict—probably related to the financial pressures of the stepfather's job loss, and the beginning of a new academic year in a new school. Per the family's report, there are no previous behavioral concerns. She has had a history of migraines from an early age that were usually well controlled with prophylactic medication. There are also no other medical problems, and there was no pattern of recurring somatic complaints other than the migraines. There is a strong family history of migraines, and mother notes that her own migraines began during childhood.

In your individual interview with Hau'oli, she admits that she has been feeling sad, "bummed out," and "a little worried" over all of the "money problems" their family has been having. She believes that her migraines may be worse whenever she feels stress. While she says that she likes the new baby, she "never really liked the idea of mom getting re-married." She recalls that in the previous marriage, "my real dad was always drunk, and he used to hit her, so that's why they got a divorce." While she reports being afraid whenever she witnessed violence, she denies any nightmares, flashbacks, or significant distress upon reexposure to reminders of previous trauma. She denies any previous or current physical or sexual abuse. She denies excessive worry about her mother's safety or anxiety upon separating from her family to attend school and other activities. While she has had poor appetite and sleep for the past 2 days, since the migraine difficulties began, she denies any previous sleep, appetite, or energy-level changes and denies any definite anhedonia or suicidal or homicidal ideations. While cooperative with your interview, she does appear uncomfortable, and she prefers to have the lights off. Vital signs are significant for mild tachycardia.

Table 29.2 Characteristics of malingering, factitious disorder, and other somatic symptom disorders

Disorder	Intentional production of symptoms?	Motivation for behavior	Presentation of symptoms	Clinical findings
Malingering	Yes	External incentive (e.g., economic gain, avoiding legal responsibility, etc.) "Secondary gain"	Often dramatic demonstrations of disability or symptoms	History may be internally inconsistent Physical and/or mental status findings may be inconsistent with known presentations of illness or plausible physiological mechanisms
Factitious disorder	Yes	To assume the sick role "Primary gain"		
Other somatic symptom disorders (e.g., somatic symptom disorder, conversion disorder, etc.)	No	Not applicable	Often less dramatic demonstrations of disability or symptoms; indifference may be present	

Based on the above presentation, various differential possibilities appear to have been ruled out. Of note, even though there may have been neurovegative symptoms to suggest depression (e.g., with sleep and appetite changes), these symptoms did not occur in the absence of the migraine headaches and did not last for 2 weeks or longer.

With the other possibilities in the list above ruled out, the diagnosis of adjustment disorder, acute, with mixed anxiety and depressed mood, is most probable, along with psychological factors affecting other medical conditions (migraine headaches, in this case). Diagnostic criteria for the latter diagnosis include the presence of another medical condition and evidence that psychological factors adversely affected the general medical condition through either the physiological sequelae of the psychological factors *(which may be applicable in this case)* or interference of the psychological factors with prevention or treatment of the general medical condition. It is also worth noting the several other potential conditions that may be a focus of clinical attention as they may affect the diagnosis, course, prognosis, or treatment.

Beyond just DSM-5 diagnosis, this case illustrates the importance of biopsychosocial formulation in insuring optimal treatment—as is often the case when managing adjustment disorders, either on its own or in the context of a general medical condition.

Please take this opportunity to do a biopsychosocial formulation for this case.

Case Vignette 29.1.3

You work collaboratively with the pediatric team to optimize medical management of acute pain. You provide individual and family supportive counseling and psychoeducation, and you address the family's concern that someone might be thinking that this is "all in her head." You "prescribe" an expected course of recovery while still allowing the patient to express the pain that likely goes along with her migraine headaches. You also consult with your team psychologist on relaxation and other behavioral techniques that might help with pain management. On outpatient follow-up, you provide individual and family psychotherapy, which proves to be very effective. You encourage the parents to spend individual time with the patient, even in the face of the demands of the new baby. Several months later, her headaches are under stable control, and there are no further hospitalizations.

As depicted in Table 29.3, with the construction of a biopsychosocial formulation, it will be possible to target interventions to optimally manage all mechanisms leading to the adjustment disorder with impact on the general medical condition. In most situations, because of the acute and (by definition) environmentally influenced nature of adjustment disorders, time-limited psychotherapy that improves individual coping and addresses environmental contributors to the symptoms is usually what is

Table 29.3 Biopsychosocial–cultural–spiritual formulation of the case vignette, "Hau'oli"

	Biological		Psychological		Social–Cultural–Spiritual	
	Factor	Intervention	Factor	Intervention	Factor	Intervention
Predisposing factors	Genetic predisposition to migraines	Continued migraine prophylaxis	Previous family transitions—parental divorce, witness to domestic violence	Individual counseling, safety education	Previous family transitions—parental divorce, witness to domestic violence	Family counseling to effectively manage conflicts
Precipitating factors	Acute migraine with pain	Medication management per pediatric team, relaxation and behavioral techniques to assist with pain management	Stressors: new baby, worry about parental conflict, new school	Individual counseling	Parental conflict affecting patient	Family counseling to effectively manage conflicts and to insure optimal parental support through other transitions
Perpetuating factors	Sensitization to pain	Effective treatment of acute pain, continued migraine prophylaxis	Pain being a route to receiving attention	Family counseling to insure regular attention to patient	Pain being a route to focusing attention on patient rather than other family conflicts	Family counseling to effectively manage conflicts

indicated. Prognosis is generally favorable, depending on the nature, pervasiveness, and chronicity of the precipitating circumstances.

The case above presented a diagnostic challenge in which many other conditions were considered. The following case presents a further diagnostic challenge:

Case Vignette 29.2.1 (Presenting Situation)
Mr. John Flame is a 25-year-old male who is brought into the emergency room by the police, who reported that he was "acting suspicious" around the scene of a fire. The police officer also told you that one of his colleagues recalled this gentleman from the scene of another fire several weeks earlier and therefore was worried that this patient may be a "pyromaniac." They noticed that he was not making sense when initially questioned but wondered whether or not he was faking his psychotic symptoms to avoid going to cell block.

Please proceed with the problem-based approach using the worksheet located in the appendix of Chap. 1!

Pyromania belongs to a series of disorders in the DSM-5 called disruptive, impulse control, and conduct disorders, some of which you may have already encountered in previous chapters (think, child and adolescent disorders.) The disorders in this category and the general characteristics of the impulse control disorders are summarized in Table 29.4:

Of historical note, disorders that previously had been included in this category include gambling disorder (now a non-substance-related disorder, under Substance-Related and Addictive Disorders, Chap. 19) and trichotillomania (hair-pulling disorder, now under Anxiety Disorders, Obsessive-Compulsive and Related Disorders, Trauma- and Stressor-Related Disorders, Chap. 22)

Therefore, before we conclude that this patient has either pyromania or another impulse control disorder, we should further analyze the differential possibilities, which for this case should include:

- Psychotic disorders (with disorganized thoughts and behavior)
- Mood disorders, including bipolar disorder, with psychotic features
- Substance use disorders, including substance intoxication and substance-induced psychotic disorders
- Psychotic disorder secondary to another medical condition
- Malingering (to avoid arrest or incarceration, as suggested by the police officer in this case)

Table 29.4 Characteristics and treatments of the disruptive, impulse control, and conduct disorders

Impulse control disorder	Key characteristics	Possible treatments
Oppositional Defiant Disorder	See Chap. 18	
Intermittent explosive disorder	Discrete episodes of aggressive and/or destructive behavior, out of proportion to precipitating psychosocial stressors (differentiated from seizure phenomena, which more commonly manifest as repetitive and/or purposeless behaviors)	Psychotherapy, anticonvulsants, lithium, antipsychotics, serotonin-selective reuptake inhibitors, propranolol
Conduct disorder	See Chap. 18	
Antisocial personality disorder	See Chap. 24	
Kleptomania	Stealing objects that are not personally or monetarily valuable	Psychotherapy, serotonin-selective reuptake inhibitors
Pyromania	Purposeful, repetitive fire setting	Psychotherapy, insure safety
Other specified disruptive, impulse control, and conduct disorder		
Unspecified disruptive, impulse control, and conduct disorder	Not meeting criteria for any other condition listed above	
General characteristics of the impulse control disorders		
Failure to resist impulses that lead to the behaviors described above Symptoms are not better explained by another disorder, including substance use disorders and general medical conditions (Implied) impairment in functioning		

Once again, we are challenged to recall the various conditions from previous chapters. Did you remember to never forget, in your list of differential possibilities, conditions secondary to either substance use or other medical conditions? ☺ Like with the first case vignette, the possibility of malingering is once again raised. At this point, given that we have not yet explored the other differential possibilities, it would be clinically unsound (and potentially a reflection of the stigma of mental illness—do you remember Chap. 13?) to assume that this patient is malingering.

Case Vignette 29.2.2

Mr. Flame states that he is a "highly intelligent and gifted grand master spirit." Notwithstanding his claim that he has been "specially chosen to chant away the fire demons and stop them from entering the mortal universe," he denies any recollection of having been near a fire recently as he has "been in a spiritual trance." He denies any history of fire setting or particular excitement upon seeing fires. He gives the history of having been treated several times at a facility located in another state. You find the history difficult to obtain because of his tangential thought processes, but you maintain your composure and ability to be empathic as you recall from a textbook you once read (Chap. 17) that, often, a challenging interview often reflects the effects of the very illness that one should be attempting to treat. Besides the tangentiality, your mental status examination is significant for poor hygiene and bizarre dress, continuous speech that is difficult to interrupt, flat affect, religious preoccupations, auditory hallucinations, and proverb interpretations that are either very bizarre or very concrete. He performs adequately on basic tests of concentration and memory. You conclude to yourself that if he were, in fact, malingering, he would need to be a very skilled and knowledgeable actor. He appears to be physically healthy, and screening laboratory studies, including a urine toxicology, are negative.

At this point, given the extensive psychopathology observed, it would seem that malingering and pyromania are less likely as possibilities. One new possibility that might be considered at this point is a dissociative disorder. Table 29.5 presents the general characteristics of the dissociative disorders.

Table 29.5 General characteristics of the dissociative disorders

Dissociative disorder	Key characteristics
Dissociative identify disorder (a.k.a., multiple personality disorder)	More than one distinct identity or personality state that recurrently control a person's behavior
Dissociative amnesia	Episodes of inability to recall important personal information (usually associated with traumatic events)
Depersonalization disorder	Recurrent feelings of detachment from one's mind or body
Other specified dissociative disorder	Chronic and recurrent syndromes of mixed dissociative symptoms, identity disturbance due to prolonged and intense coercive persuasion, acute dissociative reactions to stressful events, dissociative trance
Unspecified dissociative disorder	Dissociative symptoms not meeting criteria of any of the above disorders
Other characteristics of the dissociative disorders	
Symptoms are not better explained by another disorder psychiatric disorder (including psychotic and post-traumatic stress disorders), substance use disorders, and general medical conditions (particularly, transient global amnesia, which affects ability to learn new information)	
(Implied) impairment in functioning	
Relative preservation of other mental processes (e.g., ability to register new information, unlike in certain neurological conditions)	
Treatment considerations for the dissociative disorders	
Psychotherapy and psychopharmacotherapy targeted towards comorbid conditions and/or specific impairments and symptoms	
Medication-assisted interviews (e.g., amobarbital or benzodiazepine) may assist in uncovering traumatic memories; however, it is not clear that psychotherapeutic interventions done while under the effect of medications may be effective	

Once again, without further collateral information, and with significant evidence for other psychiatric syndromes that could explain his symptoms, it is not clear that this patient meets the criteria for any of the dissociative disorders.

Case Vignette 29.2.3 (Continuation)
With his permission, you are able to gather collateral information from Mr. Flame's family and from his previous psychiatrist. They confirm that he has the diagnosis of bipolar disorder, type I, and that he functions very well when he is stable on his medication, valproic acid. In fact, he is a well-respected research scholar who recently relocated in order to pursue doctoral-level studies. You admit him for further treatment, and he stabilizes very nicely on valproic acid and an atypical antipsychotic. He regrets that he allowed his medications to run out. He explains that, since his move, it was difficult to secure health insurance. He notes that many of the health-care plans significantly restrict behavioral health and/or medication benefits. You ponder the lessons you learned in this case and you resolve to become an advocate for accessible mental health care for everyone.

Of note, in order to comprehensively manage this patient and prevent recurrence of illness, it may be helpful for the clinician to identify problems related to access to medical and other health care in the list of conditions that may affect his course and prognosis and deserve clinical attention. It may be helpful to review the overall mental health-care system and barriers to access in the "Healthcare 101 and Systems-Based Practice" (Chap. 12).

Although this chapter may seem like the one that covers "miscellaneous" conditions, we believe that the conditions we have introduced in this chapter are excellent ones to discuss at the conclusion of this book for the following reasons. Firstly, because adjustment disorders and psychological factors affecting other medical conditions along with the section "Other Conditions That May Be a Focus of Clinical Attention" (all illustrated in the first case) and impulse control and dissociative disorders (both of which were considered in the second case) typically are not associated with any one underlying neurobiological mechanism, they illustrate the importance of treatment planning according to (can you guess what?) the biopsychosocial–cultural–spiritual matrix. Secondly, because these conditions tend to have lengthy lists of differential diagnoses, discussion of these conditions also illustrates the usefulness of the problem-based learning approach, which helps the clinician to thoughtfully consider other possibilities. Finally, these conditions illustrate the wide spectrum of psychiatric illnesses, ranging from the very common, potentially underrecognized, and generally self-limiting (e.g., adjustment disorders with the section "Other Conditions That May Be a Focus of Clinical Attention") to the relatively rare, potentially over-publicized by the media, and often chronic (e.g., impulse control disorders such as pyromania, dissociative disorders such as dissociative identity disorder). We hope that, like the clinician illustrated in the last vignette, you will become a physician who is knowledgeable about the scope of psychiatric illnesses and empathetically responsive to the behavioral health needs of patients.

29.1 Review questions

1. Which of the following is *not* classified as an "Other Condition That May Be a Focus of Clinical Attention"?
   a. Child physical abuse
   b. Homelessness
   c. Antidepressant discontinuation syndrome
   d. Overweight or obesity
   e. None of the above
2. A high school student with bronchial asthma tends to have exacerbations of illness around significant stress. Prior to final exams, and also coinciding with cold weather, he suffers from a particularly severe attack, resulting in hospitalization in the intensive care unit and significant wheezing, respiratory distress, and hypoxia. The patient is a high-achieving student who regrets needing to have the exams rescheduled. From a psychiatric perspective, the most appropriate diagnosis would be:
   a. Psychological factors affecting other medical conditions
   b. Malingering
   c. Factitious disorder
   d. Conversion disorder
   e. None of the above

For questions 3–5, please match the following illness with its associated clinical presentation.

   a. Depersonalization disorder
   b. Dissociative amnesia
   c. Intermittent explosive disorder

3. Discrete episodes of aggressive and/or destructive behavior
4. Recurrent feelings of detachment from one's mind or body
5. Episodes of inability to recall important personal information

Answers to review questions:

1. c
2. a
3. c
4. a
5. b

Further Readings

American Psychiatric Association. (2013). Diagnostic and statistical manual of mental disorders (5th ed.) Washington, D.C.: Author.
Sadock, B. J., & and Sadock, V. A. (2015). Kaplan & and Sadock's synopsis of psychiatry: Behavioral sciences/clinical psychiatry (11th ed.). New York: Lippincott Williams & Wilkins.

Index

D. Alicata et al. (eds.), *Problem-based Behavioral Science and Psychiatry*,
DOI 10.1007/978-3-319-23669-8

Lightning Source UK Ltd.
Milton Keynes UK
UKOW06n1909090816

280309UK00001B/23/P

9 783319 23668